Lecture Notes in Computer Science 905

Edited by G. Goos, J. Hartmanis and J. van Leeuwen

Advisory Board: W. Brauer D. Gries J. Stoer

Nicholas Ayache (Ed.)

Computer Vision, Virtual Reality and Robotics in Medicine

First International Conference, CVR Med '95
Nice, France, April 3-6, 1995
Proceedings

With Numerous Halftones and 9 Pages in Colour

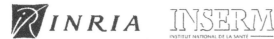 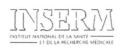 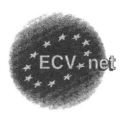

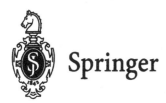 Springer

Series Editors

Gerhard Goos
Universität Karlsruhe
Vincenz-Priessnitz-Straße 3, D-76128 Karlsruhe, Germany

Juris Hartmanis
Department of Computer Science, Cornell University
4130 Upson Hall, Ithaca, NY 14853, USA

Jan van Leeuwen
Department of Computer Science, Utrecht University
Padualaan 14, 3584 CH Utrecht, The Netherlands

Volume Editor

Nicholas Ayache
INRIA
B. P. 93, F-06902 Sophia-Antipolis, France

CR Subject Classification (1991): I.5, I.3.5-8, I.2.9-10, I.4, J.3

ISBN 3-540-59120-6 Springer-Verlag Berlin Heidelberg New York

CIP data applied for

© Springer-Verlag Berlin Heidelberg 1995
Printed in Germany

Typesetting: Camera-ready by author
SPIN: 10485529   06/3142-543210 - Printed on acid-free paper

Preface

This book contains the written contributions to the program of the First International Conference on Computer Vision, Virtual Reality, and Robotics in Medicine (CVRMed'95) held in Nice during the period April 3-6, 1995.

The articles are regrouped into a number of thematic sessions which cover the three major topics of the field: medical image understanding, registration problems in medicine, and therapy planning, simulation and control.

The objective of the conference is not only to present the most innovative and promising research work but also to highlight research trends and to foster dialogues and debates among participants.

This event was decided after a preliminary successful symposium organized in Stanford in March 1994 by E. Grimson (MIT), T. Kanade (CMU), R. Kikinis and W. Wells (Chair) (both at Harvard Medical School and Brigham and Women's Hospital), and myself (INRIA).

We received 92 submitted full papers, and each one was evaluated by at least three members of the Program Committee, with the help of auxiliary reviewers. Based on these evaluations, a representative subset of the Program Committee met to select 19 long papers, 29 regular papers, and 27 posters.

The geographical repartition of the contributions is the following: 24 from European countries (other than France), 23 contributions from France, 20 from Northern America (USA and Canada), and 8 from Asia (Japan and Singapore).

All contributions are presented in a single track, leaving time for two poster sessions, a panel discussion, and a technical tour in Sophia-Antipolis. A number of stands are reserved for industrial exhibitions and research demonstrations.

This conference promises to be an exciting event based upon such a fascinating new research field.

Sophia-Antipolis, January 1995 Nicholas Ayache

CVRMed'95: a special acronym: the letters of this acronym share a double meaning: *C* for Conference and Computer, *V* for Vision and Virtual, *R* for Reality and Robotics, and *Med* for Medicine and ... Mediterranean. It might be hard to preserve this last *Nice* property in the future!

Acknowledgement

The members of the program committee deserve special acknowledgements for their superb job in reviewing all the papers in due time, and for their support in the organisation of the conference. This acknowledgment applies also to the auxiliary reviewers.

We want to acknowledge the outstanding work of Grégoire Malandain, who was in charge of the scientific coordination of this conference, in particular for the reviewing process and the compilation of the book, and whose help remains inestimable.

Special thanks are due to Monique Simonetti for her wonderful work at local arrangements with the assistance of the "Bureau des Colloques" of INRIA, and also to Jean-Philippe Thirion who (besides his role in the Program Committee) played a crucial role in the original setting and planning of this conference.

Finally, we wish to thank Francoise Pezé and Sandrine Chevris for their help in the mailing work, and Catherine Martin for her help in organizing the Program Committee meeting.

Conference Organized by

INRIA
Institut National de Recherche en Informatique et en Automatique
Sophia Antipolis - France

with financial contribution from

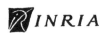 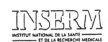 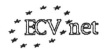

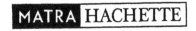

and supported by

DIGITAL EQUIPMENT CORPORATION
FOCUS MEDICAL
GENERAL ELECTRIC MEDICAL SYSTEMS EUROPE

Conference Chairman
Nicholas Ayache   INRIA, France

Scientific Coordinator
Grégoire Malandain   INRIA, France

Program Committee
Fred Bookstein	University of Michigan, USA
Michael Brady	Oxford University, UK
Grigore Burdea	Rutgers University, USA
Philippe Cinquin	Grenoble Hospital, France
Jean-Louis Coatrieux	INSERM, Rennes, France
Alan Colchester	Guy's Hospital, London, UK
James Duncan	Yale University, USA
Henry Fuchs	University of North Carolina, USA
Guido Gerig	ETH-Z, Zurich, Switzerland
Erik Granum	Aalborg University, Denmark
Eric Grimson	MIT, USA
Karl-Heinz Höhne	University Hospital Eppendorf, Germany
Thomas Huang	University of Illinois, USA
Takeo Kanade	Carnegie Mellon University, USA
Ron Kikinis	Harvard Medical School, USA
Jean-Claude Latombe	Stanford University, USA
Tomas Lozano-Pérez	MIT, USA
Charles Pelizzari	University of Chicago, USA
Richard Robb	Mayo Clinic, Rochester, USA
Paul Suetens	KULeuven, Belgium
Richard Szeliski	DEC, Cambridge, USA
Russ Taylor	IBM, Yorktown Heights, USA
Demetri Terzopoulos	University of Toronto, Canada
Jean-Philippe Thirion	INRIA, France
Jun-ichiro Toriwaki	Nagoya University, Japan
Alessandro Verri	University of Genoa, Italy
Max Viergever	University Hospital Utrecht, The Netherlands
William Wells	Harvard Medical School, USA

Local Arrangements
Monique Simonetti   INRIA, France

Local Assistants
Sandrine Chevris   INRIA, France
Françoise Pezé   INRIA, France

Referees

Ayache N.	France	Robb R.	USA
Bardinet E.	France	Röll S.	UK
Bijnens B.	Belgium	Shimoga K.B.	USA
Bookstein F.	USA	Simon D.	USA
Brady M.	UK	Sinclair D.	Denmark
Burdea G.	USA	Subsol G.	France
Camp J.	USA	Suetens P.	Belgium
Champleboux G.	France	Szeliski R.	USA
Cinquin P.	France	Taylor R.	USA
Coatrieux J.-L.	France	Terzopoulos D.	Canada
Colchester A.C.F.	UK	Thirion J.-P.	France
Collignon A.	Belgium	Tombropoulos R.	USA
Declerck J.	France	Toriwaki J.	Japan
DiGioia A.	USA	Troccaz J.	France
Dowling K.	USA	Uenohara M.	USA
Duncan J.	USA	Van Cleynenbreugel J.	Belgium
Feldmar J.	France	Vandermeulen D.	Belgium
Gerig G.	Switzerland	Verri A.	Italy
Gourdon A.	France	Viergever M.	The Netherlands
Granum E.	Denmark	Wells III W.	USA
Griffin L.	UK	Yokokohji Y.	USA
Grimson E.	USA	Zhao J.	UK
Hanson D.	USA		
Harris C.	UK		
Hawkes D.	UK		
Henri C.	UK		
Höhne K.H.	Germany		
Huang T.S.	USA		
Jaramaz B.	USA		
Kikinis R.	USA		
Larsen O.	Denmark		
Latombe J.-C.	USA		
Lavallée S.	France		
Lozano-Pérez T.	USA		
Maes F.	Belgium		
Malandain G.	France		
McInerney T.	Canada		
Michiels J.	Belgium		
Nielsen H.	Denmark		
O'Toole III R.V.	USA		
Pelizzari C.	USA		
Pennec X.	France		

Table of Contents

3. Simulation / Robotics

4. Atlases

5. Registration

7. Segmentation II

8. Reconstruction / Vessels

9. Segmentation III

10. Augmented Reality II

Augmented Reality I

Evaluating and Validating an Automated Registration System for Enhanced Reality Visualization in Surgery

W.E.L. Grimson[123] and G.J. Ettinger[13] and S.J. White[3] and P.L. Gleason[2] and T. Lozano-Pérez[1] and W.M. Wells III[12] and R. Kikinis[2]

[1] AI Lab, MIT, 545 Technology Sq, Cambridge MA 02139, USA[†]
[2] Dept. Radiology, Brigham & Womens Hospital, Harvard Med. School, Boston, USA
[3] TASC, Inc., Reading MA, USA

Abstract. Frameless guidance systems are needed to help surgeons plan exact locations for incisions, define margins of tumors and precisely locate critical structures. We describe an automatic method for registering clinical data, such as segmented MRI or CT, with any view of the patient, demonstrated on neurosurgery examples. The method enables mixing live video of the patient with the segmented 3D MRI or CT model, supporting enhanced reality techniques for planning and guiding procedures, and for interactively, non-intrusively viewing internal structures. We detail a computational evaluation of the method's performance, and clinical experiments using the system in actual neurosurgical cases.

1 Introduction

Many surgical procedures require precise localization by the surgeon, to extract targeted tissue while minimizing damage to adjacent structures. This 3D localization often requires isolating a structure deeply buried within the body. While methods exist (e.g. MRI, CT) for imaging and displaying 3D anatomy, to solve the localization problem the surgeon must relate the display to the patient. As current methods often involve a surgeon mentally transforming 2D slices of MRI or CT imagery, there is a need for registered visualization methods, in which reconstructions of internal anatomy are exactly overlaid with the surgeon's view of the patient, so that she can directly visualize key structures and plan accordingly. We describe a method for such automatic registration and visualization. While this problem is relevant in any minimally invasive procedure, we use the problem of visualization in neurosurgery as a motivating example.

1.1 Problem Definition

The goal of this project is to develop a system that automatically registers 3D data sets, and tracks changes in a data set's position over time, without

[†] Research supported in part by ARPA under ONR contract N00014-91-J-4038 and in part by Training Grant No. T 15 LM 07092 from the National Library of Medicine.

attaching fiducials to the patient. An ideal system should support: real-time, adaptive, enhanced reality patient visualizations in the operating room; dynamic image-guided surgical planning; image guided surgical procedures; and registered transfer of *a priori* surgical plans to the patient in the OR.

In this paper, we describe an implemention of a first stage of this system. Our specific problem is to take a video view of the patient and a segmented MRI or CT model of the patient's anatomy, each defined in its own coordinate system, and to return a transformation aligning model with patient, and a transformation describing the pose of the video camera relative to the patient.

By transforming the MRI model into the patient coordinate frame, then projecting it into the camera coordinate frame, one can combine a live video view of the patient with the projected registered anatomy. This can be used to guide the marking of key structures such as the tumor's position, or the planned position of the craniotomy, as well as provide the surgeon, during surgery, with a visualization of the full area of operation, for intraoperative guidance.

2 Our Approach

We have previously described [9] an early version of our system. Here, we report on extensions, and detail computational and clinical testing of the system.

Model input: A segmented 3D reconstruction of the patient's anatomy, (e.g. CT or MRI). Current segmentation techniques typically train an intensity classifier on a user-selected set of tissue samples, where the operator uses knowledge of anatomy to identify the tissue type, after which, the scans are segmented into tissue types [4, 7], based on intensities in the scanned images. Removing gain artifacts from the sensor data [21], and correcting for distortions due to magnetic susceptibility differences between different materials [16] improves the segmentation. This 3D anatomical reconstruction defines the model, and is represented relative to a model coordinate frame, with origin at the points' centroid.

Data input: To achieve the registration, we first obtain intermediate data from the patient. We obtain a set of 3D data points from the patient's skin surface using a laser range scanner, which operates by scanning a laser beam through an optical mechanism that results in a controlled plane of light. A video camera is placed at an angle to this plane such that a portion of the plane is in the camera field of view. When an object in this visible region intersects the laser plane, points in the camera image illuminated by the laser unambiguously correspond to fixed 3D scene points. The 3D measurements of the currently used scanner (Technical Arts 100X) are accurate to within $0.08mm$. This 3D information defines the data, and is represented in a laser coordinate frame, which reflects the patient's position in a coordinate frame in the OR.

Matching: We find a transformation from model to camera coordinates, by:

(1) To initiate the matching, we have two options. First, a graphical interface (Fig. 1) can be used to roughly align the laser data with the 3D model. One selects a standard view from a menu, then estimates the orientation of the patient's nose in the view. This determines a rough rotation of the model, which is

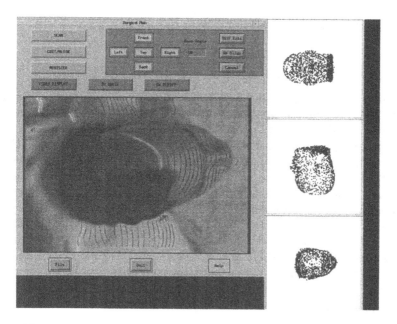

Fig. 1. Example of graphical interface used to obtain initial alignment.

then displayed on three orthogonal 2D views, together with the laser data. The user can refine the initial transformation by rotating and translating the data in any of these views. This initial alignment can be inaccurate: rotational errors of several degrees, and translational errors of several centimeters are permissible, since the subsequent stages reliably remove these misalignments.

For a totally automatic system, we instead sample a set of evenly spaced directions on the view sphere. This point on the view sphere determines the rotation needed to roughly align this temporary model with the data. For each such model and its associated alignment, we execute the following process.

(2) Next, we separate laser data of the patient's head from background data. While this can be done automatically, currently we use a simple user interface (Fig. 1), in which the data is projected onto the view from the laser's video camera. The user uses a mouse to block out laser points from the patient's skin. This laser data is displayed overlaid on the MRI model, via the rough transformation of step (1). Using any of the views of the two data sets, the laser data can be furthered edited using a mouse interface. This process can be imperfect, we simply want to remove gross outliers from the data.

(3) We refine the transformation by minimizing an evaluation function that measures the amount of mismatch between the two data sets. In particular, we sum, for all transformed laser points, a term that is a sum of the distances from the transformed point to all nearby model points, where the distance is weighted by a Gaussian distribution [19]. If vector ℓ_i is a laser point, vector m_j is a model

point, and T is a coordinate transformation, then the evaluation function is

$$E_1(T) = \sum_i \sum_j -e^{-\frac{|T\ell_i - m_j|^2}{2\sigma^2}}. \tag{1}$$

This function is similar to the posterior marginal pose estimation (PMPE) method [19]. The objective function is quite smooth, and thus facilitates "pulling in" solutions from moderately removed locations in parameter space.

In earlier versions, we used Powell's method to iteratively minimize (1). It is more efficient, however, to use the Davidon-Fletcher-Powell quasi-Newton method [13]. This requires an estimate of the gradient of the objective function, which is easily obtained. Minimizing (1) yields an estimate for the pose of the laser points in model coordinates.

We execute this minimization stage with a multiresolution set of Gaussians. A large σ (e.g. 8 *mms*) allows influence over large areas, resulting in a coarse alignment that can be reached from a wide range of starting positions. Narrower Gaussians ($\sigma = 1$) are used to focus on nearby model points to derive the pose.

(4) Starting from the resulting pose, we repeat the evaluation process, using a least squares distance measure. We use the DFP method to minimize:

$$E_2(T) = \sum_i \min \left\{ d_{\max}^2, \min_j |T\ell_i - m_j|^2 \right\} \tag{2}$$

where $d_{\max}$ is a preset maximum distance. This objective function is essentially the maximum a posteriori model matching scheme [19]. It acts much like a robust chamfer matching scheme (e.g. [11]). Equation (2) is locally more accurate, but it is also susceptible to local minima. Hence we add another stage.

(5) To avoid being trapped in local minima of E_2, we take the pose returned by step (4), perturb it randomly, then repeat the minimization. We iterate, keeping the new pose if its associated RMS error is better than our current best. This process terminates when the number of trials since the RMS value was last improved becomes larger than some threshold. The result is a pose, and the residual deviation of the fit to the model.

(7) Instead of all the laser data, we can use only "distinctive" laser data. We estimate the curvature, in the laser plane, at each data point, and keep only a predefined fraction of the most highly curved laser points. Initial experiments show that using only highly curved points improves the residual RMS error.

(8) Given the final solution, each point's residual error is measured, and laser points with large residuals are removed, automatically deleting possible outliers. Step (5) is then rerun with the remaining data, yielding a tighter surface fit.

We keep the solution, over all views, with smallest RMS measure, yielding a highly accurate transformation of MRI data into laser coordinate frame.

Camera Calibration: Given a registration, we must relate it to a view of the patient. A video camera is roughly positioned in the surgeon's viewpoint, i.e. looking over her shoulder. By calibrating this camera's pose relative to laser coordinates, we can render the aligned MRI or CT data relative to the camera view, and mix this rendering with the live video signal, giving the surgeon an enhanced reality view of the patient's anatomy [2, 20].

If the laser video camera is used for mixing, finding the camera model is easy. Points in the laser scan of any object in the camera field have unique correspondences with image plane points. During calibration, scan points from a calibration object are used to generate a close approximation of the camera pose. When scanning a patient, corresponding 3D laser data and image points from the skin are used to refine the camera pose model using Powell's method.

If an independent camera is used for video capture from the surgeon's view, a similar method uses scene objects with flat surface facets. Images of the laser slices are taken with the video camera. Straight 2D line segments are located in the video images and matched to corresponding straight 3D line segments in the laser data. Three matching segments are used to solve for the perspective projection transformation, i.e. the pose of the camera. With this starting point, Powell's method is used to optimize the pose estimate to best bring all the laser line segment data into projective alignment with the corresponding video data.

Visualization: We combine the camera calibration and the registration of the data sets into a visualization of the data. We apply the transformation to bring the MRI or CT model into alignment with the patient, in the laser system's coordinate frame. We then project that model into the video camera's coordinate frame, by applying the computed camera model. This gives a virtual view of the MRI model, as seen by that camera, which can then be mixed with a live video view, and used as a visualization tool by the surgeon.

3   Testing and Applications

We have run the system in a series of trials with actual neurosurgery patients. Example registrations of laser data to MRI models are shown in Figure 2. The tumor and the ventricles of the patient are highlighted. The RMS errors in these cases were typically on the order of $1.5mms$.

We are using this registration and visualization method to transfer presurgical plans to the patient. Currently, we use our method to provide a visual overlay, on a live video monitor, of the view of the patient with internal structures selected by the surgeon, allowing her to mark key structures on the patient's scalp [8]. This enables the surgeon to mark locations for planned surgical steps, prior to surgery. To date, we have used this procedure on eight neurosurgical patients at Brigham & Women's Hospital, Boston, MA (see Sec. 5).

Besides applications for surgical planning and guidance, the method has other applications, including the registration of multiple clinical data sets such as MRI versus CT. For example, we have registered sequences of MRI scans of the same patient, taken over a period of several months, and used differences in the registered scans to visualize and measure changes in anatomy [6]. In this testing, we have automatically registered 20 sets of 50 MRI scans each, using the fully automatic version of the initial registration.

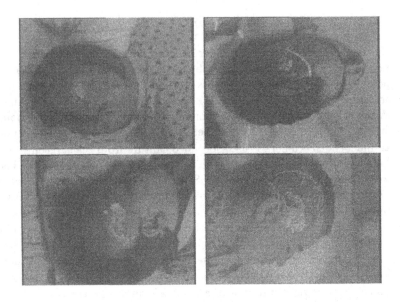

Fig. 2. Examples of combining the registration of MRI to laser data and the calibration of a video camera relative to the laser to provide an enhanced reality visualization of patients. The tumor and the ventricles are displayed in registration with the patient.

4   Computational Evaluation

We have examined a series of issues relating to the computational performance of our system. The results of our testing are described in this section.

Minimization error: It is worth commenting on the interpretation of the RMS error, in particular, on what an RMS error of 1.5 mm implies. First, there are several factors that may increase the RMS beyond the actual fit to the surface. The method we use to extract a surface model from the MRI or CT data simply computes the isosurface of the thresholded sensor data and represents the skin surface points as the vertices of the isosurface triangles. This technique may displace the surface points from their true position by up to the diameter of a voxel, thus contributing to the RMS error. Second, the RMS error will clearly be a function of the density of the model points. For efficiency, we often run the method with a subsampling of the MRI model. To explore the effect of this sampling on the residual error, we ran experiments on two patients, in which we varied the sampling of the MRI and recorded the final RMS error. This is graphed in Figure 3. One can see that as more model points are included the RMS error declines to roughly 1 mm. Note that the voxel size is $0.9375 \times 0.9375 \times 1.5mms$ so that the expected RMS error just due to the discrete size of the voxels is $.578mm$. When combined with the fact that we are measuring distance to the nearest vertex of an isosurface triangle, not to the actual surface itself, one can see that the method is close to the limit of RMS accuracy. Perhaps the most important question, however, is whether a minimum RMS error actually corresponds to the true alignment. This is difficult to test since we do not have "ground truth" for the transformation, and would probably be best tested using phantom studies. As an alternative, we examine the reliability of the RMS measure and the impact of applying the computed transformation to the model.

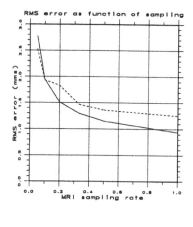
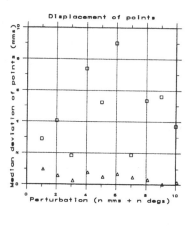

Fig. 3. Left: RMS error as a function of the sampling of the MRI data. Patient 071594 had an MRI model of 123,725 points, which were matched against 956 laser points. Patient 070194 had an MRI model of 109,641 points, which were matched against 949 laser points. The graphs show the RMS error (in mms) as a function of the fraction of the model actually sampled. Right: Graph of maximum deviation of a transformation cluster, for registration solutions obtained by successively larger initial perturbations. Each perturbation involved a translation of n mms and a rotation of n degrees.

Repeatability and Capture Radius: A key issue with any registration algorithm based on minimizing an evaluation function is the question of local minima. Since most realistic objective functions will have complex associated energy landscapes, it is important to test that the algorithm avoids getting trapped in local minima, and instead is reliable at finding the best global minimum.

To explore this issue, we ran the following test. We took a real patient case, and found a transformation close to what appears to be the correct alignment. Starting with a rough initial registration of laser data to a patient's MRI scan (RMS error of 6 mms), we perturbed that solution by successively larger translations and rotations. We then let the registration algorithm reconverge to a local minimum. We collected the final transformations for each such trial. For each size of perturbation, we ran 10 random trials. To test the variability in the results, we applied each transformation in a cluster to a set of sample points along a ray parallel to the optic axis of the camera and through the principal point of the camera, and recorded the median deviation of any such set of transformed points. This is graphed in Figure 3. Note that this is an upper bound on deviation. For points near the surface of the skull closest to the laser data, the deviation will be much smaller. The plots are flat, indicating that there is no trend for larger deviations as a function of initial perturbation. This supports the notion that the algorithm is robust in finding a consistent minimum. Finally, the deviation between solutions is on the order of one or two voxels.

Table 1 lists the number of trials (for patient 070194) in which the system terminated without finding a solution with an acceptably low RMS value (set to 2.5 mms in the current system). One can see that for larger perturbations, the system occasionally fails to find a solution, but does not get trapped into false local minima.

Table 1. Table of trials (out of 10) for which system found an acceptable solution

Perturbation size (mms of offset & degs of rotation)	1	2	3	4	5	6	7	8	9	10
Solutions found (out of 10 trials)	10	10	10	10	10	9	10	9	7	7

5 Clinical Testing

We have tested our system on neurosurgery patients[5] at Brigham & Women's Hospital for the purpose of accurately planning craniotomy locations. Each patient had an MRI scan performed a few days prior to surgery. Clinicians at the Surgical Planning Lab segmented the MRI scan into skin, brain, tumor, ventricles, and other structures of interest. Once the patient's head was shaved for surgery, he was brought for laser registration by our system. The registration procedure consisted of the following steps:

1. Place the laser scanner over the patient's head such that the camera is positioned at the expected angle of approach to the tumor.
2. Scan the patient's head with the laser.
3. Use the method of Sec. 2 to register the laser data with the MRI model.
4. Verify the registration through a visual animation of the transformed MRI skin overlaid on the video image, as well as a color coded examination of residual errors of transformed laser data overlaid on the MRI skin.

---

[5] Eight patients tested as of September, 1994.

5. Render the internal structures in their registered locations relative to the camera, and mix with the video signal into an enhanced reality visualization.
6. The surgeon draws the position of the tumor and other structures directly on the scalp while looking at the visualization. The selection and opacity of the different anatomical structures is dynamically controlled to provide as much geometric information as possible from the given viewpoint.

Each of the steps in the process can be repeated to refine the surgical plan. Elapsed time for steps 2 through 4 is approximately five minutes. Previously performed *manual* alignment aimed at achieving such visualizations took about 45 minutes with an accuracy of 10-30 mms. Our registration thus achieves an order of magnitude improvement in both efficiency and accuracy, two factors which are critical to the neurosurgeons. Feedback from the surgeons has been highly positive as they have found this easily accessible form of 3D geometric knowledge to prepare them well for the surgeries. Current work involves migrating the use of the laser registration system into the OR for neurosurgery guidance as well as for planning and guiding other types of surgery.

6 Related Work

Several other groups have reported methods similar to ours. Pelizzari et al. [12] have developed a method that matches retrospective data sets, (MRI, CT, PET), to one another, using a least squares minimization of distances between data sets, although with a different distance function. Szeliski et al. [3, 17] also do a least-squares minimization of a distance function to match data sets, with distance weighted by an estimate of the inverse variance of the measurement noise, and using a Levenberg-Marquardt method is used to find the minimum. Ayache et al. [10, 18] performs automatic rigid registration of 3D surfaces by matching ridge lines which track points of maximum curvature along the surface. Colchester et al. perform registration and video compositing using stereo data, rather than laser scanning. Other methods for matching sparse data sets include [1, 22, 15] and other examples of enhanced reality visualization include [5, 14, 15].

7 Summary

We have reported on a method to register MRI or CT reconstructions of a patient's anatomy to video views of the patient. Computational experiments show that the method is robust, in that it consistently finds the same solution over a wide range of starting positions. Clinical experiments demonstrate that the solutions found by the system are of considerable utility to the surgeon.

References

1. Besl, P., N. McKay, "A method for registration of 3D shapes" *IEEE Trans. PAMI* **14**(2):239–256, 1992.

2. Black, P. et al., "A New Virtual Reality Technique for Tumor Localization" *Cong. Neurological Surgeons*, 1993.
3. Champleboux, G. et al. "From accurate range imaging sensor calibration to accurate model-based 3D object localization", *CVPR*, 1992, pp 83–89.
4. Cline, H. et al. "3D Segmentation of MR Images of the Head Using Probability and Connectivity." *JCAT* 14(6), 1990, pp 1037–1045.
5. Colchester, A.C.F., et al., "Craniotomy simulation and guidance using a stereo video based tracking system (Vislan)", *Proc. 3rd Conf. Visualiz. in Biomed. Comp.*, 1994.
6. Ettinger, G. et al. "Automatic Registration for Multiple Sclerosis Change Detection", *IEEE Workshop Biomed. Image Anal.*, Seattle, 1994, pp. 297–306.
7. Gerig, G. et al. "Medical Imaging and Computer Vision: an Integrated Approach for Diagnosis and Planning," *Proc. 11'th DAGM Symp.*, Hamburg, Springer, 1989, pp 425–443.
8. Gleason, L. et al. "A New Virtual Reality Technique for Non-Linkage Stereotactic Surgery" *Society for Stereotactic & Functional Neurosurgery, Ixtapa, Mexico*, 1993.
9. Grimson, E. et al. "Automated Registration for Enhanced Reality Visualization in Surgery", *1st Int. Symp. Med. Robotics & Comp.-Assisted Surgery*, Pittsburgh, Sept., 1994.
10. Gueziec, A., N. Ayache, "Smoothing and Matching of 3-D Space Curves", *Second ECCV*, May 1992, pp 620–629.
11. Jiang, H., et al., "A New Approach to 3D Registration of Multimodality Medical Images by Surface Matching", *Visualiz. in Biomed. Comp.*, 1992, pp 196–213.
12. Pelizzari, C. et al. "Accurate three-dimensional registration of CT, PET, and/or MR images of the brain", *J. Computer Assisted Tomography* 13(1), 1989, pp 20–26.
13. Press, W.H. et al. *Numerical Recipes in C, The Art of Scientific Computing, 2nd Ed.*, Cambridge University Press, 1992.
14. Shweikard, A. et al., "Planning for image guided radiosurgery", *Proc. IEEE Conf. Rob. Autom.*, 1994.
15. Simon, D., et al., "Techniques for fast and accurate intrasurgical registration", *1st Int. Symp. Med. Robotics & Comp.-Assisted Surgery*, Pittsburgh, Sept., 1994.
16. Sumanaweera, T.S. et al. "MR Susceptibility Misregistration Correctoin", *IEEE TMI* 12, 1993, pp 251–259.
17. Szeliski, R., S. Lavallee, "Matching 3D Anatomical Surfaces with Non-Rigid Deformations using Octree-Splines", *IEEE Wk. Biomed. Im. Anal.*, June, 1994, pp. 144–153.
18. Thirion, J.P., "Extremal Points: Definition and Application to 3D Image Registration", *CVPR*, June 1994, pp. 587–592.
19. Wells, W. M., *Statistical Object Recognition*, Ph.D. Thesis, MIT, 1993. (MIT AI Lab TR 1398)
20. Wells, W. et al. "Video Registration using Fiducials for Surgical Enhanced Reality" *Proc. 15th Conf. IEEE Engin. in Med. Biol. Soc.*, 1993, pp. 24–25.
21. Wells, W. et al. "Statistical Intensity Correction and Segmentation of Magnetic Resonance Image Data", *Proc. 3rd Conf. Visualiz. in Biomed. Comp.*, 1994.
22. Zhang, Z., "Iterative point matching for registration of free-form curves and surfaces", *IJCV* 13(2):119-152, 1994.

Vision-Based Object Registration for Real-Time Image Overlay

Michihiro Uenohara[1] and Takeo Kanade[2]

[1] Toshiba R&D Center, Kawasaki, Japan
mue@mel.uki.rdc.toshiba.co.jp
[2] The Robotics Institute, Carnegie Mellon University,
Pittsburgh, PA 15213, U.S.A.
tk@cs.cmu.edu

Abstract- This paper presents computer vision based techniques for object registration, real-time tracking, and image overlay. The capability can be used to superimpose registered images such as those from CT or MRI onto a video image of a patient's body. Real-time object registration enables an image to be overlaid consistently onto objects even while the object or the viewer is moving. The video image of a patient's body is used as input for object registration. Reliable real-time object registration at frame rate (30 Hz) is realized by a combination of techniques, including template matching based feature detection, feature correspondence by geometric constraints, and pose calculation of objects from feature positions in the image. Two types of image overlay systems are presented. The first one registers objects in the image and projects pre-operative model data onto a raw camera image. The other computes the position of image overlay directly from 2D feature positions without any prior models. With the techniques developed in this paper, interactive video, which transmits images of a patient to the expert and sends them back with some image overlay, can be realized.

Category - on line tracking of patient or organ motion

1 Introduction

Due to the significant improvements in computer vision techniques in recent years[1][2][3], real-time and interactive imaging of complex biomedical systems have become a great priority within medicine.

One major application is to integrate the precise pre-operative information currently found within CT and MRI into intra-operative surgical procedures. The display of correctly registered medical images on a patient provides a new method of surgical guidance which can enhance human perception and skills [4]. Most previous methods of registration, however, are either off-line or assume that the patient does not move during the surgery. Real-time computer vision techniques for object registration can realize a new type of non-intrusive image overlay without using special positioning devices. The overlaid image can be kept at the same position of the patient in the image as if the overlay were physically attached to the patient. The overlay remains fixed to the patient even with movement of the patient and the camera.

Interactive video is another application. In telemedicine, rural surgeons would send patient records, X-rays and CT scans to an expert surgeon at a center who would use them to plan the operation on a surgical simulator. The expert would send the surgical plan to the remote doctor or medic and guide him through the surgery. The interactive video, which transmits images of a patient to the expert and sends them back with some image overlay, enables the expert to guide surgeons as if the expert were across the operating table from him. It could keep showing the surgeon the place on the patient's body to which the expert points, while the patient and the camera are moving in three dimensions.

This paper presents object registration and tracking techniques appropriate for the realization of real-time image overlay. Two image overlay systems are shown. The first one registers objects in the image and projects pre-operative model data onto a raw camera image. The other computes the position of image overlay directly from 2D feature positions without any prior models.

2 Object Registration for Image Overlay

Object registration is required to superimpose pre-operative model data onto a raw camera image accurately at the right place. Registration is the process of computing the object pose parameters in camera-centered coordinates. Camera-centered coordinates have the origin at the optical center of the camera with which raw camera image is taken. When the pose of the object has been computed, the remaining step is to generate an image of prestored data, such as a pre-operative bone model derived from CT, appropriately projected onto the image plane, and add it to a raw camera image.

Most previous work on object registration in medicine utilizes 3D image data (as from a scanning laser rangefinder) and searches their best match with 3D model data sets by using a least squares minimization of distances between data sets [4][5].

In the computer vision area, a few methods have been developed for visual tracking of known three-dimensional objects using only 2D images. They locate and track predefined features, such as edges and corners, on the object in the images, and use these measurements to calculate the estimate of position and orientation of the object [6][7][8][9]. In the case where we have object-centered coordinates of features in the models, the problem is formulated as an inverse problem to solve the nonlinear relationship between object pose and feature positions in the image. This problem can be solved by recursive methods.

The system described in this paper utilizes 2D intensity images and detects feature points by template matching. The change of intensity patterns due to view change is compensated by skewing reference images with computed object pose parameters. The system has been implemented on multiple DSPs and performs tracking at the frame rate.

3 Initial Recognition of the Object

For human interface systems, it is reasonable to assume that users can roughly locate objects at the start of the execution of the system. The system, for example, can superimpose the desired position and orientation of the object onto the raw camera image. Users can set the pose of the object as indicated by moving either the object or the camera (Fig.1).

When the rough pose of an object is set by the user, the initial recognition is carried out to precisely calculate the object location. For this purpose, reference images of feature points are precaptured in various conditions of illumination while objects are set to be the predefined pose. "Template space", which is the vector subspace involving not only the discrete reference images but also their interpolation, is computed. A set of images in the template space are considered as a template. The intensity pattern most similar to the input image in the template space is found and its normalized correlation to the input image is computed at each point in the search area. The point with the highest score is chosen, and it is recognized as a feature point when the highest score is over a threshold. When all the feature points are successfully found, the object pose is calculated and the system goes to the tracking phase.

3.1 Generation of Template Space

Precaptured reference images differ slightly from each other and are highly correlated. Therefore, the image vector subspace required for their effective representation can be defined by a small number of eigenvectors or eigenimages. The eigenimages which best account for the distribution of reference images can be derived by Karhunen-Loeve expansion [10][11][12][13].

Let the set of reference images be x_i, $i=1,2,...,P$ which are represented as vectors of dimension N^2, describing N by N image templates. The vectors e_j and scalars λ_j are the eigenvectors and eigenvalues, respectively, of the covariance matrix:

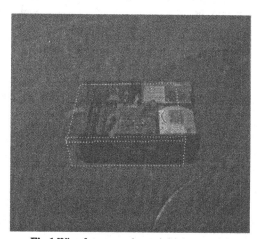

Fig.1 Wire-frame overlay at initial recognition.

$$A = \frac{1}{P}\sum_{i=1}^{P}(x_i - c)(x_i - c)^T \tag{1}$$

where $c = \frac{1}{P}\sum_{i=1}^{P}x_i$ is the average image vector. We obtain optimal approximation of reference images by selecting eigenvectors in decreasing order of magnitude of eigenvalues and representing each reference image by a linear combination of first K largest eigenvectors as

$$x_i \approx c + \sum_{j=1}^{K}p_{ij}e_j \tag{2}$$

where $p_i = [e_1, e_2, ..., e_K]^T(x_i - c)$.

The major K eigenvectors and the average image vector c span a $(K+1)$-dimensional subspace ("template space") of all possible images, and a set of images in the subspace is considered as a template to be recognized. The dimension along the average image vector is added to make the recognition insensitive to the magnitude of image patterns. A set of reference images in the template space x are therefore expressed in terms of a linear combination of a finite set of orthonormal basis:

$$x = \sum_{j=0}^{K}p_j e_j \tag{3}$$

where

$$e_0 = \left(c - \sum_{j=1}^{K}p_j^c e_j\right)\bigg/\left\|c - \sum_{j=1}^{K}p_j^c e_j\right\| \tag{4}$$

and $p^c = [e_1 e_2 ... e_K]^T c$

3.2 Normalized Correlation in the Template Space

The input image is evaluated at each location how it fits the template by extracting the region and finding the most similar pattern in the template space and computing the normalized correlation between them. The most similar pattern in the template space is the projection of the extracted region vector y into the template space (Fig. 2). Its normalized correlation to the vector y is the largest. The normalized correlation between the vector y and a reference vector x is given by $C(y,x) = x^T y / \|x\|\|y\|$. Replacing the reference image vector x with the projection $\tilde{x} = \sum_{j=0}^{K}\left(e_j^T y\right)e_j$ yields

$$C(y,\tilde{x}) = \frac{\left(\sqrt{\sum_{j=0}^{K}\left(e_j^T y\right)^2}\right)}{\|y\|} \tag{5}$$

The normalized correlation score above is the measure of similarity considering not only prestored discrete P reference images but also their interpolation. This makes

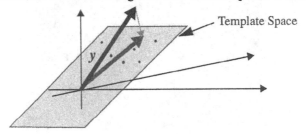

Fig.2 Template space and the projection of input image.

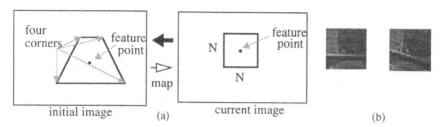

Fig.3 (a) Change of appearance of feature points. (b) Example of skewed image.

the system robust against the variation of illumination. The computation cost is greatly reduced since the original normalized correlation requires $N^2(P+1)$ operations for P reference images while (5) requires $N^2(K+2)$ operations where K can be much smaller than P.

4 Tracking of Features

Feature points that are easy to track are selected before execution, and their positions in object coordinates are given as part of the object models. When the object is recognized and the pose is calculated at the initial recognition phase, feature points are projected onto the image plane with the computed pose. A small region around each feature point is extracted as the reference image for the subsequent visual tracking. For visual tracking, normalized correlation to reference images is computed at every point in the small search areas. The positions with the best normalized correlation scores are determined as the positions of feature points in the image.

The appearance of a feature point varies during tracking due to view change. Skewing reference images using the object pose information in every cycle during tracking can compensate this effect. Reference images are small square windows of N by N pixels around feature points. Under projective transformation, straight lines are projected to straight lines and intersections are preserved in any view change. Generation of the skewed reference image is illustrated in Fig.3: first compute the skewed rectangle in the initial image which corresponds to the small square window in the current image, and then map the pixels of the initial image into the square window. The skewed rectangle in the initial image is computed from feature positions in the current image, object pose in the current and initial images, and surface orientation around feature points. Surface patches around the feature points are approximated as planar, and those equations are given as part of object models.

5 Feature Correspondence

Some features may be missed or mismatched during tracking. We need to select only those feature points which are successfully tracked. The value of normalized correlation itself can be used as the criterion, for the degree of matching at the image level. However, to cope with illumination changes and other difficulties, geometric constraints between feature points are quite useful.

5.1 Geometric Invariants

Geometric invariants [14, 15], popular in object recognition as useful descriptors of objects, are properties in the image that stay invariant under some transformation. Five coplanar points have the familiar cross ratio as their invariant. The cross-ratios I_1 and I_2 of four areas of triangles are invariant under projective transformation:

$$I_1 = \frac{S_{423}S_{125}}{S_{124}S_{523}} \qquad I_2 = \frac{S_{143}S_{125}}{S_{124}S_{153}} \tag{6}$$

where S_{ijk} is the area of a triangle with three points, i, j, and k. These values remain the same over view changes.

Another candidate is affine algebraic moment invariants [15], which are applicable to curved objects because they do not require feature points to be coplanar. If the geometric invariant values computed for tracked feature points change, it indicates that some of feature points are misrecognized.

5.2 Sensitivity of Invariants

Due to observation errors in tracking feature positions (typically 0.5 pixel), invariants vary. The sensitivity of invariants is also dependent on configuration of feature points. This makes it difficult to use constant thresholds to judge whether or not invariants are violated and thus tracking has failed. We adjust thresholds by the standard deviation of each invariant. Assume that observation errors of each feature position have a zero-means Gaussian distribution with covariance Λ_p. Invariants then have the distribution with a expected variance σ_I^2 [16]:

$$\sigma_I^2 = J\Lambda_p J^T \tag{7}$$

where J is the Jacobian matrix $[\partial I/\partial x]$ of $I = I(x)$ that relates x-y coordinates of feature points to the invariant. The threshold for each invariant is set to the standard deviation of invariants multiplied by some constant c.

Feature correspondence is carried out as follows, when cross ratios of areas of five coplanar points are used as invariants. The values I_1, I_2 in equation (6) are computed for all combinations of five points out of all feature points. The combinations whose variations of I_1 and I_2 from initial values are both below their thresholds are selected. If there is more than one combination of five feature points that satisfy the condition, we select the five feature points that produce the minimum of the maximum variation of I_1 and I_2 divided by the corresponding standard deviation. The five feature points thus selected are used to calculate the object pose.

6 Direct Computation of Image Overlay

The image invariant values help us to compute the position of points without registration. Since they are invariant to any view change, they enable us to calculate the position of one of the points from the other 2D feature positions in the current image with

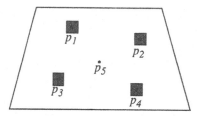

Fig.4 five coplanar points.

the value of invariants. That means that we can track a "virtual" feature point which may not have any particular pattern. We use a certain number of real trackable feature points around it, track them, and calculate the position of the virtual feature point by means of the invariant.

For example, referring to Fig. 4, with five coplanar points, the fifth point p_5 on the surface can be tracked. The values of two invariants I_1, I_2 in the first frame are calculated from the positions of p_5 and four other coplanar points. They remain constant over frames. Since they are functions of the positions of the five points, the unknown parameters are (x_5, y_5), x-y coordinates of the fifth point p_5 when we keep tracking four points p_1, p_2, p_3, p_4. We have two invariants I_1, I_2, so that we can calculate the position of the p_5 by solving these two linear equations in terms of (x_5, y_5).

7 Experimental System for Real-Time Image Overlay

We will present a real-time image overlay system. It is used for three example tasks. The first example is the tracking of a desktop PC and image overlay of the image of an I/O board. The second is the tracking of a phantom leg with some marks on it and the overlay of a bone model on its view. The third is the overlay of a virtual pin onto a leg model.

The system is implemented on multiple TMS320C40 (C40), Texas Instruments digital signal processors. We use low latency vision hardware developed at CMU[13] which has a digitizer with the high-speed data link. Image data are transferred through this high-speed data link into C40 communication ports, and then transferred to the local memory of the processor and other processors' communication ports by DMA in order to minimize the delay.

7.1 Overlay of an Image on a PC

Visual tracking of objects without attaching specific marks is tested on a desktop PC. The hypothetical task is to consistently overlay the word "Board" to indicate the I/O board that the repair person should service. At the beginning of the operation, the system displays a wire frame of the PC on the monitor and requires a user to move the camera so that the PC and the wire frame are approximately aligned (Fig.1). When the PC is roughly aligned to the wire frame, the system recognizes it, "latches" onto it, and starts tracking it. Initial recognition is executed by template matching of three regions

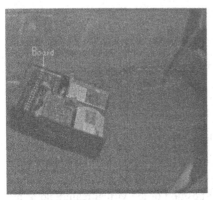 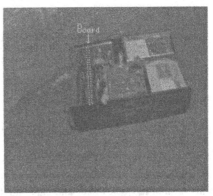

Fig.5 Real-time overlay of information ("Board") on a desktop PC image.

on the PC. Eleven images of the PC under different illumination conditions had been precaptured. Three 32 x 32 regions are extracted from each image as reference images, and template spaces are generated by four major eigenvectors.

When the three regions are successfully found, the pose of the PC is calculated from three feature positions in the image by Newton's method [8]. Feature points for tracking are projected onto the image with the computed pose. Small windows of size 16 x 12 of eight feature points are extracted from the image and are then used as reference images in the tracking phase (Fig. 5). In the tracking phase, the maximum normalized correlation of the extracted window image is searched for in 14 x 14 a region whose center position of the search area is usually set to the feature position in the last frame. In the case where the feature point is missed in the last frame, the projected feature position in the image, computed using the pose of the PC in the last frame, is used to define the center position of the search area. This allows for the recovery of tracking.

The tracking results of eight features are checked by calculating cross ratios of areas of five coplanar points. The best five points which have minimum change are selected, and the pose of the PC is computed with these five points. Feature points whose normalized correlation value is less than 0.7 are rejected before the computation of invariants. A check by geometric invariants, combined with the normalized correlation peak score, makes the tracking much more robust. The system can track the PC and superimpose the information as the camera and the PC translates and rotates in 3D, even when up to three feature points are occluded by other objects such as human hands. The system operates at the video frame rate (30 Hz). Three C40s are used in parallel: two C40s for tracking eight feature points and one for checking tracking results, pose calculation, and image overlay.

7.2 Overlay of an Image of a Bone onto a Leg

The task is to overlay a bone surface model derived from CT data on a phantom leg (Fig. 6(a)). Since there are no complex features around marks, the normalized correla-

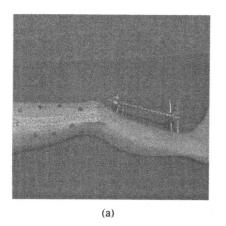 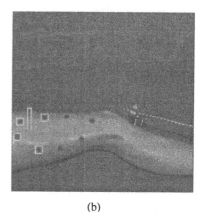

(a)   (b)

Fig.6 (a) Overlay of a bone on a leg.   (b) Overlay of a virtual pin on a leg.

tion gives us reliable matching and we did not use invariants for feature selection. As in the PC case, the overlaid image of the bone appears to remain attached to the leg despite three-dimensional motions of the leg, camera, and certain occlusions.

7.3 Pin Overlay without Models

The last task is to overlay a virtual pin onto a phantom leg (Fig.6 (b)). In the case of interactive video, when experts touch the screen to indicate the specific position of patients' bodies, the touched position is transferred to the remote site as the given pin tip position and the virtual pin is superimposed on the image of patients. Surgeons can recognize the place on patients to which the experts point, even after some motion of the patients' bodies.

The initial pin tip position is given in advance in this experiment. An overlaid image of the pin remains fixed onto the image of the leg over some motion of the leg. The tip of the pin is supposed to be attached on the leg. Four marks around the pin tip are kept tracking and the position of the pin tip is computed directly from these 2D mark positions as described before.

8 Conclusions

This paper has presented an image overlay system that uses real-time object registration and tracking. The system utilizes intensity images and detects feature points by template matching by normalized correlation. The change of intensity patterns due to view change is compensated by skewing reference images with computed object pose. Use of geometric invariants increases robustness in the feature correspondence between features in the image and the model. Real-time tracking of objects and overlaying image at frame rate (30 Hz) is achieved by the multiple DSP system with low latency vision hardware. It should be noted that no explicit model of object or display position was used in the experiment of overlaying a virtual pin on a phantom leg. This is made possible by using geometric invariants. Capable, real-time image overlay will have a broad application to interactive communication between rural surgeons and experts, which helps the delivery of expert care to geographically or socioeconomically isolated areas.

References

1. E.R. John, L.S. Prichep, J. Fridman and P. Easton, Neurometrics: computer-assisted differential diagnosis of brain disfunction, Science Vol. 239, pp.162-169 (1988).

2. L.S. Hibbard, J.S. McGlone, D.W. Davis, R.A. Hawkins, Three-Dimensional Representation and Analysis of Brain Energy Metabolism, Science, Vol. 236, pp.1641-1646 (1987).

3. C. Nastar and N. Ayache, Non-Rigid Analysis in Medical Images: a Physically Based Approach, Proc. 13th Int. Conf. on Information Processing in Medical Imaging, Berlin, Germany, pp. 17-32 (1993).

4. W.E.L. Grimson, T. Lozano-Perez, W.M. Wells , G.J. Ettinger, S.J. White, R. Kikinis, An Automatic Registration Method for Frameless Stereotaxy, Image Guided Surgery, and Enhanced Reality Visualization, Proc. CVPR'94, pp.430-436, Seattle, WA (1994).

5. C. Pelizzari, K. Tan, D. Levin, G. Chen, J. Balter, Interactive 3D Patient - Image Registration, Proc. 13th Int. Conf. on Information Processing in Medical Imaging, Berlin, Germany, pp.132-141 (1993).

6. D. Gennery, Tracking known three-dimensional objects, Proc. 2nd Nation. Conf. Artif. Intell., Pittsburgh, pp.13-17 (1982).

7. D.G. Lowe, Robust Model-Based Motion Tracking Through the Integration of Search and Estimation, Int. J. Computer Vision, Vol. 8, No.2, pp. 113-122 (1992).

8. D.G. Lowe, Fitting Parameterized Three-Dimensional Models to Images, IEEE Trans. Patt. Anal. Mach. Intell. Vol. 13, No.5, pp. 441-450 (1991).

9. D.B. Gennery, Visual Tracking of Known Three-Dimensional Objects, Int. J. Computer Vision, Vol. 7, No. 3, pp. 243-270 (1992).

10. M. Turk and A. Pentland, Face Recognition Using Eigenfaces, Proc. CVPR'91, pp.586-591, Maui, U.S.A. (1991).

11. H. Murase and S. Nayar, Parametric Eigenspace Representation for Visual Learning and Recognition, Tech. Rep. CUCS-054-92, Columbia University, NY (1992).

12. S. Yoshimura and T. Kanade, Fast Template Matching Based on the Normalized Correlation by Using Multiresolution Eigenimages, Proc. IROS'94, Munchen, Germany (1994).

13. O. Amidi, Y. Mesaki, T. Kanade, and M. Uenohara, Research on an Autonomous Vision-Guided Helicopter, Proc. RI/SME Fifth World Conf. on Robotics Research, Cambridge, Massachusetts (1994).

14. I. Weiss, Geometric Invariants and Object Recognition, Int. J. Computer Vision, Vol.10, No.3, pp. 207-231 (1993).

15. J. Munday and A. Zisserman, Introduction-Towards a New Framework for Vision. In Geometric Invariance in Machine Vision, MIT Press, Cambridge, MA (1992).

16. H. F. Durrant-Whyte, Uncertain Geometry in Robotics, IEEE J. Robotics and Automation, Vol.4, No.1, pp.23-31 (1988).

Using a 3D Position Sensor for Registration of SPECT and US Images of the Kidney

Olivier Péria[1], Laurent Chevalier[1], Anne François-Joubert[2],
Jean-Pierre Caravel[2], Sylvie Dalsoglio[3], Stéphane Lavallée[1], Philippe Cinquin[1]

[1] TIMC-IMAG, Faculté de Médecine de Grenoble, 38706 La Tronche, France
[2] Service de médecine nucléaire, C.H.U. A. Michallon, 38043 Grenoble
[3] Service de radiologie, C.H.U. A. Michallon, 38043 Grenoble

Abstract. The correlation of functional images of the kidney with anatomical images is important to improve diagnosis and treatment. We propose a method to register SPECT (Single Photon Emission Computed Tomography) and US (ultrasound) images of the kidney that consists in tracking the US probe in the space thanks to an optical three-dimensional position sensor. This method has been experimented on three patients and has provided very promising results.

1 Introduction

The complementary nature of renal nuclear medecine allows to add a physiological dimension to other image modalities [1]. The correlation of these functional images with anatomical ones would be very useful for improving diagnosis and treatment. Several techniques are available for image correlation. Good overviews of registration methods are described in [2] and [3]. All are based on the matching of external markers or reference anatomical structures visible in the involved modalities. We present a new method to register SPECT (Single Photon Emission Computed Tomography) and US (ultrasound) images of the kidney by using an intermediary sensor between the two image modalities. We already applyed this principle for registration of SPECT and MR brain images where the intermediate sensor was a range imaging system [4],[5]. In the case of US/SPECT correlation, we use a three-dimensional (3D) position sensor that provides the real time position of the US probe inside the SPECT volume.

2 Materials and Methods

2.1 Registration method

The basic idea is to have spatially referenced ultrasound images in relation with the SPECT camera. Our approch consists in using a three-dimensional localization sensor capable of providing the position of specific markers attached to the US probe. The system we use in the SPECT room consists of a workstation including a fast video digitizer board, a 3D optical localizer, rigid bodies made of infrared markers, and calibration objects.

The US/SPECT registration problem involves two calibration problems which are detailed in sections 2.4 and 2.5.

2.2 The 3D position sensor

We use an accurate 3D motion measurement sensor: the $OPTOTRAK^{TM}$ system of Northen Digital Inc. Utilizing three one-dimensional CCD cameras (figure 1), this unit can record 3D coordinates of individual infrared markers attached to the object to be measured, with an accuracy of about 0.2 mm inside a 1 m^3 volume. Several markers can be fixed on an object to build a rigid body (RB) and an intrinsic calibration procedure allows to define a local coordinate system associated with RB.

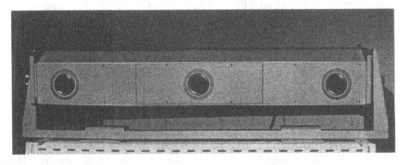

Fig. 1. The Optotrack sensor is made of three one-dimensional CCD cameras.

This sensor can then compute in real time the geometric transform between a coordinate system linked to a moving rigid body and a reference coordinate system linked to a fixed rigid body.

2.3 Localization of the US probe

A first rigid body RB0 is attached to the US probe. It is made of 18 infrared emitters and defines the coordinate system Ref_track. A second rigid body RB1 is used as a fixed reference. It is made of 6 markers and defines the coordinate system Ref_loc (figure 2). The position sensor computes in real time the rigid transform between Ref_track and Ref_loc (figure 3).

Two calibration phases are now necessary: the first one to determine the transform between Ref_track and the coordinate system Ref_us associated with the US image, the second one to determine the transform between Ref_loc and the coordinate system Ref_spect corresponding to the SPECT volume.

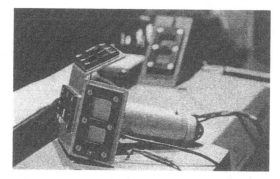

Fig. 2. A rigid body (RB0) made of 18 infrared markers is attached to the US probe. An other one (RB1) made of 6 markers is a fixed reference.

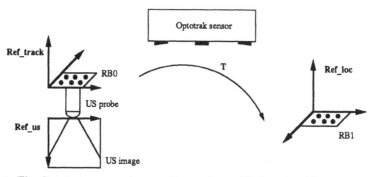

Fig. 3. The Optotrak sensor observes the motions of Ref_track with respect to Ref_loc and the transform T is real-time computed.

2.4 US / Localizer calibration

The purpose is to find the geometric transform between Ref_us and Ref_track. The method is based on the acquisition of the vertices of a triangle by the US probe (figure 4). The triangle is made of small wires stretched in a water tank to be detected by the US probe.

The vertices coordinates (3 reference points) are known in Ref_loc thanks to a 3D pointer equipped with a rigid body. An US image of the triangle is digitized and the three points are manualy segmented. The localization system provides the rigid transform T between Ref_track and Ref_loc. Therefore, the three reference points are known both in Ref_us and Ref_track. To find a rigid transform between two sets of points, simple and direct solutions exist. The problem is to estimate the transform X that minimizes the sum of squared distances between the two sets of points. It has been solved by using the Arun noniterative method [6] modified by Umeyama [7], wich is based on a singular value decomposition (SVD) algorithm. We obtain an average error on the order of 0.8 mm.

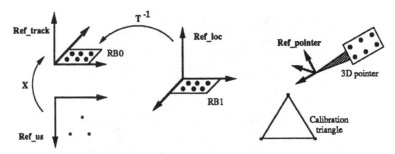

Fig. 4. The calibration triangle defines three reference points both in ref_us and Ref_track. The calibration transform X is computed by solving a point patterns registration problem.

This calibration procedure is done once only as long as the rigid body RB0 remains mounted on the US probe.

2.5 Localizer / SPECT calibration

The goal is to estimate the geometric transform H between Ref_loc and Ref_spect. These two coordinate systems are in a fixed position in the SPECT room.

The position sensor and the SPECT imager provide information that are very different by nature, that's why we have designed a calibration phantom composed with two parts (figure 5):

- A rigid body RB2 that defines the coordinate system Ref_phantom,
- Four small straight line catheters filled with Tc^{99m} that are visible by the SPECT imaging system. Their position is known in Ref_phantom with an accuracy of 0.2 mm.

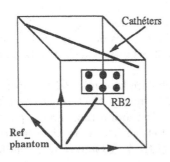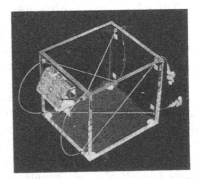

Fig. 5. The calibration phantom is made of a rigid body and four straight line catheters.

The calibration phantom is put on the SPECT couch and the calibration process is decomposed into two stages (figure 6):

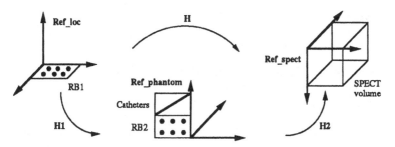

Fig. 6. The phantom is detected both by the optical sensor and the SPECT camera. The calibration transform H is the combination of the two transforms H1 and H2.

• First, the 3D position sensor directly computes the rigid transform H1 between Ref_phantom and Ref_loc with an accuracy of 0.2 mm.

• Second, a SPECT scan is performed on the phantom and the catheters are automatically segmented on the SPECT slices. We obtain four sets of points that describe the four lines in Ref_spect. To match two sets of lines, no direct solution is known [8]. The rigid transform H2 between Ref_phantom and Ref_spect is computed by a nonlinear least squares minimization method that minimizes the sum of squared distances between the points in Ref_spect and the lines in Ref_phantom. The Levenberg-Marquard algorithm is used because of its good convergence properties [9]. The average error is about 0.4 mm.

The calibration transform H is given by the combination of H1 and H2.

This calibration procedure is accomplished once for ever, on condition that the reference rigid body RB1 remains fixed in the examination room. The fact that we use a rigid body as reference instead of the Optotrak sensor allows to move the Optotrack unit without requiring a recalibration process.

2.6 Operative image processing

The patient is on the SPECT couch. First, a SPECT scan is performed with a standard one head gamma-camera (SOPHA DSX) supplied with a general purpose collimator. Reconstructed slices are obtained from the 128 pre-filtered projections (matrix size 128x128). The tracer used is DMSA-Tc^{99m}.

Second, a set of ultrasound images is obtained with a sectorial US probe (Kretz Combison 320). Each time an image is digitized on the workstation, the corresponding transform T between Ref_track and Ref_loc is acquired synchronously and stored.

For each US image, the rigid transform W between Ref_us and Ref_spect is given by the combination of the three transforms H,T and X. Therefore, the 3D position of the echographic plane is known with respect to the SPECT system.

3 RESULTS

3.1 US / SPECT registration

As soon as the SPECT images are available, they are transfered onto the workstation via the network, and the US images can be registered with the SPECT ones.
Our SPECT system takes about 20 minutes to reconstruct the images, that's
why we store the US data and display the results later. With recent SPECT
systems, reconstructed images are available immediatly after the acquisition. In
this case, it is possible to display registered US and SPECT images in real time,
during the US acquisition.

3.2 Images display

For each digitized US image, the corresponding SPECT image is reformatted
into the SPECT volume. The reformatted functional images are displayed in
pseudo color with a transparency effect on the black and white US images. It
is also possible to display them next to the anatomical images. In this case, a
linking cursor allows to identify corresponding regions of interest on the two
images (figure 7).

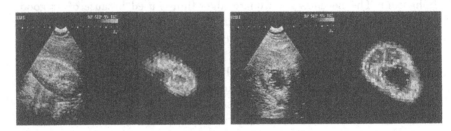

Fig. 7. Two examples of image correlation. The SPECT reformatted images are displayed next to the US slices. On the right example, white cross show corresponding
areas on the two images.

3.3 Experiments

Experiments have been performed on three patients. SPECT images has been
acquired two hours after DMSA-Tc^{99m} injection. The first one suffered from a
Wegener. The second was in a rejection phase of a transplant. The third patient
had an internal Kyst in the left kidney. In all the cases, the correlation between
SPECT and US images was approved by the physicians.

The accuracy of the whole system (transform W betwenn Ref_us and Ref_spect)
depends on the accuracy of the two calibration procedures (transforms X and

H) and on the accuracy of the Optotrak sensor (transform T). These individual accuracies are known and are better than the SPECT accuracy. We are planning to evaluate the global accuracy by using a specific phanthom.

4 CONCLUSION

We have developed a method to register SPECT and US images of the kidney that uses an intermediary sensor between the two image modalities. This registration technique is fully automated and it requires no external landmarks neither segmentation of anatomical structures. This method had been tested on three patients and has provided very promising results.

References

1. M. McBiles. Correlative Imaging of the Kidney. In *Seminars in Nuclear Medecine*, volume 14(3), pages 219–233, july 1994.
2. S. Lavallee. Registration for Computer Integrated Surgery : methodology, state of the art. In R. Taylor, S. Lavallee, G. Burdea, and R. Mosges, editors, *Computer Integrated Surgery (to appear)*. MIT Press, 1995.
3. P.A. van den Elsen, E.J. Pol, and M.A. Viergever. Medical Image Matching - A Review with Classification. In *IEEE Eng. Med. Biol.*, volume 12(1), pages 26–39, march 1993.
4. O. Peria, S. Lavallee, G. Champleboux, A.F. Joubert, J.F. Lebas, and P. Cinquin. Millimetric registration of SPECT and MR images of the brain without headholders. In *IEEE Engineering Medicine Biology Society (EMBS)*, volume 1, pages 14–15, San Diego, november 1993.
5. O. Peria, A. Francois-joubert, S. Lavallee, G. Champleboux, P. Cinquin, and S. Grand. Accurate registration of SPECT and MR brain images of patients suffering from epilepsy or tumor. In *MRCAS 94, Medical Robotics and Computer Assisted Surgery*, volume 1, pages 58–62, Pittsburgh, PA, september 1994.
6. K.S. Arun, T.S. Huang, and S.D. Blostein. Least-squares fitting of two 3-D point sets. *IEEE Trans. Pattern Anal. Machine Intell.*, PAMI-9(5):698–700, 1987.
7. S. Umeyama. Least-squares estimation of transformation parameters between two point patterns. *IEEE Trans. Pattern Anal. Machine Intell.*, PAMI-13(4):376–380, 1991.
8. O.D. Faugeras and M. Hebert. The representation, recognition and locating of 3D objects. *Int. J. Robotic Res.*, 5(3):27–52, June 1986.
9. W. H. Press, B. P. Flannery, S. A. Teukolsky, and W. T. Vetterling. *Numerical Recipes in C : The Art of Scientific Computing*. Cambridge University Press, Cambridge, England, second edition, 1992.

A New Framework for Fusing Stereo Images with Volumetric Medical Images

Fabienne Betting*, Jacques Feldmar*, Nicholas Ayache*, Frédéric Devernay+

INRIA SOPHIA, *Projet Epidaure,+Projet Robotvis
2004 route des Lucioles, B.P. 93
06902 Sophia Antipolis Cedex, France.
Email : Jacques.Feldmar@sophia.inria.fr

Abstract. Some medical interventions require knowing the correspondence between an MRI/CT image and the actual position of the patient. Examples are in neurosurgery or radiotherapy, but also in video surgery (laparoscopy). Recently, computer vision techniques have been proposed to find this correspondence without any artificial markers. Following the pioneering work of [GLPI+94], [CZH+94], [CDT+92], [SHK94] and [STAL94], we propose in this paper an alternative approach.

We propose to trade the laser range finder for two cameras. Hence, we get dense reconstruction of the patient's surface and this allows us to compute the normals to the surface. We present a new method for rigid registration when surfaces are described by points and normals. It does not depend on the initial positions of the surfaces, deals with occlusion in a strict way and takes advantage of the normal information.

Results are presented on real images.

1 Introduction

Medical images are commonly used to help establish a correct diagnosis. As they contain spatial information, both anatomical and functional, they can also be used to planify therapy, and even in some cases to control the therapy.

A recent overview of these fields of research can be found in [Aya93] and in [TLBM94], a spectacular use of planification and control of therapy using medical images and robots can be found in [Tay93, CDT+92, LSB91, LC90] for surgery and [STAL94] for radiotherapy.

More recently, the possibility of helping the surgeon to control the therapy with a projection of some pre-operative images directly onto the patient during surgery, was presented in [GLPI+94, CZH+94, SHK94].

The idea is to present on the patient some anatomical or pathological structures segmented onto pre-operative images, which are difficult to observe during surgery because they are still hidden, or simply because they are not immediately visible under normal lighting conditions (a tumor may be much more visible on a particular MRI image than with direct observation). This process is called *enhanced visualization* or *augmented reality*.

To project an image on a patient, a future solution will probably be the use of semi-transparent glasses or screen, allowing both the direct observation and the chosen image projection. A somewhat simpler solution consists in acquiring a video image of the patient from a point of view similar to the surgeon's one, and to fuse the chosen pre-operative image with this video image. Such a solution was described in [GLPI⁺94].

The difficult task is then to register, if possible in real time, the video image of the patient (intra-operative image) with the pre-operative image. This problem could be solved with artificial marker visible in both images, but this produces unacceptable constraints (e.g. pre-operative images must be taken the same day as the intervention, stereotactic frames are very painful to bear and can prevent a free access to the surgeon, etc...).

The registration problem is solved without any artificial marker by [GLPI⁺94] and [SHK94] with an intermediate laser range finder, which provides a 3D description of the patient's surface. This surface is then matched against the surface of the segmented corresponding surface in the volumetric medical image. As the laser range finder is calibrated with respect to the camera, the medical image can be fused with the video image.

In this paper we propose an alternative solution, where we would change the laser range finder for two cameras, and build the patient's surface with passive stereovision [DF94, Kan93]. Note that [CZH⁺94] also uses a stereo system.

The advantages of such an approach are the following: first, we use passive vision, instead of a laser beam, which can be annoying in the surgery room. Second, having stereo cameras, the final enhanced visualization can be done in stereovision, providing a much more vivid representation of the patient's anatomy. Third, we get a dense reconstruction of the patient's surface and this allows us to compute the normals to the surface. Thanks to these normals, we may introduce a completely new method for rigid registration when surfaces are described by points and normals as it can often be the case in medical imaging. Fourth, thanks to the density of the surface descriptions, we believe that we can get a more accurate registration than the techniques using sparse data.

The paper is organized as follows: in section 2 we briefly describe the geometry of the registration problem. In section 3, we introduce our new algorithm to find an estimate of the rigid displacement based on bitangent segments and we analyze the complexity of this algorithm. In section 4, we present a new distance minimization algorithm, which is an extension of the iterative closest point algorithm, dealing with occlusion in a strict manner and taking advantage of the normal information. Experimental results are presented in section 5. Finally, future work is presented in conclusion.

2   Geometry of the registration problem

Before the intervention, an MRI/CT image of the patient's head is acquired. This image contains the skin and the brain of the patient and also a possible tumor. The goal is to find, during the intervention, the projective transformation which maps this MRI/CT image on a video image of the patient's head.

Following the approach presented in [GLPI⁺94, CZH⁺94, SHK94], we also split the problem in two stages: reconstruction and rigid registration. But the

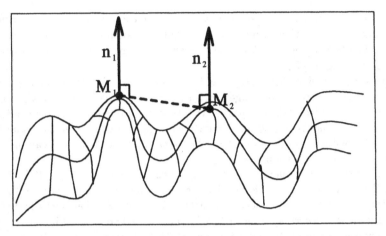

Fig. 1. A surface and two bitangent points M_1 and M_2. Let n_1 and n_2 be the normals at these points. M_1 and M_2 are bitangent if the plane defined by (M_1, n_1) and the plane defined by (M_2, n_2) are the same. Another definition is that n_1 and n_2 are identical and that the line $M_1 M_2$ is orthogonal to these two vectors.

way we perform the surface reconstruction is different. We use passive stereo as described in [DF94]. The result is a dense description of the patient's surface by points and normals. The coordinates of these points and normals are expressed in the camera frame. Because the transformation which maps the reconstructed image to the camera image is known, the problem is to find the transformation between the MRI/CT image and the reconstructed surface.

In order to find this transformation, we extract in the MRI/CT image the patient's surface and we get a description by points and normals. The rigid registration problem is the following:
Given two surfaces described by points and normals, find the rigid displacement that best superposes these two surfaces.

As mentioned in [GLPI+94], this algorithm must not depend on the initial relative positions of the surfaces, it must be accurate and robust.

3 Finding an initial estimate of the rigid displacement

The basic idea is to compute independently on each surface the set of pairs of points sharing the same tangent plane (see figure 1). We call such pairs **bitangent points**. They correspond to semi-differential invariants [GMPO92]. The technique for computing these pairs is described in [FAF94]. We simply note here that the algorithm is quasi-linear in the number of points describing the surface, and, because it involves only derivatives of order 1, the bitangent points calculation is quite stable.

In the ideal case, because the distance between the two bitangent points is invariant under rigid displacement, the following algorithm would be very efficient to rigidly superpose a surface S_1 on a surface S_2:

(1) choose a pair P_1 of bitangent points on S_1. Let $d(P_1)$ be the distance between the two points.

(2) Compute the set $SameDistance(P_1)$ of pairs of bitangent points on S_2 such that the distance between the two bitangent points is equal to $d(P_1)$.

(3) For each pair P_2 in $SameDistance(P_1)$, compute the two possible rigid displacements corresponding to the superposition of the two pairs P_1 and P_2 and of their normals. Stop when the rigid displacement which superposes S_1 on S_2 is found.

In practice, corresponding pairs of bitangent points cannot be exactly superposed because of the point discretization error and because of the error in the computation of the normal. Moreover, only a part of the reconstructed surface S_1 may be superposed on the patient's surface extracted from the MRI image S_2. So, the actual algorithm is slightly more complex, but is basically as stated. A detailed description and an analysis of the complexity can be found in [FAF94]. We simply note that the complexity of the algorithm is quasi-linear in the number of points on the surfaces and that the risk of stopping the algorithm with a wrong initial estimate decreases extremely quickly with the number of points (when the two surfaces actually show some overlapping regions up to a rigid displacement).

4 The new distance minimization algorithm

4.1 The Iterative Closest Point algorithm

Using the pairs of bitangent points as described in the previous section, we get an estimate $(\mathbf{R}_0, \mathbf{t}_0)$ of the rigid displacement to superpose S_1 on S_2. In order to find an accurate rigid displacement we have developed an extension of an algorithm called "the Iterative Closest Point algorithm" which was introduced by several researchers ([BM92], [Zha94], [CM92], [CLSB92]). We sketch the original ICP algorithm, which searches for the rigid displacement $(\mathbf{R}, \mathbf{t})$ which minimizes the energy

$$E(\mathbf{R}, \mathbf{t}) = \sum_{M_i \in S_1} \|\mathbf{R}M_i + \mathbf{t} - ClosestPoint(\mathbf{R}M_i + \mathbf{t})\|^2,$$

where $ClosestPoint$ is the function which associates to a space point its closest point on S_2.

The algorithm consists of two iterated steps, each iteration i computing a new estimation $(\mathbf{R}_i, \mathbf{t}_i)$ of the rigid displacement.

1. The first step builds a set $Match_i$ of pairs of points: for each point M on S_1, a pair (M, N) is added to $Match_i$, where N is the closest point on S_2 to the point $\mathbf{R}_{i-1}M + \mathbf{t}_{i-1}$.

2. The second step is the least squares evaluation of the rigid displacement $(\mathbf{R}_i, \mathbf{t}_i)$ to superpose the pairs of $Match_i$.

The termination criterion depends on the approach used: the algorithm stops either when a) the distance between the two surfaces is below a fixed threshold, b) the variation of the distance between the two surfaces at two successive iterations is below a fixed threshold or c) a maximum number of iterations is reached.

This ICP algorithm is efficient and finds the correct solution when the initial estimate $(\mathbf{R}_0, \mathbf{t}_0)$ of the rigid displacement is "not too bad" and when each point on S_1 has a correspondent on S_2. But in practice, this is often not the case. For example in our application, as explained in the previous section, the reconstructed surface usually only describes partially the patient's surface and often includes a description of the patient's environment. The next two subsections explain how we deal with these two problems.

4.2   Working with incomplete surfaces

In step 1 of the iterative algorithm, we map each point of S_1 to a "closest point" on S_2. But when the two surfaces are partially reconstructed, some points on S_1 do not have any homologous point on S_2. Thus, given a point M on S_1, $(\mathbf{R}_{i-1}, \mathbf{t}_{i-1})$, and $ClosestPoint(\mathbf{R}_{i-1}M + \mathbf{t}_{i-1})$, we have to decide whether $(M, ClosestPoint(\mathbf{R}_{i-1}M + \mathbf{t}_{i-1}))$ is a plausible match. This is very important because, if we accept incorrect matches, the found rigid displacement will be biased (and therefore inaccurate), and if we reject correct matches, the algorithm may not converge towards the best solution.

As proposed in [Aya91], we make use of the extended Kalman filter (EKF). This allows us to associate to the six parameters of $(\mathbf{R}_i, \mathbf{t}_i)$ a covariance matrix $\mathbf{S}_i$ and to compute a generalized Mahalanobis distance δ for each pair of matched points (M, N). This generalized Mahalanobis distance, under some assumptions on the noise distributions and some first-order approximations, is a random variable with a χ^2 probability distribution. By consulting a table of values of the χ^2 distribution, it is easy to determine a confidence level ϵ for δ corresponding to, for example a 95% probability of having the distance δ less than ϵ. In this case, we can consider the match (M, N) as *likely* or *plausible* when the inequality $\delta < \epsilon$ is verified and consider any others as *unlikely* or *unplausible*.

This distinction between plausible and unplausible matches implies a change in the second step of the iterative algorithm. Given $Match_i$, instead of computing the rigid displacement $(\mathbf{R}, \mathbf{t})$ which minimizes the least squares criterion

$$\sum_{(M,N) \,\in\, Match_i} \|\mathbf{R}_i M + \mathbf{t}_i - N\|^2,$$

we recursively estimate the six parameters of $(\mathbf{R}, \mathbf{t})$, and the associated covariance matrix which minimizes the criterion

$$\sum_{(M,N) \,\in\, Match_i \text{ and } (M,N) \text{ is plausible}} (\mathbf{R}_i M + \mathbf{t}_i - N)^t \mathbf{W}_i^{-1} (\mathbf{R}_i M + \mathbf{t}_i - N),$$

where $\mathbf{W}_i$ is a covariance matrix which allows us, for example, to increase the importance of high curvature points.

More details about the meaning of "plausible or not" and about the EKF can be found in [FAF94].

4.3 Using the normal information

As is commonly encountered with any minimization algorithm, the ICP algorithm may become trapped in a local minimum. To reduce this problem, we propose in this subsection to make use of the normal information and to define a new criterion to minimize. In our formulation, surface points are no longer 3D points: they become 6D points. Coordinates of a point M on the surface S are (x, y, z, n_x, n_y, n_z) where (n_x, n_y, n_z) is the normal to S at M. For two points $M(x, y, z, n_x, n_y, n_z)$ and $N(x', y', z', n'_x, n'_y, n'_z)$ we define the distance:

$$d(M, N) = (\ \alpha_1(x - x')^2 + \alpha_2(y - y')^2 + \alpha_3(z - z')^2 + \\ \alpha_4(n_x - n'_x)^2 + \alpha_5(n_y - n'_y)^2 + \alpha_6(n_z - n'_z)^2)^{1/2}$$

where α_i is the inverse of the difference between the maximal and minimal value of the ith coordinate of points in S_2. Using this definition of distance, the closest point to P on S_2 is a compromise between the 3D distance and the difference in normal orientation[1].

This new definition of the distance between points naturally implies modifications to steps one and two of the ICP algorithm in order to minimize the new energy:

$$E(\mathbf{R}, \mathbf{t}) = \sum_{M \in S_1} d(\ (\mathbf{R}M + \mathbf{t}, \mathbf{R}n_1(M)), \\ ClosestPoint\_6D((\mathbf{R}_{i-1}M + \mathbf{t}, \mathbf{R}_{i-1}n_1(M)))^2,$$

where $n_1(M)$ is the normal on S_1 at point M and $ClosestPoint\_6D$ is the new 6D closest point function.

In step one, the closest point now has to be computed in 6D space. We use the kd-tree technique first proposed by Zhang ([Zha94]) for the 3D case. The second step also has to be modified: the criterion which defines the best rigid displacement must use the new 6D distance. Otherwise, it is not possible to prove the convergence of our new ICP algorithm (see [FAF94]). Hence, the rigid displacement $(\mathbf{R}_i, \mathbf{t}_i)$ is now defined as the minimum of the function

$$f(\mathbf{R}, \mathbf{t}) = \sum_{(M, N) \in match_i} d(\mathbf{R}M + \mathbf{t}, N)^2,$$

where, the coordinates of the point $\mathbf{R}M + \mathbf{t}$ are $(\mathbf{R}M + \mathbf{t}, \mathbf{R}n_1(M))$.

In practice, we use extended Kalman filters to minimize this new criterion at step 2. Even though it is is non linear, the minimization works very well. Note that this use of extended Kalman filters allows us to compute Mahalanobis distances and to determine if a match is plausible or not as explained in the previous subsection.

---

[1] Of course, only two parameters are necessary to describe the orientation of the normal (for example the two Euler angles). But we use (n_x, n_y, n_z) because the Euclidean distance better reflects the difference of orientation between the normals (that is not the case with the Euler angles because of the modulo problem) and we can use kd-trees to find the closest point as explained later.

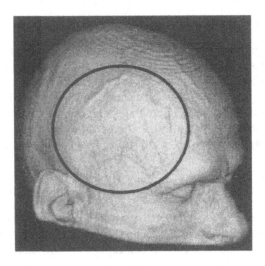

Fig. 1. Rendered view of POPR skin surface illustrating extracted IOPR patch.

surfaces. Figure 1 illustrates the surface patch extracted from the POPR that was used as the IOPR. The position of the IOPR was perturbed from its correctly registered position by adding random uniformly distributed translations and rotations (simultaneously) ranging from $\pm 1 - 14mm$ and $\pm 2 - 28^{\circ}$ (about the IOPR centre-of-mass). The automatic registration procedure then sought to recover the original position of the IOPR. At each 'level' of perturbation, 100 trials were performed. Figure 2 shows the resulting errors for this experiment. The seemingly odd behaviour of Tx and Ry can be explained by orientation and symmetry relationships between the two surfaces. The POPR x, y, z coordinate axes were right-left, anterior-posterior, and inferior-superior, respectively.

3.2 Experiment 2: Sensitivity to IOPR size

This experiment studied the extent to which an accurate registration could be achieved using IOPR surfaces of different size. Each was centred at the same position as the one illustrated in Figure 1. Perturbations of $\pm 10mm$ and $\pm 20^{\circ}$ were employed, and the basic perturbation-registration experiment was repeated 100 times. The resulting errors are shown in Figure 3 where they are plotted as a function of IOPR patch size. This size was expressed as a percentage of the 'total' segmented skin surface extracted from the MR data. For example, the patch illustrated in Figure 1 was 26% of the total POPR skin surface.

3.3 Experiment 3: Sensitivity to surface overlap

In practice it may be difficult to assure that the IOPR extracted using the video cameras overlaps completely the POPR. Points in the IOPR that extend beyond

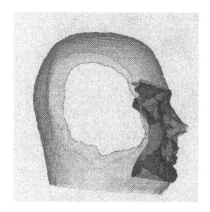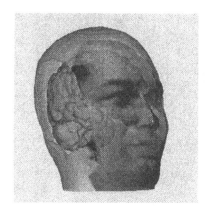

Fig. 3. Left: The result of the rigid registration. The MRI surface is clearer and the stereo surface is darker. The alternation dark/clear shows that the registration is quite accurate. **Right:** The colorized MRI head surface obtained by attaching to each matched point the gray level of its corresponding point on the stereo surface. Thanks to the transparency effect, one can observe the brain...

Using this estimate of the rigid displacement, we run the modified iterative closest point algorithm. The MRI head surface is described by 15000 points and the stereo surface by 10000 points. It takes 20 seconds. Applying this new rigid displacement, 85% of the points on the stereo surface have their closest point at a distance lower than $3mm$. The average distance between matched points is $1.6mm$. The result is presented in figure 3, left.

Because we know the point-to-point correspondences between the MRI head surface and the stereo face surface (this is the result of the registration), and because for each point of the stereo surface we know the grey level from the video image, we can map the video image onto the MRI surface (figure 3, right). The fact that the points on the MRI surface have the right grey levels qualitatively demonstrates that the MRI/stereo matching is correct.

Finally, we projected the brain onto the video image (see figure 4) using the computed projective transformation. In fact, we now have enough geometric and textural parameters to produce a stereo pair of realistic images from a continuous range of viewpoints and provide the surgeon the feeling of seeing inside the patient's head and guide him/her during the intervention.

6 Conclusion and future work

We proposed to use passive stereovision and a new rigid matching algorithm to register pre-operative with intra-operative images. Though we have presented results on real data, a lot of work still has to be done. We would like to compare the techniques described in this paper with respect to the techniques presented by others. For example, we plan to develop procedures to validate rigorously

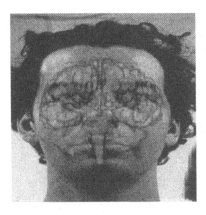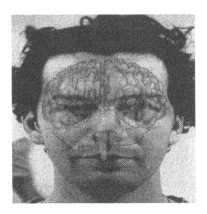

Fig. 4. The projection of the brain in the two video images using the projective transformation computed as explained in this paper. A stereoscopic display could provide the surgeon with the feeling of seeing inside the patient's head. The two presented images cannot be visually fused in this position, because the baseline between the two optical centers of the video cameras was vertical in this experiment: one can notice that the camera of left image was bellow the camera of the right one. This will be corrected in further experiments.

the accuracy of the methods. We also have to validate our approach on a larger scale, if possible in hospital environment.

We believe that it should be possible to perform real time tracking of the patient and enable the surgeon to move either patient or the 2D sensor. Indeed, for tracking we just need to correct a rigid displacement which is quite close to the right solution. Hence, because the initialization would be good, it should be possible to use the iterative closest point algorithm with just a few reconstructed points without local minimum problem and to get fast convergence. We hope and believe that it should be possible to perform the loop reconstruction/registration/visualization at a $1Hertz$ frequency using still existing fast stereo systems (as [DF94, Kan93]) and efficient graphic hardware (as Kubota or Silicon Graphics).

The passive video system should also allow us to build a system to visualize the surgeon's instruments in the MRI/CT image. Indeed, assume that on each instrument a few points (at least three) are easily identified in the two camera images. We can triangulate these points and find the position of the instruments with respect to the MRI/CT image. We believe that this could be helpful for surgeons, especially for interventions requiring high accuracy.

Acknowledgments: *we wish to thank G. Malandain and M. Brady for practical help and stimulating discussions. Thanks are also due to* **General Electric Medical System Europe (GEMS)** *for providing us with some of the data presented here. Thanks to Dr Michel Royon (Cannes Hospital) and Dr Jean-Jacques Baudet (La Timone Hospital) for fruitful discussions. This work was supported in part by a grant from* **Digital Equipment Corporation** *and by the European Basic Research Action* **VIVA**.

References

[Aya91]   N. Ayache. *Artificial Vision for Mobile Robots — Stereo-Vision and Multisensory Perception.* Mit-Press, 1991.

[Aya93]   N. Ayache. Analysis of three-dimensional medical images - results and challenges. research report 2050, INRIA, 1993.

[BM92]   Paul Besl and Neil McKay. A method for registration of 3−D shapes. *PAMI*, 14(2):239–256, February 1992.

[CDT+92]   P. Cinquin, P. Demongeot, J. Troccaz, S. Lavallee, G. Champleboux, L. Brunie, F. Leitner, P. Sautot, B. Mazier, A. Perez M. Djaid, T. Fortin, M. Chenin, and A. Chapel. Igor: Image guided operating robot. methodology, medical applications, results. *ITBM*, 13:373–393, 1992.

[CLSB92]   G. Champleboux, S. Lavallée, R. Szeliski, and L. Brunie. From accurate range imaging sensor calibration to accurate model-based 3−D object localization. In *CVPR*, Urbana Champaign, June 1992.

[CM92]   Y. Chen and G. Medioni. Object modeling by registration of multiple range images. *Image and Vision Computing*, 10(3):145–155, 1992.

[CZH+94]   A.C.F. Colchester, J. Zhao, C. Henri, R.L. Evans, P. Roberts, N. Maitland, D.J. Hawkes, D.L.G. Hill, A.J. Strong, D.G. Thomas, M.J. Gleeson, and T.C.S Cox. Craniotomy simulation and guidance using a stereo video based tracking system (vislan). In *Visualization in Biomedical Computing*, Rochester, Minnesota, October 1994.

[DF94]   F. Devernay and O. D. Faugeras. Computing differential properties of 3d shapes from stereoscopic images without 3d models. In *CVPR*, Seattle, USA, June 1994.

[FAF94]   J. Feldmar, N. Ayache, and F.Betting. 3d-2d projective registration of free-form curves and surfaces. research report 2434, INRIA, 1994. Available via ftp anonymous on zenon.inria.fr, file /pub/rapports/RR-2434.ps and via WWW ftp://zenon.inria.fr/pub/rapports.

[GLPI+94] W.E.L. Grimson, T. Lozano-Perez, W.M. Wells III, G.J. Ettinger, S.J White, and R. Kikinis. An automatic registration method for frameless stereotaxy, image guided surgery, and enhanced reality visualization. In *CVPR*, Seattle, USA, June 1994.

[GMPO92]   Luc Van Gool, Theo Moons, Eric Pauwels, and André Oosterlinck. Semi-differential invariants. In Joseph L. Mundy and Andrew Zisserman, editors, *Geometric Invariance in Computer Vision*. Mit-Press, 1992.

[Kan93]   T. Kanade. very fast 3d sensing hardware. *Internationnal Symposium on Robotic Research*, October 1993.

[LC90]   S. Lavallée and P. Cinquin. *Computer assisted medical intervention*, volume 60. Hohne K.H. et al ed, Imaging in Medicine. Springer Verlag, 1990.

[LSB91]   Stéphane Lavallée, Richard Szeliski, and Lionel Brunie. Matching 3-d smooth surfaces with their 2-d projections using 3-d distance maps. In *SPIE, Geometric Methods in Computer Vision*, San Diego, Ca, July 1991.

[SHK94]   D. Simon, M. Hebert, and T. Kanade. Techniques for fast and accurate intra-surgical registration. In *First international symposium on medical robotics and computer assisted surgery*, Pittsburgh, September 1994.

[STAL94]   A. Shweikard, R. Tombropoulos, J. Adler, and J.C. Latombe. Planning for image-guided radiosurgery. In *AAAI 1994 Spring Symposium Series. Application of Computer Vision in Medical Image Processing*, Stanford University, March 1994. Also in Proc. IEEE Int. Conf. Robotics and Automation.

[Tay93]   R. Taylor. An overview of computer assisted surgery research. *Internationnal Symposium on Robotic Research*, October 1993.

[TLBM94]   R.H. Taylor, S. Lavallee, G.C. Burdea, and R.W. Mosge. *Computer integrated surgery*. Mit-Press, 1994. To appear.

[Zha94]   Z. Zhang. Iterative point matching for registration of free-form curves and surfaces. *IJCV*, 13(2):119–152, 1994. Also RR No.1658, INRIA, 1992.

Visualisation of Multimodal Images for Neurosurgical Planning and Guidance

J. Zhao[1], A.C.F. Colchester[1], C. J. Henri[1], D. Hawkes[2] and C. Ruff[2]

Department of Neurology[1], Radiological Sciences[2], UMDS, Guy's Hospital, London, SE1 9RT

Abstract. This paper describes two new methods of rendering multimodal images developed for a neurosurgical planning and guidance system (*VISLAN*). In our volume rendering technique we introduce a colour dependent filtering mechanism that enhances the representation of objects and improves the visualisation of spatial relationships. To achieve a good compromise between rendering speed and image quality, surface rendering is divided into two processes, a fast surface voxel projection and a surface refining and shading process. By considering the reflections from voxels both near to and on a surface in shading calculations, renderings become less sensitive to small surface extraction errors. A scheme which intermixes the volume rendering for some objects and surface rendering for others in the same scene is also presented. We show examples to illustrate each method in the context of preoperative surgical planning and intraoperative guidance.

1. Introduction

Medical imaging plays an increasingly important role in neurosurgery, both preoperatively in the planning phase and intraoperatively with traditional stereotaxy or with various types of pointing devices [1]. Because the image data are typically obtained as a stack of 2D slices representing sections of the 3D object, understanding spatial relationships within the data can sometimes be difficult even for an expert, and becomes even more problematic when multimodal image data are acquired. This problem combined with the rapid advance of computer hardware has stimulated research into the 3D display of medical volumetric data [2-5].

Recently, we presented preliminary results from a new frameless stereotatic neurosurgical planning and guidance system (*VISLAN*) based on intraoperative video imaging[6]. In this paper we detail the 3D display (rendering) techniques in the system.

2. Rendering Techniques

Since the two types of rendering methods (surface rendering and volume rendering) are well suited to display different types of data under different conditions, we have implemented each one in *VISLAN*. However, our implementation incorporates a number of new features and includes a simple graphical user interface to facilitate rendering and visualisation.

2.1 Volume Rendering

Volume rendering comprises two main processes, voxel classification and volume compositing. The purpose of the first process is to determine the percentage of each material of interest in each voxel, i.e. to build an occupancy map. A simple but commonly used classification scheme is to map the intensity of a voxel into occupancy values linearly [3,4]. Problems can arise when spatially adjacent structures are not adjacent in intensity space or where each voxel contains more than two types of tissue. In a CT image, where air, fat, soft tissue and bone are often classified by their intensity ranges, this means that any mixtures other than air and fat, or fat and soft tissue, or soft tissue and bone may produce tissue misclassification at boundaries. To avoid this, a more sophisticated scheme has to be used, which usually involves manual segmentation. Even though, theoretically, a non-binary occupancy map (i.e. a map allowing spatial overlapping of different types of structures) can also be created by manual segmentation, a binary occupancy map is often preferred for simplicity. These ideas have been used previously in the volume rendering of multiple objects from both a single [7,8] and multimodal images [9]. In our implementation, we use linear intensity mapping to classify the bony structure from a CT image and the vessels from a MRA image. Interactive segmentation tools are used for binary classification of other structures.

The task of volume compositing is to project classified structures from a 3-D image onto an image plane. An efficient way to perform volume compositing is ray casting, whose principles are as follows. One ray per display pixel is cast into the volume along the view direction. Assuming that the volume is uniformly illuminated through its depth, reflections are estimated at evenly spaced locations along the ray. Each reflection is attenuated by the volume it encounters as it travels back to the image plane and then accumulated. The sum gives the colour and intensity of the pixel. To composite multiple objects, each object is assigned a unique colour and opacity. Afterwards, there are two ways to form an image. One is to first combine the colours and opacities of multiple objects at each sampled position, then treat this combination as a single object [3,4]. The other is to calculate reflections from each object independently, then accumulate all the reflections along the ray [8,9]. It is yet unclear which method is better. We use the second. In addition to some common procedures for improving computational efficiency in ray casting (such as using a bounding box to avoid casting rays into an empty volume; casting rays from front to back and stopping rays when they are completely attenuated; keeping intermediate results; and using look-up tables wherever possible), an important new feature, which we term "colour-dependent filtering" has been incorporated. The basic idea behind the colour-dependent filtering is that a voxel attenuates each colour component (red, green and blue) of reflected light passing through it differently depending on the assigned colour of the voxel: *a colour component (e.g. red) is more severely attenuated if the assigned colour of the voxel does not have that component.* The significance of colour-dependent filtering can be seen from the following two examples.

Example 1: Suppose there are two objects, say, a piece of bone and a thin blood vessel. The vessel is assigned the colour red and is closer to the viewpoint than the bone which is assigned the colour white. In traditional volume rendering, the vessel attenuates each colour of the reflected light from the bone equally. Since the vessel is thin, it reflects little light and also attenuates little of the light passing through it. This can lead to a rendered image whose colour is dominated by white (the colour of bone), and a false impression could occur that the vessel is within or behind the bone. The left image of Figure 1 illustrates this problem, In the outlined areas, the vessels, which are actually in front of the bony structure, appear within it. "Colour dependent filtering" solves this problem: we make the attenuation of transmitted light dependent on the assigned colour of an object causing the attenuation. This means, in this example, that the blue and green components of the reflected light from the bone are more severely attenuated when passing through the vessels than red . As a result, the colour of the rendered image is no longer dominated by the colour of the bone, and the true spatial relationship of the structures is correctly perceived. This is shown in the right image of Figure 1.

Example 2: Suppose there are two objects, say, a blood vessel and a tumour. The vessel is assigned the colour red and the tumour green. If the attenuation is not colour dependent, the accumulation of the reflections from these two objects could result in some yellow pixels in a rendered scene. If there happened to be a third object in the scene assigned the colour yellow, the observer might be misled or confused. With colour dependent filtering, the reflection from one of the objects is severely attenuated when it passes through the other object since the two objects do not have any common colour component, thus avoiding obvious yellow pixels in a rendered image.

2.2 Surface Rendering

An important aspect to be considered in developing a surface rendering technique is how to represent the surface of an object. The three most common ways to do so are a) by a list of polygons[10], b) by a list of surface voxels or faces of surface voxels[5] , and c) by labelling all voxels in the volume with a binary label or attaching an attribute to each grey level voxel[11]. In the *VISLAN* system, we use a list of surface voxels to represent the surface mainly because this is more economic in terms of disk and memory space and an object can potentially be quickly displayed.

We use a scheme similar to one suggested by Udupa[5] to encode a list of surface voxels. This coupled with pre-calculated and digitised grey level gradients at each surface voxel position can achieve very fast rendering through voxel projection on a general purpose workstation[5]. However, we found that the rendered images produced in this manner do not have satisfactory quality, mainly because of the following reasons:
1) The resolution of a rendered image is limited by the voxel size. Even though this problem can be solved by supersampling the data set before segmentation and construction of the data structures, this solution will dramatically increase the number of voxels to be processed, and thus the amount of memory required and computational cost.
2) Shading solely depends on the reflections from surface voxels. These reflections are very sensitive to surface voxel locations which are in turn sensitive to segmentation limitations.

In order to overcome these two problems, we perform surface rendering through two stages. First, the surface voxels extracted from the original data set (without any supersampling) are projected in the view direction onto a Z-buffer without any shading calculation. By using neighbourhood information and a number of lookup tables, this process is very fast. This first stage gives an approximate z value for each pixel. In the second stage, each value in the Z-buffer is refined by searching for the nearest surface point of the object in the view direction through supersampling. Since an approximate z value is already known, this search is much faster than conventional ray tracing techniques. Once the Z-buffer is refined, the local grey level gradient at the refined surface position and the positions nearby are calculated from the original grey level data. The reflection from each position is calculated by applying the Phong model. The reflections are weighted and summed to give the shading of the object at that position. The reflections from the refined surface positions are weighted more heavily than the reflections from the nearby positions. With such an arrangement, the partial volume effects and other small segmentation errors are reduced.

2.3 Intermixing surface and volume rendering

Since each type of rendering technique is suitable for displaying certain types of objects which can coexist in the same image, it is often desirable to mix surface and volume rendering. This is accomplished as follows:

1) The objects to be surface rendered are processed first and one full resolution shaded image is created for each object.

2) Ray casting is then employed for volume rendering from front to back along the view direction. When the ray reaches any surface rendered object, the shading of the object is accumulated in a similar way as the reflected light from a volumetric voxel.

3. Pre-operative Visualisation and Surgical Planning

3.1 Data

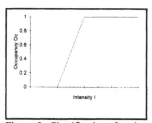

MR and MRA were acquired from a volunteer. These two data sets were co-registered. The skin and brain surfaces were segmented from the MR data using a hierarchical segmentation tool[12]. The occupancy map of the blood vessels was built from the MRA data using the function shown in Figure 2. To illustrate the concept of surgical planning, a imaginary tumour was implanted in the MR data of the volunteer.

Figure 2 Classification function used in forming occupancy map of blood vessels and bony structure.

3.2 Preoperative Visualisation

Figure 3 shows a combined display of MRA data and brain surface. The vessels are volume rendered, and the brain is surface rendered. Both objects are assigned full opacities. By displaying the two objects in the same image, their spatial relationship is more easily appreciated. In Figure 4, both the brain and tumour are surface rendered. Since a low opacity is selected for the brain surface, the tumour which is in the middle of the brain becomes visible. This type of semi-transparent display is useful for understanding hidden objects.

3.3 Cranial Window Planning

Figure 5 shows an example of cranial window planning using the *VISLAN* system which benefits from the 3D display. Different rendered scenes are displayed side by side at a view angle the surgeon selects. He can then move the mouse to draw a cranial window on the rendered scene of vessels and tumour based on the criterion that there were no major vessels on the path to the target. The same window is shown simultaneously in other rendered scenes (the brain surface and the skin surface), at the corresponding position. This allows the user to balance several constraints including the avoidance of critical brain structures and cosmetic considerations in planning the craniotomy, as well as avoiding major blood vessels. Such a preoperative planned cranial window is used in the *VISLAN* system at the start of an operation to tell the surgeon where to make the incision for the craniotomy.

4. Intra-operative Guidance

4.2 Examples of 3D Display in Intraoperative Guidance

Figure 6 shows the pre-operatively planned cranial window superimposed on the intra-operative video frame of the volunteer. Within the cranial window are shown surface rendered brain surface and volume rendered blood vessels from the POPR. The optical distortion of the camera and the perspective transformations are taken into account in the rendering. Such a display can help the surgeon in two ways. Firstly, it allows the surgeon to draw the outline of the planned cranial window on the real patient using visual feedback from the video monitor. Secondly, the surgeon can anticipate the underlying structures which will be revealed if he proceeds with this approach, and by comparing the actual structures made visible during surgery with the predicted appearances he can confirm the accuracy of registration.

Figure 7 illustrates the real time tracking of a hand held locator using our intraoperative system. The left picture is a video frame where the locator is pointing to the simulated tumour in the skull phantom. The right picture shows the graphic representation of the locator superimposed on the rendered scene in which the bony structure is volume rendered and the vessels, nerves and tumour are surface rendered. The right image intuitively tells the surgeon where he is pointing, what structures are nearby and how far away he is from the target.

5. Discussions

The main advantage of volume rendering is that it allows varying degrees of confidence in classification of voxel content to be represented, so that the uncertainty and fuzziness in object definition can be reasonably well visualised. However, it is not a trivial task to perform proper continuous classification, especially for multimodal images. In our current implementation, voxels in each image are independently classified. This could cause conflict at some spatial positions. In the further development of our volume rendering, this issue will be addressed.

6. Conclusions

Two rendering techniques have been described. A number of new features are incorporated including a method of calculating the attenuation of a transmitted ray which depends on the colours of the ray and of the object through which it passes. Some examples were given to illustrate the application of the rendering techniques in preoperative planning and in intraoperative guidance. The software is currently in trial and refinement work continues.

7. Acknowledgments

VISLAN is a joint academic - industrial project supported by the Department of Trade and Industry of the UK. The authors express our gratitude to the team lead by Richard Evans from our industrial partner, the Roke Manor Research Ltd, for their technical help and to Derek Hill for various helpful discussions. We would also like to thank our clinical collaborators, Mr Anthony Strong at the Maudsley Hospitals and Professor David Thomas at the National Hospital for Neurology and Neurosurgery, for their valuable comments on the *VISLAN* system.

8. References

1. Maiunas R (ed), Interactive Image-Guided Neurosurgery. *American Association of Neurological Surgeons*, 1993.
2. Höhne K , Bernstein R. Shading 3D images from CT using gray level gradients. *IEEE Transactions on Medical Imaging* 1986;5:45-47.
3. Drebin R , Carpenter L, Hawahan P. Volume Rendering. *Computer Graphics* 1988;22:65-74.
4. Levoy M. Display of Surface from Volume Data. *IEEE Computer Graphics & Applications* 1988;29-37.
5. Udupa JK, Odhner D. Fast visualization, manipulation, and analysis of binary volumetric objects. *IEEE Computer Graphics And Applications* 1991;11:53-62.
6. Colchester ACF, Zhao J, Henri C, et al. Craniotomy Simulation and Guidance Using a Stereo Video Based Tracking System. *Visualiazation in Biomedical Computing 1994*, R. Robb(ed), SPIE, volume 2359, 541-551.
7. Hanson D , Larson A , Karwoski R , Camp J , Robb R . Simultaneous and Interactive Rendering of Multiple Objects. *3D Advanced Image Processing in Medicine -- RENNES'92*, France, 1992;9-11.
8. Gilchrist R. A Multi-Mode 3D Render for Clinical and Scientific Visualisation. *Visualisation in Biomedical Computing 1992*, R. Robb (ed), SPIE 1808, 362-373.
9. Ruff CF, Hill DLG, Robinson GP, Hawkes D . Volume Rendering of Multimodal Images for the Planning of Skull Base Surgery. *Computer Assisted Radiology '93*, Herausgegeben Von (ed), Springer-Verlag, 1993;574-579.
10. Boissonnat J . Shape reconstruction from planar cross-sections. *Comp Vis Graph and Image Processing* 1988;44(1):1-29.
11. Höhne K , Bomans M, Pommert A, Riemer M, et al. 3D Visualization of tomographic volume data using the generalized voxel model. *Visual Computer* 1990;6:28-36.
12. Griffin L , Colchester ACF, Roll SA, Studholme CS. Hierarchical Segmentation Satisfying Constraints. *British Machine Vision Conference 94*, E. Hancock (ed), BMVA Press, 1994;

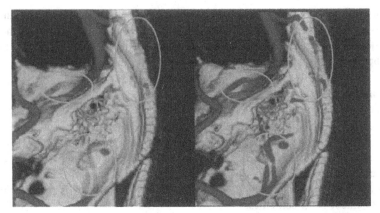

Fig. 1 Volume rendered scenes with (right image) and without colour dependent filtering (left image). Note the differences between two images, particularly at those circled areas.

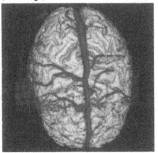

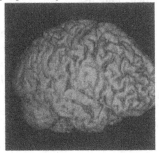

Fig. 3 Rendered scene of brain surface and blood vessels.

Fig. 4 Rendered scene of brain surface and tumour.

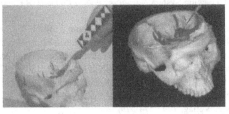

Fig. 5 Preoperative planning of cranial window based on a number of rendered scenes.

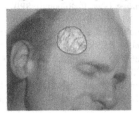

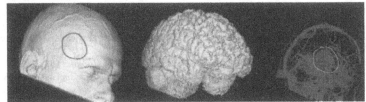

Fig. 6 Compositing image of cranial window & live video. Within the window is the rendered scene of brain surface and blood vessels.

Fig. 7 Tracking of a hand held locator. Left image is a video frame. Right image is the rendered scene with the graphical representation of the locator superimposed.

Registration of 3-D Surface Data for Intra-Operative Guidance and Visualization in Frameless Stereotactic Neurosurgery

Christopher J. Henri[1], Alan C.F. Colchester[1], Jason Zhao[1], David J. Hawkes[2], Derek L.G. Hill[2] and Richard L. Evans[3]

[1] Department of Neurology, UMDS Guy's Hospital, London SE1 9RT
[2] Division of Radiological Sciences, UMDS Guy's Hospital, London SE1 9RT
[3] Roke Manor Research Ltd, Romsey, Hants SO51 0ZN

Abstract. We describe a technique for registering 3-D multimodal image data, acquired preoperatively, with intraoperative surface data derived from stereo video during neurosurgery. Ultimately, our aim is to provide a system that supplants traditional frame-based stereotactic techniques while achieving comparable accuracy. For registration we employ chamfer-matching in conjunction with a cost function that is robust to 'outliers'. To balance robustness and computation speed, we employ a quasi-stochastic search of parameter space that includes pursuing multiple start points. This paper describes the registration problem as it pertains to our application. We discuss our approach to optimization and carry out a computational evaluation of the technique under various conditions.

1 Introduction

This paper addresses the issue of registration between 3-D image data acquired pre- and intraoperatively for neurosurgery planning and guidance. Ultimately, our aim is to provide a cost efficient and reliable system to supplant traditional (i.e., frame-based) stereotactic methods while assuring that the required accuracies are maintained. In so doing, we have chosen to avoid the use of mechanical pointing devices and magnetic, sonic or LED-based tracking systems to obtain a greater freedom of movement without being 'tethered' to cables that can be bothersome or a risk to the sterile environment. We have recently presented details of the prototype of our system, *VISLAN*[1]. Aside from registration, there are components responsible for 1) the segmentation of image data acquired preoperatively (eg, CT, MRI); 2) visualization of these data in 2-D and 3-D with tools to plan the surgical procedure; 3) the extraction of a patient surface intraoperatively via stereo video cameras; 4) the tracking of a passive hand-held pointer, and 5) the compositing of live video during surgery with either preoperative data or plans (eg, a cranial window, tumour outline, 3-D rendered images, etc.). Registration is an essential part of this system since it is necessary to relate (and update during surgery) the coordinate systems of the pre- and intraoperative patient representations (POPR and IOPR, respectively). For this purpose we employ chamfer matching in conjunction with a robust estimator. Although several groups have described the use of chamfer matching in both 2-D and 3-D medical image registration problems[2, 3, 4], until now it has not been described in intraoperative contexts.

In addition to our system, two others have been described recently that employ video intraoperatively in frameless surgical applications[5, 6]. Differences between these systems lie in the roles played by the video imaging. In *VISLAN*, for example, it is used to obtain the intraoperative patient surface; track a passive hand-held locator, and composite real-time intraoperative scenes with matching views of the preoperative data[4]. The systems described by Grimson *et al*[5] and Heilbrun *et al*[6] include only this last feature (which Grimson refers to as 'enhanced reality'). While Heilbrun relies on fiducial markers, Grimson employs a laser range scanner during surgery in conjunction with an ad hoc surface fitting method to achieve registration. Neither of these systems provide a pointer for real-time feedback and guidance during surgery.

In the following sections, we describe our approach to registration, including a number of computational evaluations, and we illustrate its use through an example.

2 Methods

2.1 Image Acquisition and Pre-processing

The patient is scanned prior to surgery using either or both CT or MRI covering as much of the head as possible. The skin surface is segmented along with any other relevant objects that may be useful in planning the surgery (eg, blood vessels in MRA, brain surface, tumour, etc.). The neurosurgeon then plans his approach using several 3-D display tools, as described in our companion paper[8].

A distance transformation applied to the skin surface data yields the 3-D distance map required for chamfer matching[2, 3, 9]. First, however, additional slices may be interpolated from the segmented data using a shape based method[9] to obtain a volume sampled isotropically (i.e., with cubic voxels).

Prior to making any incisions or draping the surgical site, two video cameras mounted overhead are used to extract the patient's 3-D skin surface. The stereo reconstruction technique uses patterned light and takes approximately 30 seconds on a SUN SPARC IPX workstation. RMS errors in this surface (the IOPR) are typically less than $0.5mm$ in 3-D.

2.2 Registration

The POPR and IOPR coordinate systems are assumed to be related by rigid body transformations (3 rotations and 3 translations) with a fixed scale factor.

---

[4] In *VISLAN*, video distortions are corrected as described by Harris and Teeder[7].

An initial registration is obtained by identifying three or more roughly corresponding landmarks on the two surfaces and computing a least-squares transformation using the 'Procrustes' algorithm[10]. This takes less than 15 seconds. In a 3-D display that combines the two surfaces as different coloured point-clouds, it is straightforward then to determine visually if there are portions of the IOPR that are not present in the POPR. These can be discarded easily via manual editing, but since we use a robust estimator in the fitting procedure (described below), the influence of these points is suppressed anyway.

The automatic registration procedure then seeks to determine the set of rotations, R, and translations, T, that minimize the cost function, C (see [11]):

$$C(R,T) = \sum_{i=1}^{N} log\left(1 + \tfrac{1}{2}\mathbf{d}_i(R,T)^2\right), \qquad \mathbf{d}_i(R,T) = min\left[t_{max}, \mathbf{p}_i(R,T) - \mathbf{q}(\mathbf{p}_i)\right],$$

where $\mathbf{p}_i(R,T)$ is the position of a point on the IOPR surface after being transformed via R and T; $\mathbf{q}(\mathbf{p}_i)$ is its closest point on the POPR surface, and their difference is a distance in mm. This distance, in fact, is found by 'looking-up' the value in the 3-D distance map at the position specified by $\mathbf{p}_i(R,T)$. t_{max} is a threshold distance that we have set to $10mm$ and is intended to limit the influence of points in the IOPR that are artifacts or have no corresponding surface represented in the 3-D distance map. Jiang et al[2] and Grimson et al[5] also employ a threshold, but use different cost functions.

The cost function, C, is a robust estimator that suppresses the influence of 'outlier' points more than functions employing, for example, least-square or RMS distance measures[11]. The attraction of such estimators was noted by Van Herk and Kooy[4] who found that 'maximum' and RMS distance measures performed worse than a mean.

2.3   Optimization

The goal of the multi-parameter minimization process is to determine the 'global' minimum which we then take as the correct solution. The difficulty lies in avoiding local minima while conducting a search that is efficient computationally. Others have employed relatively standard minimization techniques (eg, a downhill simplex[4, 11] or powell's method[4, 11]), and tackled the issue of local minima using either or both a multi-scale approach[2, 3, 4] or a stochastic search method[3]. We have chosen to employ a quasi-stochastic search strategy with multiple 're-starts'.

With six independent parameters each having a fixed step size, there is a total of $3^6 - 1$ (728) possible steps that can be taken from a given 'position' in parameter-space (i.e., each parameter can either remain unchanged, or take a $\pm$ step). Given our initial registration (i.e., a position in parameter-space), we initialize the translation parameters step size, t_{ss}, to t_{ss_start} and set the rotation parameters step size, r_{ss}. We then proceed as follows:

1. From the current position in parameter-space, evaluate a subset, N_r, (selected randomly) of the 728 possible $C(R,T)$s.

2. Select a small number, N_s, of the lowest cost evaluations and treat the corresponding parameter vectors as independent 'start-points'.

3. From each 'start-point', minimize $C(R, T)$ to obtain C_i; $i = 1..N_s$. (The minimization process is described below.)

4. Set the current position in parameter-space to $min(C_i)$; $i = 1..N_s$.

5. Reduce the step size t_{ss}, and set r_{ss}.

6. If $t_{ss} < t_{ss\_minimum}$, polish the result and quit; else go to 1. (The process of 'polishing' is described below.)

We have set N_s to 8 and N_r to 300. These values were chosen after experimentation to yield an acceptable comprise between the thoroughness in searching parameter space and speed of computation. The initial step size, t_{ss_start}, is set typically to 8-9 times the POPR data voxel size. The step size, r_{ss}, is set to a value that would move a point through a distance equal to t_{ss} when rotated on a lever-arm of $50mm$ (the typical radius of an IOPR surface patch). The minimum translation step size, $t_{ss\_minimum}$ is set to half the POPR voxel size.

In step 3, we attempt to minimize $C(R, T)$ by exploring the twelve positions in parameter space that can be reached by a positive or negative step in any one of the six parameters. The step yielding the lowest cost is taken if it improves upon the current value.

The 'polishing' process in step 6 takes the best result found and iteratively explores the 728 surrounding positions in parameter space using $t_{ss\_minimum}$ (and the corresponding r_{ss}) until no reduction in $C(R, T)$ can be obtained. Clearly, this is the most computationally intensive part of the registration process.

While more sophisticated minimization techniques could be employed (eg, downhill simplex or powell's method[11]), stopping criteria become complicated, and some control is lost over the balance of computational accuracy and speed. Our scheme is relatively simple and provides a robust approach that balances these considerations.

3 Experiments

A comprehensive study of our technique employing phantoms and models is currently underway. In this paper we describe five simulation experiments. Each employed a MR data set from a volunteer comprising $256 \times 256 \times 80$ slices with pixel dimensions of $0.94 \times 0.94mm$, and a slice thickness of $2mm$. The data were segmented to obtain the skin surface (i.e., the POPR) then interpolated to obtain cubic voxels ($0.94mm$ sides). In every experiment but one, a synthetic IOPR surface was obtained by extracting a patch of voxels from the POPR then 'smoothing' the resulting points using a 3-D Gaussian-weighted kernel ($\sigma = 2mm$), and adding uniformly distributed random perturbations of $\pm 2mm$ in 3-D.

3.1 Experiment 1: Sensitivity to initial registration

The object of this experiment was to examine the robustness of our method to errors of increasing magnitude in the initial starting position between the two

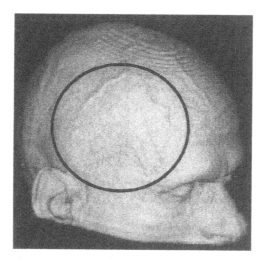

Fig. 1. Rendered view of POPR skin surface illustrating extracted IOPR patch.

surfaces. Figure 1 illustrates the surface patch extracted from the POPR that was used as the IOPR. The position of the IOPR was perturbed from its correctly registered position by adding random uniformly distributed translations and rotations (simultaneously) ranging from $\pm 1 - 14mm$ and $\pm 2 - 28^o$ (about the IOPR centre-of-mass). The automatic registration procedure then sought to recover the original position of the IOPR. At each 'level' of perturbation, 100 trials were performed. Figure 2 shows the resulting errors for this experiment. The seemingly odd behaviour of Tx and Ry can be explained by orientation and symmetry relationships between the two surfaces. The POPR x, y, z coordinate axes were right-left, anterior-posterior, and inferior-superior, respectively.

3.2 Experiment 2: Sensitivity to IOPR size

This experiment studied the extent to which an accurate registration could be achieved using IOPR surfaces of different size. Each was centred at the same position as the one illustrated in Figure 1. Perturbations of $\pm 10mm$ and $\pm 20^o$ were employed, and the basic perturbation-registration experiment was repeated 100 times. The resulting errors are shown in Figure 3 where they are plotted as a function of IOPR patch size. This size was expressed as a percentage of the 'total' segmented skin surface extracted from the MR data. For example, the patch illustrated in Figure 1 was 26% of the total POPR skin surface.

3.3 Experiment 3: Sensitivity to surface overlap

In practice it may be difficult to assure that the IOPR extracted using the video cameras overlaps completely the POPR. Points in the IOPR that extend beyond

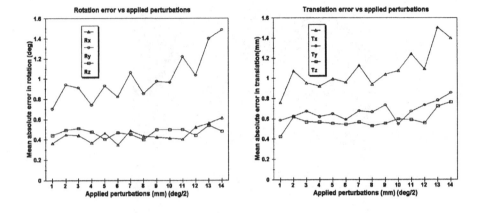

Fig. 2. Results of Experiment 1. Perturbations of increasing magnitude were applied to the IOPR, and its correct position was sought with respect to the POPR. The resulting errors in the translation and rotation parameters are plotted as a function of the perturbations.

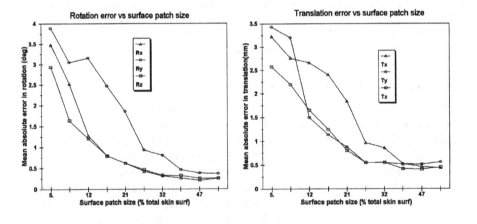

Fig. 3. Results of Experiment 2. IOPR size was varied while perturbations of $\pm 10mm$ and $\pm 20°$ were employed. The resulting errors in translations and rotations are plotted as a function of IOPR size.

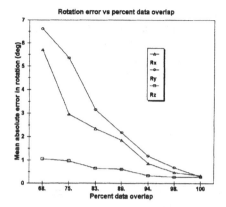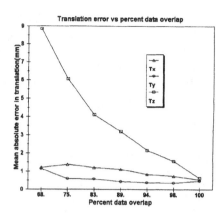

Fig. 4. Results of Experiment 3. The IOPR used here was the same as the one used in Experiment 1. Perturbations of $\pm 10mm$ and $\pm 20°$ were employed. The resulting errors in the translation parameters are plotted as a function of IOPR/POPR overlap.

the POPR might then corrupt the fitting process by contributing to the cost function when they should not be included at all. This experiment employed a different IOPR from Experiment 1 (lower on the side of the head) and used perturbations of $\pm 10mm$ and $\pm 20°$ to examine the effect of progressively cropping the POPR data. For each level of cropping, the registration exercise was repeated 100 times. The resulting errors in the are shown in Figure 4. As expected, the larger errors in Tz are a result of the POPR data being cropped from its inferior side (progressively along the z-axis).

3.4 Experiment 4: Sensitivity to cost function

This experiment repeated Experiments 1 and 3 using a cost function based on a RMS measure[5]. The results were interesting in that the errors in Experiment 1 were slightly smaller than they were for our 'robust' cost function ($RMS_{err} \approx 0.8 * ROBUST_{err}$), but gave errors that were virtually twice the magnitude in Experiment 3. This behaviour was predictable since, in Experiment 1, there were no true 'outliers' in the IOPR.

3.5 Experiment 5: Tests with real video data

This experiment used the same volunteer's POPR data, but employed an IOPR obtained from our stereo video cameras. The IOPR comprised 2501 points covering approximately 25% of the POPR skin surface. To provide a 'gold standard'

---

[5] $C(R,T) = \sqrt{\frac{1}{N-1} \sum_{i=1}^{N} d_i(R,T)^2}$

with which to compare results, parameter space was searched without regard to computational expense for a registration that minimized $C(R,T)$. We then ran 100 trials in which the IOPR was perturbed by $\pm 10mm$ and $\pm 20^{o}$ and its 'correct' position sought as usual. Table 1 lists the results. The mean time taken per registration was 153 seconds on a HP 9000/715 (50 MHz) workstation.

Table 1. Results for Experiment 5. Listed are the means and standard deviations of the errors in each parameter before and after the registration process (computed over 100 trials). Absolute values were taken prior to computing these statistics.

	t_x	t_y	t_z	r_x	r_y	r_z
Before	4.8 (± 3.0)	4.7 (± 2.8)	4.6 (± 2.9)	10.0 (± 5.6)	10.4 (± 6.0)	10.0 (± 6.1)
After	0.3 (± 0.6)	0.5 (± 0.5)	0.9 (± 0.3)	0.8 (± 0.4)	0.9 (± 0.4)	0.4 (± 0.5)

3.6 Example

We illustrate the use of registration in our application with an example that shows how pre- and intraoperative image data may be combined. Figure 5 shows the live video image of a volunteer overlayed with a wire-frame mesh (and simulated cranial window) derived from a portion of his earlier MRI scan. The mesh lies approximately over the same area of surface extracted by the two video cameras. After the registration procedure, a mean distance of $0.4(\pm 0.5)mm$ was obtained between the two surfaces with a maximum separation of $2.2mm$. When inspected visually in 3-D, no deviations were apparent between the two surfaces.

4 Discussion and Conclusions

In developing our approach to registration it became apparent that the common minimization techniques employed by others (eg, [3, 4]) were either more susceptible to local minima or computationally too complex when applied to our problem. Furthermore, there appeared to be no apparent benefit in using methods which employ blurring of the data at multiple scales[2, 3, 4]. Our use of multiple restarts with successively finer step sizes in parameter space provides a minimization strategy that is adequately robust in seeking global extrema. The ineffectiveness of a multi-scale approach when applied to our problem seems to be due to the relative sparsity of distinct surface features present in the IOPR. Since these features are easily lost at coarser resolutions, the effort in seeking a match may be wasted if not misguided. The limited size of the IOPR, together with its lack of visually distinct features, means that local minima are more widespread. It is possible, therefore, to obtain reasonable fits in terms of surface-to-surface separations that are distant from the desired match. For this reason, like Van Herk and Kooy[4], we strongly advocate checking the result visually.

The problem of dealing with 'outliers' in the data has been handled in a number of ways, most commonly by manual editing or introducing a threshold

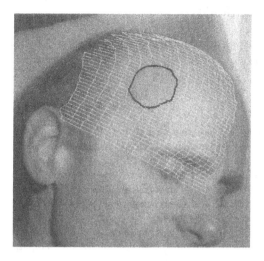

Fig. 5. Live video image of a volunteer overlayed with a wire-frame mesh (including simulated cranial window) derived from the POPR.

distance above which no greater contribution is made to the cost function[2, 5]. We do employ these techniques as well, but in conjunction with a 'robust estimator'[11] whose value was demonstrated in Experiment 4. Strategies to handle structured artifacts (eg, gross segmentation errors, skin surface swelling, etc.), are more difficult to envisage and will require more sophisticated experiments to assess their effects and develop solutions.

The issue of tracking patient or camera movement during surgery has not yet been addressed in the literature. In *VISLAN*, we are exploring two solutions to this problem; one using external fiducials attached to, for example, a Mayfield clamp, and one using surgically fixed intraoperative marker pins similar to those of Maciunas *et al*[12]. In each case, the positions of the fiducials are determined relative to IOPR, then tracked periodically to detect any movement. Solutions like these are essential in applications requiring a high degree of accuracy and must form an integral part of any such system.

The perturbations simulated in our experiments were intentionally quite severe, and the selected IOPR patch was relatively featureless. Nevertheless, our results are satisfying. Given that some groups rely solely on point based registration methods[6, 12], we anticipate initial registrations that are more accurate than those simulated here. We have begun more thorough experiments, using phantoms, to quantify accuracies in each component of the *VISLAN* system; from surface extraction, through registration, to tracking the hand-held locator. Together with clinical trials, we expect to obtain experience that will be valuable in making further refinements.

5 Acknowledgments

VISLAN is a joint academic-industrial project supported by the Department of Trade and Industry of the UK.

References

1. A.C.F. Colchester, J. Zhao, and C. Henri et al. Craniotomy simulation and guidance using a stereo video based tracking system (vislan). In *Visualization in Biomedical Computing 1994*, volume 2359, pages 541–551. SPIE, October 1994.
2. H. Jiang, R.A. Robb, and K.S. Holton. A new approach to 3-d registration of multimodality medical images by surface matching. In Richard A. Robb, editor, *Visualization in Biomedical Computing 1992*, pages 196–213, Chapel Hill, N.C., October 1992. Proc. SPIE, 1808.
3. D.L.G. Hill and D.J. Hawkes. Medical image registration using knowledge of adjacency of anatomical structures. *Image and Vision Computing*, 12(3):173–177, 1994.
4. M. van Herk and H.M. Kooy. Automatic three-dimensional correlation of CT-CT, CT-MRI, and CT-SPECT using chamfer matching. *Medical Physics*, 21(7):1163–1178, 1994.
5. E. Grimson, T. Lozano-Perez, W. Wells, G. Ettinger, S. White, and R. Kikinis. Automated registration for enhanced reality visualization in surgery. In G.M. Wells, editor, *Applications of Computer Vision in Medical Image Processing*, pages 26–29. Working Notes, AAAI, Menlo Park, CA, 1994.
6. M.P. Heilbrun, S. Koehler, P. McDonald, W. Peters, V. Sieminov, and C. Wiker. Implementation of a machine vision method for stereotactic localization and guidance. In Robert J. Maciunas, editor, *Interactive Image-Guided Neurosurgery*, pages 169–177. American Association of Neurological Surgeons, 1993.
7. C.G. Harris and A. Teeder. Geometric camera calibration for vision-based navigation. In *Proc. IFAC International Conference on Intelligent Autonomous Vehicles*, pages 77–82. Univ. of Southampton, Pergamon Press., 1993.
8. J. Zhao, A.C.F. Colchester, and C.J. Henri. Visualisation of multimodal images for neurosurgical planning and guidance. In *First International Conference on Computer Vision, Virtual Reality and Robotics in Medicine*, page submitted, Nice, France, April 3-5 1995.
9. G.T. Herman and C.A. Bucholtz. Shape-based interpolation using a chamfer distance. In A.C.F. Colchester and D.J. Hawkes, editors, *Information Processing in Medical Imaging - Lecture Notes in Computer Science*, pages 314–325. Springer, Heidelberg, 1991.
10. R. Sibson. Studies in the robustness of multidimensional scaling: Procrustes statistics. *JR Statist. Soc.*, 40:234–238, 1978.
11. W.H. Press, S.A. Teukolsky, W.T. Vetterling, and B.P. Flannery. *Numerical Recipes in C*. Cambridge University Press, New York, 1992.
12. R.J. Maciunas, J.M. Fitzpatrick, R.L. Galloway, and G.S. Allen. Beyond stereotaxy: Extreme levels of application accuracy are provided by implantable fiducial markers for interactive image-guided neurosurgery. In Robert J. Maciunas, editor, *Interactive Image-Guided Neurosurgery*, pages 259–270. American Association of Neurological Surgeons, 1993.

Segmentation I / Telemedicine

Adaptive Segmentation of MRI Data

W. M. Wells III[123] , W.E.L. Grimson[24] , R. Kikinis[15] and F. A. Jolesz[16]

[1] Harvard Medical School and Brigham and Women's Hospital, Department of
Radiology, 75 Francis St., Boston, MA 02115
[2] Massachusetts Institute of Technology, Artificial Intelligence Laboratory, 545
Technology Square, Cambridge, MA 02139
[3] sw@ai.mit.edu [4] welg@ai.mit.edu [5] kikinis@bwh.harvard.edu
[6] jolesz@bwh.harvard.edu

Abstract. Intensity-based classification of MR images has proven problematic, even when advanced techniques are used. Intra-scan and inter-scan intensity inhomogeneities are a common source of difficulty. While reported methods have had some success in correcting intra-scan inhomogeneities, such methods require supervision for the individual scan. This paper describes a new method called *adaptive segmentation* that uses knowledge of tissue intensity properties and intensity inhomogeneities to correct and segment MR images. Use of the EM algorithm leads to a fully automatic method that allows for more accurate segmentation of tissue types as well as better visualization of MRI data, that has proven to be effective in a study that includes more than 1000 brain scans.

1   Introduction

Medical applications that use the morphologic contents of MRI frequently require segmentation of the imaged volume into tissue types. Such tissue segmentation is often achieved by applying statistical classification methods to the signal intensities [1, 2], in conjunction with morphological image processing operations [3, 4].

Conventional intensity-based classification of MR images has proven problematic, however, even when advanced techniques such as non-parametric, multichannel methods are used. Intra-scan intensity inhomogeneities due to RF coils or acquisition sequences (e.g. susceptibility artifacts in gradient echo images) are a common source of difficulty. In addition, the operating conditions and status of the MR equipment frequently affect the observed intensities, causing significant inter-scan intensity inhomogeneities that often necessitate manual training on a per-scan basis. While reported methods [5, 6, 7, 8, 9, 10] have had some success in correcting intra-scan inhomogeneities, such methods require supervision for the individual scan.

This paper describes a new method called *adaptive segmentation* that uses knowledge of tissue properties and intensity inhomogeneities to correct and segment MR images. Use of the expectation-maximization algorithm leads to a method that allows for more accurate segmentation of tissue types as well as better visualization of MRI data. Adaptive segmentation has proven to be an effective fully-automatic means of segmenting brain tissue in a study including more than 1000 brain scans.

2 Description of Method

2.1 Bias Field Estimator

We use a Bayesian approach to estimating the bias field that represents the gain artifact in log-transformed MR intensity data. We first compute a logarithmic transformation of the intensity data as follows,

$$Y_i = g(X_i) = (\ln([X_i]_1), \ln([X_i]_2), \ldots, \ln([X_i]_m))^T \ , \tag{1}$$

where X_i is the observed MRI signal intensity at the i-th voxel, and m is the dimension of the MRI signal.

Similar to other statistical approaches to intensity-based segmentation of MRI [3, 4], the distribution for observed values is modeled as a normal distribution (with the incorporation of an explicit bias field):

$$p(Y_i \mid \Gamma_i, \beta_i) = G_{\psi_{\Gamma_i}}(Y_i - \mu(\Gamma_i) - \beta_i) \ , \tag{2}$$

where

$$G_{\psi_{\Gamma_i}}(x) \equiv (2\pi)^{-\frac{m}{2}} |\psi_{\Gamma_i}|^{-\frac{1}{2}} \exp\left(-\frac{1}{2} x^T \psi_{\Gamma_i}^{-1} x\right)$$

is the m-dimensional Gaussian distribution with variance ψ_{Γ_i}, and where

Y_i is the observed log-transformed intensities at the ith voxel
Γ_i is the tissue class at the ith voxel
$\mu(x)$ is the mean intensity for tissue class x
ψ_x is the covariance matrix for tissue class x
β_i is the bias field at the ith voxel.

Here Y_i, $\mu(x)$, and β_i are represented by m-dimensional column vectors, while ψ_x is represented by an m-by-m matrix. Note that the bias field has a separate value for each component of the log-intensity signal at each voxel.

A stationary prior (before the image data is seen) probability distribution on tissue class is used, it is denoted $p(\Gamma_i)$. If this probability is uniform over tissue classes, our method devolves to a maximum-likelihood approach to the tissue classification component. A spatially-varying prior probability density on brain tissue class is described in [11]. Such a model might profitably be used within this framework.

The entire bias field is denoted by $\beta = (\beta_0, \beta_1, \ldots, \beta_{n-1})^T$, where n is the number of voxels of data. The bias field is modeled by a n-dimensional zero mean Gaussian prior probability density. This model allows us to capture the smoothness that is apparent in these inhomogeneities:

$$p(\beta) = G_{\psi_\beta}(\beta) \ , \text{where } G_{\psi_\beta}(x) \equiv (2\pi)^{-\frac{n}{2}} |\psi_\beta|^{-\frac{1}{2}} \exp\left(-\frac{1}{2} x^T \psi_\beta^{-1} x\right) \tag{3}$$

is the n-dimensional Gaussian distribution. The $n \times n$ covariance matrix for the entire bias field is denoted ψ_β. Although ψ_β will be too large to manipulate directly in practice, we will show below that tractable estimators result when ψ_β is chosen so that it is banded.

We assume that the bias field and the tissue classes are statistically independent, this follows if the intensity inhomogeneities originate in the equipment. Using the definition of conditional probability and computing a marginal over tissue class leads to the conditional probability of intensity alone:

$$p(Y_i \mid \beta_i) = \sum_{\Gamma_i} p(Y_i, \Gamma_i \mid \beta_i) = \sum_{\Gamma_i} p(Y_i \mid \Gamma_i, \beta_i) p(\Gamma_i) \ . \tag{4}$$

Thus, our modeling has led to a class-independent intensity distribution that is a mixture of Gaussian populations (one population for each tissue class). Since this model is a Gaussian mixture, rather than a purely Gaussian distribution, the estimators that we derive below will be non-linear.

We assume statistical independence of the voxel intensities (in other words, the noise in the MR signal is spatially white).

Bayes' rule may then be used to obtain the posterior probability of the bias field, given observed intensity data as follows, $p(\beta \mid Y) = \frac{p(Y \mid \beta) p(\beta)}{p(Y)}$, where $p(Y)$ is an unimportant normalizing constant.

Having obtained the posterior probability on the bias field, we now use the maximum-a-posteriori (MAP) principle to formulate an estimate of the bias field as the value of β having the largest posterior probability,

$$\hat{\beta} = \arg \max_\beta p(\beta \mid Y) \ . \tag{5}$$

A necessary condition for a maximum of the posterior probability of β is that its gradient with respect to β be zero. We use an equivalent zero-gradient condition on the logarithm of the posterior probability,

$$\left[\frac{\partial}{\partial [\beta_i]_k} \ln p(\beta \mid Y) \right]_{\beta = \hat{\beta}} = 0 \qquad \forall_{i,k} \ , \tag{6}$$

where $[\beta_i]_k$ is the k-th component of the bias field at voxel i. Installing the statistical modeling of (2-5) yields the following expression for the zero gradient condition:

$$\left[\frac{\partial}{\partial [\beta_i]_k} \left(\sum_j \ln p(Y_j \mid \beta_j) + \ln p(\beta) \right) \right]_{\beta = \hat{\beta}} = 0 \qquad \forall_{i,k} \ .$$

Equations 2 and 4, and the fact that only the i-th term of the sum depends on β_i leads to:

$$\left[\frac{\sum_{\Gamma_i} p(\Gamma_i) G_{\psi_{\Gamma_i}}(Y_i - \mu(\Gamma_i) - \beta_i) \left[\psi_{\Gamma_i}^{-1}(Y_i - \mu(\Gamma_i) - \beta_i) \right]_k}{\sum_{\Gamma_i} p(\Gamma_i) G_{\psi_{\Gamma_i}}(Y_i - \mu(\Gamma_i) - \beta_i)} + \frac{\frac{\partial}{\partial [\beta_i]_k} p(\beta)}{p(\beta)} \right]_{\beta = \hat{\beta}} = 0$$

$\forall_{i,k}$.

This expression may be written more compactly as

$$\left[\sum_j W_{ij} \left[\psi_j^{-1}(Y_i - \mu_j - \beta_i) \right]_k + \frac{\frac{\partial}{\partial[\beta_i]_k} p(\beta)}{p(\beta)} \right]_{\beta=\hat{\beta}} = 0 \qquad \forall_{i,k} \; , \qquad (7)$$

with the following definition of W_{ij}, (which are called the *weights*),

$$W_{ij} \equiv \frac{\left[p(\Gamma_i) G_{\psi_{\Gamma_i}}(Y_i - \mu(\Gamma_i) - \beta_i) \right]_{\Gamma_i = tissue\text{-}class\text{-}j}}{\sum_{\Gamma_i} p(\Gamma_i) G_{\psi_{\Gamma_i}}(Y_i - \mu(\Gamma_i) - \beta_i)} \; , \qquad (8)$$

where subscripts i and j refer to voxel index and tissue class respectively, and defining $\mu_j \equiv \mu(tissue\text{-}class\text{-}j)$ as the mean intensity of tissue class j. Equation 7 may be re-expressed as follows,

$$\left[\left[\bar{R}_i \right]_k - \left[\overline{\psi^{-1}}_{ii} \beta_i \right]_k + \frac{\frac{\partial}{\partial[\beta_i]_k} p(\beta)}{p(\beta)} \right]_{\beta=\hat{\beta}} = 0 \qquad \forall_{i,k} \qquad (9)$$

with the following definitions for the mean residual, and the mean inverse covariance,

$$\bar{R}_i \equiv \sum_j W_{ij} \psi_j^{-1}(Y_i - \mu_j) \; , \quad \overline{\psi^{-1}}_{ik} \equiv \begin{cases} \sum_j W_{ij} \psi_j^{-1} & \text{if } i = k \\ 0 & \text{otherwise} \end{cases} . \qquad (10)$$

The mean residuals and mean inverse covariances defined above are averages taken over the tissue classes, weighted according to W_{ij}.

Equation 9 may be re-expressed in matrix notation as

$$\left[\bar{R} - \overline{\psi^{-1}}\beta + \frac{\nabla_\beta p(\beta)}{p(\beta)} \right]_{\beta=\hat{\beta}} = 0 \; .$$

After differentiating the last term, the zero-gradient condition for the bias field estimator may be written concisely as

$$\hat{\beta} = H\bar{R} \; , \qquad (11)$$

where the linear operator H is defined by

$$H \equiv \left[\overline{\psi^{-1}} + \psi_\beta^{-1} \right]^{-1} \; , \qquad (12)$$

that is, the bias field estimate is derived by applying the linear operator H to the mean residual field, and H is determined by the mean covariance of the tissue class intensities and the covariance of the bias field.

The bias field estimator of 11 has some resemblance to being a linear estimator in Y of the bias field β. It is not a linear estimator, however, owing to the fact that the W_{ij} (the "weights") that appear in the expression for $\bar{R}$ and H are themselves non-linear functions of Y (8).

The result of the statistical modeling in this section has been to formulate the problem of estimating the bias field as a non-linear optimization problem embodied in (11).

2.2 EM Algorithm

We use the expectation-maximization (EM) algorithm to obtain bias field estimates from the non-linear estimator of (11). The EM algorithm was originally described in its general form by Dempster, Laird and Rubin [12]. It is often used in estimation problems where some of the data are "missing." In this application, the missing data is knowledge of the tissue classes. (If they were known, then estimating the bias field would be straightforward.)

In this application, the EM algorithm iteratively alternates evaluations of the expressions appearing in (11) and (8).

In other words, (8) is used to estimate the weights given an estimated bias field, then (11) is used to estimate the bias, given estimates of the weights.

As frequently occurs in application of the EM algorithm, the two components of the iteration have simple interpretations. Equation (8) (the *E-Step*) is equivalent to calculating the posterior tissue class probabilities (a good indicator of tissue class) when the bias field is known. Equation (11) (the *M-Step*) is equivalent to a MAP estimator of the bias field when the tissue probabilities W are known.

The iteration may be started on either expression. Initial values for the weights will be needed to start with (11), and initial values for the bias field will be needed to start with (8).

It is shown in [12] that in many cases the EM algorithm enjoys pleasant convergence properties – namely that iterations will never worsen the value of the objective function. Provided that the bias estimates are bounded, our model satisfies the necessary conditions for guaranteed convergence (although there is no guarantee of convergence to the global minimum).

In principle, given $\mu(\Gamma_i)$, ψ_β, and ψ_j, we could use the EM algorithm to obtain the needed estimates. In practice, we cannot directly measure ψ_β, and thus we will seek other estimates of ψ_β (in Sect. 2.3).

Although the covariance matrix ψ_β that characterizes the prior on bias fields is impractically large in general, tractable estimation algorithms may yet be obtained.

ψ_β may be chosen to be a banded matrix. If it is then factored out of H, the bias estimation step (11) may be implemented as the solution of a banded linear system (note that $\overline{\psi^{-1}}$ is diagonal).

2.3 Determination of the Linear Operator H

We have taken a Bayesian approach to estimating the bias field and tissue classes, and a formal prior model on bias fields has been assumed. This approach has allowed us to derive a version of the EM algorithm for this application. The operator H is related to the prior on the bias field via ψ_β^{-1} and to the measurement noise via $\overline{\psi^{-1}}$ (12) . Ideally, H would be determined by estimating the covariance ψ_β, but given the size of this matrix, such an approach is impractical.

As pointed out above, H is the MAP estimator of the bias field when the tissue probabilities are known, (the "complete-data" case with the EM algorithm).

As such, H is an optimal estimator (with respect to the Gaussian modeling), and is also the optimal *linear* least squares estimator (LLSE) for arbitrary zero-mean models of the bias field whose second-order statistics are characterized by ψ_β.

A frequent problem that arises in filter design (the present complete-data case included) is that of estimating a slowly-varying signal that has been contaminated with white noise. The optimal filter in such situations will be a low-pass filter [13, Sect. 9.2].

In practice, it is difficult to obtain *the* optimal linear filter. H may be instead chosen as a good engineering approximation of the optimal linear filter (this approach is described in more detail below). In this case, (8) and (11) are still a useful estimator for the missing data case, and the good convergence properties of the EM algorithm still apply. This is the approach we have taken in our implementations, where the filter was selected empirically.

While the low-pass filters H we have used in practice are not the optimal filters for estimating these bias fields, they are reasonable choices, and may correspond to reasonable subjective estimates of the unknown probability law for bias fields, in the sense described by Friden [14, Chapt. 16]. In the end, they are justified empirically by the good results obtained via their use. Because ψ_β is required to be positive definite, not all choices of low-pass filter H will correspond to formally valid prior models on the bias field.

Computationally Efficient Filter. As argued above, the optimal H will be a linear low-pass filter, when tissue class is constant. We have employed a particularly efficient filter that is characterized as follows

$$\hat{\beta}_i = \frac{[F\overline{R}]_i}{[F\psi^{-1}\mathbf{1}]_i} \quad \text{where} \quad \mathbf{1} \equiv (1, 1, 1, \ldots, 1)^T \tag{13}$$

The filter specified above is clearly linear in the mean residual, and it will be a low-pass filter when the tissue class is constant, provided that F is a low-pass filter. It has been designed to have unity DC gain – a spatially constant shift in Y induces the same constant shift in $\hat{\beta}$. If F is chosen to be a computationally efficient low-pass filter, then the filter specified by (13) will also be computationally efficient.

2.4 Equal Covariance Case

The formalism simplifies somewhat when the tissue classes have the same covariance. This case, for scalar data, was previously reported in [15], along with scalar formulas for the weights. The bias estimator is then particularly simple when the bias model is stationary. It is a shift-invariant linear low-pass filter applied to the difference between the observed intensities and a prediction of the signal that is based on the weights (which are a good estimator of tissue class).

2.5 Non-Parametric Extension

The method that was described in previous sections has two main components: tissue classification and bias field estimation. Our approach in the extended method has been to use the same basic iteration, and to replace the tissue classification component with the technique described in [16]. The classifier described in [16] uses the *Parzen Window* representation for non-parametric probability densities [17] that are derived from training data

The non-parametric tissue class conditional intensity models are derived from training in the "natural" MR intensities. In view of our logarithmic transformation of the intensity data (1), we use the standard formula for transforming probability densities.

In the expressions for the average residual (10) and average covariance (10) we approximate with the empirical tissue class means and covariances from the log transformed training data.

The resulting iterative algorithm is a simple generalization from the Gaussian theory developed in the previous sections. Results obtained using the method are described in Sect. 3.

3 Results

This section describes results recently obtained for segmenting MR images from a large, longitudinal study of several dozen patients with multiple sclerosis (MS) [18].

All of the MR images shown in this setion were obtained using a General Electric Signa 1.5 Tesla clinical MR imager [19]. An anisotropic diffusion filter developed by Gerig et al. [20] was used as a pre-processing step to reduce noise.

We used an implementation of the non-parametric extension that is described in Sect. 2.5. This implementation is coded in the C programming language. It accommodates 2 channel data (typically registered proton-density and T2-weighted images), and multiple (more than two) tissue classes having un-equal covariances. Because it can model the important intensities in the imagery (including the background signal) it is able to correct and segment brain images without the need for a previously generated ROI. It uses the computationally-efficient filter described in Sect. 2.3, F is implemented as a moving average filter. Both uniform and non-uniform distributions have been used for the prior on tissue class.

In a typical case, the program was run until the estimates stabilized, typically in 5 – 10 iterations, requiring approximately 2 seconds per iteration (per 256^2 slice pair) on a Sun Microsystems Sparcstation 10 [21].

The method has been found to be substantially insensitive to parameter settings. For a given type of acquisition, intensity variations across patients, scans, and equipment changes have been accommodated in the estimated bias fields without the need for manual intervention. In this sense, the method is fully automatic for segmenting healthy brain tissue.

The data comprised registered proton-density and T2-weighted images for a single multiple-sclerosis patient with multiple white matter lesions. These images represented the same section from 20 scans over time after they were spatially registered using the method described in [22, 23]. The same tissue class conditional intensity models were used to segment all sections.

As expected, the results without intensity correction were dissapointing. These results are equivalent to those which would be obtained using conventional non-parametric intensity-based segmentation (which would more typically be used with per-scan manual training). They showed many gross misclassifications and demonstrated that conventional intensity-based segmentation is unfeasible in this application, at least without per-scan training. Even with per-scan training, significant asymmetries remained in the results due to the spatial intensity inhomogeneities present in the data.

Results using adaptive segmentation are shown in Fig. 1. Tissues are encoded from black to white as follows: background, subcutaneous fat, gray matter, CSF, lesions, white matter. Good stability and symmetry of the cortical gray matter structures are apparent. Similar results have been obtained in processing 23 complete scans for each of 47 patients participating in the study mentioned above, without the need for retraining or manually-generating regions-of-interest. This has facilitated monitoring the evolution of specific white matter lesions over time. Thus, fully automatic segmentation of clinical MRI data has been demonstrated in more than 1000 complete scans, without the need for per-patient or per-scan training or adjustments. The exams occurred over a 2.5 year period that included a major MR equipment upgrade.

The algorithm embodies an interative solver for a non-linear optimization problem, and like other local methods, there is no guarantee of convergence to the global solution. We have found that in practical applications, such as the one described here, the algorithm will reliably converge to a satisfactory solution once the appropriate tissue model has been identified.

4 Discussion

The use of multi-channel statistical intensity classifiers was pioneered by Vannier et al.[1]. The classification component of adaptive segmentation is similar to the method described by Gerig et al. and Cline et al. [3, 4]. The classification component of the non-parametric extended method is equivalent to that described [16].

The bias field estimation component of adaptive segmentation method is somewhat similar to homomorphic filtering (HMF) approaches that have been reported. Lufkin et al. [5] and Axel et al. [6] describe approaches for controlling the dynamic range of surface-coil MR images. Lim and Pfferbaum [7] use a similar approach to filtering that handles the boundary in a novel way, and apply intensity-based segmentation to the result.

When started on the "M Step", and run for one cycle, adaptive segmentation is equivalent to HMF followed by conventional intensity-based segmentation. We

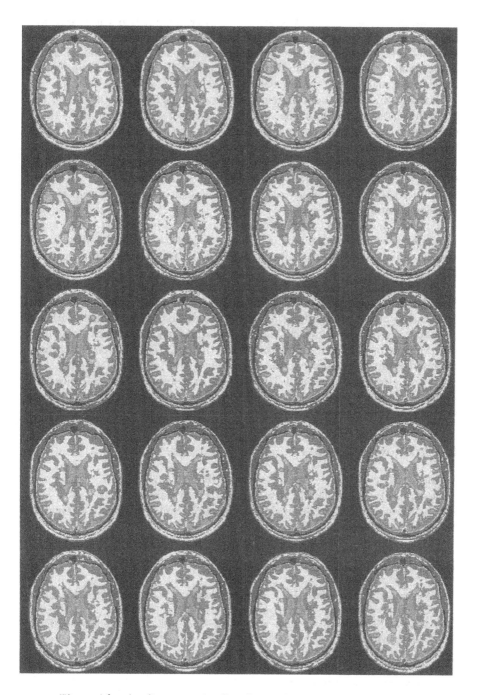

Fig. 1. Adaptive Segmentation Results (without Per-Scan Training)

have discovered, however, that more than one iteration are frequently needed to converge to good results – indicating that adaptive segmentation is more powerful than HMF followed by intensity-based segmentation. The essential difference is that adaptive segmentation utilizes evolving knowledge of the tissue type to make increasingly accurate estimates of the gain field.

Dawant, Zijdenbos and Margolin describe methods for correcting intensities for tissue classification [8]. In one variant, an operator selected points of a tissue class are used to regress an intensity correction. In the other method, a preliminary segmentation is used in determining an intensity correction, which is then used for improved segmentation. This strategy is somewhat analogous to starting adaptive segmentation on the "E step" and running it for one and a half cycles. As in the previous case, our results demonstrate improvement with additional iterations.

Aylward and Coggins describe a two-stage approach that first uses a band-pass intensity corrector. Remaining inhomogeneities are handled by using supervised training to obtain spatially-varying statistics for classifying the corrected MR data [10].

Several authors have reported methods based on the use of phantoms for intensity calibration [6, 9]. This approach has the drawback that the geometric relationship of the coils and the image data is not typically available with the image data (especially with surface coils). Fiducial markers were used to address this problem in [9]. In addition, the calibration approach can become complicated because the response of tissue to varying amounts of RF excitation is significantly non-linear (see [24, Equations 1-3 and 1-16]). In addition, phantom calibration cannot account for possible gain inhomogeneities induced by the interaction of anatomy and the RF coils.

5 Acknowledgments

We thank Maureen Ainsle, Mark Anderson, Ihan Chou, Gil Ettinger, Langham Gleason, Charles Guttmann, Steve Hushek, Hiroto Hokama, Tina Kapur, Sanjeev Kulkarni, Robert McCArley, Martha Shenton, Simon Warfield and Cynthia Wible for contributions to this paper.

References

1. M. Vannier, R. Butterfield, D. Jordan, W. Murphy, et al. Multi-Spectral Analysis of Magnetic Resonance Images. *Radiology*, (154):221 – 224, 1985.
2. M. Kohn, N. Tanna, G. Herman, et al. Analysis of Brain and Cerebrospinal Fluid Volumes with MR Imaging. *Radiology*, (178):115 – 122, 1991.
3. G. Gerig, W. Kuoni, R. Kikinis, and O. Kübler. Medical Imaging and Computer Vision: an Integrated Approach for Diagnosis and Planning. In *Proc. 11'th DAGM Symposium*, pages 425–443. Springer, 1989.
4. H.E. Cline, W.E. Lorensen, R. Kikinis, and F. Jolesz. Three-Dimensional Segmentation of MR Images of the Head Using Probability and Connectivity. *JCAT*, 14(6):1037–1045, 1990.

5. R.B. Lufkin, T. Sharpless, B. Flannigan, and W. Hanafee. Dynamic-Range Compression in Surface-Coil MRI. *AJR*, 147(379):379–382, 1986.

6. L. Axel, J. Costantini, and J. Listerud. Intensity Correction in Surface-Coil MR Imaging. *AJR*, 148(4):418–420, 1987.

7. K.O. Lim and A. Pfferbaum. Segmentation of MR Brain Images into Cerebrospinal Fluid Spaces, White and Gray Matter. *JCAT*, 13(4):588–593, 1989.

8. B. Dawant, A. Zijdenbos, and R. Margolin. Correction of Intensity Variations in MR Images for Computer-Aided Tissue Classification. *IEEE Trans. Med. Imaging*, 12(4):770 – 781, 1993.

9. J. Gohagan, E. Spitznagel, W. Murphy, M. Vannier, et al. Multispectral Analysis of MR Images of the Breast. *Radiology*, (163):703 – 707, 1987.

10. S. Aylward and J. Coggins. Spatially Invariant Classification of Tissues in MR Images. In *Proceedings of the Third Conference on Visualization in Biomedical Computing*. SPIE, 1994.

11. M. Kamber, D. Collins, R. Shinghal, G. Francis, and A. Evans. Model-Based 3D Segmentation of Multiple Sclerosis Lesions in Dual-Echo MRI Data. In *SPIE Vol. 1808, Visualization in Biomedical Computing 1992*, 1992.

12. A.P. Dempster, N.M. Laird, and D.B. Rubin. Maximum Likelihood from Incomplete Data via the EM Algorithm. *J. Roy. Statist. Soc.*, 39:1 – 38, 1977.

13. J.S. Lim. *Two-Dimensional Signal and Image Processing*. Prentice Hall, 1990.

14. B.R. Frieden. *Probability, Statistical Optics, and Data Testing*. Springer-Verlag, 1983.

15. W. Wells, R. Kikinis, W. Grimson, and F. Jolesz. Statistical Intensity Correction and Segmentation of Magnetic Resonance Image Data. In *Proceedings of the Third Conference on Visualization in Biomedical Computing*. SPIE, 1994.

16. R. Kikinis,   M. Shenton, F.A. Jolesz, G. Gerig, J. Martin, J. Anderson, D. Metcalf, C. Guttmann, R.W. McCarley, W. Lorensen, and H. Cline. Quantitative Analysis of Brain and Cerebrospinal Fluid Spaces with MR Imaging. *JMRI*, 2:619–629, 1992.

17. R.O. Duda and P.E. Hart. *Pattern Classification and Scene Analysis*. John Wiley and Sons, 1973.

18. Ron Kikinis et al. in preparation.

19. General Electric Medical Systems, Milwaukee, WI.

20. G. Gerig, O. Kübler, and F. Jolesz. Nonlinear Anisotropic Filtering of MRI data. *IEEE Trans. Med. Imaging*, (11):221–232, 1992.

21. Sun Microsystems Inc., Mountain View, CA.

22. G. Ettinger, W. Grimson, T. Lozano-Pérez, W. Wells, S. White, and R. Kikinis. Automatic Registration for Multiple Sclerosis Change Detection. In *Proceedings of the IEEE Workshop on Biomedical Image Analysis*, Seattle, WA., 1994. IEEE.

23. W.E.L. Grimson, T. Lozano-Pérez, W. Wells, et al. An Automatic Registration Method for Frameless Stereotaxy, Image Guided Surgery, and Enhanced Realigy Visualization. In *Proceedings of the Computer Society Conference on Computer Vision and Pattern Recognition*, Seattle, WA., June 1994. IEEE.

24. D. Stark and Jr. W. Bradley, editors. *Magnetic Resonance Imaging*. Mosby Year Book, 1992.

Virtual Space Editing of Tagged MRI Heart Data

Luis Serra, Tim Poston, Ng Hern,
Heng Pheng Ann, and Chua Beng Choon

Centre for Information-Enhanced Medicine
Institute of Systems Science
National University of Singapore
Heng Mui Keng Terrace
Singapore 0511
{luis@iss.nus.sg}, {http://ciemed.iss.nus.sg/people/luis.html}

Abstract. To estimate local contraction from tagged MRI heartbeat images, and deduce the presence of non-contributing muscle (usually ischæmic), it is necessary to map the heart contours accurately in each slice at each imaged time. Neither an algorithm nor a human has been found able to do this on the evidence contained in a single slice; machine estimates must be corrected by humans, using criteria of 4D (space and time) consistency. This has taken a full working day per heartbeat, using only a 2D interface; in our Virtual Workbench environment for dextrous 'reach-in' work in virtual spaces, this time is reduced to less than an hour, making it practical to analyze larger numbers of cases.

1 The Problem of Heart Strain Estimation

We[1] are using a 'reach-in' VR environment to edit computer estimates of the heart boundary for strain analysis, for the purpose of revealing ischæmic muscle.

Magnetic Resonance Imaging (MRI) has made it possible to construct 3D datasets that distinguish tissues in ways that X-rays cannot; in particular, to distinguish heart muscle from its surroundings. MRI is not fast enough to track heart motion in real time, but recording from multiple beats enables reconstruction of a 3D cine-loop of a full beat. This makes the beating heart visible, with volume rendering; but change in overall shape does not reveal clearly how individual parts of the heart muscle are moving. (Analogously, surface wave motion does not reveal the circles in which fluid particles move.) Since it is the contraction or not of a section of muscle that reveals whether it is functioning properly, this is important information. Often, defective motion is due to ischæmia (inadequate blood supply); if the defective blood vessel(s) can be properly located, corrective measures such as surgery or angioplasty become practical.

The recent development of 'tagged' MRI has made it possible to track motion in more detail (Zerhouni et al. 1988, McVeigh and Zerhouni 1991). Planes (or other marker forms) across the tissue are prepared in nuclear magnetic states which leaves them dark, independent of composition (Fig. 1a), and these 'tags' move with the muscle.

---

1. That is, the Centre for Information-enhanced Medicine (CI$_E$MED) established jointly by Johns Hopkins University and the Institute of Systems Science of the National University of Singapore.

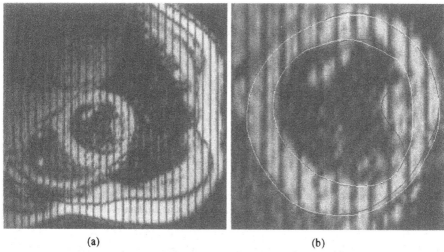

(a)   (b)

Fig. 1. (a) A section of the left ventricle of a human heart, showing MRI tag lines. (b) Detail showing computer estimated contours (dark) for the inner and outer surface. The white curve is a hand correction by the team at Johns Hopkins.

The task is to track and quantify the heart motion from tagged MRI data. Our current starting point is the FindTags program developed at Johns Hopkins (Guttman et al. 1994, McVeigh et al. 1994), which simultaneously locates the tag lines and estimates the inner and outer contours of the heart, in individual slices. Given the resolution and quality of the MRI data, this estimation produces results that are not always correct. In the example in Fig. 1b, the output of the automatic contour is wrong (the dark line), and must be manually corrected. After correction, the contours become input to an analysis program (see Moore et al. 1992 for details) that estimates geometric strains in the heart. Our concern in this paper is with the contouring step.

The estimated contour in Fig. 1b is not *obviously* wrong. The human correcting it used the context provided by neighbouring slices, above/below in space, before/after in time, and a knowledge of heart anatomy and pathology. (Higher resolution would reveal this 'inward bulge of the heart wall' to be a blurred view of the papillary muscles, of no concern here.) The interface to date for this work has been a standard 2D X/Motif display, so that this context becomes available only by switching between the current slice and its neighbours, and comparing them by visual memory. This makes the contour editing job a long one; on the order of eight to ten hours per complete heartbeat record, with ten frames of seven slices each. Such an investment of time is possible in preliminary investigations, but not for an experimental series of 100 heartbeat records, let alone eventual clinical use.

Merely displaying contours together in a 3D view (stacked by time or space) in a monoscopic display does not improve comparison. One sees a jumble of lines, as in either half of Fig. 2. In stereo, however, the curves are readily distinguished, and the false curve is immediately obvious.

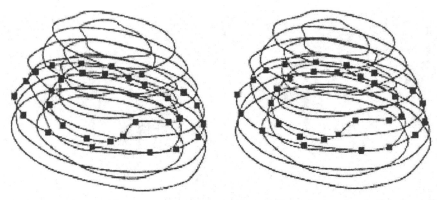

Fig. 2. In this stereoscopic pair for the bad contour shown in Fig. 2, is clear that the dots (control points used in editing the contours) lie on an inner and an outer contour in the same plane.

It is a step forward to display the contours in stereo; the point, however, is to change them. One needs a 3D environment in which it is as easy to act as to perceive--- and an environment in which one can work comfortably for many hours, at such tasks as correcting contours for a whole series of heartbeat cine-loops. These criteria are not met by currently available immersive VR environments.

2 The Virtual Workbench

We have prototyped a 'Virtual Workbench' (Poston and Serra 1994), a form of VR workstation modelled less on the immersion paradigm than on the binocular microscope familiar to medical workers, but allowing 'hands on' manipulation. The Virtual Workbench consists of a computer screen, a pair of stereo glasses, a mirror and one or more 3D sensors. The user looks into the mirror through the glasses and perceives the stereo virtual image within the work volume, where the sensors and hands lie. This produces a stereo view of a virtual volume in which a hand can move a sensor, its position known through the arm, without obscuring the display. Our display configuration, schematically, is:

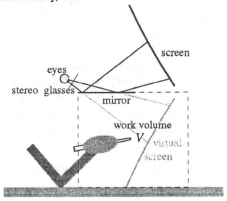

Fig. 3. The Virtual Workbench.

The system supports fixed and head-tracked viewpoint. A fixed viewpoint requires less computation and is excellent for objects within the skilled worker's natural work volume, where for most people stereo fusion appears to be the dominant cue. Currently the Virtual Workbench is based on an SGI Reality Engine, but we intend soon to have a version based on a high-end PC.

We have experimented with acoustic, electro-magnetic and mechanically-linked 3D input sensors. The acoustic and the mechanical (the Immersion Probe™) both had serious spatial restriction problems that made them unsuitable for full dextrous manipulation. The electro-magnetic sensor (the Polhemus FastTrak™), which had no such restrictions, was also lighter than the mechanical sensor and only suffered from a minor susceptibility to noise, became the 'tool' of choice.

3 The 3D Contour Editor

In the 3D Contour Editor, the user can make fine adjustments in computer-estimated curves, using their neighbours in space or time as a guide to help distinguish fact from artefact. It facilitates and speeds up the adjustment of contours by providing:

- the stereo viewing and the hand-eye coordination of the Virtual Workbench.
- simultaneous views of the slice being edited with all the other slice contours in a stack: of the slices simultaneous with it at different levels, or of the same slice at different moments.
- for a particular slice, quick context switches between the spatial arrangement and the temporal arrangement.

Figure 4 shows a snapshot of the complete environment, in which the editing tool (referred to as 'stylus'), is editing a control point. The stylus has a built-in switch. The function and appearance of the stylus change with each different operation, so at different times it becomes a slice-selector, a point-picker, a rotator, etc. The stylus interacts with the stack of MRI slices and with a 3D widget called the 'tool rack', which holds the buttons to enable tools and activate different modes of operation.

Central to the editor is the stack of slices under inspection. Each slice is a 2D MRI density map, converted into an image and texture-mapped over a polygon. In each stack, there is always a 'working slice' or slice of interest, in which the contour editing takes place. Its background opacity can be interactively controlled from totally opaque (useful to concentrate on a slice at a time) to totally transparent (to bring into context the rest of the stack).

3.1 The Tool Rack

The tool rack consists of a row of buttons, each with an icon showing its function (Fig. 4). The tool rack becomes active when the stylus moves close to it. Then, as the user moves the stylus over it, the button nearest to the tip is highlighted and displays a short piece of text identifying its function (in Fig. 5a, the button 'edit' displays an "Edit the Slice" message). When the stylus switch is pressed and the button is highlighted, the button's function is enabled. To control this 1D row of buttons, a constrained mouse allows selection with the other hand.

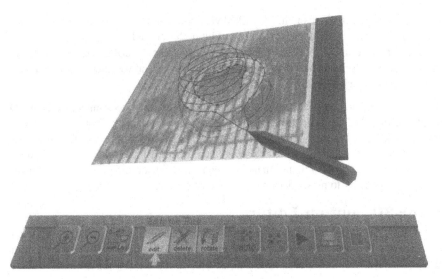

Fig. 4. The 3D Contour Editor: a view of the complete environment.

The tool rack allows a hierarchy of functions to be activated: each new level in the hierarchy replaces itself in the rack. A 'return' button is provided to go back to the calling level. Figure 5 shows three different levels of the tool rack. In Fig. 5a the button labelled rotate enables the rotation tool which controls the orientation of the stack of slices by means of a 'rubber-band' interaction scheme. When the button is pressed, the stack rotates to follow a 'rubber' string attached from the centre of the stack C to the stylus tip, each step being a rotation in the plane formed by C and two successive stylus positions. Intuitively, the feel is 'reach in and turn it about its centre'.

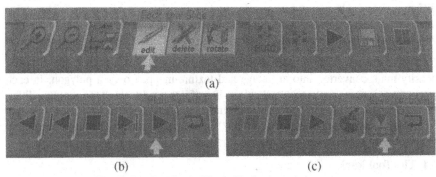

Fig. 5. The Tool Rack. Hierarchical sub-menus.

The edit and delete buttons control the placement of the control points that give shape to the contour. Set into each slice are the two contours, for the inside and the outside of the ventricle. Using direct manipulation, the stylus allows to reach into them and drag them to the correct position. The contour is supplied by FindTags as a sequence of 64 points; we convert it to a cardinal spline cubic curve. To make the direct manipulation of the control points more efficient and comfortable rather than control 64 points directly, we apply an adaptive dominant point detection algorithm (Kankanhalli 1993) to capture the same curve ---within an appropriate tolerance--- with many fewer parameters.

The control points and the MRI data are shown only for the working slice; for the other slices, we display only the contours. The working slice can be changed by selecting its handle with the stylus, and raising or lowering it through the stack. The slices are arranged in either spatial or temporal sequence, showing a set of slices at a particular instant (in geometrically correct spacing), or the time variation of a particular slice. Switching between these stacks is done by pressing the hourglass icon; this leaves the working slice fixed at the current position and orientation. The stack can be re-centred automatically at every space/time switch (the auto button), or moved to the centre explicitly by pressing the icon to the right of the auto button.

The tool rack provides access to several functions: The Magnifying Glass (+/-) enlarges or reduces the view of the stack of slices to enable finer or coarser adjustment of the control points; The Playback sub-menu (Fig. 5b) controls the playback of the heart motion sequence (the sequence can be played continuously, backwards and forwards, or step by step); The File Management sub-menu (Fig. 5c) allows the editor to invoke a 3D file loader to load and save the contour data from files, and also to record stylus movements for later playback (a feature useful in producing 'canned' demos and also in the help system).

4 Results

Preliminary tests show that contour estimates from a full 7-slice, 10-instant, 140-curve heartbeat record can be edited by a technician with minimal practice (and lacking the anatomical and MRI expertise of the JHU group) in less than an hour, against the full working day required in the previous system. The results appear comparable to those of the editing at JHU (Fig. 6); we expect soon to run joint tests with the medical group, so that we can report how quickly they can achieve the specific editing to their specific standards, in this new environment.

Work is continuing on speedier tools. At present it is necessary to select control points and move them individually, but we expect that a repelling head for the stylus that can be run along a contour, pushing it sideways in the plane of its slice, will significantly speed the editing process. Adding a 'deformation energy' term to such forces acting on the contour will enable it to remain smoother while being deformed; this smoother behaviour, again, will make fast editing easier. Several such improvements have recently been implemented in the 2D environment by the Hopkins team, and an integrated version will combine these sources of speedup.

5 Discussion

Hand-eye coordination in a stereo environment with an intuitive set of interactions can greatly speed the dextrous manipulation of 3D structures. This is easier and less costly to achieve in a 'reach-in' setting rather than an immersive one, which is more applicable to experience (such as an architectural walk-through) than to crafting, and whose latency, low resolution and narrow field of view still make simulator sickness a

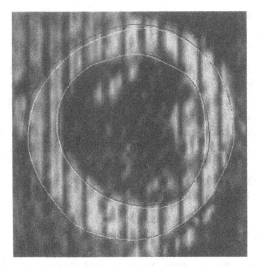

Fig. 6. ISS hand-corrected contours (white) for the inner and outer surface of the same 2D slice of Fig. 3. The black curve is a hand correction by the medical research team at Johns Hopkins.

problem for painstaking applications where the user must work for hours rather than minutes. For delicate constructive work where the criteria of success are set by the nature of a scientific, medical or engineering problem, the Virtual Workbench is a promising environment. The 3D Contour Editor described here is an example of this.

6 References

Guttman, M., Prince, J. L., and McVeigh, E. R. Contour estimation in tagged cardiac magnetic resonance images. IEEE Trans. on Med. Imag. **13**, 1 (1994), pp. 74-88.

Kankanhalli, M. An adaptive dominant point detection algorithm for digital curves. Pattern Recognition Letters **14**, 5 (1993), pp. 385-390.

(a) McVeigh, E. R., Guttman, M., Poon, E., Chandrasekhar, P., Moore, C., Zerhouni, E. A., Meiyappan, S., and Heng, P. A. Visualization and analysis of functional cardiac MRI data. World Wide Web at URL http://jmi.gdb.org/JMI/ejourn.html, 1994.

(b) McVeigh, E. R., Guttman, M., Poon, E., Chandrasekhar, P., Moore, C., Zerhouni, E. A., Meiyappan, S., and Heng, P, A. Visualization and analysis of functional cardiac MRI data. In Medical Imaging 94, SPIE conference Proceedings. (1994), **2168**, SPIE.

McVeigh, E. R., and Zerhouni, E. A. Non-invasive measurement of transmural gradients in myocardial strain with MR imaging. Radiology **180** (1991), pp. 677-683.

Meiyappan, S., Heng, P. A., and Poston, T. Strain visualization in the beating heart. World Wide Web at URL http://ciemed.iss.nus.sg/research/heart/strain.html, 1994.

Moore, C. C., O'Dell, W. G., McVeigh, E. R., and Zerhouni, E. A. Calculation of three-dimensional left ventricular strains from biplanar tagged MR images. J. Magn. Reson. Imag. **2** (1992), pp. 165-175.

Poston, T. and Serra, L. The Virtual Workbench: Dextrous VR. In proceedings of VRST'94 - Virtual Reality Software and Technology (Singapore, August 23-26, 1994). G. Singh, S.K. Feiner, D. Thalmann (eds.). World Scientific. Singapore (1994), pp. 111-122.

Zerhouni, E. A., Parish, D. M., Rogers, W. J., Yang, A., and Shapiro, E. P. Human heart: tagging with MR imaging---a method for non-invasive assessment of myocardial motion. Radiology **169** (1988), 59.

Computer-Aided Interactive Object Delineation Using an Intelligent Paintbrush Technique

Frederik Maes*, Dirk Vandermeulen, Paul Suetens, Guy Marchal

Laboratory for Medical Imaging Research**,
Katholieke Universiteit Leuven, Belgium.
Department of Electrical Engineering, ESAT,
Kardinaal Mercierlaan 94, B-3001 Heverlee, Belgium.
Department of Radiology, University Hospital Gasthuisberg,
Herestraat 49, B-3000 Leuven, Belgium.

Abstract. A method for fast generic object segmentation is presented that allows the user to quickly paint the object of interest in the image using an intelligent paintbrush. This intelligence is based on a partitioning of the image in segmentation primitives, which are computed automatically by merging watershed regions with similar image intensity distribution using the Minimum Description Length principle. We show results for Magnetic Resonance images of the heart and of the brain and for Computerized Tomography images of the abdomen.

1 Introduction

Segmentation of medical images is a necessary requirement for three-dimensional (3D) visualization and quantification of the anatomical structures of interest. There are numerous clinical applications, for instance in surgery and radiotherapy treatment planning and in quantitative diagnosis. Because completely manual object delineation on large 3D datasets is very tedious and time-consuming, computer-assistance is needed to facilitate the segmentation task in clinical routine. Fully automatic methods, relying on a priori knowledge such as shape and intensity models, are precluded by the complexity of the images, the diversity of the objects of interest and the occurrence of pathological deformations.

In this paper, we present a semi-automatic segmentation method, whereby the user, assisted by the computer, interactively segments the object of interest by colouring it in the image using an intelligent paintbrush [1]. This approach is based on a partitioning of the image in primitive regions and assumes that the object of interest is the union of one or more of these regions. In that case, only one point of each region that belongs to the object needs to be selected to completely segment it, which dramatically speeds up the interactive segmentation process.

---

* Frederik Maes is Aspirant of the Belgian National Fund of Scientific Research (NFWO). Corresponding author. Email: frederik@uz.kuleuven.ac.be
** Directors: André Oosterlinck & Albert L. Baert.

Section 2 describes how a relevant partitioning is computed automatically using a fast watershed-like procedure. In order to reduce the need for user interaction in the paintbrush tool, regions that are likely to belong to the same object need to be merged selectively while maintaining the relevant object boundaries. Section 3 describes how this is achieved using the Minimum Description Length (MDL) criterion [9]. Section 4 illustrates the power of the method by showing results for Magnetic Resonance (MR) images of the heart and of the brain and for Computerized Tomography (CT) images of the abdomen.

2 Construction of primitive image regions

Boundaries between different objects in an image are often characterised by a significant change in image intensity across the boundary. Such boundaries correspond to ridges in the gradient magnitude image and the contours of the objects coincide with the crest lines of these ridges. Therefore, a partitioning of the image in meaningful segmentation entities can be obtained by detecting these crest lines using the watershed of the gradient magnitude image. A true watershed transformation, however, is intractable, because it is a computationally expensive operation [10]. Instead, we construct pseudo-watershed regions by tracking downhill Maximum Gradient Paths (MGP) [6], starting from each point in the image and terminating in a local gradient minimum.

The gradient of the image intensity is computed using the Sobel [4] operator, after Gaussian smoothing of the original image in order to reduce the influence of noise on the gradient computation. The downhill MGP of each pixel p is tracked by recursively selecting the pixel q in the 8-connected (in 2D, or 26-connected in 3D) neighbourhood of p for which the gradient magnitude is minimal. If more than one such pixel q exists, we systematically select the first one found. The MGP terminates in the pixel m if there is no pixel in its neighbourhood with strictly smaller gradient magnitude. Each such pixel m is marked as a local minimum of the gradient magnitude and given a distinct label. If a minimum is reached in whose neighbourhood another minimum with the same gradient magnitude value has already been detected, the new minimum is disregarded by giving it the same label as the neighbouring one in order to reduce the number of regions. Each pixel in the image is assigned the label of the minimum its downhill MGP terminates in.

A pixel p is a boundary pixel of the region $R(p)$ it belongs to if there is at least one pixel q in the 4-connected (in 2D, or 6-connected in 3D) neighbourhood of p that does not belong to $R(p)$. This pixel q is a boundary pixel of its region $R(q)$ and the common pixel boundary of p and q is a boundary line element (in 2D, or surface element in 3D) of $R(p)$ and $R(q)$. The boundary between two regions is the union of all their common boundary elements. We now argue that the so-defined region boundaries coincide with the crest lines of the gradient magnitude. Indeed, if the pixel p is located on the crest line of a gradient ridge, the gradient of the image gradient magnitude points in opposite directions on both sides of the ridge, flipping direction in p. Therefore, the neighbourhood of

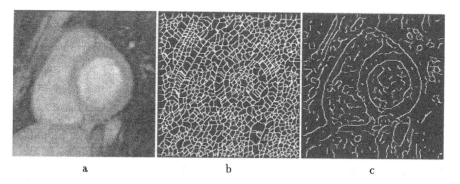

a   b   c

Fig. 1. (a) Short-axis MR cross-section of the heart at diastole (200×200). (b) Watershed regions of the gradient magnitude of the smoothed image ($\sigma = 2$). (c) Canny edges thresholded at 10% of the maximum edge strength ($\sigma = 2$).

p will contain at least two pixels that are mapped on two different local minima on opposite sides of the crest and p is a boundary pixel of its downhill region.

The result of this algorithm is an oversegmentation of the image, as illustrated in Fig. 1. The correspondence of the watershed boundaries to object contours can be compared with the result of an edge detector, such as the Canny edge detector [2] (Fig. 1c). A typical problem of Canny edge detection is that the edges found are not closed and that additional processing for explicit detection of junctions and linking of edge segments is usually required. The watershed method on the contrary, has no problem detecting junctions and, because of the region based approach, all boundaries are closed implicitly, regardless of noise or low intensity contrast.

3   Selectively merging primitive regions

Because the image intensity is often rather homogeneous within one object and significantly different between objects, the oversegmentation of the watershed can be reduced while preserving the relevant object boundaries by selectively merging regions with similar intensity distributions. Apart from intensity similarity, merging small regions that have a large common boundary compared to their size should be preferred, because this reduces the oversegmentation more than merging large regions that only share a small common boundary.

These criteria can be formulated mathematically as an optimization problem using the Minimum Description Length (MDL) principle: the optimal image partitioning is the one for which the total number of bits required to describe the image data in terms of a specified descriptive language is minimal [8, 9]. In our case, such a description consists of the number of bits needed to code the image intensity of each pixel in each region and the number of bits needed to code the region boundaries. In this section, we only discuss the 2D case, but extension to 3D regions is straightforward.

We code the image data using separate code alphabets for each region R_i by treating the image intensity x of all pixels in R_i as a stochastic variable with distribution $p_{R_i}(x)$. According to information theory [3], the number of bits $B_I(R_i)$ required to code the image intensity of all pixels in R_i using an optimal coding scheme is given by $B_I(R_i) = n(R_i)H(R_i)$, with $n(R_i)$ being the number of pixels in R_i and $H(R_i)$ the entropy of $p_{R_i}(x)$. The image intensity distribution $p_{R_i}(x)$ is estimated from the histogram of the original image in the region R_i as the convolution of the histogram with a Gaussian Parzen-window [4].

The boundary line of each region is coded by specifying one starting point and a chain code of boundary line elements, such that the total number of bits needed to code the region boundary information of the partitioning R is $B_B(R) = N_R(R) \times b_1 + N_b(R) \times b_2$, with $N_R(R)$ being the number of regions in R, $N_b(R)$ the total boundary length, b_1 the number of bits required to code the starting point and b_2 the number of bits required to code each element of the boundary chain code. We take $b_1 = 2 \times 8 = 16$ for a 2D 256×256 image and $b_2 = \log_2 4 = 2$, as each 2D boundary element corresponds to one of 4 possible directions. The total number of bits to code the image data from the image partitioning R using this coding scheme is $B(R) = B_I(R) + B_B(R) = \sum_i B_I(R_i) + B_B(R)$.

If two neighbouring regions R_1 and R_2 are merged into a new region R_3, more bits will be required to code the image intensity information of R_3 than of R_1 and R_2 separately. However, the total description length might decrease because no bits are needed to code the common boundary segment of R_1 and R_2. The description length gain $\delta B(R_1, R_2)$ of merging R_1 and R_2 into $R3$ is given by $\delta B(R_1, R_2) = n(R_1)H(R_1) + n(R_2)H(R_2) - n(R_3)H(R_3) + b_1 + n_b(R_1, R_2) \times b_2$, with $n_b(R_1, R_2)$ being the length of the common boundary of R_1 and R_2.

The merging process proceeds iteratively by selecting at each step the couple of neighbouring regions with the largest positive description length gain, merging these into a new region and updating the neighbour relations. This procedure is repeated as long as regions can be merged with positive description length gain and merging terminates at a local minimum of the description length function. Figure 2 shows the result of this procedure on the partitioning of Fig. 1b. This partitioning is used as input to the intelligent paintbrush tool.

4 Results obtained with the intelligent paintbrush tool

The original image and the region label image of the primitive region partitioning are used as input to the intelligent paintbrush tool. Only the original image is presented to the user, while the label image remains hidden. When the user selects a point on the screen by clicking the left mouse button, the region the selected point belongs to is extracted from the label image and shown in colour overlay on the screen. The user can erase coloured regions by clicking the right mouse button. Dragging the mouse with the left or the right mouse button pressed, colours or erases all regions the mouse pointer hits.

In the current implementation of this tool, the colour overlay is opaque and hides the underlying image, which might make it difficult for the user to assess

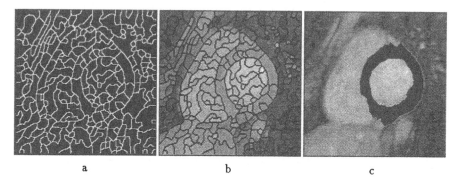

Fig. 2. (a) Merged region boundaries for the image of Fig. 1. (b) Overlay of (a) on the original image. (c) The myocardium segmented with the intelligent paintbrush tool.

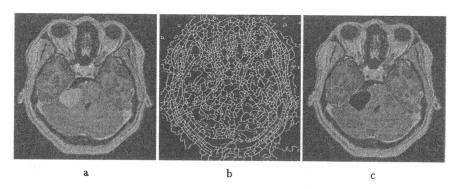

Fig. 3. (a) Original MR image of the brain (400 × 400). (b) Merged watershed partitioning. (c) Tumor segmented with the intelligent paintbrush tool.

the result of the segmentation. For clinical use, the colourings should be transparent and the user should be offered the choice of displaying the filled coloured regions or only the boundary of their union. Manual editing of the contour of the delineated region might also be needed to correct segmentation errors.

Figure 2c shows the segmentation of the myocardium in the image of Fig. 1, using the partitioning of Fig. 2a. This partitioning was computed automatically from the original image in less than 5 seconds on an IBM RS/6000 workstation. It takes the user about 5 seconds to complete the segmentation with the intelligent paintbrush tool. Figure 3 shows the segmentation of a tumor in one slice of a transversal 3D MR image of the brain. Slice by slice segmentation of the tumor on all 33 slices takes the user less than 3 minutes. Figure 4 shows one slice of a 3D 512 × 512 CT image of the abdomen and the segmentation of the prostate in this image.

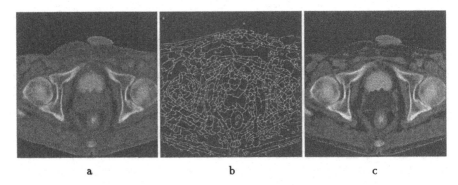

a   b   c

Fig. 4. (a) Original CT image of the abdomen (512 × 512). (b) Merged watershed partitioning. (c) Prostate segmentation with the intelligent paintbrush.

5 Discussion

The accuracy of the intelligent paintbrush segmentation depends on the overlap of boundaries in the image partitioning with the contours of the object of interest. First results show that the pseudo-watershed procedure is able to detect small intensity differences in the image, as long as these correspond to a ridge in the gradient magnitude image. This might not be the case for the boundaries of thin line-like (or plate-like) structures, which are likely to be blurred with the background due to the smoothing needed for the gradient computation. Other image partitionings can be obtained that are based on another ridge definition. Griffin [6] describes a method to partition the image in districts by growing MGP's both uphill and downhill from the saddle points of the gradient magnitude image, computed at different scales from a continuous representation of the original image. Eberly [5] uses a ridge flow model, whereby ridges, corresponding to medial structures, are computed from the image intensity itself.

The MDL criterion requires estimation of the image intensity distribution in each region. For small regions, the number of samples might be too small to obtain reliable statistics. However, the image intensity is likely to be rather homogeneous within each region, such that the average number of samples per histogram bin might still be significant. Region merging is favored by histogram binning, because all region intensity distributions will be more compact and therefore more similar. Other optimization strategies to minimize the description length function, such as simulated annealing [7], might result in more optimal partitionings with lower description length, but are computationally more expensive than the procedure used here.

Instead of using one single image partitioning as input to the intelligent paintbrush tool, several partitionings of the same original image could be used with different granularity. A hierarchy of different image partitionings is constructed implicitly during merging. One partitioning with larger granularity could be used for fast, but rough, colouring of the object of interest, while another with smaller granularity could be used for erasing and more detailed editing.

6 Conclusion

Partitioning of the image in segmentation primitives is a powerful technique. It allows fast and robust computer-aided interactive segmentation of the object of interest using the intelligent paintbrush tool. Further work includes extension of the merging procedure to 3D with the purpose of true 3D object segmentation, and evaluation of the accuracy of the method on clinical applications by medical experts.

Acknowledgements

This research is supported by the Belgian National Fund for Scientific Research (NFWO). The algorithms were developed with AVS (Application Visualization System) on an IBM RS/6000 workstation. We thank Dr. J. Bogaert and Dr. F. Demaerel for providing the images and D. Delaere and E. Bellon for their contribution to the implementation of the intelligent paintbrush tool.

References

1. Beard, D. V., Eberly, D., Hemminger, B., Pizer, S., Faith, R., Kurak, C., Livingston, M.: Interacting with image hierarchies for fast and accurate object segmentation. Proc. SPIE Newport Beach, CA, **2167** (1994) 10–17
2. Canny, J.: A computational approach to edge detection. IEEE Trans. PAMI **11** (1986) 679–698
3. Cover, T. M., Thomas, J. A.: Elements of information theory. John Wiley & Sons (1991)
4. Duda, R. O., Hart P. E.: Pattern classification and scene analysis. John Wiley & Sons (1973)
5. Eberly, D., Pizer, S. M.: Ridge flow models for image segmentation. Proc. SPIE Newport Beach, CA, **2167** (1994) 54–64
6. Griffin, L. D., Colchester, A. C. F., Robinson, G. P.: Scale and segmentation of grey-level images using maximum gradient paths. Image and Vision Computing **10** (1992) 389–402
7. Kirkpatrick, S., Gelatt, C. D., Vecchi, M. P.: Optimization by simulated annealing. Science **220** (1982) 671–680
8. Leclerc, Y. G.: Constructing simple stable descriptions for image partitioning. Intern. J. Computer Vision **3** (1989) 73–102
9. Rissanen, J.: Minimum-description-length principle. Encyclopedia of Statistical Sciences, Wiley, New York **5** (1987) 425–527
10. Vincent, L., Soille, P.: Watersheds in digital spaces: an efficient algorithm based on immersion simulations. IEEE Trans. PAMI **13** 583–598

Biomedical Data Exploration Meets Telecollaboration

Gudrun Klinker[1], Ingrid Carlbom[2], William Hsu[3], Demetri Terzopoulos[4]

[1] ECRC, Arabellastrasse 17, 81925 Munich, Germany; email: klinker@ecrc.de
[2] Digital Equipment Corporation, Cambridge Research Lab, One Kendall Square, Cambridge, MA 02139, USA; email: carlbom@crl.dec.com
[3] Microsoft Corporation, One Microsoft Way, Redmond, WA 98052, USA; email: whsu@microsoft.com
[4] Computer Science Department, University of Toronto, 10 Kings College Road, Toronto, Ontario, CANADA M5S 1A4; email: dt@vis.toronto.edu

Category: therapy planning, simulation and control: telepresence in medicine.

Abstract. In many biomedical applications, several researchers need to collaborate on extracting or validating models from empirical and simulation data. Often these collaborators do not reside at the same location, making collaboration and consultation difficult and costly. We present a system, TDE, which integrates sophisticated data exploration and telecollaboration capabilities. It runs in a heterogeneous distributed computing environment, supporting a wide variety of displays around a centralized compute server. It offers the users customizable views of the data. Pointing and cursor linking are based in n-dimensional object space, rather than screen space. We demonstrate TDE's telecollaborative data exploration facilities in three biomedical applications: user-assisted, boundary-based segmentation of an embryo heart, multi-spectral segmentation of thyroid tissue, and volume probing of a CT scan.

1 Introduction

Many biomedical applications use models extracted from and validated by empirical and simulation data. Data collected from one or more sources is analyzed and combined to form models containing both geometric and non-geometric information. These models are then used for measurement, for simulation, and for understanding the structures and relationships that may exist among the data. Data extraction, validation, and simulation are rarely performed by one individual, but rather by a group of collaborators. Often the collaborators do not reside at the same location, making collaboration and consultation difficult and costly. Unfortunately, current scientific visualization and data exploration environments [11, 12, 15] do not provide telecollaboration.

The TDE (Telecollaborative Data Exploration) system [8] combines sophisticated scientific data exploration tools with telecollaboration. For example, a physician or biomedical researcher can use TDE to share results from medical image registration or segmentation with distant collaborators. All collaborators can also control the registration and segmentation parameters and modify the results. This is in contrast to other existing systems, where collaborators have to switch back and forth between two systems, one to analyze and explore the data, and a second to share the results with distant colleagues, thus limiting the collaboration to viewing the end result of some registration or segmentation task.

TDE imposes only minimal system requirements. Users can collaborate by merely sending an X-window across the network - even to PCs or laptops. Other telecollaboration systems [1, 2, 3, 5, 10, 13, 14] typically expect all collaborators to use the same software package and similar computer hardware.

TDE provides a rich set of data exploration functions. It is relatively easy to set up complex applications with these functions, such as telecollaborative, physically based data segmentation using snakes, multi-spectral statistical color image segmentation using three-dimensional histograms, and volume-probing. Other systems offer only a rather limited set of data exploration facilities; typically, remote users are restricted to tele-pointers for image annotation.

2 TDE Architecture

Figure 1 summarizes TDE's approach to telecollaborative data exploration. The left side (a) describes TDE's client-server architecture. The right side (b) shows the visual programming interface.

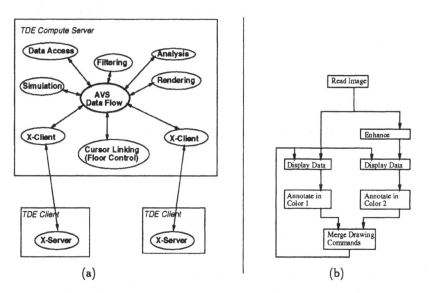

Fig. 1. a) TDE client-server architecture, b) data flow graph

We now discuss four key features in TDE: its heterogeneous distributed collaboration architecture, its integration into an existing visualization environment, view customization, and n-dimensional cursor linking.

2.1 Heterogeneous Distributed Collaboration Environment

TDE consists of several independent components: a *TDE Compute Server*, and one or more *TDE Clients* (see Figure 1a). The compute server executes all data exploration tasks. It also has a set of X-clients that display image and geometric data at remote sites. From a user's perspective, the X-servers at the remote sites function as TDE clients, connected to a remote compute server.

The TDE clients do not require any special-purpose hardware or software – just an X-server. TDE adapts to different frame buffer technology at different sites. If possible, TDE uses either full-color display capabilities or a locally compatible color mapping algorithm. Yet, users can also request special color maps to maintain a required level of color or grayscale fidelity. Furthermore, the rendered image is stored at the remote site so that the screen can be refreshed quickly to support simple interactive data exploration tasks like telepointing and annotation.

The TDE architecture is particularly useful when slow remote systems, such as laptops, are connected to a fast centralized compute server. We expect increasingly to encounter such centralized server architectures when one expert needs to consult another expert in a different organization that is not using the same collaboration software. Other televisualization systems replicate data and computational services at all collaborative sites, thus reducing the data bandwidth needed during interaction at the expense of requiring a homogeneous distributed computing environment [2]. We observe that in many cases, applications perform a significant amount of data exploration, such as data probing, annotation and segmentation, on a stable view. While the view does not change, very low data transfer bandwidth is required to synchronize user interaction. Thus, users can often exploit our architecture even across moderate bandwidth data networks, such as ISDN, while operating in a much less homogeneous computing environment.

2.2 An AVS-based Data Exploration Server

TDE's compute server uses AVS [15] to provide a large, user-extensible collection of tools to access, filter, analyze and render image, volume, and geometric data. Users can interactively access these tools via a visual programming interface, selecting modules and assembling them into data flow networks. The visual programming interface depicts data flow networks as graphs, with boxes connected by lines to indicate the data flow connections (see Figure 1b).

The visual programming interface of AVS is an essential component of TDE. Yet, TDE surpasses standard AVS functionality in several important ways: AVS uses only one screen to display images, and it does not allow users to link cursors between several windows. TDE's extensions to multiple screens and cursor linking enable whole new classes of applications, as seen in the subsequent sections.

2.3 View Customization

In TDE, users can customize their views and windows individually at each site. For example, users may individually reposition and resize their windows or customize the data presentation style and data content by selecting different color maps, image enhancement operators, and viewing orientations (for three-dimensional data). To this end, TDE exploits AVS's visual programming interface [15] to include any number of data processing steps in the data flow path before the image is rendered on a particular display (see Figure 1b).

In contrast, window-sharing systems [1, 5] duplicate communication from one X-client to several X-servers. Sharing at this later stage in the data rendering pipeline can lead to irrevocable loss of precision and flexibility in data display. It is hard for such tools to adapt to varying display technology between the collaborators, or to their different viewing preferences.

2.4 *N*-Dimensional Cursor Linking

Cursor linking allows users to simultaneously explore data in several views; when they move the cursor in any one view, all other views are updated accordingly. To maintain geometric consistency between the cursor positions in all views, TDE has to ensure that the cursors undergo the same transformations as the data. To this end, TDE modules send a *log record* along with the data which records the history of geometric transformations performed on the data.

We can link cursors between any number of windows [8]. Linked cursors can show corresponding pixels in images of identical dimensions and size, such as an image and its edge-enhanced counterpart, or they can link images of different sizes, such as images at different levels of a pyramid, or an image and an enlarged subimage. The linking mechanism can also be used to help visualize the relationship between data sets of different dimensions, such as an image and its histogram (see Section 4). In fact, a user can establish any transformation between two data sets. Any such windows can be duplicated, cross-linked and forwarded to remote collaborators for remote exploration.

Figure 1b shows how collaborators can use TDE to jointly annotate an image in different colors. Module "Merge Drawing Commands" provides the floor control: all collaborators are treated equally on a first-come-first-served basis. Other floor control schemes can be installed by replacing this module [9].

3   User-Assisted Boundary-Based Segmentation

Snakes, or interactive deformable contours, are a model-based image-feature localization and tracking technique [7]. The user traces a contour which approximates the desired boundary and then starts a dynamic simulation that enables the contour to locate and conform to a nearby boundary in the image. Where necessary, the user may guide the contour by using a mouse to apply simulated forces. Snakes exploit the coherence between adjoining images to quickly find corresponding regions in an image sequence.

Snakes have been used to segment several types of biomedical image data [4]. Figure 2 shows four phases of a snake simulation applied to one section of an embryo heart from a serial light micrograph: the initial manual trace, the initial equilibrium position of the snake (top); interactive manipulation of the snake, and the final snake boundary (bottom).

TDE's telecollaborative snakes allow each collaborator to trace the initial contour on duplicated windows and to guide the contour during simulation. When the simulation module generates a new snake contour, the outline is updated on both windows. Each collaborator can adjust the viewing contrast of the input image and select to view either the original or the contrast enhanced heart data. The data flow diagram of Figure 2 provides this functionality by parallel tracks, each track having its own modules for enhancement, data selection and display.

User interaction from either site is multiplexed and fed back to the snakes simulation module. For general n-way telecollaboration, n parallel display tracks would exist, with user interaction being combined through a cascade of multiplexers.

4   Multi-Spectral Segmentation

The second application employs multi-spectral segmentation to quantify tissue vascularity from a serial section of a rat thyroid [8]. The tissue is stained so that blood capillaries appear bluish. The segmentation is difficult to achieve because the boundaries of the blood vessels are sometimes imprecise, and the stained capillaries do not exhibit a color shift large enough to isolate the colors into a separate cluster. The top row of Figure 3 shows a picture of the thyroid image and of its three-dimensional color histogram.

Each color pixel in the thyroid image constitutes an index $[r, g, b]$ into the histogram. The value of each slot in the histogram indicates how often this particular color occurs in the image. On the thyroid image is a crosshair accompanied by the index and the red, green, and blue color values of a selected pixel. The corresponding color slot in the color histogram is also marked with a crosshair and text indicating the color index and the histogram count. We show several other crosshairs on the thyroid image and on the histogram to demonstrate how users can employ cursor linking to visualize color similarities between several selected pixels.

Conversely, users can also relate areas of the color histogram to the thyroid data. When a user outlines an area of the histogram, all image pixels with such colors are highlighted (bottom row of Fig. 3). Two or more users can collaborate on this segmentation task, editing the regions in the histogram until the optimum segmentation is found.

Collaborators can each select individual viewing angles for the histogram. The selected color pixel and the color mask are still shown in their correct three-dimensional positions.

5 Volume Probing

The third application demonstrates the exploration of three-dimensional volume data. It uses a volume ray-caster, where rays are cast from each pixel in the projection plane through the volume data. The value for each pixel is calculated by integrating sample values along the ray [6]. While this tool can be used to view the volume and its internal structures, it can also be used to find locations with particular values (densities) in the volume. To aid in this process, we extract data along a ray, and display the density profile of the ray. We use linked cursors to explore the location of selected density values along the ray.

The data flow graph in Figure 4 shows how the two windows with the volume data and the density profile can be displayed at two sites. In this example, we have selected a data probe piercing from the nose through the head. When the cursor is positioned on the profile, the corresponding voxel is marked with a green crosshair in the volume window. Telecollaborative volume rendering allows all collaborators to rotate the volume and to position new data probes.

6 Conclusions

TDE is a system which integrates scientific data exploration tools with telecollaborative capabilities. We have demonstrated the use of TDE in several applications. In each case, collaborators are able to interact with the system and explore the data using n-dimensionally linked cursors. Individual collaborators are able to customize their views.

TDE offers a framework within which researchers can integrate various interactive segmentation, registration, and other image analysis algorithms to design telecollaborative medical applications. We have successfully demonstrated telecollaborative arrangements between Chicago and Boston as part of the Innovation Showcase at SIGGRAPH '92, across the U.S., and between the U.S. and Sweden, displaying windows on workstations and laptops.

TDE is complementary to other teleconferencing and groupware technology. Sophisticated telemedicine systems will require a well-integrated mix of all telecommunications capabilities: a teleconferencing system to see and hear the participants, telecollaborative data exploration tools to explore multi-modal data with high data fidelity, general-purpose window-sharing tools to interact with data bases containing patient records, and hyperlinked browsers to interrogate remote data repositories, such as national libraries. We expect this work to inspire the next generation of telecollaboration and telemedicine tools, which will allow true collaboration – for example, neuro-surgery planning by a surgeon and a radiologist, where the two physicians are not co-located, or remote consultation by the radiologist with the surgeon in the operation room.

Acknowledgments

The embryo heart is part of the Carnegie Collection in the National Library of Medicine, courtesy of Adrianne Noe. The thyroid data was provided by Michael Doyle at UCSF. The CT data is from the North Carolina Memorial Hospital.

References

1. M. Altenhofen, J. Dittrich, R. Hammerschmidt, T. Kaeppner, C. Kruschel, A. Kueckes, and T. Steinig. The BERKOM multimedia collaboration service. In *ACM Multimedia'93*, pages 457–463. ACM Press, 1993.

2. V. Anupam and C.L. Bajaj. Collaborative multimedia scientific design in SHAS-TRA. In *Proc. ACM Multimedia'93*, pages 447–456. ACM Press, August 1993.

3. D.V. Beard, B.M. Hemminger, P.H. Brown, J.R. Perry, and R. Thompson. Remote consultation with a multiple screen filmplane radiology workstation. In *Conference on Image Capture, Formatting, and Display*, pages 310–315. SPIE (vol. 1653), 1992.

4. I. Carlbom, D. Terzopoulos, and K.M. Harris. Computer-assisted registration, segmentation and 3D reconstruction. *IEEE Transactions on Medical Imaging*, 13(2):351–362, June 1994.

5. E. Craighill, R. Lang, M. Rong, and K. Skinner. CECED: A system for informal multimedia collaboration. In *ACM Multimedia'93*, pages 437–443. ACM, 1993.

6. W.M Hsu. Segmented ray casting for data parallel volume rendering. In *Visualization'93, Parallel Rendering Symp.*, pages 7–14. IEEE Comp. Soc. Press, 1993.

7. M. Kass, A. Witkin, and D. Terzopoulos. Snakes: Active contour models. *International Journal on Computer Vision (IJCV)*, 1(4):321–331, 1988.

8. G.J. Klinker. An environment for telecollaborative data exploration. In *Visualization '93*, pages 110–117. IEEE Computer Society Press, 1993.

9. G.J. Klinker. Coroutine synchronization in AVS. In *Proc. of the 3rd Int. AVS User Group Conference*, pages 225–232, Boston, MA, May 2-4 1994.

10. E. A. Krupinski, R.S. Weinstein, K.J. Bloom, and L.S. Rozek. Progress in telepathology: System implementation and testing. *Advances in Pathology and Laboratory Medicine*, 6:63–87, 1993.

11. J. Mundy, T. Binford, T. Boult, A. Hanson, R. Beveridge, R. Haralick, V. Ramesh, C. Kohl, D. Lawton, D. Morgan, K. Price, and T. Strat. The image understanding environment program. In *IEEE Conference on Computer Vision and Pattern Recognition (CVPR'92)*, pages 406–416, 1992.

12. R.A. Robb and D.P. Hanson. ANALYZE: A software system for biomedical image analysis. In *Proc. 1st Conference on Visualization in Biomedical Computing (VBC)*, pages 507–518. IEEE Computer Society Press, 1990.

13. D.D. Stark and J.V. Crues III. Teleradiology. *Diagnostic Imaging*, page 91, November 1993.

14. S.T. Treves, E.S. Hashem, B.A. Majmudar, K. Mitchell, and D.J. Michaud. Multimedia communications in medical imaging. *IEEE Journal on Selected Areas in Communications*, 10(7):1121–1132, September 1992.

15. C. Upson, T. Faulhaber Jr., D. Kamins, D. Laidlaw, D. Schlegel, J. Vroom, R. Gurwitz, and A. van Dam. The Application Visualization System: A computational environment for scientific visualization. *IEEE Computer Graphics and Applications*, 9(4):30–42, July 1989.

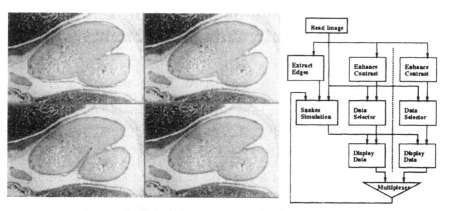

Fig. 2. Snake-based segmentation (embryo heart)

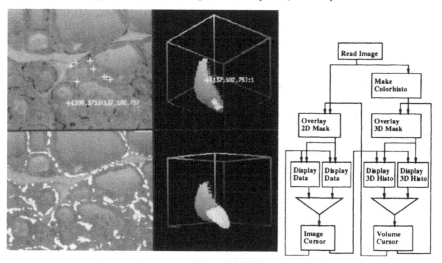

Fig. 3. Multi-spectral segmentation (thyroid)

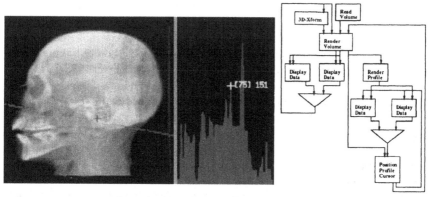

Fig. 4. Volume probing (human head)

Medical Image Segmentation Using Topologically Adaptable Snakes

Tim McInerney and Demetri Terzopoulos

Dept. of Computer Science, University of Toronto, Toronto, ON, Canada

Abstract. This paper presents a technique for the segmentation of anatomic structures in medical images using a topologically adaptable snakes model. The model is set in the framework of domain subdivision using simplicial decomposition. This framework allows the model to maintain all of the strengths associated with traditional snakes while overcoming many of their limitations. The model can flow into complex shapes, even shapes with significant protrusions or branches, and topological changes are easily sensed and handled. Multiple instances of the model can be dynamically created, can seamlessly split or merge, or can simply and quickly detect and avoid collisions. Finally, the model can be easily and dynamically converted to and from the traditional parametric snakes model representation. We apply a 2D model to segment structures from medical images with complex shapes and topologies, such as arterial "trees", that cannot easily be segmented with traditional deformable models.

1 Introduction

The segmentation and quantification of anatomic structures is an essential stage in the analysis and interpretation of medical images. Image interpretation tasks such as registration, quantitative analysis, labeling, and motion tracking require anatomic structures in the original image to be reduced to a compact, geometric representation of their shape. Recently, segmentation techniques which combine a local edge extraction operation with the use of active contour models, or snakes [4], to perform a global region extraction have achieved considerable success (see, eg., [3, 2, 1, 6]). These models simulate elastic material which can dynamically conform to object shapes in response to internal forces, external image forces and user-provided constraints. The result is an elegant method of linking sparse or noisy local edge information into a coherent free-form object model.

The application of active contour models to extract regions of interest is, however, not without limitations. The models were designed as interactive models and are sensitive to their initial conditions. Consequently, they must be placed close to the preferred shape to guarantee good performance. The internal energy constraints of the models can limit their geometric flexibility and prevent a model from representing long tube-like shapes or shapes with significant protrusions or bifurcations. Furthermore, the topology of the structure of interest must be known in advance since classical snakes models are parametric and are incapable of topological transformations without additional machinery.

Several researchers have attempted to address some of these limitations. Terzopoulos [7] and Cohen [3] used an internal "inflation" force to expand the deformable surface or snake past spurious edges towards the real edges of the structure, making the model less sensitive to initial conditions. Samadani [6] used a heuristic technique based on deformation energies to split and merge active contours. Similar split and merge operations were done interactively in [2]. More recently, Malladi *et al.* [5] developed a topology independent active contour scheme based on the modeling of propagating fronts with curvature dependent speeds, where the propagating front is viewed as an evolving level set of some implicitly defined function.

Most active contour models are parametric models whose parameterization is pre-specified and does not change automatically throughout the deformation process. If the topology of an object is fixed and known a priori, such models are preferable in that they provide the greatest constraint. Implicit models on the other hand, such as the formulation used in [5], provide topological and geometric flexibility through their level sets. They are best suited to the recovery of objects with complex shapes and unknown topologies. Unfortunately, implicit models are not as convenient as parametric models in terms of mathematical formulation, for shape analysis and visualization, and for user interaction.

This paper presents a new snakes model formulation that is set in the framework of domain subdivision using simplicial decomposition. This framework allows the model to maintain the traditional properties associated with snakes, while overcoming the limitations described above. We develop a parametric model that has the power of an implicit formulation by using a superposed simplicial grid to quickly and efficiently reparameterize the model during the deformation process, allowing it to flow into complex shapes and dynamically sense and change its topology as necessary. Multiple instances of the model can be dynamically created or destroyed, can seamlessly split or merge, or can simply and quickly detect and avoid intersections with other models. The result is a simple, convenient and flexible model that considerably extends the geometric and topological adaptability of snakes.

We apply our topologically adaptable snakes model to segment structures from medical images with complex shapes and topologies that cannot easily be segmented with traditional snakes models. In this paper, we consider the 2D case only, although the model is readily extensible to three dimensions.

2 Model Implementation

We begin by defining our model as a closed elastic contour (in 2D) consisting of a set of nodes interconnected by adjustable springs [2]. The elastic contour model is a discrete approximation to the traditional snakes model and retains all of the properties of snakes. That is, an "inflation" force pushes the model towards image edges until it is opposed by external image forces, the internal spring forces act as a smoothness constraint, users can interact with the model using spring forces, and the deformation of the model is governed by discrete Lagrangian equations of motion.

Unlike traditional snakes, the set of nodes and interconnecting springs of our model does not remain constant during its motion. That is, we decompose the image domain into a grid of discrete cells. As the model moves under the influence of external and internal forces, we reparameterize the model with a new set of nodes and springs by efficiently computing the intersection points of the model with the superposed grid. By reparameterizing the model at each iteration of the evolutionary process, we create a simple, elegant and automatic model subdivision technique as well as an unambiguous framework for topological transformations. This allows the model to be relatively independent of its initial placement and "flow" into complex shapes with complex topologies in a stable manner. Furthermore, conversion to and from a traditional parametric snakes model representation is simply a matter of discarding or superposing the grid at any time during the evolutionary process.

2.1 Discrete Snake Model

We define a discrete snake as a set of N nodes indexed by $i = 1, \ldots, N$. We associate with these nodes time varying positions $\mathbf{x}_i(t) = [x_i(t), y_i(t)]$ and a mass m_i along with compression forces which make the snake act like a series of unilateral springs that resist compression, rigidity forces which make the snake act like a thin wire that resists bending, and external forces that act in the image plane. We connect the nodes in series using nonlinear springs. This forms a discrete dynamic system whose behavior is governed by the set of ordinary differential equations of motion

$$m_i \ddot{\mathbf{x}}_i + \gamma_i \dot{\mathbf{x}}_i + \boldsymbol{\alpha}_i + \boldsymbol{\beta}_i = \mathbf{f}_i \ , \tag{1}$$

where $\ddot{\mathbf{x}}_i$ is the acceleration of node i, $\dot{\mathbf{x}}_i$ is its velocity, m_i is its mass, γ_i is a damping coefficient that controls the rate of dissipation of the kinetic energy of the node and $\mathbf{f}_i$ is an external force that attracts the model toward salient image edges [4]. The force

$$\boldsymbol{\alpha}_i = a_i e_i \hat{\mathbf{r}}_i - a_{i-1} e_{i-1} \hat{\mathbf{r}}_{i-1} \tag{2}$$

makes the snake resist expansion or compression, where $\mathbf{r}_i = \mathbf{x}_{i+1} - \mathbf{x}_i$ and the caret denotes a unit vector, a_i is the spring stiffness and $e_i = \|\mathbf{r}_i\| - L_i$, where L_i is the spring "rest" length. Since a new set of model nodes and springs is computed during every iteration, we update these rest lengths by setting them equal to the new spring lengths. The "rigidity" forces

$$\boldsymbol{\beta}_i = b_{i+1}(\mathbf{x}_{i+2} - 2\mathbf{x}_{i+1} + \mathbf{x}_i) - 2b_i(\mathbf{x}_{i+1} - 2\mathbf{x}_i + \mathbf{x}_{i-1}) + b_{i-1}(\mathbf{x}_i - 2\mathbf{x}_{i-1} + \mathbf{x}_{i-2}) \ , \tag{3}$$

act to make the snake resist bending. When computing this force, we "normalize" the spring lengths to account for the uneven node spacing. Finally, an "inflation" force, $\mathbf{h}_i = k\mathbf{n}_i$, is used to push the model towards image edges until it is opposed by external image forces, where k is the force scale factor and $\mathbf{n}_i$ is the unit normal to the contour at node i. The use of an inflation force essentially eliminates the need for an inertial force term. For this reason, we have simplified the equations of motion, while still preserving useful dynamics, by setting the mass density m_i in equation (1) to zero to obtain a model which has no inertia and which comes to rest as soon as the applied forces vanish or equilibriate. We integrate this first-order dynamic system forward through time using an explicit Euler method.

2.2 Domain Decomposition

The grid of discrete cells used to approximate the deformable contour model is an example of space partitioning by simplicial decomposition. There are two main types of domain decomposition methods: non-simplicial and simplicial. Most nonsimplicial methods employ a regular tessellation of space. These methods are fast and easy to implement but they cannot be used to represent surfaces or contours unambiguously without the use of a disambiguation scheme.

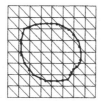

Fig. 1. Simplicial approximation of a contour model using a Freudenthal triangulation. The model nodes (intersection points) are marked.

Simplicial methods, on the other hand, are theoretically sound because they rely on classical results from algebraic topology. In a simplicial decomposition, space is partitioned into cells defined by open simplicies (an n-simplex is the simplest geometrical object of dimension n). A simplicial cell decomposition is also called a triangulation. The simplest triangulation of Euclidean space $\mathcal{R}^n$ is the Coxeter-Freudenthal triangulation (Fig. 1). It is constructed by subdividing space using a uniform cubic grid and the triangulation is obtained by subdividing each cube in $n!$ simplicies.

Simplicial decompositions provide an unambiguous framework for the creation of local polygonal approximations of the contour or surface model. The set of simplicies (or triangles in 2D) of the grid that intersect the contour (the boundary triangles) form a two dimensional combinatorial manifold that has as its dual a one dimensional manifold that approximates the contour. The one dimensional manifold is constructed from the intersection of the true contour with the edges of each boundary triangle such that a line segment approximates the contour inside this triangle (Fig. 1) and such that the contour intersects each boundary triangle in 2 distinct points, each one located on a different edge. The set of all these line segments constitute the combinatorial manifold that approximates the true contour.

The cells of the triangulation can be classified in relation to the partitioning of space by the closed contour model by testing the "sign" of the cell vertices during the each time step. If the signs are the same for all vertices, the cell must be totally inside or outside the contour. If the signs are different, the cell must intersect the contour (Fig. 2).

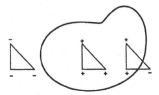

Fig. 2. Cell classification.

2.3 Topological Transformations

When a deformable model collides with itself or with another model, or when a model breaks into two or more parts, a topological transformation must take place. In order to effect consistent topological changes, consistent decisions must be made about disconnecting and reconnecting model nodes. The simplicial grid provides us with an unambiguous framework from which to make these decisions. Each boundary triangle can contain only one line segment to approximate a closed snake in that triangle. This line segment must intersect the triangle on two distinct edges. Furthermore, each vertex of a boundary triangle can be unambiguously classified as inside or outside the snake. When a snake collides with itself, or when two or more snakes collide, there are some boundary triangles that will contain two or more line segments. We then choose two line segment end-points on different edges of these boundary triangles and connect them to form a new line segment. The two points are chosen such that they are the closest points to the outside vertices of the triangle and such that the line segment joining them separates the inside and outside vertices (Fig. 3). Any unused node points are discarded. With this simple strategy, topological transformations are handled automatically, consistently and robustly.

To determine inside and outside vertices of a boundary triangle, we use a simple, efficient, and robust ray casting technique. That is, we count the number of intersections that a ray cast from a cell vertex along its grid row makes with the enclosing snake. An odd number of intersections indicates that the vertex is inside the snake. Counting the number of intersections is simply a matter of a look-up into an active edge-list table, constructed during each time step when a snake is projected onto the grid.

Once the topological transformations have taken place, we can run through the list of nodes generated by the procedure above and perform contour tracings via the grid cells, marking off all nodes visited during the traversals. In this fashion we find all new snakes generated by the topological transformation phase

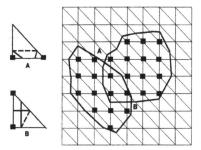

Fig. 3. Intersection of two models with "inside" grid cell vertices marked. Model nodes in triangles A and B are reconnected as shown.

and assign each a unique identifier. The result is that at any time during the evolutionary process, we can track, control, and interact with each model created.

2.4 Tracking Interior Regions for Model Collision Detection

We can keep track of the interior regions of our closed contour models as they deform. Interior region information can be used to perform efficient collision detections among multiple models or potentially to aid in a region analysis of the structures extracted by the models. We track the interior region of a model using an efficient update mechanism. As a closed snake deforms, new interior regions of the snake are defined, usually encompassing all or part of the old interior. We then use an efficient region filling algorithm to "turn on" all new cell vertices and turn off vertices in regions no longer encompassed by the snake. In practice, the increased (or decreased) area encompassed by the new snake boundary is usually small compared to the current area, meaning that few vertices require "filling" or "emptying".

When segmenting multiple objects with common or adjacent boundaries using multiple models, an efficient collision detection scheme could be utilized as an extra constraint in the segmentation process. By keeping track of the interior regions of our models, we can perform efficient collision detection between models. Each snake simply fills the grid vertices of its interior with a unique value, effectively giving these vertices an identifier (Fig. 4). As a snake deforms, it may attempt to move into new grid triangles. A simple and efficient check can then be performed to see if any of the vertices of these new grid cells are already filled with a value different from the value of the interior vertices of the current snake. If so, various "avoidance" strategies can be used such as applying a force to the intersecting nodes of the colliding model to push the model out of the already occupied region.

3 Segmentation Results

Currently our topologically adaptable snakes model based segmentation procedure requires the user to draw an initial contour (or multiple contours, if desired)

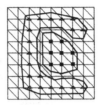

Fig. 4. Collision detection and avoidance using model interior region "identifiers". A model cannot deform into "territory" already occupied by another model.

within the objects of interest. These contours are then closed and converted to a parametric model representation using the superposed grid. The snakes are then updated during each time step by: calculating the forces on each snake node and updating the node positions using the simplified equation (1), reparameterizing each snake (computing a new set of nodes and springs) by finding the intersection points of the snake with the grid, computing the new spring rest lengths L_i, performing topological transformations within grid cells as needed, and traversing each snake via the grid cells, identifying all new snakes.

3.1 Experiments with Synthetic Data

In the first experiment we demonstrate the "flowing" property of the snake by segmenting a spiral shaped object (Fig. 5a–d). We superposed a 40 × 40 square cell grid, where each cell is divided into two triangles, onto a 128 × 128 pixel image. The parameter values for all of the experiments with synthetic data sets are: $\Delta t = 0.002, a_i = 10.0, b_i = 5.0, k = 20.0, \kappa = 20.1$ (note: κ is the external image force scale factor):

In the second set of experiments we demonstrate the topological transformation capabilities of the model. In Figure 5e–h, a snake flows around two "holes" in the object, collides with itself and splits into three parts. In Figure 5i–l, several snakes are initialized in the protrusions of the object, flow towards each other, and seamlessly merge. In Figure 5m–p, the snake shrinks, wraps and finally splits to segment each object.

3.2 Experiments with 2D Medical Images

In the first experiment we use several 256 × 256 image slices of a human vertebra phantom. We overlay these images with a 64 × 64 square cell grid, with each cell divided into two triangles. The parameter values are: $\Delta t = 0.001, a_i = 30.0, b_i = 15.0, k = 60.0, \kappa = 62.0$. Once the snake collides with itself in Figures 6a–d, it automatically splits into three parts, two parts segmenting the inner boundary of the vertebra and one for the outer boundary. In Figures 6e–h, the snake shrinkwraps itself around the objects and splits to segment the different parts.

In the second set of experiments, we apply the model to a 128 × 128 portion of a retinal image (Figs. 7a–d) to segment the vascular "tree", a structure with extended branches and bifurcations. Note that the arteries and veins do not

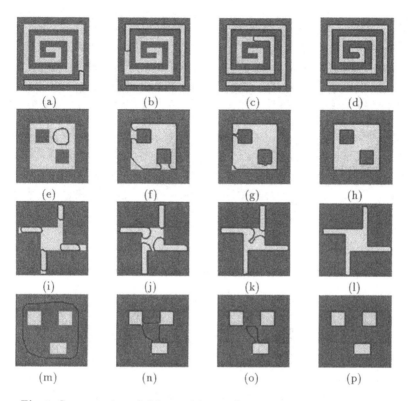

Fig. 5. Segmentation of objects with complex geometries and topologies.

physically intersect as they appear to do in this 2D image projection. Currently, we do not attempt to identify vessel intersections or bifurcations. A 64×64 square cell grid is used and the parameter values are: $\Delta t = 0.001, a_i = 30.0, b_i = 30.0, k = 60.0, \kappa = 70.0$. In Figures 7e–h we have initialized several models in various branches, demonstrating the potential for automating and parallelizing the segmentation process.

In the final experiment we demonstrate the use of the model collision detection property. A sagittal slice of an MR brain image was manually segmented into four anatomical regions and the pixels in each region were assigned a constant intensity level. We initialized two snakes in regions 4 and 3 and recovered the shapes of these regions (Fig. 8). We then initialized two snakes in regions 1 and 2 and allowed the snakes to flow, using only a minimum intensity threshold as the external image force. When these snakes attempt to flow into the brighter regions 4 and 3 they collide with the initial snakes and are forced to assume the shape of the common boundary regions (Fig. 8c).

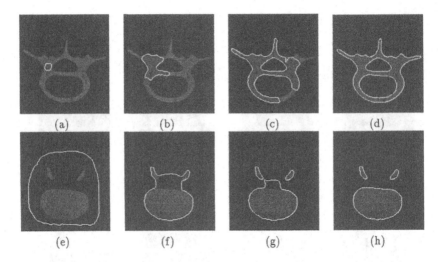

Fig. 6. Segmentation of two cross sectional images of a human vertebra phantom.

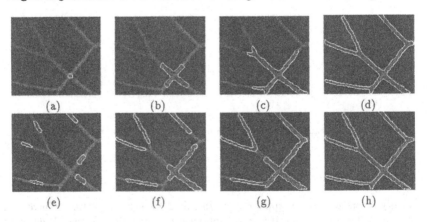

Fig. 7. Segmentation of the blood vessels in angiogram of retina. Top row: using a single snake. Bottom row: using multiple snakes.

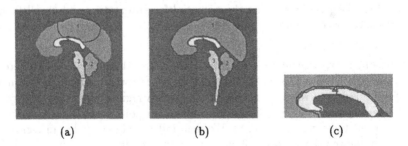

Fig. 8. Segmentation of anatomical regions of the brain using multiple models. The collision detection property was used as an extra constraint when segmenting regions 1 and 3.

4 Conclusion

We have developed a topologically adaptable snakes model that can be used to segment and represent structures of interest in medical images. By combining a domain decomposition technique with snakes, we have considerably extended the snake capabilities and overcome many of the limitations while keeping all of the traditional properties associated with these models. By iteratively reparameterizing the snake using the superposed grid, we have created a simple and efficient automatic subdivision technique as well as an unambiguous framework for topological transformations. Furthermore, the model has all of the functionality of the implicit level set techniques described in [5], but does not require any mathematical machinery beyond the basic formulation of classical snakes. Since the model retains a parametric formulation, users can control and interact with it as they would with traditional snakes. We have applied the model to various 2D synthetic and medical image datasets in order to segment structures of interest that have complicated shapes and topologies. We are currently extending the model to a three dimensional surface representation based on a tetrahedral decomposition of the image domain.

Acknowledgements

The segmented MR brain image was provided courtesy of Stephanie Sandor and Richard Leahy of the Signal and Image Processing Institute, Dept. of Electrical Engineering Systems, University of Southern California. TM is grateful for the financial support of an NSERC postgraduate scholarship. DT is a Fellow of the Canadian Institute for Advanced Research. This work was made possible by the financial support of the Information Technologies Research Center of Ontario.

References

1. M. O. Berger and R. Mohr. Towards Autonomy in Active Contour Models. In *Proc. of Tenth International Conference on Pattern Recognition*, pages 847–851, 1990.
2. I. Carlbom, D. Terzopoulos, and K. Harris. Computer-assisted registration, segmentation, and 3D reconstruction from images of neuronal tissue sections. *IEEE Transactions on Medical Imaging*, 13(2):351–362, 1994.
3. L.D. Cohen. On active contour models and balloons. In *CVGIP: Image Understanding*, volume 53(2), pages 211–218, March 1991.
4. M. Kass, A. Witkin, and D. Terzopoulo. Snakes: Active contour models. *International Journal of Computer Vision*, pages 321–331, 1988.
5. R. Malladi, J. Sethian, and B. Vemuri. Shape modeling with front propagation: A level set approach. *IEEE Trans. Pattern Analysis and Machine Intelligence*. In Press.
6. R. Samadani. Changes in connectivity in active contour models. In *Proceedings of the Workshop on Visual Motion*, pages 337–343, March 1989.
7. D. Terzopoulos, A. Witkin, and M. Kass. Constraints on deformable models: Recovering 3D shape and nonrigid motion. *Artificial Intelligence*, 36(1):91–123, 1988.

Simulation / Robotics

SOPHOCLE:
A Retinal Laser Photocoagulation Simulator Overview

Philippe Meseure[1], Jean-François Rouland[3], Patrick Dubois[2],
Sylvain Karpf[1] and Christophe Chaillou[1]

[1] Laboratoire d'Informatique Fondamentale de Lille
Université des Sciences et Technologies de Lille
UFR d'IEEA - Bât M3
F-59655 Villeneuve d'Ascq Cedex, France
[2] CLARC-Laboratoire de Biophysique
Pavillon Vancostenobel - CH&U Lille, France
[3] Clinique ophtalmologique, Hôpital Huriez, CHU Lille, France

Abstract. Retinal laser photocoagulation has been used for a decade, but no real improvement in results has been observed.The simulator described in this paper, by separating actual practice from apprenticeship, allows one both to learn how to manipulate the equipment and to train oneself for making a diagnosis and operating. It has been designed as close as possible to the actual operation conditions and gives the opportunity to deal with a large library of current or rare cases. An actual slit-lamp is supplied with sensors measuring all the degrees of freedom of the system. The images are calculated by a PC computer and are displayed on a miniature screen placed inside the binocular. A user interface is provided through a Computer Assisted Training software, which allows users to manage the pigmentations and pathologies data base, to follow the students skill level and to prepare critical operations.

Introduction

Retinal laser photocoagulation is a widely spread surgical technique. It has become one of the most important part of the ophthalmic area (about 3000 operations are performed in a year at the Regional Hospital Center of Lille). The therapeutic effects of photocoagulation are no more to be demonstrated in retinal detachment prevention, diabetic retinopathy, A.R.M.D. (Age Related Macular Degeneration), etc... However, despite the number of installed equipments, no real improvement of complications which should have been solved has been observed. These can, in worst cases, lead to a complete blindness. One of the reasons is undoubtedly the population aging, but one has the right to wonder whether the teaching of this technique is not to be improved. Today teaching is indeed based on two points: on one hand, theoretical knowledge is taught authoritatively or from books, on the other hand, gestures apprenticeship is learned by watching the teacher and practicing on actual patients.

Medicine always gains from the incoming of advanced new technologies: therapeutic laser, phakoemulsificators, diagnosis tools (video-photokeratoscope, visual field, electrophysiology...). Their consequence is a constant change of therapeutic methods. Why not take advantage of these new technologies to improve apprenticeship?

A retinal laser photocoagulation simulator provides a good answer to the apprenticeship problem. It is defined by two steps. First, a diagnosis step means the recognition of pathologies requiring a treatment or not. The second step consists in the treatment of the disease, taking account of the different settings like dosage or impacts locations. The interest of such a simulator lies inside the opportunity that it gives to the student to train as often as he wants and to deal with very rare pathologies which he would have had little chance to meet during his relatively short training course (5 semesters with one half day in a week for photocoagulation). Moreover, it allows ophthalmologists to improve their technique during their continuous education or to prepare critical operations. Finally, it gives the ability to separate actual practice from apprenticeship, and therefore to lower the risks for the patients.

The simulator has been designed as close as possible to the actual operation conditions. The slit-lamp is kept, all the other tools and the patient are simulated. Sensors measure the position of the different degrees of freedom and send the results to a PC computer, which calculates the images. These images are displayed in the binocular by means of a miniature screen. The simulator comes with a user interface (a computer assisted training software), which makes the simulator easy to use and allows the students level to be followed.

After a quick state of the art in medical simulators, we will see a description of the laser photocoagulation. Then, all the sensors, mathematical models and visualization algorithms will be presented, followed by a complete description of the simulator and its user interface.

1 Previous Works

Medical simulators have been a recent research area. Compared to driving simulators, medical simulators utilization increases quite slowly. One of the reasons may be the reserve of the surgeons. Another reason is undoubtedly the complexity of algorithms required within the medical area. Indeed, the surgeon not only visualizes the environment, but also interacts with it. That is why most simulators demand powerful workstations. [6] study laparoscopic gall-bladder surgery simulator, and try to generalize their model to other organs. [16] have designed a complete immersive simulator (including sensors, modeling, real-time deformations, visualization and force feedback) allowing anterior segment of the eye operation to be simulated. Their goal is to find new operation techniques. Other teams (Chapel-Hill, Georgia) are working on complete virtual environments. New domains are visited like childbirth [3][4], cardiology [17]... Cinquin's team in Grenoble is working on subjects like data acquisition, simulation, critical operation preparation and computer assisted intervention in areas like stereostatic neurosurgery, knee surgery, plastic and maxillo-facial surgery, rigid endoscopy [1]... Some other teams are working on 2D-data acquisition and 3D reconstitution which can be used for teleoperation, for instance [8] on stereostatic MRI.

Since the equipment required for complete environments is costly, some teams are working on cheaper simulators. For instance, [2] use images recorded on CD-ROM. [10] have designed a cranofacial surgery simulator, with intend to predict the result of an operation.

Some areas like observation, laser or endoscopy do not require very costly hardware [13], for the surgeon watches the organ through a binocular or a screen, and there is not or few mechanical interactions between the surgeon and the organ. Our simulator is lying in this frame, since it has been implemented on a general purpose PC, the vision of the surgeon is limited by the binocular and only a laser is used for the therapy.

2 Retinal Laser Photocoagulation

The goal of laser photocoagulation is to heal retinal diseases. The ophthalmologist beams a high power laser in order to create a barring around the lesion. The equipment includes a binocular, a slit-lamp, which provides the surgeon with light for the fundus observation, and the laser outfit.

A 3-mirror lens is placed on the patient's eye. It is made of three mirrors, spaced at 120 degree intervals, around a central lens. These mirrors have different inclinations so that the surgeon can observe different retina zones.

The operation and simulator description is showed on Fig. 1. The surgeon looks through the binocular, at the eye, which is lit by means of a slit, located at the back of the apparatus. A control lever enables the user to move the slit-lamp horizontally, and vertically by rotating it. A micro-manipulator can make a mirror rotate around two axes, in order to choose the orientation of the laser. A control panel allows the settings of the laser to be changed (power, fire duration).

The surgeon makes the 3-mirror lens slip around the eye, and looks at the fundus through the central lens or through one of the mirrors. In the same way, the laser beam can reflect onto a mirror before passing through the central lens. A low power laser sets the target site for the surgeon to fire the high power laser by pressing a pedal.

In an actual operation, about one hundred impacts are fired.

3 Mechanical Features

In our simulator, only the slit-lamp is kept. The patient and the lens are completely simulated. So, what the surgeon sees in the binocular has to be synthetized. The image depends upon the degrees of freedom of the system, which are measured by sensors. Here is the list of the degrees of freedom:

1. 3 translations (2 horizontal, 1 vertical) of the slit-lamp, which are measured by linear potentiometers, fixed on the observation statif.

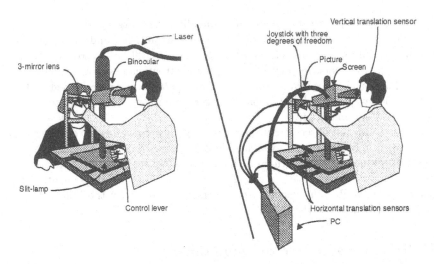

Fig. 1. Real and virtual operation description

2. 3 rotations (2 around the patient's eye and 1 around the lens axis), which are measured by an analogical 3-axis joystick. An exact copy of the lens is placed onto the stick part of the joystick. Two joysticks are used to simulate both right and left eyes and are inserted into the eyes slits of a mask.
3. 2 rotations of the laser mirror, which are measured by an analogical joystick.
4. The slit width and spot size are controlled by potentiometers.
5. The power of the laser and the firing duration are modified with the help of +/- interrupters located on the control panel. Their values and the number of laser impacts during the operation are displayed with three 7 segments LED.
6. The slit height, the magnifying level and the power of the lamp are controlled by means of multi-position interrupters.
7. Firing is controlled by an interrupter.

Data from the analogical and digital sensors are sent to the computer by means of a conversion interface. This card encodes values in 12-bit format.

4 Modeling

4.1 Lens Modeling

A 3-mirror lens is simulated since it is a good generalization of all ophthalmic lenses. It allows the eye to be observed directly or indirectly. The proposed model can therefore be adapted to other types of lenses. The three mirrors enable the surgeon to observe different zones of the eye. The lens is represented on Fig. 2.

1. The mirror 2, with a low inclination, allows the zones located around the central fundus to be observed.

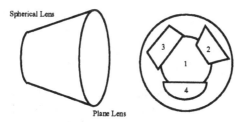

Fig. 2. The 3-mirror lens

2. The mirror 3, with an average inclination, allows the peripheral retina to be observed.

3. The mirror 4, with a high inclination, allows the regions, located just behind the iris to be observed.

The 3-mirror lens is modeled by a cone, and the (spherical) central lens is approximated by a planar circle. Each mirror is modeled by a plane (an equation) and four points belonging to the plane, which delimit the mirror edges. A local coordinates system which is centered on the cornea sphere, is used.

The model must be parameterized by the joystick data, in order to define the orientation of the virtual lens. These data are converted into angles: the 2 rotations around the eye are defined just as the spherical system coordinates (a latitude and a longitude). A space transformation matrix (from the local to the global coordinates) is calculated from the angles and is used to calculate the position of the lens elements. This matrix also allows the new equations of the mirrors planes to be determined and therefore, the image of space, seen through the mirrors, to be calculated by an orthogonal symmetry.

4.2 Eye Modeling

The eye is modeled by a sphere, the cornea by a half-sphere. The center of the eye and of the cornea are not the same: the cornea center is translated, along the visual axis, toward the pupil. The iris is modeled by a flat ring, orthogonal to the visual axis. As the lens, a local coordinates system is used, and a transformation matrix is calculated, to simulate any movement of the eye. But, this time, the angles are chosen by the computer, depending upon how "nervous" the virtual patient is: random numbers with Gauss distribution give realistic effects.

In order to get a realistic image of the eye, a photomapping is used. Thus, a complete map of an eye is created. At least 20 photographs of an actual fundus are taken and placed side by side with a specific software. Blood vessels continuity is used for the assembly. A complete 2D map is obtained thanks to spherical coordinates.

In order to visualize a textured eye, we decided to use a tessellated sphere representing the eye and associate a texture map to each face. The tessellation triangles do not need to be small: the smaller the triangles, the more faces will have to be processed, so processing time will increase, but the display time will not change (the same number of pixels will be colored). The tessellation must embody the sphere. Indeed, the surgeon looks at the interior of the eye, and some parts of the eye will not be displayed if the surgeon looks along a skimming direction.

The tessellation we choose is a regular icosahedra, which is a polyhedron with 20 equilateral triangles. The texture map of each triangle is put into an array, the color of each point is obtained by projecting the icosahedra onto the sphere, with a projection whose center is the central point of the sphere.

Only one resolution of the texture is used for the map, for it is optimized for the usually used magnifying level. If the surgeon increases the magnifying level, several pixels on the screen will be displayed with the color of the same texel[1], if he decreases the magnifying level, several texels will not be used.

4.3 Operation Modeling

An absolute coordinates system is chosen: it is located on the center of the surgeon's eye. So the patient's eye is supposed to move and not the surgeon's eye, although it is actually the contrary. The entire laser path is calculated: it reflects first onto the deflection mirror, then, possibly on one of the mirrors of the lens, and reaches the fundus, if it has not met any obstacle like the lens or the iris. The impact point is then calculated on the icosahedra. Impacts are put in memory for evaluation purpose and in the texture map for display. Impacts color depends upon the type of the fundus, the firing duration, the laser power and focus.

5 Visualization

5.1 Image Drawing

All the objects are projected onto the screen plane with a perspective projection. No usual algorithms for 3D synthesis such as Z-buffer have been used. We preferred instead to use 2D algorithms. Indeed, according to depth order, the objects are always arranged the same way. So, no sort is needed. Objects are displayed sequentially, first the central lens, iris, fundus, then each mirror and image of what is seen through the mirror. In order not to display the hidden parts, we chose to use Sutherland-Hodgman polygons clipping algorithm (see [11]).

An efficient algorithm for texture mapping has been implemented on the PC: a bilinear interpolation has been used [12].

5.2 Rendering

In actual operation, sharpness is controlled by the depth translation which focuses the different lenses. A good focus is required for a good photocoagulation,

---

[1] Texture element.

for the focus of the image causes the focus of the laser, which is only effective for a good focus. So it was important to implement a real-time depth of field simulation. Four texture maps of the eye, with increasing blurring level are put in memory. The color of a point is obtained by interpolating between the colors of this point in two blurring levels.

Only the part of the eye which is lit by the slit is visible, the rest is too dark to be seen. The light from the slit looks like a rectangle on the screen. In order to suppress the discontinuous transition between the lit part and the dark one, a gradation on the edge of the rectangle has been implemented (the distance between the point and the edge determines the loss of brightness).

As far as the laser is concerned, the impact point on the icosahedra is known. The spot can be drawn, if it is seen through the central lens and/or through a mirror. In order to draw a translucent spot, it is filled with a grid bitmap: one point out of two are displayed with the color of the laser, the other points are kept unchanged (screen-door transparency).

6 Design

The software has been implemented on a PC with a 80486DX2.66. The video card is a Local Bus one, which makes a 32-bit access at the frequency of the processor possible. The algorithms have been implemented in C and run in protected mode. Images are displayed both on a control screen and on a miniature screen, located in the binocular. In the first prototype, a CGA-resolution LCD screen was used. However, we are now working on a new implementation using a Textronix VGA field sequential color display which give best results. At every step, the PC gets the sensors data, calculates the image with them, and, using a double buffer, displays this image on the two screens. A second PC, called master, runs the user interface under the Windows environment. This interface is described in next section. The Master PC sends orders to the simulation PC (also called slave-PC) by means of a serial link. Any fundus, pathology or fluorography is displayed on the simulation PC screen, on one hand, to take advantage of higher resolutions and number of colors, independently of Windows, and on the other hand, to make the access to the data base easier, since the data base is centralized on the slave PC (the amount of information passing through the serial link is lowered). Figure 3 shows the complete configuration.

7 User Interface - Computer Assisted Training Software

The user interface consists in a succession of explicit menus, which are easy to use, even for people with little knowledge of computers. The first step is the recognition of the user to assume access security. This means that the user types a name and a password. If the authentication succeeds, the software can know what kind of user he is. Three classes has been implemented: *system manager*, *experts* and *students*.

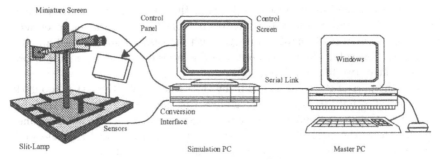

Fig. 3. Configuration

The *system manager* is responsible for the well-running of the simulator and for the data base coherency. Several options are proposed to help making a diagnosis of the simulator, but this is far beyond the scope of this paper. The *experts* are the ophthalmologists who are in charge of students. The software allows them to create photocoagulation exercises for their students, by choosing fundus, pathology, eye side and mobility... The software can help them to prepare a critical operation too.

The *students* can also register, in order to train on their own or to inspect their improvement since their last operation simulations.

Any operation simulation is called a session. Every sessions are recorded and can be reviewed (by means of the simulator), if required by the user, with the help of a video tape-like interface. This film allows an expert to evaluate a session, even if he was not present at that time.

In order to accommodate each *school of therapy*, no standard is imposed. The expert chooses the appropriate treatment, called reference session. The software can then give some pieces of information for the evaluation of the students (number, localization, settings of the impacts). However, only the expert can validate a session.

The data base is put in the hard drive of the simulation PC and consists in the set of fundus and pathologies. Some pathologies (A.R.M.D., diabetic retinopathy) can come with a fluorography, which is also put in the data base. Finally, all the films which have been kept by the users, are recorded into the data base. Each fundus and pathology belongs to an expert, who can therefore have personalized data.

Results - Perspectives

An example of image is given on Fig.4.The current frame rate is about 8 images per second in a 640x400 resolution and 32768 colors and 10 images per second, in a 640x480 resolution and 256 colors. About 35% of time is used for processing, 65% for displaying. The new PC technologies (Pentium, PCI) can improve the frame rate (new processors lower the calculation time, new buses lower the displaying time), and the simulator is soon to be adapted on pentium PCI with a faster video card. A satisactory frame rate would be between 15 to 20 images per second.

The current work are the improvement of impacts treatment and rendering (iris texture, light interferences...). Some sounds will be added. Long-term project is the inclusion of the entire eye semiology, in order to simulate other diseases (pathologies located in the anterior segment, for instance).

A prototype is being validated by the students at the hospital of Lille. Some other ophthalmologists team will be contacted to criticize and complete the data base. This project has been patented [7] and is aimed to be industrialized.

Acknowledgments

The simulator is supported by DRED and CHR&U credits and by a grant from ANVAR (Agence Nationale de la Valorisation de la Recherche).

References

1. Bainville, E., Chaffanjon, P., Cinquin, P., Troccaz, J., and Lavallée, S., "Computer Augmented Medecine". Troisième séminaire du groupe de travail "Animation et Simulation" Lille 1994, 163-170.
2. Beer-Gabel, M., Delmotte, S., and Muntlak, L., "Computer Assisted Training in Endoscopy (CATE) - From a Simulator to a Training Station" Endoscopy vol 24 suppl 2, 1992,534-538.
3. Boissonat, J.D., and Geiger, B., "Modélisation 3D et Simulation de Mouvements". Premières Journées AFIG-GROPLAN, Labri Bordeaux 1993, 187-191.
4. Boissonat, J.D., and Geiger, B., "3d Simulation of Delivery". Proceedings of Visualization'93, 416-419.
5. Bier, E.A., and Sloan, K.R., "Two part Texture Mappings". IEEE Computer Graphics & Applications 6,10 September 1986,40-53.
6. Cover, S.A., Ezquerra, N.F., O'Brien, J., Rowe, R., Gadacz, T., Palm, E., "Interactively Deformable Models for Surgery Simulation". IEEE Computer Graphics & Applications 13,6 november 1993.
7. Chaillou, C., Dubois, P., Karpf, S., Meseure, P., and Rouland, J.F., "Dispositif et Procédé de simulation d'un examen ou d'une opération chirurgicale effectuée sur un organe simulé". Dépôt de brevet no 9405487.
8. Clarysse, P., Gibon, D., Rousseau, J., Blond, S., Vasseur, C., and Marchandise, X., "A Computer-Assisted System for 3D Frameless Localization in Stereostatic MRI" IEEE Transactions on Medical Imaging 10,4 (1991).
9. Chen, D.T., and Zeltzer, D., "Pump it up: Computer Animation of a Biomechanically Based Model of Muscle using the Finite Element Method". SIGGRAPH'92 Conference Proceedings 26,2 (1992) 89-98.
10. Delingette, H., Subsol, G., Cotin, S. and Pignon, J., "A craniofacial Surgery Simulation Testbed". Rapport de recherche INRIA no 2199 february 1994.
11. Foley, J.D., van Dam, A., Feiner, S.K., and Hughes, J.F., Computer Graphics: Principles and Practice, Addison Wesley 1990.
12. Heckbert, P.S., "Survey of Texture Mapping". IEEE Computer Graphics & Applications 6,11 November 1986. 56-67.

114

13. Haritsis, A., Gillies, D.F., and Williams, C.B., "Realistic Generation and Real Time Animation of Images of the Human Colon". Proceedings of the EUROGRAPHICS'92 11,3 (1992) 367-379.

14. Jouve, F., Modélisation de l'œil en élasticité non linéaire, Masson.

15. Meseure, P., Karpf, S., Chaillou, C., Dubois, P., and Rouland, J.F., "Sophocle : un simulateur de photocoagulation rétinienne par laser". Troisième séminaire du groupe de travail "Animation et Simulation" Lille 1994, 145-152.

16. Sagar, M. A., Bullivant, D., Mallinson, G. D., Hunter, P. J, and Hunter, J. W., "A Virtual Environment and Model of the Eye for Surgical Simulation". SIGGRAPH'94 Conference Proceedings (1994).

17. Schwartz, S.L., Cao, Q. L., Azevedo, J., and Pandian, N.G., "Simulation of Intraoperative Visualization of Cardiac Structures and Study of Dynamic Surgical Anatomy with Real-Time Tridimensional Echocardiography". Am. J. Cardiol., vol 74(7), 1994, 501-7.

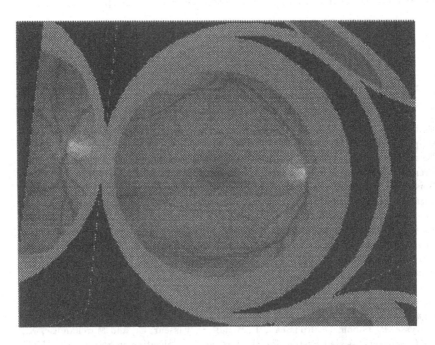

Fig. 4. Synthetized image of the 3-mirror lens and the eye

A New Robot for High Dexterity Microsurgery

Paul S. Schenker, Hari Das, and Timothy R. Ohm

Jet Propulsion Laboratory, California Institute of Technology
4800 Oak Grove Drive / MS 198-219
Pasadena, CA 91109
Email: schenker@telerobotics.jpl.nasa.gov

Abstract. We report the development of a new six degree-of-freedom (d.o.f.) manipulator. This robot and its task-space controls enable relative tip positioning to better than 25 microns over a singularity-free work volume exceeding 20 cubic centimeters. By virtue of an innovative cable drive design, the robot has zero backlash in five joints and can sustain full extent loads of over three pounds. The robot is applicable to both fine motion manipulation of microsurgical tools and also dexterous handling of larger powered devices for minimally invasive surgery. Our current development emphasis is a teleoperated system for dexterity-enhanced microsurgeries; we believe the new robot will also have useful applications in computer assisted surgeries, e.g. image-guided therapies. In this brief paper, we outline the robot mechanical design, controls implementation, and preliminary evaluations. Our accompanying oral presentation includes a five minute videotape that illustrates engineering laboratory results achieved to date.

1 Introduction

Robotics researchers are exploring several new medical applications thrusts, as surveyed in proceedings of recent special interest meetings and workshops [1]. These applications include robot-assisted stereotaxic interventions (imaging-guided biopsy), orthopedic preparations by robot (precision joint emplacements), endoscopic & laparoscopic assists (minimally invasive procedures), teleoperative remote surgeries (telesurgery), and recently, robotically-enhanced microsurgery (high dexterity, scaled operations under microscopic viewing). Our primary interest is the last area. Building on our recent work in high dexterity telerobotics [2], we have begun development of a *Robot Assisted MicroSurgery* (RAMS) workstation for procedures of the eye, ear, brain, face, and hand. Jet Propulsion Laboratory is conducting this work in cooperation with MicroDexterity Systems, Inc., a USA-based medical products and microsurgical tools venture. Collectively, JPL/MDS plan to evaluate the RAMS developments in clinical microsurgery procedures circa 1996, and initiate some basic medical laboratory experimentation in 1995. The JPL-based work is closest in spirit to prior pioneering efforts of Hunter et al., who to date have performed significant engineering development and quantitative characterization of a force-reflecting teleoperator for microsurgery [3]. By comparison to this more mature light-weight parallel-link robot system, RAMS design targets a comparatively lower position scaling (~1:3), larger force regimes (fractions of an oz. sensitivity), a large included work angle of surgical access (>120 degree cone), and mechanically stiff precision tracking at low speeds and higher payloads (viz. minimized backlash, stiction, deflections, inertia, etc.). We note also the related efforts of Salcudean et al., Grace et al. and Green et al. to develop force-reflecting teleoperative systems for medical applications including telesurgery, as they have reported in recent IEEE conference papers [4]. In particular, while addressing surgeries of conventional scale (e.g., laparoscopy), the SRI telepresence system of Green et al. is a mature R&D effort that has been demonstrated in simulated surgeries.

2 Robot Design

2.1 Motivation

The RAMS workstation is conceived as a dual-arm 6-d.o.f. master-slave telemanipulator with programmable controls, one arm handling primary surgical tooling, and the other auxiliaries (suction, cauterization, imaging, etc.). The primary control mode is to be teleoperation, including task-frame referenced manual force feedback and possibly a cross-modal textural presentation. Later sensor-related developments include *in situ* imaging modes for tissue feature visualization and discrimination. The operator will also be able to interactively designate or telerobotically "share" automated control of robot trajectories, as appropriate. RAMS is intended to refine the physical scale of manual microsurgical procedures, while also enabling more positive outcomes for the average surgeon during typical procedures -- e.g., the RAMS workstation controls include features to enhance the surgeon's manual positioning and tracking in the face of the 5-10 Hz band myoclonic jerk and involuntary tremor that limit many surgeons' fine-motion skills. The first RAMS development, now completed and undergoing engineering evaluation, is a small six-d.o.f. surgical robot ("slave"), the configuration of which is a torso-shoulder-elbow (t/s/e) body with non-intersecting 3-axis wrist. This robot manipulator is approximately 25 cm. full-extent and 2.5 cm. in diameter. Robot actuation is based on a new revolute joint and cable-drive mechanism that achieves near zero backlash, constant cable length excursions, and minimized joint coupling. The robot design and controls currently allow relative positioning of tools to at least 25 microns over a non-singular work volume of ~20 cm^3. Note this resolution is several times better than that observed in the most exceptional and skilled manual medical procedures to date (e.g., vitreo-retinal manipulations of ~50-100 micron tissue features).

2.2 Design

We describe the robot design in this section, briefly outlining related design requirements, as motivated both by kinematic control objectives and robot suitability to re-usable and safe application in a sterile medical environment. *Figure 1* highlights some recent robot mechanical developments, e.g., the integrated six-d.o.f. robot slave (manipulator and motor-drive base), a 3-d.o.f. wrist (close-up view), and the highly novel double-jointed tendon drive rotary joint mechanization used in shoulder-and-elbow actuation. In the presentation that follows we list a design objective (*in italics*) and its definition; we then provide a brief technical description of the technical approach we took to meet the objective. Where appropriate, and known to date, we give quantitative information. We have as yet done relatively little modeling or quantitative experimental analysis of the robot kinematics & dynamics (explicit calibration, inertial properties, impedance/mechanical response, etc.).

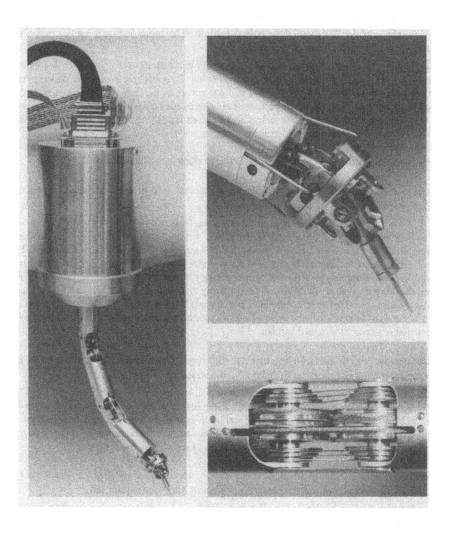

Fig. 1. Robot Assisted MicroSurgery (RAMS) manipulator: on *left* the six-degree of freedom cable-driven robot arm (length ~25 cm, outer diameter ~2.5 cm), with motor-drive base and sterile containment (torso rolls 165 degrees within); at *upper right* the Rosheim-derived three degree-of-freedom wrist enabling 180 degrees pitch-and-yaw and 540 degrees continuous roll; and at *lower right* the cable-driven double-jointed mechanism enabling full 360 degree rotary motions in the shoulder and elbow, while decoupling interactions between the primary robot actuation joints.

Drive Unit Separability. Autoclaving of the robot is possible by removing the motor/encoder units at the base prior to sterilization. The motor/encoder units can be re-attached in a quick and simple procedure.

This is done by integrating the motors/encoders into two distinct sets of three on a common mount and registering these packages via alignment pins. The resulting two motor packages can be easily removed by undoing two screws and one connector on each set. The mechanism can then be autoclaved. The two motor packages can be reinstalled quickly by reversing the removal procedure. In normal operation the motors are contained inside the robot's base, protecting anything they might contaminate. An added advantage obtained with this design is that debugging of servo and kinematics control systems can be done while the motors are not attached to the robot, thereby sparing the robot damage during software development and validation.

Zero/Low Backlash. Low backlash (free play) is essential to fine manipulation, especially when position sensors are on the motor shafts.

Five of the robot's six degrees of freedom have zero backlash and the sixth has about 20 microns. Zero backlash is achieved by using dual drive-trains that are pre-loaded relative to one another. These dual drive-trains are coupled together at only the motor shaft and the joint output. The steel cables which actuate each joint also act as springs to pre-load the gear-train. The drive-train's pre-load can be easily adjusted by disengaging the motor, counter-rotating the dual drives until the desired pre-load is reached, and re-engaging the motor. This also allows for easy cable adjustment as the cables stretch with time. The one axis that does not have zero backlash is a result of the wrist design which makes low backlash possible but zero backlash difficult, especially if stiction is a concern as with this robot.

Low Stiction. Stiction (stick/slip characteristic) must be minimized to achieve small incremental movements without overshooting or instability.

Stiction was minimized by incorporating precision ball bearings in every rotating location of the robot (pulleys, shafts, joint axes, etc.), so as to eliminate metal-to-metal sliding. Due to severe size and loading constraints, some of these bearings had to be custom designed. Indeed, there is only one location in the wrist where such direct contact exists, because size constraints therein restricted use of bearings. Backlash was allowed here to reduce stiction, per above.

Decoupled Joints. Having all joints mechanically decoupled simplifies kinematics computations as well as provides for partial functionality should one joint fail.

Developing a six axis, tendon-driven robot that has all joints mechanically decoupled is very difficult. Decoupling requires driving any given joint without affecting any other joint. The shoulder and elbow joints incorporate a unique double-jointed scheme that allows passage of any number of activation cables completely decoupled from these joints. The three axis wrist is based on a concept (as originated by Mark Rosheim, Ross-Hime Designs, Inc., Minneapolis, MN) that not only decouples the joints, but also has no singularities. Further, the torso simply rotates the entire robot base to eliminate coupling. *If any one of the joints were to fail mechanically, the remaining five would be unaffected.*

Large Work Envelope. A large work volume is desirable so that the arm's base will not have to be repositioned frequently during tasks.

To achieve a large work envelope, each joint needs to have a large range of motion. The torso was designed with 165 degrees of motion while both the shoulder and elbow have a full 360 degrees. This high range of motion in the shoulder and elbow is attained by the unique double-jointed scheme mentioned above. The wrist design (utilizing the Rosheim concept) has 180 degrees of pitch and yaw with 540 degrees of roll. Such large motion ranges greatly reduce the chance of a joint reaching a limit during operation, thus increasing the work volume.

High Stiffness. A stiff manipulator is necessary for accurate positioning under gravitational or environmental loads, especially when position sensing is at the motor drives.

When a robot changes its orientation relative to gravity, it will deflect due to its own weight. Likewise, if a force acts on the arm, it will also deflect. Furthermore, if position sensing is done at the motor drive, this deflection will not be known. Therefore, such deflections must be minimized by increasing stiffness. The stiffness of RAMS arm is about 15 lb./inch at the tip. This high stiffness is achieved by using high spur gear reductions off the motors, combined with large diameter, short path length stainless steel cables to actuate each joint. The pitch and yaw axes also include an additional 2:1 cable reduction inside the forearm (near the joint) for added stiffness.

Compact/Lightweight. In some applications, a restricted work-space warrants a small serial manipulator to minimize both geometric and visual interference.

The physical size of the arm is about one inch in diameter and about 25 cm long. The robot base, containing the motor drives and electrical interfaces, has a 12 cm diameter and is 17.75 cm long. The entire unit (arm and base) weighs about 5.5 lbs. All electrical cables connect to the bottom of the base so as to not protrude into the robot's work-space.

Fine Incremental Motions. Human dexterity limitations constrain surgical procedures to feature sizes of about 50-to-100 microns. This arm is designed to achieve 10 microns relative positioning.

By combining many of the features mentioned above (low backlash, low stiction, high stiffness, etc.), this arm is designed to make very small incremental movements. This means that the manipulator can make incremental steps of 10 microns. Note conversely this does not necessarily mean that the arm is repeatable to within 10 microns absolute position accuracy.

Tool Wiring Provisions. Some tools require electrical or pneumatic power which can be routed through the arm in some cases.

The arm is designed to allow running a limited amount of wiring or hoses from the base to the arm's tip (where the tool is mounted). This passageway is about .35 cm in diameter through the wrist and exits through the center of the tooling plate. The wiring can be passed out the base of the robot so that it does not interfere with its work-space, as would be the case if such wiring was routed externally.

Configuration Management and Control. It is necessary to sense, monitor, and control basic failure conditions (e.g., to implement corrective motion control/braking actions)

A Programmable Logic Device (PLD) controls power and braking relays through an optically isolated interface, and allows fault detection and error recovery. The major features of this electronic system are: 1) power up and down button, manual start-stop buttons to switch motor power from a brake mode to control mode, panic button to stop motors, and brake relay fault detection, 2) watchdog timer fault detection to insure control processors are functioning, 3) amplifier power supply & fuse fault detection, and 4) PLD logic fault detection.

3   RAMS System Computing and Control

Operator-robot interaction is at present implemented through a *graphics user interface* (GUI) that resides on a UNIX workstation. This workstation also is host for a VxWorks real-time control environment. The VxWorks-based *kinematic & joint controls* are in turn implemented on a MC 68040 board installed in a VME chassis. A Delta Tau Data Systems PMAC board, also on the VME chassis, controls the six axes of the robot by directly reading the robot sensor outputs and driving the motors through amplifiers.

3.1   Graphics User Interface

The GUI is based on the X Windows and OSF/Motif libraries. We have developed a number of GUI-driven demonstration modes to show and evaluate the robot capabilities:

- a *manual joint control mode* wherein the user moves individual joints manually by selecting buttons in a control window, incrementing and decrementing a desired joint position

- an *autonomous joint control mode* demonstrating the workspace of the robot. In this mode, the robot simultaneously moves each of its joints in a sinusoidal motion between set limits

- a *manual teleoperated mode* in which the robot is controlled either by using a mouse (or by selecting buttons on a display), incrementing or decrementing motion along single axes of a world-referenced coordinate frame, or by using the spaceball input device to simultaneously move all six axes of the robot

- an *autonomous world space control mode* in which the robot moves its end effector in a sinusoidal motion about one or more Cartesian-defined axes simultaneously.

3.2   Kinematic and Joint Controls

The control software of the robot resides on the VME-based system. *Figure 2* sketches the control flow for the manual and autonomous world coordinate frame-referenced control modes. The general scheme by which the operator currently commands forward control to the robot is as follows: he inputs to the system from the GUI and this input is passed forward using the UNIX socket facility over an Ethernet link. Data thus passed into the control system is specified as desired changes in the robot tip position. We relate these world frame tip coordinate changes to commanded robot joint motions through a Jacobian inverse matrix, which is computed using a JPL-developed Spatial Operator Algebra [5]; this inverse is then multiplied with the input tip displacement vector to determine a corresponding joint position change vector. The primary advantage afforded by the Spatial Operator Algebra for this application is its concise recursive formulation of the kinematics equations, allowing rapid software development and testing -- a simple addition of the joint position change vector to the actual position of the joints results in the desired joint positions for the robot. The desired joint positions are then downloaded to the PMAC controller board wherein joint servo control is performed using a PID loop for each joint axis. In the manual and autonomous joint control modes, the PMAC controller correspondingly receives the joint position change vector as its input. The vector is added to the actual joint positions of the robot and the resulting vector is the desired joint position vector sent to the servo controller.

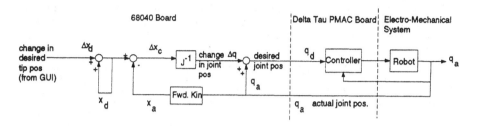

Fig. 2: RAMS control flow diagram

4 Results and Future Plans

As of end-year, 1994, we have integrated the slave robot system described above and demonstrated its successful operation in all control modes. On initial integration, without benefit of significant mechanical tuning or refitting of the robot mechanisms, we achieved repeatable relative positioning of the robot tip to 25 microns or less. This measurement, verified in a number of calibrated and videotaped [6] experiments, was performed both mechanically and optically. In the former case, we utilized calibrated mechanical dial indicators on three orthogonal axes of a wrist-tip-mounted needle; for the latter, we utilized a calibrated viewing field microscope with integrated CCD camera, and programmed and visually monitored a number of different free space, small motions within a 800 micron full-extent reticle. Cumulatively, we observed that both small (micron) and large (centimeter) free space motion trajectories are smooth. Impromptu tests in which a leading microsurgeon compared his free hand motions with that of the robot indicate that the desired scaling will be possible and highly beneficial, given an appropriate hand master interface. Development of such a non-replica master is one immediate project focus, as is also continuing, more quantitative evaluation of the robot, including its loaded (contact) motion performance. Another planned activity is development of control compensation techniques to reject feed-forward "disturbances" arising from the surgeon's involuntary tremor and jerk. And of course, we want to begin evaluation of the robot design in medical laboratory settings at appropriate opportunities.

5 Acknowledgments

The Robot Assisted Microsurgery (RAMS) task is being carried out at the Jet Propulsion Laboratory, California Institute of Technology, under a contract with the National Aeronautics and Space Administration. Related New Technology Notices have been filed, and a JPL-Industry Technology Cooperation Agreement with MicroDexterity Systems (MDS), Inc., exists. MDS Chief Officer Steven T. Charles, M.D., is an instrumental partner in defining RAMS system operational requirements, elements of the engineering conceptual design, and strategies & practice for subsequent medical evaluation.

References

1. Report on **NSF Workshop on Computer Assisted Surgery**, February 28-March 2, 1993, Washington, D.C. (Orgs., R. H. Taylor and G.A. Bekey). **Proc. Medicine Meets Virtual Reality III**, January 19-22, 1995, at San Diego, California, sponsored by the Univ. Calif. San Diego (Publisher: Aligned Management Consultants, San Diego, CA.). Proc. First Intl. Symp. **Medical Robotics and Computer Assisted Surgery (MRCAS'94)**, September 22-24, Pittsburgh, PA (Eds., A.M. DiGioia, III, T. Kanade, and R. Taylor); NCI-NASA-**SCVIR Workshop on Technology Transfer in Image Guided Therapy**, August 5, 1994, San Francisco, CA (Chr., H. Y. Kressel). **Virtual Reality: Scientific and Technological Challenges**, a report of the Committee on Virtual Reality Research & Development (Chr., N. Durlach), National Research Council, NAS Press (1994), Washington D.C.

2. **S. Schenker**, A. K. Bejczy, W. S. Kim, and S. Lee, "Advanced man-machine interfaces and control architecture for dexterous teleoperations," in Proc. Oceans `91, pp. 1500-1525, Honolulu, HI, October, 1991, and references therein. **H. Das**, H. Zak, W. S. Kim, A. K. Bejczy, and P. S. Schenker, "Operator performance with alternative manual modes of control," *Presence*, Vol. 1, no. 2, pp. 201-218, Spring 1992; see also, **H. Das**, P.S. Schenker, H. Zak, and A. K. Bejczy, "Teleoperated satellite repair experiments," in Proc. 1992 IEEE-RSJ Intl. Conf. IROS, Raleigh, NC, July. **P. S. Schenker** and W. S. Kim, "Remote robotic operations and graphics-based operator interfaces," in Proc. 5th Intl. Symp. on Robotics and Manufacturing (ISRAM `94), Maui, HI, August 14-17, 1994, and references therein. **P. S. Schenker**, W. S. Kim, and A. K. Bejczy, "Remote robotic operations at 3000 miles -- dexterous teleoperation with time-delay via calibrated virtual reality task display," in Proc. Medicine Meets Virtual Reality II, San Diego, CA, January, 1994. **P. S. Schenker**, S. F. Peters, E. D. Paljug, and W. S. Kim, "Intelligent viewing control for robotic & automation systems," in Sensor Fusion VII, in Proc. SPIE 2355, Boston, MA, October, 1994.

3. **Hunter**, T. Doukoglou, S. Lafontaine, P. Charette, L. Jones, M. Sager, G. Mallinson, P. Hunter, "A teleoperated microsurgical robot and associated virtual environment for eye surgery," *Presence*, Vol. 2, no. 4, pp. 265-280, fall, 1993.

4. **Salcudean** and J. Yan, 'Towards a force-reflecting, motion-scaling system for microsurgery," in Proc. 1994 IEEE Intl. Conf. Robotics and Automation, May, San Diego, CA; see also, **S. Salcudean**, N.M. Wong, and R.L. Hollis, "A force-reflecting teleoperation system with magnetically levitated master and wrist," in Proc. 1992 IEEE Intl. Conf. Robotics and Automation, Nice, France, May. **K. W. Grace**, J. E. Colgate, M. R. Glucksberg, and J. H. Chun, "A six degree-of-freedom manipulator for ophthalmic surgery," in Proc. 1993 IEEE Intl. Conf. Robotics and Automation, Atlanta, GA, May. J. W. Hill, **P. S. Green**, J. F. Jensen, Y. Gorfu, and Ajit S. Shah, "Telepresence surgery demonstration system," in Proc. 1994 IEEE Intl. Conf. Robotics and Automation, San Diego, CA, May

5. **Rodriguez**, "Kalman filtering, smoothing and recursive robot arm forward and inverse dynamics," *Journal of Robotics and Automation*, Vol. 3, No. 6, pp. 624-639, 1987; **G. Rodriguez**, K. Kreutz, and A. Jain, "A spatial operator algebra for manipulator modeling and control, *International Journal of Robotics Research*," Vol. 10, No. 4, pp. 371-381, 1991.

6. "Robot Assisted Microsurgery project accomplishments for FY94 -- demonstration of robot joint motion, Cartesian control, and precise tip control," Production **AVC-94-228 (VHS Videotape), September 1, 1994, Audiovisual Services Office, Jet Propulsion Laboratory**: E. Barlow, C. Boswell, H. Das, S. Lee, T. Ohm, E. Paljug, G. Rodriguez, and **P. Schenker**(PI), for NASA Headquarters.

Towards More Capable and Less Invasive Robotic Surgery in Orthopaedics

R.V. O'Toole III[1,2], D.A. Simon[2],
B. Jaramaz[1,2], O. Ghattas[3], M.K. Blackwell[2], L. Kallivokas[1],
F. Morgan[2], C. Visnic[1], A.M. DiGioia III[1,2,3], and T. Kanade[2]

[1] Center for Orthopaedic Research, Shadyside Hospital
[2] The Robotics Institute, Carnegie Mellon University
[3] Department of Civil Engineering, Carnegie Mellon University
Pittsburgh, PA

Abstract. Current surgical robotic systems in orthopaedics lack realistic pre-operative simulations and utilize invasive methods to register bone intra-operatively. A multidisciplinary group of researchers is addressing these deficiencies in the context of robotic cementless hip replacement surgery. In this paper we outline our current research progress and a road-map for the short-term future of our research agenda. This paper addresses four components of this effort: (1) realistic anatomical modeling, (2) biomechanics-based simulations, (3) surface-based registration, and (4) surgical robotics. We are integrating these components with the goal of developing more capable and less invasive robotic systems for use in orthopaedic surgery.

1 Introduction

The field of orthopaedics presents excellent opportunities for the incorporation of robotic and computer-based technologies to improve surgical techniques. Procedures such as total joint replacement are performed in large numbers and at significant cost each year. Over 300,000 total hip and knee replacements occur annually in the U.S. alone [3]. The short and long term clinical success of these surgical procedures depends strongly on the proper alignment, placement, and fit of the implant within the bony structure [9]. The clinical importance of precision and accuracy, along with the large number and high cost of the surgical procedures, indicates that important contributions can be made through the use of surgical robots and computer-based pre-operative planning and simulation in orthopaedics.

Figure 1 outlines the four basic components of our research effort: (1) realistic anatomical modeling, (2) biomechanics-based simulations, (3) surface-based registration, and (4) surgical robotics. We are integrating these components with the goal of developing more capable and less invasive robotic systems for use in orthopaedic surgery.

In biomechanics, our goal is to allow a surgeon to simulate the mechanical consequences of a proposed surgery, and to change surgical strategies based

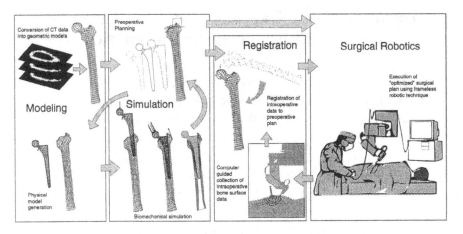

Fig. 1. Interaction of Research Topics

upon these consequences. By coupling this realistic simulation and planning capability with precise surgical robots, the surgeon can not only plan an "ideal" surgery, but also ensure that it is carried out. To execute a surgical plan with a robot, the system must possess the ability to register (determine the position and orientation) a bone in the clinical environment. Surface-based registration is desirable because it does not require fiducials to properly align the pre-operative plan with the patient's anatomy. The success of both surgical registration and pre-operative simulation is highly dependent upon the realism of geometric and physical models. As such, anatomic modeling has also emerged as a distinct research area. Our work attempts to join these four seemingly disparate research topics into one integrated effort to improve techniques in orthopaedic robotics.

2 Modeling

While algorithms exist for the creation of geometric models from volumetric medical data, little work has been published on the validation of these models. One reason for this lack of research is that until recently, geometric surface models have been used primarily for visualization tasks that do not demand highly accurate models. With the increased use of surface models for pre-operative planning and intra-operative guidance, geometric model accuracy has taken on new importance. Physical modeling issues subsume those associated with geometric modeling. In addition to difficulties in generating the geometry of the bone and implant, physical models must appropriately represent the underlying constitutive laws.

2.1 Geometric Model Creation and Validation

The primary geometric model in our work is the polyhedral surface mesh. It is used for visualizing 3D surface geometries and for surface-based intra-surgical registration. A variety of techniques are available for reconstructing polyhedral surface meshes directly from CT or MRI data [6]. We currently generate surface meshes using several of these methods [2][8][1].

Geometric surface model validation is complicated since errors can be introduced at several stages of model creation: during imaging, segmentation, and surface creation. Furthermore, there are multiple measures of error that can be used (e.g. Hausdorff distances, difference volumes, surface normal differences). Since different tasks place different requirements upon the underlying model, validation criteria should be application dependent. For example, a geometric model used to specify pre-operative prosthesis placement may have very different accuracy requirements than one used for surface-based registration.

Geiger [2] provides an excellent discussion of surface model validation assuming idealized input data. He uses an analytical model of a torus instead of actual CT data to evaluate surfaces generated using several approaches. This work provides a first step towards the validation of surface models derived from clinically realistic CT data. The following list suggests a progression of experiments (in order of increasing complexity and realism) that could be performed to reach this goal:

1. Analytic model of a solid (cylinder, torus) — no CT data
2. CT images of physical objects that can be analytically modeled (cylinder, torus), constructed from bone analog
3. CT images of anatomical phantoms (femur, pelvis) made from bone analog
4. CT images of cadaver anatomy (femur, pelvis)

A fundamental issue in model validation is determining the "ground truth" to which the reconstructed model will be compared. Ground truth can either be determined by accurately sensing an existing object, or by accurately manufacturing an object based on an existing model. In Experiments 2 and 3, we can use either method for obtaining ground truth, whereas in Experiment 4 we must rely on accurate sensing.

An important measure of clinical realism in the above experiments is the ease with which an object of interest can be segmented from surrounding objects. In order to study this issue at early stages of experimentation, we are using CT soft tissue analogs. By surrounding an object with soft tissue analog during imaging, we complicate the segmentation process and make the resulting images closer to clinical reality. A second measure of experimental realism is the spatial density variation within an object. Density variations, like that in real bone, complicate segmentation by reducing the effectiveness of simple thresholding schemes. Cadaver studies allow us to study both of the above effects. In cadaver studies, bones would be imaged within the cadaver and then dissected out and used to build highly accurate ground truth models. We are currently investigating Experiment 2 and plan to progress to Experiments 3 and 4.

2.2 Physical Model Creation

The geometric modeling of biological surfaces is a fairly well understood process. This is not the case for the accurate *physical* modeling of complex biological systems such as the bone-implant systems in total joint replacements. Fundamental research is still needed to create computer models that realistically mimic the biomechanical properties of the bone-implant construct.

In contrast to bone, physical modeling of an implant is relatively straightforward since the material properties are well known and a geometric description can be obtained from CAD models. The situation is much more difficult for a biological material such as bone. To simulate the mechanical consequences of a total hip replacement surgery, the bone model must accurately represent the geometric complexity and spatial distribution of material properties of a patient's femur and pelvis. Furthermore, bone exhibits a complex constitutive law with significant anisotropy, viscoelasticity, and nonlinearity. Additional nonlinearity arises from the contact between the implant and bone, with the interface depending on numerous geometric, material, and loading parameters.

When developing biomechanical models, there are a variety of options which progressively add realism to the resulting physical models. The types of models we are currently investigating fall into one of the following four broad categories:

1. Idealized (e.g axisymmetric) geometry, and complex material properties — both based upon the literature.
2. Idealized geometry, and complex material properties — both derived directly from CT scan data.
3. Full 3D geometry based on CT data, but with idealized material properties.
4. Full 3D geometry, and complex material properties — both derived directly from CT scan data.

The categories range from least (1) to most (4) clinically realistic. There is a tradeoff between model complexity and the computational resources required to perform a simulation with a given model. The simplest model that accurately captures patient-specific mechanics is the best; however, more detailed models are still useful to help validate simplified approaches. As such, we are examining models that fall into all of the above categories.

Our initial approach was to develop simplified axisymmetric models to simulate the implantation of femoral and acetabular components (Category 1 above). These models incorporated idealized material properties with bi-linear elastic stress response and contact elements [10] [16]. While the bone geometries and material properties were not derived from CT data, these models incorporated many of the biomechanical complexities. Next, to help validate the results derived with the first set of models, full 3D irregular mesh FEM models were developed with geometry based upon CT scan data, but using material properties from the literature (Category 3 above).

Ideally, we wish to create realistic physical models directly from CT scans (Category 4). One option for such models is an irregular tetrahedral mesh that is grown directly from the CT data. Although potentially yielding a very realistic simulation, the disadvantage of this approach is the difficulty in growing and solving large irregular meshes. A second option is the use of a regular grid to represent the CT data, while embedding the unstructured implant model within the regular bone grid. Material properties can be based on the CT numbers using experimentally derived relations. The disadvantage of this approach is that it may yield a mesh that is too large unless the resolution is lowered. On the other hand, special fast algorithms that exploit the regular structure can be derived. Currently we are pursuing both the irregular and regular mesh options.

3 Simulations

Software systems exist that allow a surgeon to plan a surgery on the computer before entering the operating room. In orthopaedics, a clinical system now exists that can carry out a pre-operative plan precisely for the femoral part of total hip replacements [15]. In such systems, the surgeon can no longer rely on intra-operative feedback to determine the proper placement and fit of a press-fit implant. Instead, the surgeon must make these decisions by interacting with geometric implant models and the CT data to plan the surgery on a computer. By adding simulations of the mechanical consequences of a proposed surgery, it may be possible to compensate for the lack of intra-operative feedback in the current scenario.

We have simulated the press-fit insertion of cementless acetabular and femoral components for total hip replacements. Unlike previous efforts which have assumed an initial line-to-line fit between the implant and bone, our models and simulations have included contact coupling to simulate the actual implantation process [10] [16] . We argue that since the short term success of the implants depends strongly on the post-operative mechanical environment, this type of simulation provides valuable information in planning the surgery.

Currently, we are working towards simulations using more realistic models of the bone-implant system, as described above. These simulations will also incorporate contact coupling between bone and implant that occurs during the forceful insertion of the oversized implant into the bone cavity. The choice of model will dictate which solvers we ultimately use. For unstructured meshes we are developing preconditioned conjugate gradient methods. We are also developing fast multigrid methods that exploit the structure of the regular meshes.

A surgical simulation must be realistic, but must also run fast enough that the information is useful clinically. Currently our analyses require between several hours (simple models), to several weeks (full 3D models), using commercial code and low-end workstations. By incorporating the latest algorithms and using high-end workstations, we anticipate performing biomechanical simulations in near real-time.

Once realistic surgical simulations exist, work can progress on parametric studies of total joint replacement. Variables include the implant size and placement, and the shape of the bone cavity. The long-term goal of this work is not only to model the consequences of a surgery, but to create a system that can suggest optimal parameters to the surgeon.

4 Registration

Intra-surgical registration is the process of establishing a common reference frame between pre-surgical data and the corresponding patient anatomy. Once a common reference frame is established, pre-surgical data can be used to guide robotic tool movements [7], superimpose graphical overlays of internal anatomy upon a surgeon's view of the patient [4], position radiosurgical equipment [13], or guide a surgeon's tool movements [12]. Recent clinical approaches to intra-surgical registration assume a known correspondence between points in the two data sets being registered [15]. This is usually achieved by attaching *fiducials* to the underlying object, and extracting the locations of these markers in both data sets. Unfortunately, attachment of fiducials typically require an additional surgical procedure prior to the collection of pre-surgical data. Furthermore, these fiducials are invasive and cause added trauma to the patient in sites far from the primary surgical field.

An alternative to fiducial-based registration is to use surfaces that are intrinsic to the data itself. If data from the bounding surface of an object can be extracted pre- and intra-surgically, these data sets can be matched to perform registration. Several research groups have investigated such *surface-based* methods in medical registration [14][4][11][5]. A benefit of these techniques is that they do not require the use of costly and invasive external markers. Surface-based methods, however, place a heavy burden on sensing and modeling technology since accurate pre- and intra-surgical surface data are needed. This is a much more difficult sensing task than acquiring 3D fiducial locations as required by previous approaches.

As we demonstrated in [14], the accuracy resulting from surface-based registration depends highly on the underlying data. These data include the geometric surface models from pre-operative CT scans, as well as data collected intra-surgically using digitizing probes, ultrasound, fluoroscopes or CT. We are currently developing methods for planning the acquisition of potentially costly intra-surgical registration data using pre-operative geometric models as input. The goal of this work is to select data that will result in the best possible registration accuracy, while minimizing the quantity of data required.

5 Robotics

In total hip replacement surgery, the modeling, simulation, and registration components manifest themselves in the robotic milling of a bone cavity. The focus of our work is on the milling of the acetabulum (socket in the pelvis) to prepare for the implantation of a cementless acetabular component. We have developed a robotic testbed to demonstrate registration and cutting strategies. The testbed is not designed for clinical use, so issues of sterility, sensor redundancy, and clinical safety have not been addressed. Our system consists of a 5 DOF SCARA direct drive manipulator (Adept, San Jose, CA) with an attached 6 axis force-torque sensor (JR3 Inc, Woodland, CA) and pneumatic milling tool. The overall system configuration is conceptually similar to that used by Taylor [15].

A pre-operative plan is defined using our custom planner and models of the implants. There are three reference frames of interest: (1) the CT reference frame (where the pre-operative plan is defined), (2) the intra-operative sensor reference frame (where bone surface data are defined), and (3) the robot reference frame (where the actual robot paths are defined). Intra-operative surface data and a surface model from the CT data are used to determine the transformation between sensor and CT reference frames (as described in Section 4). The transformation between the sensor and the robot frames is derived by repeatedly moving the robot and sensor to the same point in space, recording the locations, and then calculating an average transformation matrix.

The above process yields the pose of the bone and a cutting plan in the robot's coordinates. Shapes in the bone can be milled by first making broad cuts to remove large amounts of material in a short time, and then returning to finish the cavity with finer passes. We have demonstrated (on pelvis bone phantoms) milling of hemispherical cavities that match the shape of the implants, but are undersized to allow varying amounts of press-fit. These shapes are high precision versions of the cavities created with standard hand-held tools, but arbitrary shapes could be generated should the biomechanics simulations predict that a non-hemispherical cavity is preferable.

Current work centers on milling less-rigidly fixed bones. With high speed tracking it may be possible to do away with rigid fixation and allow some small (millimeters) motion of the bone. The robotic system would compensate for this motion. The accuracy and bandwidth requirements of such a system are strenuous, and much work is needed to evaluate the clinical efficacy of the concept.

6 Conclusion

The value of surgical robots is greatly enhanced by realistic surgical simulations, less invasive registration methods, and accurate modeling. Surgical simulations will enhance the surgeon's ability to investigate the implications of pre-operative plans. Surface-based registration will eliminate invasive and costly fiducials which limit the clinical application of orthopaedic robotics. Accurate modeling is a prerequisite for realistic simulations and precise intra-operative registration. Each of these components are worthy research efforts on their own; together, they form a framework for advancing the clinical utility of medical robotics.

References

1. H.N. Christiansen and T.W. Sederberg. Conversion of complex contour line definitions into polygonal element mosaics. *Computer Graphics*, 8:658–660, August 1978.

2. B. Geiger. *Three-dimensional modeling of human organs and its application to diagnosis and surgical planning*. PhD thesis, Ecole des Mines de Paris, April 1993.

3. E.J. Graves. 1992 summary: National hospital discharge survey. In *Advance Data from Vital Health and Statistics*, page 45. National Center for Health Statistics, 1992.

4. E Grimson, T. Lozano-Perez, W. Wells, G. Ettinger, S. White, and R. Kikinis. Automated registration for enhanced reality visualization in surgery. In *AAAI 1994 Spring Symposium Series, Applications of Computer Vision in Medical Image Processing*, pages 26–29. AAAI, March 1994.

5. H. Jiang, R.A. Robb, and K.S. Holton. A new approach to 3-d registration of multimodality medical images by surface matching. In *Visualization in Biomedical Computing - SPIE Vol 1808*, pages 196–213. SPIE, 1992.

6. A.D. Kalvin. A survey of algorithms for constructing surfaces from 3D volume data. IBM Reseach Report RC 17600, IBM, January 1992.

7. J.T. Lea, D. Watkins, A. Mills, M.A. Preshkin, T.C. Kienzle, and S.D Stulberg. Registration and immobilization for robot-assisted orthopaedic surgery. In *Proceedings of the First International Symposium on Medical Robotics and Computer Assisted Surgery*, pages 63–68, Pittsburgh, PA, September 1994.

8. W.E. Lorensen and H.E. Cline. Marching cubes: A high resolution 3D surface construction algorithm. *Computer Graphics*, 21:163–169, July 1987.

9. V.C. Mow and W.C. Hayes. *Basic Orthopaedic Biomechanics*. Raven Press, 1991.

10. R.V. O'Toole, B. Jaramaz, A.M. DiGioia, C.D. Visnic, and R.H. Reid. Biomechanics for pre-operative planning and surgical simulation in orthopaedics. *Computers in Biology and Medicine*, 1994.

11. O. Peria, A. Francois-Joubert, S. Lavallee, G. Champleboux, P. Cinquin, and S. Grand. Accurate registration of SPECT and MR brain images of patients suffering from epilepsy or tumor. In *Proceedings of the First International Symposium on Medical Robotics and Computer Assisted Surgery*, pages 58–62, Pittsburgh, PA, September 1994.

12. K. Radermacher, H.W. Staudte, and G. Rau. Computer assisted orthopedic surgery by means of individual templates - aspects and analysis of potential applications. In *Proceedings of the First International Symposium on Medical Robotics and Computer Assisted Surgery*, pages 42–48, Pittsburgh, PA, September 1994.

13. A. Schweikard, R. Tombropoulos, J.R. Adler, and J. Latombe. Planning for image-guided radiosurgery. In *AAAI 1994 Spring Symposium Series, Applications of Computer Vision in Medical Image Processing*, pages 96–101. AAAI, March 1994.

14. D.A. Simon, M. Hebert, and T. Kanade. Techniques for fast and accurate intrasurgical registration. In *Proceedings of the First International Symposium on Medical Robotics and Computer Assisted Surgery*, pages 90–97, Pittsburgh, PA, September 1994.

15. R.H. Taylor, B.D. Mittelstadt, H.A. Paul, W. Hanson, P. Kazanzides, J.F. Zuhars, B Williamson, B.L. Musits, E. Glassman, and W.L. Bargar. An image-directed robotic system for precise orthopaedic surgery. *IEEE Transactions on Robotics and Automation*, 10(3):261–275, June 1994.

16. C.D. Visnic, R.H. Reid, A.M. DiGioia, B. Jaramaz, and O. Ghattas. Finite element pre-operative simulation of cementless hip replacement. In *Proceedings of the 1994 Winter Simulation Conference*, 1994.

Treatment Planning for Image-Guided Robotic Radiosurgery

Rhea Tombropoulos[1,2], Achim Schweikard[2,3], Jean-Claude Latombe[2], and John R. Adler[3]

[1] Section on Medical Informatics
[2] Department of Computer Science Robotics Laboratory
[3] Department of Neurosurgery
Stanford University, Stanford CA 94305, USA, rhea@flamingo.stanford.edu

Abstract. Radiosurgery is a non-invasive procedure that uses focused beams of radiation to destroy brain tumors. Treatment planning for radiosurgery involves determining a series of beam configurations that will destroy the tumor without damaging healthy tissue in the brain, particularly critical structures. A new image-guided robotic radiosurgical system has been developed at Stanford University in a joint project with Accuray, Inc. It has been in clinical use at Stanford since July, 1994, and thus far three patients have been treated with it. This system provides much more flexibility for treatment planning than do traditional radiosurgical systems. In order to take full advantage of this added flexibility, we have developed automatic methods for treatment planning. Our planner enables a surgeon to specify constraints interactively on the distribution of dose delivered and then to find a set of beam configurations that will satisfy these constraints. We provide a detailed description of our treatment planning algorithms and summarize our first experiences using the system in a clinical setting.

1 Introduction

In radiosurgery, a moving beam of radiation is used as an ablative surgical instrument to destroy brain tumors [2, 3]. The goal of radiosurgery is to deliver a necrotic dose of radiation to the tumor while minimizing the amount of radiation to healthy brain tissues, particularly critical or dose-sensitive tissues (such as the brain stem or optic nerves). This goal is usually accomplished by *crossfiring* at the tumor: rather than aiming one powerful beam of radiation directly at the tumor, which would destroy not only the tumor but everything on its path, several weaker beams are aimed from different directions. Though none of these weaker beams can destroy tissue by itself, the sum of the radiation in the regions where they intersect is severely lethal to tissues.

Treatment planning involves determining a series of beam configurations (position and orientation) such that the beams will intersect to form a region of high dose at the tumor. The dose distribution produced by the beams should match the shape of the tumor, with the entire tumor region receiving at least 80% of the maximum dose delivered to any one location. The fall-off of the dose around the tumor should be rapid, to minimize radiation to healthy tissues, and there should be little or no dose within the critical structures.

Recently, a new system capable of image-guided robotic radiosurgery was developed at Stanford University Medical Center in a joint project with Accuray, Inc. This system was developed to overcome many of the limitations of conventional radiosurgery [1, 7]. It uses a six-degree-of-freedom GMF robotic manipulator arm to position the radiation source and a real-time imaging system to monitor the patient's motion continuously. The system has been described previously [1]. In [7] we propose a new method for treatment planning that takes advantage of the flexibility offered by this new system and enables us to create irregularly shaped dose distributions that closely match the tumor shape.

We have continued to refine the treatment planning methods described in [7]. Our new planner gives the surgeon more power to define the final dose distribution: it allows the surgeon to specify particular regions of interest, such as the tumor and critical structures, and to specify the range of dose that each of these structures can receive. Our system uses linear programming to optimize the plans and satisfy the constraints specified by the surgeon whenever feasible. A fully integrated version of the system is now installed at Stanford University Medical Center and has been in use since July 1994. Three patients have been treated to date. This paper describes our treatment planning methods and our first experiences using the system in a clinical setting.

2 Treatment Planning

The treatment planning process is divided into several steps. First, the surgeon specifies regions of interest (e.g., the tumor and critical structures) and imposes constraints on the amount of radiation that these regions should receive. The system then uses this data to construct a three-dimensional representation of the necessary geometry and to select beams that will best approximate the tumor shape. Next, linear programming is used to refine plan in terms of the amount of radiation sent along each beam and the width of each beam such that the dose distribution produced will meet the specifications of the surgeon. Finally, the dose distribution is calculated by the system and evaluated by the surgeon. If the distribution is satisfactory, treatment is delivered. Otherwise, the planning system can backtrack to several different points in the process in order to improve the plan.

2.1 User Specifications and Geometry Reconstruction

The physician first views successive CT scans of the patient's brain. The tumor and any dose-sensitive critical regions are outlined on the images. Once the physician has outlined all of the regions of interest on the CTs, the system makes a three-dimensional reconstruction of the geometry. The surgeon then sets upper and lower bounds for these regions. For example, he might specify that the tumor must get a minimum 2000 rads but no more than 2200 rads, and that the brain stem should receive a maximum of 500 rads. These constraints are crucial in defining the distribution of the dose that will result, as they are later used to optimize the plan. For example, the narrower the range of possible values for the total dose in the tumor tissues, the more homogeneous the dose will be in that region.

2.2 Beam Selection

The beam selector must find a series of *beam configurations* such that the beams will intersect to form a region of high dose that closely matches the shape of the tumor. The configurations must be chosen and ordered in such a way that the robot can move from one to the next without colliding with objects in the workspace or obstructing the view of the imaging system. By beam configuration, we refer to the position and orientation of the radiation source producing the beam. Our system uses two points to define each beam configuration: the *source point*, where the beam originates, and the *target point*, at which the beam will be aimed. The source point corresponds to the position of the radiation source and, together with the target point, defines the orientation of the beam at that position. Our beam selector first finds a set of target points and then matches these with appropriate source points on a presynthesized path that the robot can traverse. The beam selector generates several hundred beams. However, not all of these beams will ultimately be used; during the plan-refinement step, non-useful beams are removed from the path.

Target Point Selection We have experimented with several different methods for selecting target points [1]. The method that has produced the best results involves selecting target points that are evenly spaced on the surface of the tumor. To approximate the tumor surface, we use the three-dimensional reconstruction generated from the surgeon's description of the tumor. Target points are evenly spaced on this polygonal surface using Turk's algorithm [8]: first points are randomly placed on the surface of the tumor; each point repels the other points with a force proportional to its distance from them; the points thus cause each other to spread apart; and, after a certain number of iterations, they stabilize at locations that are roughly equidistant from each other.

Source Point Selection Each target point must then be associated with a source point in order to define a beam configuration. Source points are selected from a presynthesized, well-tested template path. The path is comprised of several hundred points, or *nodes*. For each node, we precompute the range of possible joint angles for the robot. We select source points from the nodes in the following manner. For each target point, we define a beam passing through it at a random orientation. We then associate that beam with the nearest node in the presynthesized path, making sure the association is possible given joint constraints of the robot. That node becomes the source point for the given target point. We have experimented with more deterministic methods for orienting the beams at the target points [1] but have found that using random orientations leads to a more homogeneous dose distribution within the tumor.

Path Generation The final step in the beam selection process is to connect all of the beam configurations into a path that is feasible for the robot to traverse without colliding with objects in the workspace or obstructing the view of the imaging system. For safety reasons, however, we do no optimization in connecting the beam configurations. Instead, we simply use the template path used to determine the source points. The robot arm will move through each node in the path when executing the treatment, but will only stop and deliver radiation at the nodes where treatment beams have been defined.

2.3 Plan Refinement

The beam configurations are chosen by the beam selector such that they will intersect to form a region of high dose in the tumor. After beam selection, shape-matching is quite good: the 80% isodose surface produced by the selected beams closely matches the shape of the tumor. However, beam selection does not guarantee that all of the constraints specified by the surgeon will be satisfied: the beam selector does not consider the location of the critical tissues, nor does it guarantee a highly homogenous distribution of the dose within the tumor.

To satisfy these constraints, we refine the plan, using *linear programming* to adjust the weights and diameters of the individual beams once they have been selected. Linear programming is a mathematical technique for solving a set of linear equalities and inequalities subject to a linear objective function. It has been successfully applied to different aspects of the treatment planning problem in radiotherapy [4, 6]. We transform the constraints specified by the surgeon into linear inequalities involving beam weights. The inequalities are input into MINOS [5], a large-scale optimization program developed at Stanford University. If it is mathematically feasible, MINOS returns optimal weights for the beams such that all of the surgeon's constraints are satisfied. The weights are used to determine how much radiation to send along each beam and also what the optimal width for each beam is. This process is described below.

Beam Weighting We define our constraints in the following manner. In order to determine the weight of each beam, we divide the regions of interest into *cells* based on the arrangement of the beams inside them.

Cells are defined by the pattern of intersection of the beams in the regions of interest. Constraints are imposed on each cell such that the sum of the weights of the beams passing through each cell must be in the range specified by the surgeon for that region of interest. For example, a cell in the tumor intersected by beams 1, 3, and 4 would give rise to the following constraint:

$$TumorMin \leq w1 + w3 + w4 \leq TumorMax$$

where $TumorMin$ is the minimum amount of radiation the tumor should receive, $TumorMax$ is the maximum amount of radiation, and $w1 - w4$ are the weights of beams 1-4 respectively. For cells in the critical regions, constraints are usually one-sided, as there is no minimum. For example, the constraint introduced by a critical cell intersected by beams 2 and 3, is

$$w2 + w3 \leq CriticalMax$$

where $CriticalMax$ is the maximum amount of radiation that can be tolerated by this particular critical structure. It is important to note that all beam weights are constrained to be positive by the system, so negative beam weights (which are physically impossible) are never assigned.

Beams assigned zero weights are discarded. Because the linear programming assigns on average a weight of zero to 60% of the beams, this method provides an effective way of pruning our initial beam selection and identifying beams that are important for obtaining the desired dose distribution. By pruning the number of necessary treatment beams, we are able to decrease the time needed to deliver the radiation.

Collimator Selection We can augment this method to determine optimal diameters for each beam. As stated previously, the diameter of the beam depends on the collimator used. We can create beams with diameters ranging from 5 mm to 60 mm, along 2.5 mm increments. For any given treatment, however, we realistically cannot use more than four different beam diameters, as the collimator must be manually set in place. Hence, our goal is to find a maximum of four optimum collimator sizes to use for a given treatment plan.

Consider case where we must pick the optimal diameter for a beam from three possibilities: narrow, medium, and wide. Instead of representing the beam as a cylinder of fixed diameter, we represent it as a set of concentric cylinders. The innermost cylinder represents the smallest diameter, and each surrounding cylindrical tube corresponds to a wider diameter. Again, we analyze the arrangements of the cylinders in the regions of interest and form constraints based on these. We create additional constraints such that outer cylinders must receive weights that are less than or equal to those assigned to their respective inner cylinders.

Let ww correspond to the weight for the widest beam diameter, wm for the medium width, and wn for the narrowest. We have the constraint $ww \leq wm \leq wn$. If the linear program outputs that ww, wm, and wn are all equal, we use the widest diameter for that beam. If wn and wm are equal, but ww is substantially smaller, then we choose the medium width diameter. And if wn is substantially larger than both wm and ww, we choose the narrow diameter.

2.4 Dosimetry Calculations and Plan Evaluation

The dose distribution for a given set of beam configurations and weights is calculated and evaluated by the surgeon. The surgeon is presented with several different methods for visualizing this dose, including three-dimensional isodose surfaces, dose-volume histograms, color washes of the dose on the CT scans, and planar cross-sectional slices through the dose volume. If the surgeon is satisfied with the resulting dose distribution, treatment is delivered. If he is not satisfied, then planning can be restarted at several different points in the process. The surgeon can delineate new regions or alter constraints to specify a distribution that will be more satisfactory. Furthermore a new series of beam configurations can be generated.

One method of evaluating plans produced by our new planner is to compare them with the actual treatment plans used with the LINAC-System. Figure 1 shows such a comparison using dose-volume histograms. The black lines correspond to our new plans and the gray lines correspond to the old plans. In terms of both delivering a homogeneous dose to the tumor (Figure 1a) and minimizing the dose to the healthy tissues (Figure 1b), the planner for our new system performed much better.

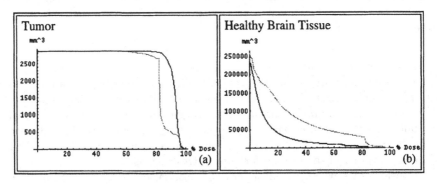

Fig. 1. Comparison of Dose-Volume Histograms

3 Clinical Use

Three patients have been treated with the system at Stanford Medical Center. In all cases, the tumor was reduced or was stabilized. Simple arc-shaped paths were used in planning for all of these cases so as to simulate treatments done with the LINAC-System and facilitate comparisons between the two. We hope to soon be able to use more complex paths in our planning system and make full use of its capabilities. All planning for these cases was done prior to the day of treatment. The robot was tested with each of the proposed paths before using it on the patient.

Treatment time for these first few cases averaged approximately 45 minutes. We expect this time to decrease as more patients are treated and we become more familiar with using the system. Even now, it is comparable to the duration of treatment with the LINAC-System, which usually takes between 30 and 45 minutes. Furthermore with this new system, the patient was able to walk into the clinic in the morning, receive treatment, and leave approximately 1 hour later. Fractionation of radiosurgical treatments will clearly be possible with this system.

4 Conclusion

A new system for frameless, robotic radiosurgery has been developed. This system is installed at Stanford University Medical Center and has been used to treat three patients. This system overcomes many of the limitations of traditional stereotaxic radiosurgery. By eliminating the need for a frame, it not only provides increased patient comfort, but also the ability to fractionate treatments and to treat extra-cranial tumors. By using a six-degree-of-freedom robotic arm to position the source of radiation, the system enables us to deliver highly accurate treatments and to create irregularly shaped dose distributions that conform closely to the shape of the tumor. In order to be able to fully utilize the advantages offered by this new system, we have implemented an automatic planner. This planner allows the surgeon to set constraints on the dose distribution produced and to find a set of beam configurations that will produce a dose distribution that satisfies these constraints. We hope the new features and abilities of our system will lead to new directions for this field and cures for previously untreatable tumors.

References

1. Adler, J. R., Schweikard, A., Tombropoulos, R., and Latombe, J. C., Image-Guided Robotic Radiosurgery. *Proc. First International Symposium on Medical Robotics and Computer Assisted Surgery*, 2:291-297, 1994.
2. Betty, O. O., Munari, C., and Rosler, R. Stereotactic Radiosurgery with the Linear Accelerator: Treatment of Arteriovenous Malformations. *Neurosurgery*, 24(3):311-321, 1989.
3. Larsson, B. et. al. The High Energy Proton Beam as a Neurosurgical Tool. *Nature*, 182:1222-1223, 1958.
4. Morrill, S. M., Lane R. G., Wong, J. A., and Rosen, I. I., Dose-Volume Considerations with Linear Programming Optimization. *Medical Physics*, 18(6):1201-1210, 1991.
5. Murtagh, B. A. and Saunders, M. A., *MINOS 5.4 User's Guide*, Technical Report SOL 83-20R, Dept. of Operations Research, Stanford University, March, 1993.
6. Rosen, Issac I., Lane, Richard G., Morrill, Steven M., and Belli, James A., Treatment Plan Optimization Using Linear Programming. *Medical Physics*, 18(2):141-152, 1991.
7. Schweikard, A., Tombropoulos, R., Kavraki, L., Adler, J. R., and Latombe, J. C., Treatment Planning for a Radiosurgical System with General Kinematics. *Proc. IEEE Int. Conf. Robotics and Automation*, 1720-1727, 1994.
8. Turk, G., Re-Tiling Polygonal Surfaces, *Computer Graphics*, 26(3):55-64, 1992.

Robotic Radiosurgery with Beams of Adaptable Shapes

Achim Schweikard[1,2], Rhea Tombropoulos[1], John R. Adler[2]

[1] Robotics Laboratory, Department of Computer Science
[2] Department of Neurosurgery
Stanford University, Stanford, CA 94305, USA, as@cs.stanford.edu

Abstract: *In radiosurgery, a moving beam of radiation acts as an ablative surgical instrument. Conventional systems for radiosurgery use a cylindrical radiation beam of fixed cross-section. The radiation source can only be moved along simple standardized paths. A new radiosurgical system based on a six degree-of-freedom robotic arm has been developed to overcome limitations of conventional systems. We address the following question: Can dose distributions generated by robotic radiosurgery be improved by using non-cylindrical radiation beams of adaptable cross-section? Geometric methods for planning the shape of the beam in addition to planning beam motion are developed. Design criteria considered in this context are: treatment time, radiation penumbra as well as transparency of interactive treatment planning. An experimental evaluation compares distributions generated with our new radiosurgical system using cylindrical beams to distributions generated with beams of adaptable shapes.*

1 Introduction

In radiosurgery, a radiation beam generated by a moving linear accelerator is used to destroy brain tumors. By combining cross-firing from multiple directions with precision targeting, the radiation beam acts as an ablative surgical instrument.

A *collimator*, typically made of heavy metal is used for focusing and shaping the radiation beam. Conventional radiosurgical systems use static collimators producing cylindrical beams [5, 6, 8]. Cylindrical beams yield adequate distributions for spherical tumors. Our previous research has demonstrated that non-spherical dose distributions can be produced by moving a cylinder beam along appropriate paths. However, collimators of non-cylindrical shape are most natural for producing non-spherical dose distributions. In addition to a substantial improvement in distribution characteristics, non-cylindrical collimators allow for reduction of treatment time. The goal of this research is the design of a collimator and corresponding planning methods suiting the requirements of robotic radiosurgery. Two types of mechanical collimator designs can be used to produce beams of adaptable shapes:

- multi-leaf collimator (fig. 1-a)
- jaw collimator (fig. 1-b)

A jaw collimator produces a beam of rectangular cross-section. Fig. 1-c shows how non-rectangular beams with given planar cross-section can be pro-

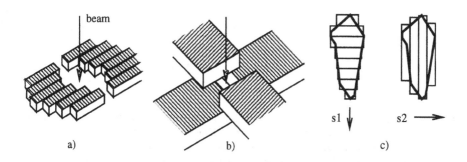

Fig. 1. a) Multi-leaf collimator: rectangular fingers can be moved under computer control. b) Jaw collimator. Jaws can be moved under computer control. Beam cross-section is rectangular. c) To produce a beam of given polygonal cross-section with a jaw collimator, the polygon is covered by a series of parallel rectangles. $s1$, $s2$ are called sweeping directions. Radiation time/number of rectangles depends on sweeping direction.

duced with a jaw collimator: A series of rectangular beams with varying size is overlaid.

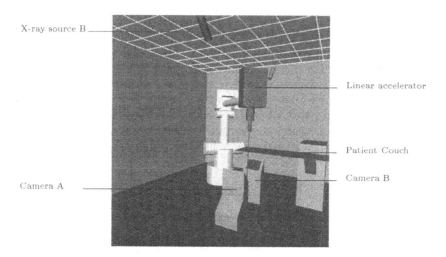

Fig. 2. N-1000 radiosurgical system; robot workspace

1.1 Previous Work

In an interdisciplinary project between the Departments of Neurosurgery and the Department of Computer Science at Stanford University, geometric treatment planning methods for conventional systems were developed [9]. This project led to the design of treatment procedures for image-guided radiosurgery with the

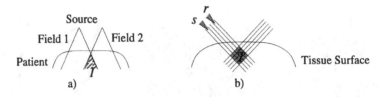

Fig. 3. a)Aligning two separate large radiation fields results in undesirable dose inhomogeneity; the intersection region I will receive high dose, since the radiation source is a point. b)To achieve homogeneity within region T, weight of beam r should be smaller than weight of s, since dose is reduced with depth in tissue.

Neurotron-1000 system in cooperation with Accuray, Inc., Santa Clara [10]. The Neurotron-1000 (N-1000) is a new radiosurgical system with the following features (fig. 2).

- The mechanical gantry is a GM-Fanuc robotic arm with 6 degrees of freedom, which allows for arbitrary spatial paths of the radiation beam. In contrast, conventional systems can only perform simple standardized motions.

- An on-line vision system (with two orthogonal X-ray cameras) determines the position of the patient's skull once a second. In this way, patient motion can be tracked.

- A treatment planning system (*inverse dosimetry*) computes beam paths for generating a dose distribution satisfying specifications input by the surgeon (homogeneous and focussed dose in the tumor, reduced doses in healthy tissues).

The on-line vision system removes the need for the painful stereotaxic frame. Consequently the vision system allows for fractionated treatment. To date, three patients have been treated with a prototype of the N-1000 system at Stanford University Medical Center. Given the flexibility of the new system, it is expected that radiosurgical procedures will replace conventional radiation methods as well as conventional surgery in many instances.

1.2 Related Research

Nedzi, Kooy et al. [7] investigate characteristics of so-called single beam field-shaping paradigms. In particular, their analysis and simulations suggest that an ideal multi-leaf collimator has significant advantages over collimation methods currently in clinical use. They also give design recommendations for an actual implementation of collimators suitable for radiosurgery. Carol [1] describes an implementation of a multi-leaf collimator for a conventional radiosurgical system. The methods in [1, 7] use a single beam for each planar field. In contrast, the approach illustrated in fig. 1-c uses a series of beams for each (planar) field. This paradigm has two advantages over single-beam field shaping, including ideal multi-leaf collimation.

• General beam shapes can be produced. In particular, the beam cross-section does not have to be monotonic. The example in fig. 3-a shows that it is generally not practical to cover fields by aligning two or more large subfields.

• The hardware required for a jaw collimator is comparatively simple and inexpensive. This reduces the cost of required safety features.

• The radiation penumbra can be controlled by using rectangles of varying widths.

• The beams for individual rectangular fields can be *weighted,* i.e. predetermined dose can be assigned to each rectangle. In this way, we can take into account the decrease of dose with depth in tissue (fig. 3-b). In addition, a very simple geometric method for generating non-convex regions of high dose is obtained. The derived algorithms are resolution-complete, i.e. at an appropriate resolution, it can be guaranteed that beam weights generating a distribution specified by the user will be found, if such a distribution can exist. In this way we can avoid problems arising with standard optimization techniques.

Experiments suggest that multiple-beam methods allow for improved dose distributions when compared to conventional collimation methods. However, the use of adaptable collimators must be supported by computer-based planning methods. The planning methods described below are based on an analysis of trade-offs between total radiation time and penumbra, methods for appropriate partitoning of planar fields as well as geometric algorithms for beam weighting.

2 Planning paradigms

We consider a jaw collimator (fig. 1-b). Two pairs of jaws, orthogonal to each other, produce a rectangular beam. The length and width of the (rectangular) beam cross-section can be changed during treatment. Instead of aligning rectangles as in fig. 1-c, we *overlay* a larger number of (parallel) rectangles with small displacement. The direction of displacement is called *sweeping direction.* This avoids problems stemming from alignment inaccuracy and yields higher dose homogeneity. Note that the collimator jaws never move during beam activation. Collimator motion during activation would require additional safety features and accurate velocity control. Our experiments for the N-1000 system show that sufficient homogeneity can be achieved with a small number of rectangles if many beam directions are used.

Fig. 4 illustrates improvements in beam characteristics achievable by combining the kinematic flexibility of a six degree-of-freedom robotic arm with adaptable collimation. Given full kinematic flexibility, the beam can translate along any given direction. Thus the motion along the sweeping direction can be performed by the radiation source (fig. 4-b). Both penumbra and conicity angle can be reduced.

2.1 Reduction of Radiation Time

The output dose rate of commercial linear accelerators is limited. The time required to deliver a fixed dose to every point within a planar field does not

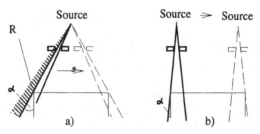

Fig. 4. a) sweeping motion (in direction s) is performed by collimator jaws; b) sweeping motion is performed by radiation source. Beam conicity angle α is reduced in case b). In addition, the size of the penumbral region R can be reduced in case b).

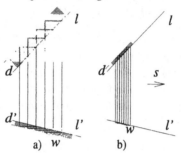

Fig. 5. Radiation penumbra is influenced by slope of polygon edges as well as rectangle width; a) Field edges l, l', widths d, d' of penumbral region, rectangle width w. Slope of edge l with respect to sweeping direction s is higher than slope of edge l'. Therefore penumbral region at edge l is wider than at edge l'. b) Reducing rectangle width w reduces width d of penumbral region.

increase with the field size. Thus, irradiating a given planar field with a series of 50 "pencil beams" of small cross-section instead of one single beam will lead to a (well over) 50-fold increase in required radiation time. Consider the example in fig. 1-c. The number of rectangles needed to cover the given polygon (at a fixed density) depends on the sweeping direction s. Direction $s2$ in fig. 1-c requires less rectangles than direction $s1$.

Large penumbra in the tissue surrounding a tumor is undesirable, and should be reduced as much as possible. Fig. 5 illustrates the trade-offs between total radiation time and penumbra. Increasing the (rectangle) width of each beam will lead to shorter radiation time but increased penumbra.

Our planning method proceeds as follows. A polyhedral reconstruction of the tumor shape is computed from the input data. This reconstruction is projected onto a series of planes through the origin. The normal vectors of these planes are chosen from a large regular grid of points on the 3D unit sphere. In each projection, we obtain a polygonal *field*.

Consider a sweeping direction s in the plane. Assume s is the horizontal direction. We divide the given polygonal field into a series of trapezoidal slabs, obtained by drawing vertical partitioning lines through all polygon vertices. Note that the decomposition into trapezoids changes as the sweeping direction s varies.

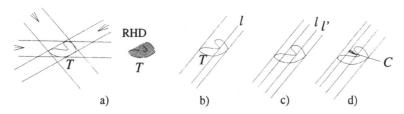

Fig. 6. a)If T is irradiated from multiple directions, such that each field is covered homogeneously, then the region of high dose is convex, and may cover a critical region surrounded by the tumor. b)-d) Partitioning fields; b) Convex-Hull subtraction. Lines passing through $Conv(T) \setminus T$ are separated from remaining lines. c) Monotonic subregions. Lines crossing boundary of T more than twice are separated from other lines. d) Partitoning induced by user defined critical regions.

For the fixed direction s, the penumbra along the upper and lower edge of a single slab is proportional to the rectangle width w.

For each (planar) field, the planning system computes a sweeping direction and a set of rectangle widths for each slab, such that the field is covered with the minimum number of rectangles. Values for the required homogeneity (density of rectangles) as well as maximum allowable (planar) penumbra are entered by the user. The rectangle width of the output path can change between trapezoids, but not within one trapezoid. The functional dependency of edge slope and penumbra is approximated by a series of linear equations with values taken from measurements.

Our current implementation computes the sweeping direction by discretizing, i.e. by considering a series of fixed orientations, and computing the number of polygons required at each such orientation. In this way, we obtain a path minimizing total radiation time, given user-defined homogeneity and penumbra values.

2.2 Non-convex Fields

By region of high dose (RHD) we denote the region (in 3-D space) receiving 80% or more of the maximum dose. As described above, we irradiate a tumor from a set of directions, given as a grid of vectors on the unit sphere. For each direction d the projection of the tumor along d is a (planar) polygon.

For many larger extra-cranial lesions, the tumor is non-convex, and there are critical healthy regions surrounded by the tumor. Such regions should not be part of the RHD, but will be covered by the RHD if we irradiate all fields homogeneously (fig. 6-a). This is undesirable in many cases. An example are tumors of the spine, growing around the spinal cord.

In addition, some of the directions thus chosen may pass through critical healthy structures. Such directions should receive lower *dose weight*.

To address the two problems mentioned, we compute distinct weights for the rectangular beams to be overlaid. Planar fields are partitioned into subregions. Each subregion can then be irradiated with an individual weight. There are several possibilities for partitioning fields. Fig. 6-b,c shows two examples. In case b), a field partitioning is obtained by considering the convex hull of T. T is subtracted from its convex hull, i.e. we set $S = Conv(T) \setminus T$. Beams (lines) passing through S are separated from the remaining beams (lines). The partitioning of each planar field induced by this separation can be computed automatically, and a distinct weight can be assigned to each sub-field thus obtained.

Case c) shows a different way to obtain a field partitioning. We call a line *monotonic* with respect to T if it crosses the boundary of T at most twice. Thus, in fig. 6-c, lines above l and lines below l' are monotonic with respect to T. Lines between l and l' are non-monotonic. To obtain a field partitioning using monotonicity we can separate monotonic beams (beams crossing the tumor boundary at most twice) from non-monotonic beams. The example shows that methods a) and b) will yield distinct partitionings in general. We thus do not fully automatize field partitioning. Instead, we use a semi-manual method (fig. 6-d). This method allows for improved user-control. The user delineates a structure C on the tomographic images. Given this (two-dimensional) delineation, we compute a three-dimensional reconstruction of C by thickening between tomographic cross-planes. Each field is then split into two sets; lines passing through C are separated from the remaining lines. After this, we compute the *arrangement* of beams thus obtained and apply the weighting method in [10] to assign weights to each (rectangular) beam. The user can change the delineation of C interactively to obtain distinct partitionings.

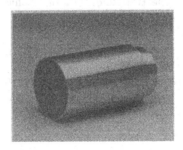

Fig. 7. Collimator for N-1000 system; conic beam with rectangular cross-section.

3 Experiments

The described methods were implemented in the context of the Neurotron-1000 system. While the characteristics of larger rectangular beams are comparatively well-known, it is difficult of provide adequate simulations for small rectangular fields. To verify characteristics of very small rectangular beams with the N-1000 system, a collimator with static rectangular cross-section (5 mm by 15 mm cross-section at target) was manufactured (fig. 7).

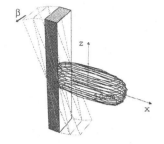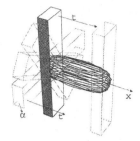

Fig. 8. Three-parameter sweep motion used for generating ellipsoidal high dose region with a static rectangular collimator. Beam is swept along translational direction t. This sweep is combined with rotational sweeps (parameters α, β).

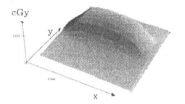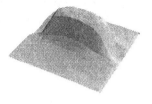

Fig. 9. 2-dimensional dose profile for ellipsoidal high dose region. a) Cylinder beam b) Rectangular beam. Height above x-y-plane represents dose. Much sharper focus of dose within ellipsoidal region is achievable with rectangular beam than with cylindrical beam.

3.1 Ellipsoidal Isodose Surfaces

A first series of experiments considers methods for generating non-spherical regions of high dose. An ellipsoidal shape is a very simple non-spherical shape. Figs. 9-12 compare two distributions with an ellipsoidal RHD. The first distribution was generated with a cylindrical collimator. The second distribution corresponds to a *static* rectangular collimator. The same motion was used in both cases. This motion is shown in fig. 8.

To evaluate the homogeneity of a distribution, one could consider the difference between maximum and minimum dose in the tumor region. However, this measure does not take into account the respective volumes of so-called hot spots and cold spots. A *dose-volume histogram* provides a more adequate way to evaluate homogeneity: for each percentage value x, the volume of tissue receiving $\geq x$ percent of dose is computed. The dose-volume histogram (DVH) shows the volume (ordinate values) absorbing dose $\geq x$ as a function of x (abscissa values). A DVH can equally be used to evaluate the distribution outside the tumor. An evaluation of the distributions for cylindrical/static rectangular collimators based on dose-volume histograms for lesion and surrounding tissue is shown in fig. 9-12. For each DVH, we compute the integral of the DVH-function and normalize to unit volume. The RHD is substantially more homogeneous for the rectangular collimator. In addition, the dose in the surrounding healthy tissue is lower for the rectangular collimator.

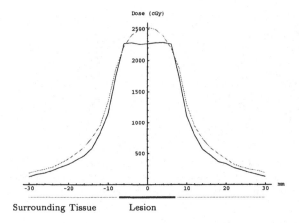

Surrounding Tissue   Lesion

Fig. 10. 1-dimensional cross-sections of dose profiles (ellipsoidal high dose region). Gray curve: cylinder beam; black curve: static rectangular beam.

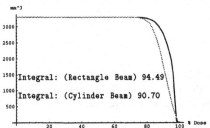

Fig. 11. Dose-volume histograms (lesion), ellipsoidal RHD. Black curve: rectangular beam; gray curve: cylinder beam.

3.2   Sample Case

Fig. 13-a shows a sample case with an arterio-vascular malformation (AVM). The malformation is delineated in the figures. The distribution generated with the described methods for a jaw collimator is shown in figs. 13-b through 15.

The dose distribution generated by a cylinder collimator (in the same case) using the planning methods in [10] was computed for comparison. Fig. 14 shows the dose-volume histograms for jaw and cylinder collimators respectively. In both cases, integrals were computed and normalized to unit volume. Substantially higher dose homogeneity is obtained for the adapatable collimator.

3.3   Non-convex shapes

The field partioning methods described in the previous section were evaluated in connection with manual and automatic beam weighting methods. Fig. 16 shows an example. The input to the planning system are the coordinates of cross-sections for the u-shaped region R (fig. 16-a). To generate a region of high dose matching this shape, a series of 600 rectangles in 40 planar projections were

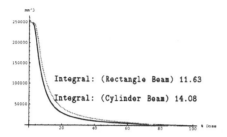

Fig. 12. Dose-volume histograms for ellipsoidal RHD (tissue surrounding lesion).

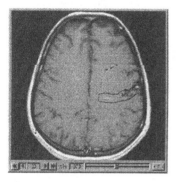 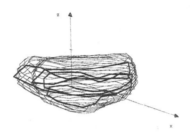

Fig. 13. a) Anatomy for sample case; arterio-vascular malformation (AVM) delineated. b) 80% isodose surface for distribution generated with adaptable jaw collimator (thin lines). Surface overlaid upon delineation of malformation. Bold lines: delineation of malformation in tomographic cross-planes.

overlaid. A constant rectangle width of 12 mm was used. The length of rectangles varies according to the projection shape. A critical region was delineated in the cavity of R. Automatic beam weighting based on arrangement computation was then applied to minimize weights of beams through the critical region while keeping the dose inside R between specified thresholds. Fig. 16-b shows the 80% isodosic surface generated in this way. Similar matching between input and output shape was unachievable with manual weighting.

4 Conclusions

We describe collimation methods for robotic radiosurgery. Paradigms for the interactive application of geometric algorithms are developed in this context. Geometric planning techniques have been combined with an algorithm for computing a path giving shortest total radiation time for a given maximum planar penumbra. The techniques include means for generating non-convex regions of high dose. Sweep methods for beam-shaping are particularly appropriate for robotic radiosurgery. Low cost, low collimator weight and high flexibility for generating complex distributions are the benefits of this approach.

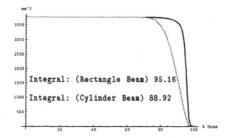

Fig. 14. Dose-volume histograms for the AVM in the sample case. Integral over histogram normalized to unit volume. Black curve: cylinder beam. Gray curve: rectangular beam

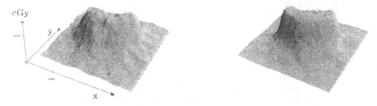

Fig. 15. Distribution cross-section for adaptable jaw collimator (AVM sample case). Height above x-y-plane represents dose. a) Cylinder beam. b) Rectangular beam.

A first series of experiments suggests that multiple-beam field shaping methods in connection with 6 degree-of-freedom beam motion can produce radiosurgical distributions with characteristics approaching the characteristics of spherical distributions.

References

1. Carol, M. An Automatic 3-D treatment planning and implementation system for optimized conformal therapy. Reprint of paper presented at 34th Annual Meeting Am. Soc. Therap. Radiology and Oncology, San Diego, Nov. 9-13, 1992.
2. Convery, D., Rosenbloom, M. The generation of intensity-modulated fields for

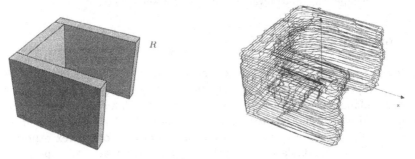

Fig. 16. a) Extruded u-shape. b) 80% isodose surface for distribution generated with jaw collimator and automatic beam weighting. RHD is an extruded u-shape

conformal radiotherapy by dynamic collimation. *Phys. Med. Biol.*, 36 (7): 1359–1374, 1992.

3. Kallman, P., Lind, A., Eklof, A., Brahme, A. Shaping of arbitrary dose distributions by dynamic multileaf collimation. *Phys. Med. Biol.*, 33 (11): 1291–1300, 1988.

4. Leavitt, D., Martin, M., Moeller, J. H., Lee, W. Dynamic wedge techniques through computer-controlled collimator motion and dose delivery. *Med. Phys.*, 17 (1): 87–91, 1990.

5. Lutz, W., Winston, K. R., and Maleki, N. A System for stereotactic radiosurgery with a linear accelerator. *Int. J. Radiation Oncology Biol. Phys.*, 14:373–381, 1988.

6. Podgorsak, E. B., et al. Dynamic Stereotactic Radiosurgery. *Intern. J. Radiation Oncology Biol. Phys.*, 14:115–126, 1988.

7. Nedzi, L. A., Kooy, H. M., Alexander, E., et. al. Dynamic Field Shaping for Stereotactic Radiosurgery: A Modeling Study. *Intern. J. Radiation Oncology Biol. Phys.*, 25:859–869, 1993.

8. Rice, R. K., et al. Measurements of Dose Distributions in Small Beams of 6 MeV X-Rays. *Phys. Med. Biol.*, 32:1087–1099, 1987.

9. Schweikard, A., Adler, J. R., and Latombe, J. C. Motion Planning in Stereotaxic Radiosurgery. *IEEE Tr. Robotics and Automation*, 9, 6, 764 - 774, 1993.

10. Schweikard, A., Bodduluri, M., Tombropoulos, R. Z., Adler, J. R. Planning, Calibration and Collision Avoidance for Image-Guided Radiosurgery. *Proc. IEEE Int. Workshop Intelligent Robots and Systems*, 854–861, 1994.

11. Starkschall, G., Eifel, P. An interactive beam-weight optimization tool for three-dimensional radiotherapy treatment planning. *Med. Phys.*, 19 (10): 155–164, 1992.

12. Webb, S. Optimization by simulated annealing of three-dimensional conformal treatment planning for radiation fields defined by a multi-leaf collimator. *Phys. Med. Biol.*, 36 (9):1201–1226, 1991.

Atlases

Automatic Retrieval of Anatomical Structures in 3D Medical Images

Jérôme Declerck, Gérard Subsol
Jean-Philippe Thirion and Nicholas Ayache

INRIA, B.P. 93, 06 902 Sophia Antipolis Cedex, France
E-mail: Jerome.Declerck@sophia.inria.fr
http://zenon.inria.fr:8003/epidaure/Epidaure-eng.html

Abstract. This paper describes a method to automatically generate the mapping between a completely labeled reference image and 3D medical images of patients. To achieve this, we combined three techniques: the extraction of 3D feature lines, their non-rigid registration and the extension of the deformation to the whole image space using warping techniques. As experimental results, we present the retrieval of the cortical and ventricles structures in MRI images of the brain.

1 Introduction

It becomes needless to emphasize the advantages of electronic atlases versus conventional paper atlases. However, even if such atlases are available [9] and even if Computer Graphic techniques are sufficiently developed to manipulate and display those atlases in real time, there remains a crucial need for *automatic* tools to analyze the variability of features between patients [11], [14]. For that purpose, we have to find correspondences between the image of any patient and the atlases.

This paper presents one possible approach to achieve this goal, usually referred to as a segmentation problem, by using a strong a priori knowledge of the human anatomy.

There are usually two complementary ways to explore, which are the region based technique using the voxel values inside the regions [3], and the feature based one only using the boundaries of those regions [5], such as the interfaces between organs, or specific lines or points of those surfaces [17], [16]

In the present paper, we concentrate on a feature line based technique to segment fully automatically the same organ in the images of different patients. We give first a global description of the method, which is then detailed into feature lines extraction using differential geometry, registration of lines using deformable models, and at last 3D space deformation using warping techniques. Finally, we present a practical example, which is the automatic extraction of the cortical and ventricle surfaces from the 3D MRI images of a patient.

2 A global description of the method

Let us assume that we have a 3D reference image I_r and an associated fully labeled image M_r, called map (figure 1) in which each voxel value specifies the type of a corresponding structure in I_r. We call *structure* a set of connected voxels of M_r having the same label. I_p is the image of a new patient to process.

We suppose also that images I_r and I_p have been acquired with the same modality and parameter settings: their intensities are very similar.

To find the correspondence between I_p and the reference map M_r, we propose to follow this scheme (figure 1):

- automatically find and label some features in I_r corresponding to a labeled structure S_r of M_r,
- automatically find the equivalent features in I_p,
- find the correspondence $C_{p,r}$ between those features,
- either deform individual structures or the global map M_r into new structures or into a new map M_p, which is exactly superimposable to I_p. This step is achieved by finding a space warping function $D_{p,r}$ and applying it to M_r. We retrieve then the structure S_p in I_p corresponding to S_r in I_r.

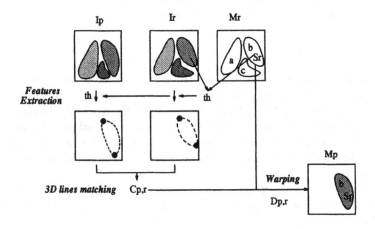

Fig. 1. *Features of the labeled structure S_r are extracted from the reference image I_r. Equivalent features are extracted from I_p. By finding the registration $C_{p,r}$ between these features, a warping function $D_{p,r}$ can be computed to obtain the map M_p superimposable on I_p and so, the structure S_p.*

3 Feature based non-rigid registration

3.1 The feature type: the crest lines

Raw medical images are stored in a discrete 3D matrix $I = f(x, y, z)$. By thresholding $I = I_0$, isosurfaces of organs are computed (for instance the brain with MRI images). To get a sparser but relevant representation of the isosurface, we propose to use the "crest lines" introduced in [10].

They are defined as the successive loci of a surface for which the largest principal curvature is locally maximal in the principal direction (see figure 2, left). Let k_1 be the principal curvature with maximal curvature in absolute value and $\overrightarrow{t_1}$ the associated principal direction, each point of a crest line verifies: $\overrightarrow{\nabla} k_1 . \overrightarrow{t_1} = 0$. These lines are automatically extracted by the "marching lines" algorithm [17].

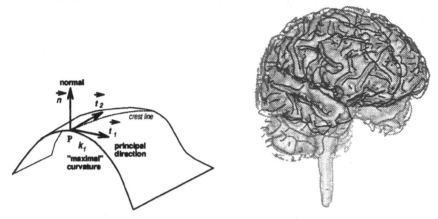

Fig. 2. *Left: mathematical crest line definition. Right: crest lines on a brain.*

In fact, crest lines turned out to be anatomically meaningful. Thus, in figure 2, right, crest lines follow the cortical convolutions, emphasizing the sulci and gyri patterns described by Ono et al. [12].

3.2 The crest lines extraction

We want to extract the crest lines of the structures S_r in I_r and their equivalent in I_p. The problem is then to find the threshold I_0. I_0 is representative of the interface between S_r and the other structures and can be computed as the mean value of the voxels of I_r labelled as S_r in M_r. As the images have the same dynamic, we can use the same threshold in I_p.

3.3 The 3D non-rigid registration algorithm

The 3D lines registration algorithm is a key point in our scheme: given two sets A and A' composed of the crest lines L_i and L'_j extracted from two different images, we want to find which lines L_i of A correspond to which lines L'_j of A'. Two difficulties arise: the number of lines of each set is quite large (several hundreds to more than a thousand) and the registration between A and A' is not rigid, preventing from using Euclidean invariant based methods as in [8].

Zhang [18] and independently Besl [1] introduced an "iterative closest points" matching method. Both authors use this algorithm to register free-form curves but only for the rigid case. Nevertheless, we can improve and generalize this method to our problem and our algorithm follows the steps of the "iterative closest point" method.

Points matching Each point of A is linked with its closest neighbour in A' according to the Euclidean distance. We plan also to use in the distance computation the differential curve parameters as the tangent, normal, curvature and torsion [8] or surface parameters as the normal, the principal directions and principal curvatures as described in [6]. This gives a lists of registered points, C_1.

But as we have curves, i.e. an *ordered* list of points, we can apply some topological constraints in order to remove non-consistent couples of registered points and then to avoid irrelevant configurations. We obtain an other list C_2.

From C_2, two coefficients can be computed: p_i^j and $p_j^{'i}$ which are the proportion of the curve i of A matched with the curve j of A' and vice versa. By thresholding, $p_i^j \geq thr$ and $p_j^{'i} \geq thr$, we can determine the curves which are "registered" at thr percent. For instance, curves can be considered completely registered when $p_i^j \geq 0.5$ and $p_j^{'i} \geq 0.5$.

Least-squares transformation We want to register A and A' with polynomial transformations. The 0th-order is a rigid transformation and 1st-order an affine one but they are not sufficient for an accurate non-rigid registration. So, we use 2nd-order polynomial transformations defined by (for the x coordinate):

$$x' = a_1 x^2 + a_2 y^2 + a_3 z^2 + a_4 xy + a_5 yz + a_6 xz + a_7 x + a_8 y + a_9 z + a_{10}$$

As these polynomials are linear in their coefficients, we can use the classical least-squares method to compute the a_i from C_2.

2nd-order polynomial transformations give accurate registration but we are not able to decompose them into intuitive physical meaning transformations such as rotation, translation or scaling. Notice that, at each iteration, we compose the transformation with a 2nd-order polynomial and so, we obtain after n iterations, a potential 2^n-order polynomial transformation.

2nd-order transformations are also used by Greitz et al. [7] to model natural deformations as brain bending.

Updating The transformation is then applied and the algorithm iterates again or stops according to some criteria (mean value of the distance distribution between matched points, stability of the registration coefficients p_i^j and $p_j^{'i}$, threshold on the matrix norm $\|T - I_d\|$ where T is the transformation and I_d the identity matrix).

Parameters adaptation By incrementing the threshold value thr at each iteration and by taking only into account the matched point couples belonging to "registered" curves at thr percent, the algorithm tends to improve the registration of already matched curves and to discard isolated ones. Moreover, we can begin to apply rigid transformations to align the two sets of lines, then affine transformations to scale them and, at last, quadratic transformations to refine the registration.

At the end, we obtain a good registration between the two sets of lines and so, a point to point correspondence between lines. These correspondences give significant landmarks to define a B-spline based warping on the whole space.

4 Space warping

4.1 The problem

Let us call F, the exact matching function, i.e. the geometric transformation that takes a point P_r in I_r and gives its anatomically equivalent P_p in I_p:

$$F : \quad \begin{aligned} I_r &\longrightarrow I_p \\ P_r(x, y, z) &\longmapsto P_p(u, v, w) \end{aligned}$$

The set of matched points $\mathcal{M}$ obtained with the feature based registration is an estimation of some pairs $(P_r, F(P_r))$. We have then a sparse estimation of F which we can extend to the whole space by a warping function $\varphi_{\mathcal{M}}$.

4.2 Calculation of the warping function

Bookstein and Green [2] define $\varphi_{\mathcal{M}}$ as a thin-plate spline interpolating function but only in 2D. Two problems raise if we apply this definition to our approach. First, it appears difficult to generalize in 3D. Second, interpolation is relevant when the matched points of $\mathcal{M}$ are totally reliable and regularly distributed (for example, a few points manually located). In our case, these points are not totally reliable due to possible mismatches of the registration algorithm and are sparsed in a few compact areas as they belong to lines.

So for $\varphi_{\mathcal{M}}$, we prefer to use an approximation function which is regular enough to minimize the influence of erroneous matched points. We choose a B-spline tensor product which is easy to define and control in 3D.

The B-spline approximation We define the coordinate functions of $\varphi_{\mathcal{M}}$, (u, v, w) as a three-dimensional tensor product of B-spline basis functions. For instance, for u:

$$u(x, y, z) = \sum_{i=0}^{n_x-1} \sum_{j=0}^{n_y-1} \sum_{k=0}^{n_z-1} \alpha_{ijk} \, B_{i,K}^x(x) \, B_{j,K}^y(y) \, B_{k,K}^z(z)$$

with the following notations:

- n_x : the number of control points in the x direction. n_x sets the accuracy of the approximation.
- α : the 3D matrix of the control points abscissae.

- $B_{i,K}^x$: the ith B-spline basis function. Its order is K. u is then a piecewise K^{th} degree polynomial in each variable x, y and z, easy to evaluate with the de Casteljau algorithm [13]. We choose cubic B-splines in our examples ($K = 3$), for their regularity properties. For the B-spline knots, we take the classic regular mesh.

For a given number of control points and a set of B-spline basis functions, u is completely defined by the α_{ijk}. They are calculated by minimizing a criterion computed with the set $\mathcal{M}$ of matched points.

The criterion We define three criteria J^x, J^y and J^z (one for each coordinate) to determine the best $\varphi_\mathcal{M}$, with respect to our data. For instance, for u, J^x splits in two parts:

- position term. For each data point P_r, $u(P_r)$ must be as close as possible to the abscissa of P_p. We choose a least-squares criterion:

$$J^x_{position}(u) = \sum_{l=1}^{N} \left(u(x_1^l, y_1^l, z_1^l) - x_2^l\right)^2$$

- smoothing term. B-splines have intrinsic rigidity properties, but it is sometimes not enough. We choose a second order Tikhonov stabilizer: it measures how far from an affine transformation the deformation is.

$$J^x_{smooth}(u) = \rho_s \int_{\mathbb{R}^3} \left[\frac{\partial^2 u}{\partial x^2}^2 + \frac{\partial^2 u}{\partial y^2}^2 + \frac{\partial^2 u}{\partial z^2}^2 + \frac{\partial^2 u}{\partial x \partial y}^2 + \frac{\partial^2 u}{\partial x \partial z}^2 + \frac{\partial^2 u}{\partial y \partial z}^2 \right]$$

where ρ_s is a weight coefficient. It is currently manually defined and some solutions to choose it automatically are under study.

The criterion to minimize is then: $J^x(u) = J^x_{position}(u) + J^x_{smooth}(u)$

The linear systems J^x is a positive quadratic function of the α_{ijk} variables. To find the coefficients that minimize J^x, we derive its expression with respect to all the α_{ijk}: it gives $n_x \times n_y \times n_z$ linear equations. Assembling those equations, we get a sparse, symmetric and positive linear system. We solve the 3 systems (one for each coordinate) to completely calculate $\phi_\mathcal{M}$.

5 Results and discussion

We apply the described process to retrieve the cortical and ventricles structures in MRI images of the brain of a patient from a reference segmented image (see figures 3 to 7).

The structures have been correctly recovered in spite of the sparse representation of the data. It shows that crest lines turn out to be significant features with few ambiguities and to be anatomically consistent. Moreover, a data point has a *local* influence: to evaluate a transformed point, we need only $(K+1)^3$ control points (to be compared with the $n_x \times n_y \times n_z$ that have been calculated). Hence, the influence of outliers is very local. At last, the regularity of the B-splines defined $\varphi_{\mathcal{M}}$ allows to get consistent correspondences everywhere in the image. In particular, we can retrieve inner structures of the brain, with a warping only based on its external surface features.

6 Conclusion and perspectives

The proposed method allows us to build fully automatically the maps associated to the 3D images of new patients, from manually designed maps of reference patients. It can be used to efficiently initialize 3D surface snakes if a more precise final segmentation of the organs is needed [4], [15].

We especially thank Dr Ron Kikinis from the Brigham and Woman's hospital, Harvard Medical School, Boston, for having provided the segmented image of the brain, and the MR images to analyse. We also thank Digital Equipment Corporation (External Research Contract) and the BRA VIVA european project who partially supported this research.

References

1. Paul J. Besl and Neil D. McKay. A Method for Registration of 3-D Shapes. *IEEE PAMI*, 14(2):239–255, February 1992.
2. F.L. Bookstein and W.D.K. Green. Edge Information at landmarks in medical images. *SPIE Vol.1808*, 1992.
3. Gary E. Christensen, Michael I. Miller, and Michael Vannier. A 3D Deformable Magnetic Resonance Textbook Based on Elasticity. In *AAAI symposium: Application of Computer Vision in Medical Image Processing*, pages 153–156, Stanford, March 1994.
4. Isaac Cohen, Laurent Cohen, and Nicholas Ayache. Using deformable surfaces to segment 3D images and infer differential structures. In *CVGIP : Image understanding '92*, September 1992.
5. Chris Davatzikos and Jerry L. Prince. Brain Image Registration Based on Curve Mapping. In *IEEE Workshop on Biomedical Image Analysis*, pages 245–254, Seattle, June 1994.
6. Jacques Feldmar and Nicholas Ayache. Rigid and Affine Registration of Smooth Surfaces using Differential Properties. In *ECCV*, Stockholm (Sweden), May 1994. ECCV.
7. Torgny Greitz, Christian Bohm, Sven Holte, and Lars Eriksson. A Computerized Brain Atlas: Construction, Anatomical Content and Some Applications. *Journal of Computer Assisted Tomography*, 15(1):26–38, 1991.
8. A. Guéziec and N. Ayache. Smoothing and Matching of 3-D Space Curves. In *Visualization in Biomedical Computing*, pages 259–273, Chapel Hill, North Carolina (USA), October 1992. SPIE.

9. K. Höhne, A. Pommert, M Riemer, T. Schiemann, R. Schubert, and U. Tiede. Framework for the generation of 3D anatomical atlases. In R. Robb, editor, *Visualization in Biomedical Computing*, volume 1808, pages 510–520. SPIE, 1992. Chapell Hill.

10. Olivier Monga, Serge Benayoun, and Olivier D. Faugeras. Using Partial Derivatives of 3D Images to Extract Typical Surface Features. In *CVPR*, 1992.

11. Chahab Nastar. Vibration Modes for Nonrigid Motion Analysis in 3D Images. In *Proceedings of the Third European Conference on Computer Vision (ECCV '94)*, Stockholm, May 1994.

12. Michio Ono, Stefan Kubik, and Chad D. Abernathey. *Atlas of the Cerebral Sulci*. Georg Thieme Verlag, 1990.

13. J.-J. Risler. *Méthodes Mathématiques Pour la CAO*. Masson, 1991.

14. Gérard Subsol, Jean-Philippe Thirion, and Nicholas Ayache. Steps Towards Automatic Building of Anatomical Atlases. In *Visualization in Biomedical Computing '94*, October 1994.

15. D. Terzopoulos, A. Witkin, and M. Kaas. Constraints on deformable models : recovering 3D shape and non rigid motion. In *AI J.*, pages 91–123, 1988.

16. J-P Thirion. Extremal Points : definition and application to 3D image regist ration. In *IEEE conf. on Computer Vision and Pattern Recognition*, Seattle, June 1994.

17. J.P. Thirion and A. Gourdon. The Marching Lines Algorithm : new results and proofs. Technical Report 1881, INRIA, March 1993. to be published in CVGIP.

18. Zhengyou Zhang. On Local Matching of Free-Form Curves. In David Hogg and Roger Boyle, editors, *British Machine Vision Conference*, pages 347–356, Leeds (United Kingdom), September 1992. British Machine Vision Association, Springer-Verlag.

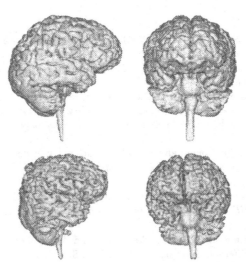

Fig. 3. *The data : top, the reference brain, bottom, the patient brain. Notice the differences in shapes and orientations.*

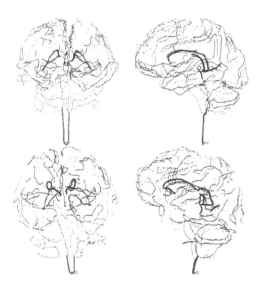

Fig. 4. *The crest lines have been automatically extracted from the reference brain (top) and from the patient brain (bottom). Some of the crest lines have been labeled (ventricles and medulla) and thickened for a better visualization.*

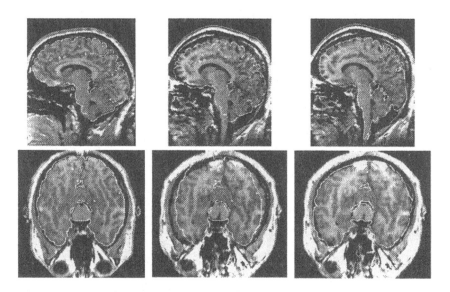

Fig. 5. *Left, the reference image I_r with the cortical surface S_r. Middle, the patient image I_p with S_r before deformation. Right, I_p with the result S_p of the found deformation applied on S_r.*

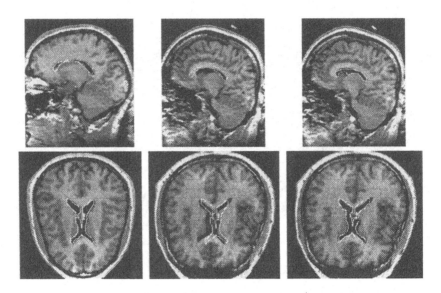

Fig. 6. *The same as figure 5, with the ventricles surface.*

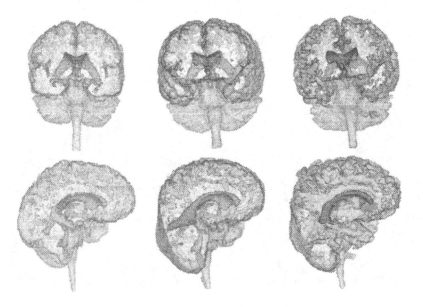

Fig. 7. *Different 3D views of the brains with their ventricle: left, the reference brain, middle, the same after warping and right, the patient brain.*

A Novel Virtual Reality Tool for Teaching Dynamic 3D Anatomy

Anantha R. Kancherla[1], Jannick P. Rolland[1],
Donna L. Wright[2], Grigore Burdea[3]

[1] Department of Computer Science,
University of North Carolina, Chapel Hill
[2] Department of Medical Allied Health Professions
University of North Carolina, Chapel Hill
[3] Department of Electrical and Computer Engineering
Rutgers–State University of New Jersey, Piscataway

Abstract. A Virtual-Reality-based tool for teaching dynamic three-dimensional anatomy may impart better understanding of bone dynamics during body movement. One application of this teaching tool is radiographic positioning instruction. We propose Augmented Reality, a technology that allows the overlay of graphically generated objects(bones in this case) on the real scenes(body in this case), as a means of visualization for such an application. In this paper we describe the design and the three stages of development of a prototype unit which demonstrates elbow movement. Preliminary results and problems encountered while developing the first stage, are also presented.

1 Introduction

Virtual Reality (VR) tools are being developed for medical diagnostics and therapy, because of their extremely powerful, but non-invasive, three-dimensional(3D) visualization, which was hitherto unavailable. This paper describes a way to harness this power to better educate radiologic science students who currently struggle to visualize 3D bone movements using 2D teaching tools and stationary teaching models.

The current teaching methods for radiographic positioning include 1)2D photographs and radiographs; 2)Memorization of standard central ray centering points and degrees of beam angle; 3)Demonstrations that are passively watched by the students; 4)Videotapes, slides, audiotapes describing positioning methods; 5)Supervised positioning of real patients in clinical setting.

Not only do the students have to correlate all these inputs to what they know about the three dimensionality of the human body, but also form an understanding of the 3D dynamics of the bones when the model patient moves. These teaching methods have limitations such as: 1)None of the current physical models realistically simulate the alignment and movement of anatomical joints; 2)None of the current models teach the compensations for patients with limited range of movements; 3)And none of the current models effectively reinforce the connection between the patient's anatomical parts being imaged and the rest of the patient.

We speculate that an innovative and effective VR teaching tool could offer several advantages including: 1)Students will be better prepared for clinical work; 2)Students will learn through multiple senses (vision, touch etc.) which will reinforce their learning experience; 3)Students get an immediate feedback about the accuracy of the positions they create; 4)Model patients in the learning situation have no risk of radiation exposure or repeated attempts to position a part correctly; 5)There are no limits on repeating a given exercise several times. 6)This tool can be potentially expanded to work for any portion of the skeleton by appropriate modeling of the desired anatomy.

In this paper, a prototype of such a tool is described. This prototype is designed to demonstrate flexion, extension, pronation and supination movements of the elbow joint while maintaining a fixed humerus position.

After describing the elbow anatomy, then the concept of Augmented Reality, including how it derives its power, and the current problems are reviewed. This is followed by a description of the three stages of development of the first working prototype of the VR positioning tool. Finally, preliminary results and problems encountered while developing the test system are described. We conclude with a brief description of future work.

2 Anatomy

The prototype is currently restricted to the elbow joint. In the initial stage of the project, directed at demonstrating a proof of concept for future use in teaching radiographic positioning, only normal cases are considered(pathological cases such as tennis elbow, arthritis, congenital malformation etc. are not considered). The general description of a normal elbow joint, and some of the anatomical terms encountered elsewhere in this paper are presented in this section. For more details on anatomy see [1].

The articulation between the upper arm and the forearm is the elbow joint. It is a hinge type of joint, allowing mainly forward and backward movement. The bones involved in this joint are the humerus(in the upper-arm), radius and ulna(in the forearm), see Fig.1. The elbow joint includes a radioulnar articulation as well as articulations between the humerus and the radius and ulna. The three joints are enclosed in a common capsule at the elbow.

The lower part of the humerus is broad and has medial and lateral condyles and epicondyles, which are bulges on the sides. On its inferior surface are two elevations(trochlea and capitellum) for articulation with the forearm bones. On its posterior and anterior sides there are depressions to accommodate the processes of the ulna when the elbow is extended and flexed. The upper extremity of ulna presents a process called the olecranon process, which forms the semilunar notch at which it articulates with the trochlea of the humerus. The flat, disk-like head at the upper extremity of the radius rotates around the capitellum of the humerus and articulates with the radial notch of the ulna on the side.

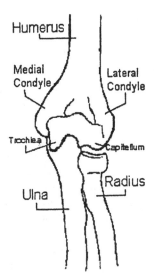

Fig. 1. Anterior aspect of elbow joint

The movements of supination (forearm outstretched with the palm facing up) and pronation (the forearm is twisted and palm facing down) of the forearm are largely the result of the combined rotary action of these two joints. In the act of pronation, the radius crosses over the ulna, while the ulna makes a slight counterrotation.

3 Augmented Reality as a New Tool

The Head Mounted Display(HMD) is a standard VR equipment. It is a helmet, worn by the user, mounted with two miniature displays, one for each eye, and a head position tracker. Stereoscopic images of the scenes of interest are painted on the displays and updated in realtime by a computer based on the position and orientation information provided by the tracker. Usually HMDs are opaque, i.e. only the computer generated graphics are visible, we call this full VR. Alternatively, the HMDs maybe see-thru. In which case the real world view is also available in addition to the computer graphics. One refers to the technique of superimposition of real and virtual information using a see-thru HMD as "Augmented Reality". If the real scene is presented as a video image then the HMD is termed "video see-thru"[2], else, if the real world is presented optically, then it is termed "optical see-thru" [3].

Based on our experience with developing see-thru HMDs and AR systems at the University of North Carolina at Chapel Hill [2], [10], it is felt that AR systems are extremely well suited for medical applications. However, research [3] [5] [10] has shown that many challenges specific to AR need to be surmounted, in addition to the problems of full VR. By far the most important one is the registration of the real image with that of the virtual one. A major component of this task is the calibration of the HMD [3].

4 VR Positioning Tool, the Scheme

The VR positioning tool will be developed in three stages, which differ in the display modality used.

- The objective of the first stage is to achieve proper modeling of motion of the bones in the elbow joint. Only the graphics will be displayed(monoscopically). No stereo will be involved.
- The second stage involves the use of Enhanced Reality for visualization. Here, the real scene is captured by a small TV camera and is displayed superimposed with the "enhancing" graphics on a flat display. The difference from the video see-thru being that the display is not stereo and no head tracking is done. This stage will enable proper testing of tracking and registration. We anticipate that the calibration problems encountered here will be common to in the next stage and hence the experience beneficial.
- Finally, in the third stage, we plan to use an optical see-thru HMD, where, instead of using video cameras, an optical viewer will merge the real and virtual scenes.

5 Apparatus

The apparatus used in the various stages of the development includes magnetic trackers, an Enhanced Reality setup used at an early stage of the prototype development and a bench prototype of the see-thru HMD that will serve as the final visualization tool of the first prototype. A good discussion on VR technology can be found in[6].

Tracker. An extended range Flock of Birds magnetic tracker developed by Ascension Technology [8] is being used to track the patient's arm movement in the second and third stages. Specifications of the tracker can be obtained in [9]. The tracker uses one transmitter and three receivers placed, one near the extremity of the humerus, close to the forearm, and two at either end of the forearm. Using the position information obtained from the trackers, the current position of the bones in the world computed and immediately displayed. To model just the flexion and extension of the arm, only one forearm receiver suffices, two of them are needed to capture the displacement of radius and ulna with respect to each other when pronation and supination take place. The receivers are mounted as accurately as possible on or around some major anatomical landmarks(eg. condyles) to enable accurate registration. They are fastened firmly to prevent sliding along the arm. However, unless the receivers can be surgically implanted on the bones themselves, the stretching of the skin will cause inconsistencies.

Enhanced Reality Setup. It will be used for the second stage. The difference from the first stage is in the visualization mechanism. Here, the graphics are superimposed over a video of the real scene captured by a miniature camera appropriately placed to simulate one of the observer's eyes. The superimposition of the graphics on the video is done in realtime.

Optical See-Thru HMD. A Bench setup of an optical see thru HMD, with no allowable head motion, will be used in the final stage, see Fig.2. The benefits of using a bench prototype comes from not being penalized by another component of tracking delay due to the head tracker. The displays are driven by an SGI Onyx's Multi Channel Option which provides two separate channels.

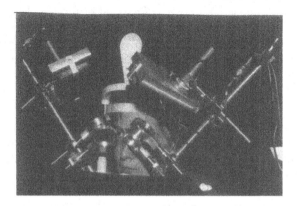

Fig. 2. The bench prototype of optical see-thru head-mounted display

6 Preliminary Results of Developing the First Stage

The major portion of the implementation of the first stage involves modeling and rendering the bones and their motion so that they can be reproduced by graphics and presented as virtual objects in the HMD. The various modeling that has been done for the first stage is presented in this section.

In the first stage, the software simply animates the graphic bones according to the motion model described previously. This stage enabled us to validate the motion model.

6.1 Modeling and Rendering of the Anatomy

A commercially available model of the bones was obtained from Viewpoint [11]. The bones were modeled as lists of polygons with a normal at each vertex. A low-resolution model with 690 vertices and 472 polygons was used. The Viewpoint model was arrived at by digitizing a representative set of bones of a specific size.

There is a wide variation in the various aspects of anatomy, not only by gender, but also among individuals of the same gender. For example, women tend to have, in general, shorter bones than men. Also, the angle subtended by the forearm to the line passing through the humerus is generally greater for women than for men.

This wide variation implies that separate modeling be done for each patient, and this provides a logistic difficulty. To avoid this problem, the model uses a unique polygonal model which is scaled appropriately to match the patient. Also, only a small subset of variation about the norms for a single sex is modeled.

An x-ray of the patient's arm was used to compute the correct scaling factor. This is achieved by applying the process of registration of the bone images obtained by x-ray with the rendered image of the computer model.

The rendering was done on an SGI ONYX platform using the OpenGL [7] library. Two views (one for each eye) were rendered in different areas of the screen for the Multi-Channel Option (video splitting mechanism provided by SGI) hardware to capture and generate from them, two different signals.

6.2 Modeling Motion

There are two elements to motion modeling of the joint: 1)dynamics and 2)kinematics. Dynamics involve modeling the various forces and the accompanying deformations that are involved during motion. Whereas, the kinematics is an aspect of dynamics which deals with aspects of motion apart from considerations of mass and forces. In the case where the arm is flexed very quickly, there are some impulse forces involved which cause some spurious motion. However, when the arm is flexed slowly, the forces involved in the joint can be considered to be at equilibrium. Hence, while modeling motion, only the kinematic aspects of the bone are considered.

Firstly, a skeleton of the arm was used to reach a better understanding of the anatomy involved. Fluoroscopy was used to deliver a good understanding of the motions of the various joint components. The pivotal points and axes were then identified using knowledge of physical anatomy and the corresponding points were located on the bone model. The following useful information about the motion was derived in this process.

- The main axis about which the ulna rotates when the arm is flexed lies roughly through the middle of the two condyles of the humerus.
- During the twisting motion (supination and pronation) the ulna rotates about an axis passing through its shaft and its head touches the trochlea of the humerus.
- In the same twisting motions, the head of the radius moves along the capitellum of the humerus, however its axis lies outside the shaft resulting in the crossover with the ulna. This axis changes too.

7 Discussion and Conclusion

The biggest stumbling block is the speed and accuracy of the tracker. Since the virtuals objects interact with the real world, the requirements on the positions are extremely strict to obtain proper registration. We hope to solve this problem by a proper motion model. The use of generic bones causes another problem since anatomy differs between people. Currently this problem is avoided by limiting the model to work for only a small subset of the possible range.

Currently, the system is in the first stage of development (ref. Sec. 4). We plan to enhance the visualization modality in two more stages as mentioned before. The current CS graph used by the program accounts for the flexion and extension motions so far. It needs to be extended to utilize the input from the second forearm receiver to model the twisting motions of the forearm. Finally, work has to be done to model the motion more accurately (this can be better understood only when the second stage of development is completed).

In this paper we have summarized the drawbacks of current teaching methods for radiographic positioning and described the concepts of a novel VR tool for teaching dynamic 3D anatomy. Different issues involving the merging of real and virtual worlds were briefly presented. The proposed three stages of a first prototype as well as its components were discussed. Preliminary results of the modeling and implementation of the first stage were presented. Finally, it is concluded with a brief discussion and a look ahead at the future work.

Acknowledgements

This work was supported by a UNC-CH Foundation Fund Award and the Office of Naval Research under Grant N00014-94-1-0503. Thanks are also due to Cheryl Rieger-Krugh whose expertise in human anatomy proved invaluable for proper modeling of the elbow joint.

References

1. Ballinger, W. Philip, *Merrill's Atlas of Radiographic Positions and Radiologic Procedures*, vol. 1, 7th edition, Mosby, 1991.
2. Bajura, M., Fuchs, H., Ohbuchi, R., "Merging virtual objects with the real world", Computer Graphics, Proc. SIGGRAPH'92, 26, pp203-1,0 1992
3. Rolland, J.P., Ariely, D., Gibson, W., "Towards quantifying depth and size perception in virtual environments", Presence, 1994, forthcoming.
4. Caudell, T.P., David, W. M., "Augmented reality: An application of heads-up display technology to manual manufacturing process", pp 659, IEEE 1992.
5. Rolland, J.P., Holloway, R.L., Fuchs, H., "A comparison of optical and video see-thru head-mounted displays", Proc. SPIE 2351, 1994.
6. Burdea, G., Coiffet, P., *Virtual Reality Technology*, John Wiley and sons, New York, 400pp, 1994.
7. Neider, J., Davis, T., Woo, M., *OpenGL Programming guide*, Addison Wesley.
8. Ascension Technology Co., P.O.Box 527 Burlington, VT 05402, USA.
9. Holloway, R., Lastra, A., "Virtual Environments: A Survey of the Technology", Tech. Report TR93-033, Univ. of North Carolina at Chapel Hill.
10. Holloway, R., " An Analysis of Registration Errors in a See-T hrough Head-Mounted Display System for Craniofacial Surgery Planning", Ph.D. dis sertation, University of North Carolina at Chapel Hill, in preparation, 1994.
11. Viewpoint Animation Engineering, 870 W Center Street, Orem, Utah 84057, USA.

A Supporting System for Getting Tomograms and Screening with a Computerized 3D Brain Atlas and a Knowledge Database

Hidetomo Suzuki[1], Keiichi Yoshizaki[1], Michimasa Matsuo[2] and Jiro Kashio[1]

[1] Mie University, 1515, Kamihama-cho, Tsu, Mie, 514, Japan
[2] Tenri Hospital, 200, Mishima-cho, Tenri, Nara, 632, Japan

Abstract. We introduce a system which includes a 3D atlas of a human central nervous system, a knowledge database which has correspondences between patient's symptoms and damaged nerves, and a display tool which has various graphical display methods to show 3D structure of damaged nerves and its adjoining organs. 3D atlas is composed of two MRI images and a labeled image whose labels stand for motor nerves and brain matters. The knowledge database includes 66 if-then rules. If a user uses this system, he will be able to acquire appropriate sectional images and the corresponding atlas data needful for screening images, diagnosing patients and planning a therapy.

1 Introduction

Recently tomographic imaging technologies like MRI (Magnetic Resonance imaging) and X-ray CT (Computed Tomography) have advanced in its quality, and they have become very important modalities for image diagnoses because they are non-invasive methods and can make cross sections sliced at arbitrary positions. Among them, MRI images are seemed to be rather useful for image diagnoses because of security against irradiation unlike X-ray CT images, images acquired in arbitrary directions, and soft tissues with high contrast.

A skilled brain surgeon diagnoses a case using patient's symptoms, medical images, knowledge about the anatomical structure in the head which he have accumulated empirically, and so on. Since motor disturbance and sensory disorder which a patient develops have the close connections with damaged nerves, he can identify the damaged part if he makes the thorough investigation. But there is a variety of the correspondence, and it is not easy to remember all of them. Furthermore, it is difficult for a brain surgeon to imagine the 3D (three-dimensional) location of a selected part of a nerve and the mutual relationship to other tissues, even if he remember the connections. One clinician said that his knowledge about the position of nerves has a close relation with the cross sections and the anatomical atlases which he have encountered empirically, so it is very difficult to recognize nerves in the sectional images obtained at untrained positions and directions.

As one of the ways to settle such problems and to assist clinical works, we made a system which consists of four parts, i.e. a 3D atlas of a central nervous system, a knowledge database which includes the connections between motor disturbances and damaged parts of motor nerves, a display tool which displays the 3D structure of objects with various ways of 3D graphic techniques, and an editing tool which manages our 3D atlas. With this system, firstly a user, like a brain surgeon or a radiologist, examines a patient, consults our knowledge database to find suspicious parts of nerves, and then uses our display tool to see the selected nerves.

Studies on making computerized 3D atlases are done by many research groups[1,2], and several clinical applications of 3D atlases are reported. However, we have not found no study like our system which utilizes a 3D atlas together with a knowledge database in order to guess the damaged nerves and to display them. Höhne et al.[2] have constructed a detailed 3D atlas which has labels related to structural regions, functional regions, and so on, and implemented a tool for exploring a head. It implies the ability to infer damaged nerves, but it is not so easy to realize functions like our system.

2 System configuration

our system consists of four parts: an editing tool, a 3D atlas, a knowledge database, and a display tool. We will explain the latter three parts.

2.1 3D atlas

We made a computerized 3D atlas using two MRI images acquired from a mild case patient. One is an image which is obtained with TR:2.5 sec. and TE:15 msec., and presents mainly the proton density. It is a popular image and easy to grasp the structure of brain matters. Another one is an image which is obtained with TR:2.5 sec. and TE:90 msec., and presents mainly T2 (spin-spin relaxation time). It is useful for following the contours of brain matters because the signal intensity of cerebrospinal fluid is rather high than that of brain matters. Each of the images has 168 slices of 256x256 2D images, i.e. 256x256x168 3D image. The distance between adjacent voxels is 1 mm, and each voxel has a two-byte word.

Many groups including us are trying to extract brain matters automatically, but there is no methods which make the sufficient classification, so that we need supplemental revision. In addition, segmentation of nerves from other organs is almost impossible due to their complicated shapes and their close signal distribution to other organs. Hence, in the construction of our 3D atlas, we segmented organs and put labels to the regions interactively with our editing tool. To enter a large region like a pons, we made contours by putting points sequentially, painted inside the contours, and then corrected their shapes by hand. For a thin region like an oculomotor nerve, we used a spline curve fitting. A user can confirm and revise 3D continuity of a region slice by slice, and also correct labels at each voxel because this tool has an ability to display cross sections and surface images viewed from various positions. In the labeling step, we used anatomical atlases[3,4] and doctor's advice.

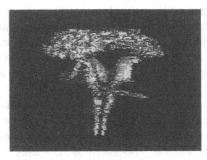

Fig.1. A surface display of pyramidal tract, thalamus, caudate nucleus and optic nerves

Our 3D atlas is a three dimensional array which has 256x256x168 elements (voxels) each of which has at most eight labels. A label is a number from 0 (background) to 255, and corresponds to a certain organ. Thus one element has eight-byte length, and the amount of the atlas is about 88 mega bytes. The limits on the number of labels and byte length of an element are sufficient for the current implementation, but we may have to remove the limitation for the future system. We are also attempting to reduce the data size of the atlas by converting its data structure, since the total of the registered labels is rather few than the maximum number registerable in the 3D array. At present, 25 labels are registered(see Table 1). Fig.1 is made through our 3D atlas. From such an image, we find that one can easily grasp the 3D structure of organs by use of our system.

Table 1. Registered organs

head	medulla oblongata	cerebellum
pons	mesencephalon	diencephalon
cerebrum	white matter (left)	white matter (right)
gray matter (left)	gray matter (right)	ventricles
pyramidal tract	optic nerve	oculomotor nerve
trochlear nerve	abducens nerve	thalamus
striatum	caudate nucleus	pallidum
claustrum	putamen	facial nerve (left)
facial nerve (right)		

2.2 Knowledge database

Motor disturbance of a patient corresponds to damages of several parts of motor nerves, so skilled surgeons and radiologists exploit such kind of knowledge when they acquire medical images and guess the areas where nerves are damaged. However, one who wishes to master such kind of knowledge and comprehend 3D structure of nerves must do a great deal of study and experience because there are many correspondences between them, whereas there are few books which treat the connections between symptoms and damaged nerves systematically. This is the reason why only the well-trained experts can remember and use such knowledge. If there was a knowledge database or an expert system which comprises such knowledge, it may carries us over the obstacles. Currently, there are many medical expert systems, but we could not find such a system.

Accordingly, we have constructed a knowledge database based on neuro-anatomical texts[5,6] and doctor's advice. The knowledge is registered as assertions of Prolog predicates and text data in the form of "if-then" type rules. Text data are written in Japanese and English, and a user can select one of them as occasional demands. Currently our knowledge database has 66 rules. Table 2 shows several examples. Connections in our knowledge database are elementary ones and have only one-to-one correspondences, so we must improve it so that the database offers enough information to specify the damaged nerves or their parts in a diagnosis. In the improvement, we will introduce a kind of certainty factor, which is popular in the current expert systems.

Table 2. Examples of rules registered in our knowledge database

	symptoms	damaged part
1	hemiparesis, paralysis at the opposite side of face	pons
2	hemiparesis, paralysis at lower left part of face	from internal capsule to cerebral peduncle
3	atetoze, gystony	putamen
4	Dejerine-Roussy syndrome	thalamus
5	conjugate deviation	(accessory) abducens nucleus

We can find nerves suspected of being damaged with this knowledge and display them with our display tool. Our system displays a table of the connections between symptoms and damaged parts, and makes a user select one of the listed items. After a user specifies an item which corresponds to or comprises patient's symptoms, he can procure the names of the nerves which seems to be damaged.

Fig.2 is a window to select symptoms. In this example, a user selects hemiparesis (paralysis at the one side of a human body) and paralysis at the lower left part of the face. The system answers the area from the internal capsule to the cerebral peduncle as a damaged part. The images at upper left corner are sectional images with two selected parts which are dark round areas located beside a ventricle.

2.3 Display tool

We can grasp the location of an organ and the adjacency among organs by exploiting the 3D atlas(**2.1**), the knowledge database(**2.2**), and 3D graphic techniques. We used a volume rendering technique to display surfaces, but more sophisticated one will be needed to produce high fidelity surfaces which are used in precise diagnoses. The followings are examples of the images made with this tool.

A superposed image of organs and an arbitrary cross section Firstly, a user selects three points in one or more cross sections to define the direction of a cutting

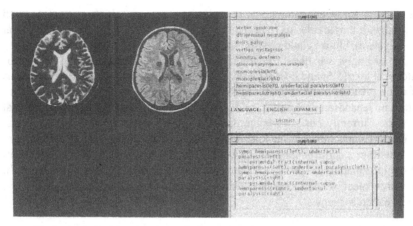

Fig.2. A window for selecting pathologies and the resultant superposed image
of a cross section and the selected organ

plane. Then our tool displays a composed image of nerves and the cross section so
that he can grasp the location of nerves in the selected cross section.

A composed image of surfaces of organs   If a user selects labels or organs which
he want to display, our tool displays the surfaces of the selected organs
simultaneously as in Fig.1. He can recognize the disposition of adjacent organs in the
form of single image and an animation which gives a rotation of organs.

A synthetic image of cross sections and surface images   This image is made by
removing a part of the head surface, pasting cross sections at the cut ends, and laying
marks and/or surfaces of the selected organs on the cut ends. With this image, a user
can imagine the arrangement on the basis of the cut ends or the whole head. Fig.3
shows a cross section and a surface of caudate nucleus.

A composed image of sequential cross sections around a specified point   This
image is made by specifying a point of attention, which may be a point inside a
damaged nerve. Our tool displays a set of sections arranging along three mutually
perpendicular axes whose intersection corresponds to the specified point. Therefore
brain surgeons and radiologists, who are accustomed to diagnose using sectional
images, can readily explore and imagine 3D arrangement of organs by viewing this
image while they move the point of attention. Moreover one can search out the best
slice position for an imaging and a diagnosis. A doctor estimated this tool as a useful
one in clinics for grasping the disposition of the watching organ and others around it.
Fig.4 is an example.

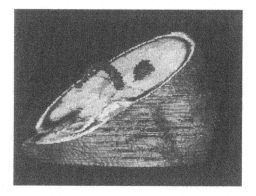

Fig.3. An example of the synthetic images of cross sections and surface images

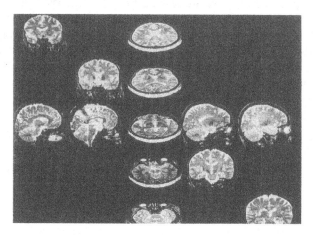

Fig.4. An example of sequential images of cross sections

2.4 Implementation of our system

We implemented our system on a Sun workstation (SPARC station 2 GX), but it does not have sufficient power to display and animate images without any delay, nor can it display a full color image. We will transfer our system to a more powerful computer system. It may be easily done because our system is written in a popular programming language, and uses a user interface widely spread, i.e. C language, X window system and XVIEW library.

3 Conclusions

We have introduced a system which includes a 3D atlas of a central nervous system, a knowledge database of the connections between motor disturbance and damaged motor nerves, and then shown its ability to assist a screening. A user can understand the location of a damaged part precisely if he selects it using the atlas, the database, and the display tool based on patient's pathologies. After the detailed observation with this system, he can obtain images at an appropriate position, and make thorough diagnosis using the appropriate sectional images which are picked up from the heap of images acquired before then. As you can see easily, this system is also applicable to a training of 3D structure of a human head in anatomy and brain surgery. If a user utilizes the atlas as a model of a human head, he will be able to develop a model-driven image processing system which extracts tumors, hematomas, and so on, which hurt or constrict nerves. So we are engaged on this work.

This system leaves something to be desired, while it has a great potential in clinical applications. Nerves in our atlas are rather rough in shape for locating a damaged part more correctly. We must exploit a multi-level resolution, that is, we must divide a voxel through which a thin nerve passes into several small voxels and put labels to them. Currently we are reorganizing the atlas based on the doctor's evaluation. Our system has the knowledge about the nerves of motor systems. It is known that the paraesthesia (sensory disorder) as well as the motor disturbance is one of good clues for a diagnosis. Thus we will improve the power of our system by adding the knowledge about sensory nerves. Our system is not evaluated in clinics. It is necessary for our system to apply to screenings and diagnoses, and then improve it based on the result.

Acknowledgements

We wish to thank our colleagues for discussion and advice. We also grateful to Dr. Jun-ichiro Toriwaki (Nagoya University) for his kind advice.

References

1. Greitz, T., Bohm, C., Holte, S., Eriksson, L.: A Computerized Brain Atlas: Construction, Anatomical Content and Some Applications. Journal of Computer Assisted Tomography Vol.15, No.1 (1991) 26-38

2. Höhne, K.H. et al.: A Volume-based Anatomical Atlas. IEEE Computer Graphics and Applications Vol.12, No.4 (1992) 72-78

3. Japanese version of "Neuroanatomie der kraniellen Computertomographie" (written by Kretschmann, H.J., Weinrich, W., translated by Kuru, Y., Mayanagi, Y.) Igaku-Shoin Ltd. (1986)

4. Japanese version of "The Human Central Nervous System" (written by Nieuwenhuys, R. et al., translated by Mizuno, N. et al.), Igaku-Shoin Ltd. (1983)

5. Sugiura, K.: Understanding of The Central Nervous System by Illustrations Ishiyaku Shuppan Ltd. (1984) (In Japanese)

6. Gotoh, F., Amano, T.,: Functional Neuroanatomy for Clinical Practice. Chugai Igaku Co. (1992) (In Japanese)

A MRF Based Random Graph Modelling the Human Cortical Topography

J.-F. Mangin[1,2], J. Regis[3], I. Bloch[1],
V. Frouin[2], Y. Samson[2] and J. Lopez-Krahe[1]

[1] Département Images, Télécom Paris, 46 rue Barrault, 75634 Paris Cedex 13, France
[2] Service Hospitalier Frédéric Joliot, Commissariat à l'Énergie Atomique, Orsay
[3] Serv. de Neurochirurgie Fonctionnelle et Stéréotaxique, CHU La Timone, Marseille

Abstract. This paper presents a project aiming at the automatic detection and recognition of the human cortical sulci in a 3D magnetic resonance image. The two first steps of this project (automatic extraction of an attributed relational graph (ARG) representing the individual cortical topography, constitution of a database of labelled ARGs) are briefly described. Then, a probabilistic structural model of the cortical topography is inferred from the database. This model, which is a structural prototype whose nodes can split into pieces according to syntactic constraints, relies on several original interpretations of the inter-individual structural variability of the cortical topography. This prototype is endowed with a random graph structure taking into account this anatomical variability. The recognition process is formalized as a labelling problem whose solution, defined as the maximum a posteriori estimate of a Markovian random field (MRF), is obtained using simulated annealing.

1 Introduction

The current revival of the Talairach stereotactic proportional system applied to magnetic resonance (MR) images reflects the need for a precise identification of brain structures in a number of domains of neurology [6]. This need appears especially urgent in the field of human brain mapping, where several programs have been recently initiated in order to create an electronic database of human functional neuro-anatomy which can mediate data communication among a network of laboratories. This need appears also crucial in the current design of increasingly precise neuro-surgical operations. Indeed, the success of micro-surgical techniques depends upon utilizing natural sulcal pathways to gain access to pathologic structures within the brain, while preserving the integrity of healthy adjacent tissues [4, 5]. Unambiguous identification of internal brain structures is possible in high resolution MR images, when the neuro-anatomist is guided by a reference atlas, thanks to a relatively low variability [6]. In return, it turns out to be much more difficult to overcome the high variability of the human cortex, even with sophisticated 3D display interfaces. Indeed, the few studies dealing with this variability are only descriptive [6, 4] and therefore provide no real identification methodology.

This paper describes a project which aims at developing robust and reproducible methods to detect and identify automatically various cortical structures, mainly the sulci (cortical folds) and the dual gyri (cortical regions delimited by sulci). In the context of human brain mapping, main sulci are reliable landmarks to guide atlas deformation or individual definition of volumes of interest. This project consists of three main parts, the last one being addressed in this paper:

1. The design of a robust method allowing the construction of a high level representation (ARG) of the individual cortex topography [2].

2. The constitution of a large database of ARGs in which the main sulci are identified via the labelling of ARG nodes [1, 5].

3. The inference of a generic model of the cortex topography from this database and the design of a method matching this model and any individual cortex.

1.1 ARG Structure: An individual ARG is inferred from the segmentation in simple surfaces (SSs) of the 3D skeleton of the union of cerebrospinal fluid and gray matter. Hence ARG nodes represent mainly cortical folds. ARG relations are of two types: first, SS pairs connected in the skeleton (ρ_T); second, SS pairs delimiting a gyrus (ρ_C) (see Fig.1). An ARG is defined by the 6-tuple $\mathcal{G} = (\mathcal{N}, \mathcal{R}, \sigma_\mathcal{N}, \sigma_\mathcal{R}, \lambda_\mathcal{N}, \lambda_\mathcal{R})$, where: $\mathcal{N}$ and $\mathcal{R}$ are respectively node and relation sets; $\sigma_\mathcal{N} : \mathcal{N} \rightarrow S_\mathcal{N} = \{SS, S_{brain}, \mathcal{P}_{med}\}$ is a function called node syntactic interpreter (S_{brain} and $\mathcal{P}_{med}$ denote respectively brain surface and inter-hemispheric plane); $\sigma_\mathcal{R} : \mathcal{R} \rightarrow S_\mathcal{R} = \{\rho_T, \rho_C\}$ is a function called relation syntactic interpreter; $\lambda_\mathcal{N} : \mathcal{N} \rightarrow E(At_\mathcal{N})$ and $\lambda_\mathcal{R} : \mathcal{R} \rightarrow E(At_\mathcal{R})$ are functions called respectively node and relation semantic interpreters; $At_\mathcal{N}$ and $At_\mathcal{R}$ are sets of semantic attributes describing respectively nodes and relations; $E(At_x)$ is the set of all semantic descriptions using semantic attributes of At_x. A semantic description of $E(At_x)$ is a set of couples (attribute, attribute value), each attribute of At_x appearing at most in one couple. A semantic attribute reserved to instances of only one syntactic type t is noted t-name: $At_\mathcal{N}=\{SS$-size, SS-center, SS-orientation, SS-depth$\}$; $At_\mathcal{R} =\{\rho_T$-length, ρ_T-direction, ρ_C-size$\}$.

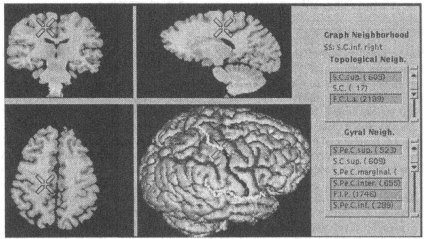

Fig. 1. *A glimpse of the interface allowing navigation in an ARG for the sulcus identification. The black SS (S.C.inf.right) neighborhood is explored. Topological neighbors are displayed in white and gyral neighbors are displayed in dark grey.*

1.2 Anatomical Variability: Unlike the case of monkey, the human cortical anatomy presents large pattern variations between individuals or even between brain hemispheres. Therefore, when trying to develop pattern recognition methods dedicated to cortical sulci, we have first to propose a coherent interpretation of this variability. Pratical results will show the validity or the weakness of this interpretation and will suggest modifications or improvements. The choice of cortical sulcus as landmarks, which may be criticized, relies on a number of anatomical and functional studies from the literature [5, 3]. An interpretation of these studies can be the following: the cortical surface may be viewed as a map of constant functional regions potentially separated by sulci. From this point of view, an individual sulcal topography is necessary a subset of the network of borderlines between these functional regions (the complete network of border-lines can be viewed as a skeleton by influence zones). This interpretation, which is clearly an abstract simplification of reality, will appear formally in our model through the notion of random graph. Another level of variability relies in potential sulcus interruptions. We think that a sulcus interruption occurs when a fiber bundle constituting a functional pathway between the two delimited gyri is especially developed. This variability aspect will be embedded in our model through a grammatical language describing usual sulcus forms in ARGs. Moreover, we have performed a first mapping of the main fiber bundles which leads to a new original description of the cortex anatomy of great help when identifying sulci [5]. We have begun the constitution of a database of labelled ARGs whose nodes are identified according to this description. A label corresponding to a brain structure of the hierarchical description introduced in Fig.2 is attached to each ARG node.

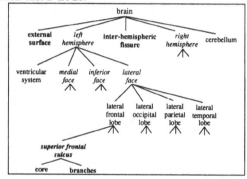

Fig. 2. *A glimpse of the hierarchical description of the cortex anatomy. The full tree will be noted* $\mathcal{A}$. *Bold fonts are used for elements involved in the web grammar describing usual sulcus patterns (see sect. 3). Italic fonts are used for nodes corresponding to random elements with empty realization (see sect. 2).*

2 Structural Framework

In an ideal case (no variability, perfect segmentation), sulcus recognition would just amount to finding an isomorphism between an ARG $\mathcal{G}$ and a structural prototype $\mathcal{P}$ whose nodes correspond to the leaves of tree $\mathcal{A}$ (see Fig.2). Because of all potential deformations of this prototype (node insertion and deletion, node split...), recognition amounts to finding a homomorphism between a subgraph of $\mathcal{G}$ and a subgraph of $\mathcal{P}$. For an accurate management of node insertion, the prototype $\mathcal{M}$ used in the following includes higher level structures of $\mathcal{A}$.

2.1 Random Graph: In order to formalize the different kinds of variabilities described previously, $\mathcal{M}$ is endowed with a structure of random graph (RG). This probabilistic framework provides then a natural adaptive similarity measure between any ARG $\mathcal{G}$ and $\mathcal{M}$: the maximum a posteriori (MAP) estimator. In order to allow node split (sulcus interruptions, branches...), the classical random graph definition proposed by Wong [7] is extended by substituting the monomorphism by a homomorphism (see Fig. 3). A random graph $\mathcal{M}$ is defined on a 4-tuple $(\mathcal{S}_{\mathcal{N}}, E(At_{\mathcal{N}}), \mathcal{S}_{\mathcal{R}}, E(At_{\mathcal{R}}))$ by the couple $(\mathcal{N}^A, \mathcal{R}^A)$ with:
$\mathcal{N}^A$ is a set $\{\alpha_1, \alpha_2, ..., \alpha_n\}$ where each α_i, called a random vertex (RV), is a random variable whose realizations are sets of couples $(s, d) \in \mathcal{S}_{\mathcal{N}} \times E(At_{\mathcal{N}})$;

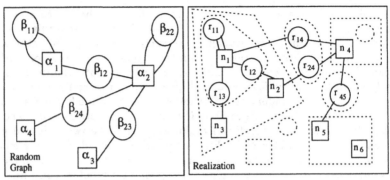

Fig. 3. *RG realization* $(h_\mathcal{N}(n_1)=h_\mathcal{N}(n_2) = h_\mathcal{N}(n_3)=\alpha_1; \ h_\mathcal{N}(n_4)=\alpha_2; \ h_\mathcal{N}(n_5)=h_\mathcal{N}(n_6)=\alpha_3).$

$\mathcal{R}^A$ is a set $\{\beta_{i_1 j_1}, \beta_{i_2 j_2}, ..., \beta_{i_m j_m}\}$ where each β_{ij}, called a random arc (RA), is a random variable whose realizations are sets of relations between elements of the realizations of the RVs α_i and α_j, each relation being described by a couple $(s, d) \in \mathcal{S}_\mathcal{R} \times E(At_\mathcal{R})$.

A realization of the random graph $\mathcal{M}$ is a couple $(\mathcal{G}, h_\mathcal{N})$, where $h_\mathcal{N}$ is a graph homomorphism between the ARG $\mathcal{G}$ and $\mathcal{M}$.

2.2 Random Graph and Set Hierarchy: Given an ARG $\mathcal{G}$, let e_i be the subset of nodes of $\mathcal{N}$ belonging to the brain structure i (element of the tree $\mathcal{A}$ defined in Fig. 2). The set hierarchy described in $\mathcal{A}$ induces naturally a partition of $\mathcal{N} = \bigcup \mathcal{N}_i$, where $\mathcal{N}_i$ is the complementary in e_i of the union of the e_j strictly included in e_i. This partition is composed by two kinds of $\mathcal{N}_i$: those corresponding to leaves of $\mathcal{A}$ and those corresponding to other elements of $\mathcal{A}$. This last subsets of $\mathcal{N}$ regroup nodes that cannot be identified according to the brain structure nomenclature defined by $\mathcal{A}$ leaves. These nodes can only be associated to higher structures in the hierarchy. In the following, we consider each set $\mathcal{N}_i$ as the realization of a RV α_i. The RA set is defined by endowing the underlying random graph $\mathcal{M}$ with a complete graph structure. Hence, we define a RA β_{ii} for each RV α_i, and a non-oriented RA β_{ij} for each pair $\{\alpha_i, \alpha_j\}$ of distinct RVs. A homomorphism $h_\mathcal{N}$ between $\mathcal{G}$ and $\mathcal{M}$ induces a mapping $h_\mathcal{R}$ between $\mathcal{R}$ (relation set of $\mathcal{G}$) and $\mathcal{R}^A$. The labelled ARGs of the database $\mathcal{B}$ are naturally considered as realizations of the random graph $\mathcal{M}$.

3 Markovian Framework

The recognition process is formalized as a labelling problem. A label l_i is associated with each RV α_i of $\mathcal{M}$, the label set being noted $\mathcal{L}$. A labelling l of $\mathcal{N}$ is equivalent to a homomorphism $h_\mathcal{N}$. The recognition will be achieved using the MAP estimator: $\arg \max_l p(l|\mathcal{G})$. This estimator is constructed from a Markovian random field (MRF) model. The main reasons which motivate this choice, which is a key feature of our model, are the following:

1. The contextual information used by a neuro-anatomist to identify a sulcus derives from a confined neighborhood of the sulcus in the brain.
2. The equivalence between MRFs and Gibbs random fields (GRFs) gives a very flexible way to introduce syntactic constraints in a MRF based discrete relaxation sheme which has not been exploited yet.
3. It has been proven that stochastic relaxation schemes like simulated annealing (SA) applied to a Gibbs distribution based MAP have very good

convergence properties.

3.1 Random Field: Let us introduce a few notations:
$\mathcal{L}_B = \{l_i \in \mathcal{L} \mid p(h_{\mathcal{N}}^{-1}(\alpha_i) = \emptyset) \neq 1\}$. Related elements of $\mathcal{A}$ are its leaves, lobes and brain (see Fig. 2). Indeed, during database $\mathcal{B}$ constitution, an ARG node is either identified (leaves) or associated to one lobe (lobes make up a cortex partition) or to the brain (segmentation error, pathology);
l_0, $l_{S_{brain}}$ and $l_{\mathcal{P}_{med}}$ denote respectively labels bound to brain, S_{brain} and $\mathcal{P}_{med}$.
$\mathcal{L}_m = \mathcal{L}_B - \{l_{S_{brain}}, l_{\mathcal{P}_{med}}\}$; $\mathcal{L}_p = \mathcal{L}_m - \{l_0\}$ and $\mathcal{L}_t = \mathcal{L}_B - \{l_0\}$;
$\mathcal{N}_x^A$ and $\mathcal{R}_{xy}^A$ denote respectively the set of RVs related to $\mathcal{L}_x$ and the set of RAs connecting a RV of $\mathcal{N}_x^A$ and a RV of $\mathcal{N}_y^A$ (x and $y \in \{m, p, t\}$);
$S = \{n \in \mathcal{N} \mid \sigma_{\mathcal{N}}(n) = SS\}$.
Since $h_{\mathcal{N}}^{-1}(\alpha_{S_{brain}})$ and $h_{\mathcal{N}}^{-1}(\alpha_{\mathcal{P}_{med}})$ are known, $p(l|\mathcal{G}) = p(l_{|S}|\mathcal{G})$. $l_{|S}$ is considered as the realization of a random field defined on the set of sites S. For $n \in S$, $l(n)$ is a random variable whose realization set is $\Omega_n \subset \mathcal{L}_m$.

3.2 State Space of the Random Field: Introduction of constraints on the localization in a reference frame $\mathcal{D}_{\mathcal{M}}$ (similar to Talairach one [6]) of the realization nodes of the RVs of $\mathcal{N}_p^A$ endowes the random field with the Markovian property. These constraints rely on the attachment of an influence domain $\mathcal{D}_i^{inf}$ to each RV $\alpha_i \in \mathcal{N}_m^A$. The state space Ω of the random field is then defined by:
$\Omega = (\Omega_n)_{n \in S}$, where $\forall n \in S, \Omega_n = \{l_i \in \mathcal{L}_m \mid \lambda_{SS}^c(n) \in \mathcal{D}_i^{inf}\}$, ($\lambda_t^n$ denotes the function which gives the value of the semantic attribute t-*name*; hence λ_{SS}^c refers to the SS-*center* attribute). The $\mathcal{D}_i^{inf}$ of the RVs of $\mathcal{N}_p^A$ are parallelepipedic boxes of $\mathcal{D}_{\mathcal{M}}$ inferred from the database $\mathcal{B}$, and $\mathcal{D}_0^{inf} = \mathcal{D}_{\mathcal{M}}$.

3.3 Markovian Random Field: The random field is a MRF defined on $(S, \Omega, \mathcal{C})$ where $\mathcal{C}$ is the set of cliques involved in the distribution of the equivalent GRF: $p(l_{|S}|\mathcal{G}) = \frac{1}{Z}\exp\{-U(l)\}$, where $U(l)$ is the energy (or Hamiltonian) of the GRF defined by $U(l) = \sum_{c \in \mathcal{C}} V[c](l)$, and Z is a normalization constant. $V[c](l)$ is a potential attached to clique $c \in \mathcal{C}$ whose value depends only on $l_{|c}$.
The set $\mathcal{C}$, defined for a given ARG $\mathcal{G}$, is constituted by five kinds of cliques:
1. Topological cliques, inferred from the graph structure of $\mathcal{G}$:
   (a) $\mathcal{C}_1$ is the set of order one cliques, noted c_n for $n \in S$.
   (b) $\mathcal{C}_2$ is the set of order two cliques, noted $c_{nn'}$ for $(n, n') \in S^2 \cap \mathcal{R}$.
2. Influence cliques, inferred from the RV influence domains:
   (a) $\mathcal{C}_p^{inf}$ is the set of RV influence cliques c_i^{inf} defined by $\forall \alpha_i \in \mathcal{N}_p^A, c_i^{inf} = \{n \in S \mid l_i \in \Omega_n\}$.
   (b) $\mathcal{C}_{pt}^{inf}$ is the set of RA influence cliques, noted c_{ij}^{inf} for $\beta_{ij} \in \mathcal{R}_{pt}^A$ when it exists. RA influence cliques are naturally induced by RV influence cliques. We point out that c_{ij}^{inf} exists only if $p(h_{\mathcal{R}}^{-1}(\beta_{ij}) = \emptyset \mid \Omega) \neq 1$, which holds for a very restricted number of RAs. Otherwise, the random field would not really be Markovian.
3. Grammatical cliques (set $\mathcal{C}^G$) associated to each cortical sulcus. For a sulcus s of the sulcus set $\mathcal{A}_s$, the grammatical clique c_s^G is the union of the two influence cliques bound to the core and to the branches of s (note that a sulcus itself is associated to a RV with empty realization (see Fig. 2)).

3.4 Gibbs Distribution: The random field distribution is estimated from the following decomposition: $p(l|\mathcal{G}) = p(l|\mathcal{G}, \Omega) = p(l|\mathcal{N}, \mathcal{R}, \sigma_{\mathcal{N}}, \sigma_{\mathcal{R}}, \lambda_{\mathcal{N}}, \lambda_{\mathcal{R}}, \Omega)$
$\propto p(\lambda_{\mathcal{N}}, \lambda_{\mathcal{R}}|l, \mathcal{N}, \mathcal{R}, \sigma_{\mathcal{N}}, \sigma_{\mathcal{R}}, \Omega)p(l|\mathcal{N}, \mathcal{R}, \sigma_{\mathcal{N}}, \sigma_{\mathcal{R}}, \Omega) = p_1 p_2$. Probability p_2 is

considered as the probability of a first MRF defined on (S, Ω, C). The energy $U_{str}(l)$ of this MRF will constitute the "structural energy" of the whole random field. In order to estimate probability p_1, the notion of indivisible random graph (IRG) is introduced. An IRG is a RG whose RVs and RAs have realizations of cardinal one or zero [7]. We assume that this "a posteriori" probability of semantic attribute values of a realization of $\mathcal{M}$ is equivalent to the "a posteriori" probability of the semantic attribute values of $\mathcal{M}$ if $\mathcal{M}$ were an IRG. Hence, we attach a set $At[\alpha_i]$ of new semantic attributes to each RV of $\mathcal{N}_m^A$ and a set $At[\beta_{ij}]$ to each RA of $\mathcal{R}_{pt}^A$ [3]. The values of this new semantic attributes are synthesized from the values of the semantic attributes of $\mathcal{G}$ using semantic rules similar to semantic rules of an attributed grammar. We assume that the respective values taken by all these synthesized attributes are independent, which allows to express p_1 as a sum of potentials attached to influence cliques of C which will constitute the "semantic energy" $U_{sem}(l)$ of the whole random field. Hence the product $p_1 p_2$ has the form of a Gibbs distribution of energy $U(l) = U_{str}(l) + U_{sem}(l)$. Therefore, the whole random field is a MRF defined on (S, Ω, C). $U_{str}(l)$ is the sum of an occurrence energy and a syntactic energy. $U_{sem}(l)$ is the sum of a recognition energy and an identification energy.

3.5 Occurrence and Recognition Potentials: These potentials are attached to cliques of C_p^{inf} and C_{pt}^{inf}. They constitute three kinds of potential families. The first kind is associated to RVs of $\mathcal{N}_p^A$, and the two other kinds are associated to sub-RAs of RAs of $\mathcal{R}_{pt}^A$ defined by the following partitions: $\forall \beta_{ij} \in \mathcal{R}_{pt}^A$, $h_{\mathcal{R}}^{-1}(\beta_{ij}) = h_{\mathcal{R}}^{-1}(\beta_{ij}^{\rho_T}) \cup h_{\mathcal{R}}^{-1}(\beta_{ij}^{\rho_C})$, where $h_{\mathcal{R}}^{-1}(\beta_{ij}^t) = \{r \in h_{\mathcal{R}}^{-1}(\beta_{ij}) \mid \sigma_{\mathcal{R}}(r) = t\}$. All the families are constructed according to the same principle. We briefly describe, for instance, the potential family related to a sub-RA $\beta_{ij}^{\rho_T}$, whose contribution to $U(l)$ is weighted by the frequence of occurrence $f_{\rho_T}^{oc}[i, j]$ of a non empty realization of $\beta_{ij}^{\rho_T}$ in the database $\mathcal{B}$. If $h_{\mathcal{R}}^{-1}(\beta_{ij}^{\rho_T}) \neq \emptyset$, occurence potential $V_{\rho_T}^{oc}[c_{ij}^{inf}](l)$ is equal to $-K_{\rho_T}^{oc} f_{\rho_T}^{oc}[i, j]$, where $K_{\rho_T}^{oc} > 0$; otherwise this potential is zero. For each synthesized semantic attribute ρ_T-*Name* of $At[\beta_{ij}^{\rho_T}]$, if this attribute can be synthesized from $h_{\mathcal{R}}^{-1}(\beta_{ij}^{\rho_T})$, the recognition potential $V_{\rho_T}^N[c_{ij}^{inf}](l)$ is a positive function of the attribute value ranging from zero to $K_{\rho_T}^N[i, j] f_{\rho_T}^{oc}[i, j]$, where $K_{\rho_T}^N[i, j] > 0$; otherwise this potential is zero. This function has a basin shape centered around a mean parameter, and with a declivity depending on a variance parameter. These two parameters are estimated from the database $\mathcal{B}$. Constants are chosen according to the following constraint: $\Sigma_{At[\beta_{ij}^{\rho_T}]} K_{\rho_T}^N[i, j] = K_{\rho_T}^{oc}$. Hence, contribution to the global energy of the family constituted by $V_{\rho_T}^{oc}[c_{ij}^{inf}]$ and the different $V_{\rho_T}^N[c_{ij}^{inf}]$ is negative and varies from $-K_{\rho_T}^{oc} f_{\rho_T}^{oc}[i, j]$ to zero.

3.6 Syntactic and Identification Potentials: The global energy includes three other kinds of potentials with positive values. Two kinds introduce syntactic constraints and the last kind manages recognition failure cost.

A. Grammatical potentials: At any step of the relaxation, a sulcus is represented by a subgraph $\mathcal{G}_s$ possibly empty. This subgraph is made up of nodes labelled as belonging to sulcus core or sulcus branches, and of relations between these nodes and with S_{brain} and $\mathcal{P}_{med}$. In order to favour sulcus patterns which respect our interpretation of variability, potentials are attached to grammatical cliques of C^G. A context-free web grammar $G_{\mathcal{G}_s}$, whose terminal set is $S_{\mathcal{N}} \cup S_{\mathcal{R}}$

describes usual patterns of subgraphs corresponding to sulci [3]. For each sulcus s, the grammatical potential $V_G[c_s^G](l)$ is zero if the subgraph $\mathcal{G}_s(l)$ can be parsed by $G_{\mathcal{G}_s}$, otherwise this potential is a rough distance to the language generated by $G_{\mathcal{G}_s}$, namely $K^G n_{cc}(\mathcal{G}_s(l))$, where $K^G > 0$ and $n_{cc}(\mathcal{G}_s(l))$ is the number of connected components of $\mathcal{G}_s(l)$. Since the node set of a subgraph $\mathcal{G}_s$ is already partitioned in two subsets, one for the core and one for branches, the parsing is unambiguous and can be performed with an efficient algorithm.

B. Potts model: A higher level constraint, induced from the hierarchical description of Fig. 2, intends to act on the realization structure of RVs and RAs which are not taken into account by the grammar $G_{\mathcal{G}_s}$. This is achieved using a Potts model (n-class Ising model) whose classes C_i^P are inferred from the partition of the brain in lobes and out of lobes leaves of $\mathcal{A}$. The class C_i^P associated with a lobe is the subset of $\mathcal{L}$ corresponding to RVs whose realizations belong anatomically to this lobe (see Fig. 2). The model expresses itself with potentials attached to cliques of $\mathcal{C}_2$: $\forall(n, n') \in S^2$, if $\exists C_i^P$ with $l(n) \in C_i^P$ and $l(n') \in C_i^P$, then $V^P[c_{nn'}] = 0$, otherwise the potential is equal to K^P ($K^P > 0$).

C. Identification Potentials: Thanks to the linearity of the semantic production yielding the single synthesized semantic attribute of the RV brain (α_0), contribution of this attribute can be decomposed in potentials attached to cliques of $\mathcal{C}_1$. $\forall n \in S$, if $l(n) = l_0$, $V^{int}[c_n] = K^{int}\lambda_{SS}^s(n)$, where $K^{int} > 0$; otherwise the potential is zero. Hence the cost of a full failure of the recognition process for a given SS increases linearly with the SS-size attribute value.

4 Conclusion

First recognition experiments using SA (Gibbs sampler) have been performed with the five first ARGs of database $\mathcal{B}$ with very satisfying results as regard the main sulci identification. The increase of $\mathcal{B}$ size will allow the study of the model hyper-parameter influence. This paper shows that the MRF framework provides an appealing way to combine syntactic and semantic constraints in a relaxation based recognition process relying on a structural prototype potentially subject to various kinds of deformations. The flexibility of the proposed construction principle with regard to the modelling of anatomical variability calls for adaptations to other similar recognition problems in the field of medical imaging.

References

1. V. Frouin, J.-F. Mangin, J. Regis, and B. Bendriem. A 3D editor of the cortical sulcal topography. In *7th. IEEE Comp. Based. Med. Syst., Winston Salem*, 1994.
2. J.-F. Mangin, V. Frouin, I. Bloch, J. Regis, and J. Lopez-Krahe. Automatic construction of an attributed relational graph representing the cortex topography using homotopic transformations. In *SPIE Mathematical Methods in Medical Imaging III, San Diego*, vol. 2299, pages 110–121, July 1994.
3. J.-F. Mangin, J. Regis, I. Bloch, V. Frouin, Y. Samson, and J. Lopez-Krahe. Modélisation structurelle de la topographie corticale: un graphe aléatoire fondé sur un champ markovien. Technical Report D016, Télécom Paris, 1994.
4. M. Ono, S. Kubik, and C. D. Abernethey. *Atlas of the Cerebral Sulci*. Georg Thieme Verlag, 1990.
5. J. Regis. Deep sulcal anatomy and functional mapping of the cerebral cortex (in french). MD Thesis, Université d'Aix-Marseille II, 1994.
6. J. Talairach and P. Tournoux. *Co-Planar Stereotaxic Atlas of the Human Brain. 3-Dimensional Proportional System: An Approach to Cerebral Imaging*. Thieme Medical Publisher, Inc., Georg Thieme Verlag, Stuttgart, New York, 1988.
7. A. K. C. Wong and M. L. You. Entropy and distance of random graph with application to structural pattern recognition. *IEEE PAMI*, 7:599–609, 1985.

Combining "Vertical" and "Horizontal" Features from Medical Images

Fred L. Bookstein

University of Michigan, Ann Arbor, Michigan 48109 USA

Abstract. Landmark points, when they can be located reliably over a sample of medical images, serve both to generate a feature space of biometric "shape variables" and also to specify an unwarping by which variation of pixel values associated with displacements of the landmarks can be corrected with respect to all landmarks simultaneously. There thus arise two separate spaces of descriptors, the "horizontal" and the "vertical." Combinations of features from this pair of spaces for prediction or discrimination can be visualized in one or the other space alone by injecting precisely calibrated crosstalk between these channels. This essay analyzes a set of brain images in this way to highlight the effect of schizophrenia upon anatomy in the midsagittal plane.

1 Introduction

The focus of computer vision extends beyond artifacts of human engineering; it incorporates as well the more natural classes that correspond to biomedical processes and clinical medical decisions. The procedures for classification that seem promising in this context typically refer not to the matching of templates within certain tolerances but instead to quantitative tools for the apprehension of natural biological variation. These tools, collectively called *biometrics*, originated a hundred years ago in the effort to found evolutionary inference upon measurements of living organisms. Over the intervening century the toolkit has expanded into a remarkably protean and sturdy adjunct to the logic of measurement across a great variety of natural sciences, from astronomy through physical anthropology—the "applied multivariate statistics" that you surely encountered in graduate school.

It may be helpful to carry analyses of this spirit, techniques for combining measured variables into composites that characterize the structure or function of whole organic systems, over to the considerably more discrete and Boolean domain of classic digital image processing. This paper pursues one such possibility: intentionally biasing the output of image analyses so as to incorporate, as it were by miscalibration, the additional predictive power of the missing biometric information for whatever task is at hand. There are partial precedents for this sort of analysis in various ad-hoc approaches to statistical analysis of samples of medical images. In Friston's "statistical parametric mapping," from a series of images presumed in adequate register (e.g., a time series on an unmoving subject), some conventional statistical parameter is produced pixel by pixel—a t-statistic within groups, a spectral analysis—and that statistic, whether scalar or vector, is then visualized as a picture in the same pixellated coordinate system, its pixels clustered into regions, etc. Regarding these tactics there is a growing literature reviewed, for example, in the chapters of Thatcher et al., eds., 1994.

To the underlying geometry of such pictures, which these simple registrations treat as invariable, correspond new, specialized biometric tools pertaining to the geometric descriptors arising out of classical comparative anatomy: sizes, shapes, and positions of the apparently discrete "parts" composing the organism. The methods suggest that information about form be encoded in *landmark configurations*, sets of discrete geometric points that can be reasonably claimed to correspond biologically across the images of a data set. Most of my work over the last decade has been devoted to the construction of one particular method for this analysis, an unexpected marriage between one technique for shape description and an apparently unrelated technique for parametric deformation. In the resulting protocol, the unwarping transformation, while highly nonlinear in the space of the original pixels, is rigorously linear in the space of landmark shape descriptions, and thus shares many properties with the more familiar sorts of "adjustment" that proceed by analysis of covariance or other linear models. I propose to combine this "horizontal" information with the sort of "vertical" analysis with which we are already familiar, **as applied, however, to the unwarped pictures only**, those that have already been horizontally registered throughout the image using whatever landmarks have been supplied by one's collaborators or by the algorithm they have trained.

The methods sketched here are not aimed at the task of detecting particular features as "absent" or "present" in single images. Nor can they easily handle the task of ascertaining whether a feature extracted separately, such as a convex blob, is "normal" or "abnormal." We need two or more classes each having a central tendency in feature space, not just one class and its complement. For the linear techniques here to predict from image to some criterion, characteristic points and the associated curves or blobs must already be known to correspond across the forms of a data set. Such knowledge, which lies at the core of the "atlas problem," is not easy to acquire or even to formalize; its accrual incorporates centuries of comparative anatomy. The most strenuous demand upon the scientist is that the training set be *biometrically homogeneous*, adequately characterized by the means and the covariance structure of all image features and criteria of the study. Such assurances are obviously not matters of theorem or algorithm.

But once all the assumptions are granted and all the prior knowledge is in place, my suggestion here becomes a simple, perhaps obvious, combination of image manipulations already familiar separately. A somewhat related technique arose in exploratory multivariate statistics in the 1970's: "Chernoff faces," intentional distortions of an anthropomorphic cartoon to convey aspects of any data set regardless of its actual domain. Another antecedent is the work at the University of North Carolina dealing with anisotropic diffusion. In the algorithms of Steve Pizer and his colleagues and students, aspects of picture content or its spatial derivatives are used to alter that content prior to a definitive analysis of the single scene. (But thus far the UNC group have emphasized the imitation of human visual processing. While a fascinating scientific project, this is not likely to be the most suitable model for criterion-driven biometric analysis per se.)

Many other groups are pursuing the production of averaged images, the representation that will here be called the "vertical." Rigorous attempts to this end likewise date back to the dawn of biometrics in the nineteenth century. Complementary to the splined unwarping demonstrated here are the approach via a hierarchy of cross-correlations (Evans's group at McGill) and the approach via diffusion of one image over another (Grenander, Miller, and their students). The method of intentional crosstalk (this paper) could apply as well to deformations generated in any of those other formalisms, so long as the corresponding "horizontal" descriptors could be developed into biometrically effective shape variates.

2   A horizontal-vertical data analysis

The example here deals with a small data set of 25 midsagittal brain images to be analyzed in detail elsewhere. As exemplified in Figure 1, these are single parasagittal images selected as "most midsagittal" after synthesis from coronal MR imaging at a standardized pulse sequence. Thirteen of the images are of patients diagnosed schizophrenic (on the basis of behavioral checklists only, without access to these images) while the other twelve are of medical students and staff. The images were selected by Dr. John DeQuardo, Adult Psychiatry Unit, University of Michigan Hospitals, who also located the thirteen landmarks shown in the figure. In itself this congeries is not a statistically representative sample of anything. Subsequent studies must carefully attend to gender, age, race, patient drug history, and behavioral symptoms. Also, it would be more useful to carry out the analysis in fully three dimensions. Neither of these design flaws affects the argument here, which concerns image analysis, not schizophrenia.

Figure 2 shows the averaged unwarped images for the normals (at left) and the schizophrenics (right), each superposed over its Procrustes-averaged mean landmark configuration (see also Figure 4). These images were produced by a publicly distributed software package, Edgewarp, that has been described in detail elsewhere (Bookstein & Green, 1994).

Begin the discriminatory analysis vertically, with the pixelwise difference image (Figure 3) of the two frames in Figure 2, left minus right, after the right side has been further unwarped to the landmark locations on the left. Even after contrast enhancement, one barely sees the contours on which the original landmarks had been located. Instead, a new feature arises, the crescent along the inner (ventricular) margin of the corpus callosum, which clearly appears "whiter" (that is, less often cerebrospinal fluid, more often neural tissue) in the normals than in the schizophrenics. It is easy to interpret this as greater thickness of the callosum in the normal subsample—but that is a horizontal description, premature until we have examined horizontal aspects of the data already collected. The straight line

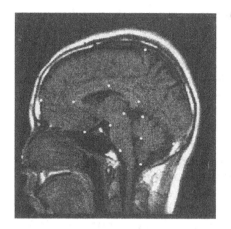

Figure 1.

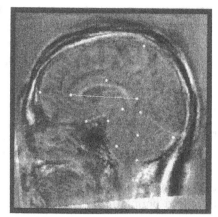

Figure 3.

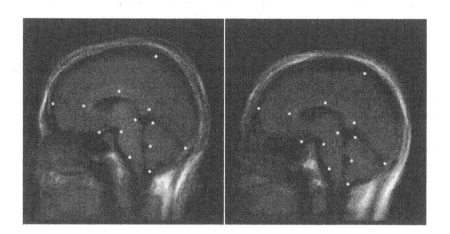

Figure 2.

that has been added to the graphic overlay, transect across the long diameter of the corpus callosum, will concern us presently.

Biometric analysis of landmark variation begins with the composite scatter at the left in Figure 4: the range of shapes after each form is translated, rotated, and scaled onto the sample average. This is the celebrated *Procrustes superposition*. This landmark configuration appears to be very well-behaved, so that the group means (at right) are representative of their central tendencies. Dots signify the mean registered landmark positions for normals; triangles, the same for schizophrenics, after a threefold exaggeration of their difference.

Regional features of the shape difference encoded in Figure 4 may be localized with the aid of a supplementary graphic, the *thin-plate spline* interpolating the landmark rearrangement (Bookstein, 1991). A square grid is put down over the mean normal form and warped by a certain optimal transformation that maps landmarks onto landmarks. See Figure 5, in which, corresponding to the right-hand graphic in Figure 4, that deformation has been magnified threefold. A region of strenuous deformation is visible here corresponding to the upper part of the cerebral aqueduct. The dominant visual feature of this complex is the primarily vertical extension representing the divergence of group differences between splenium and colliculus (Figure 4). The discrepancy corresponds to a change of mean scaled distance by about 10% between the groups, and is statistically significant. Take the scaled distance between these landmarks as a representative "horizontal" variable image by image.

To sharpen the vertical analysis we extract an informative subset of the pixels in Figure 3, those (totalling 90 in number) along the callosal diameter on the graphic overlay. The transects are normalized separately to range from 0 to 1 (cerebrospinal fluid to solid callosal tissue) and averaged again within groups. Figure 6 shows the right third of these averages—solid line for normals, dashed line for schizophrenics. The brightening we already saw in Figure 3 emerges here as the vertical shift of the curves about 15/90 of the way from right to left endpoint. The contrast is the same as the clear shape difference of the spleniums in Figure 2, but is expressed vertically. The difference between the group mean transects over this region is likewise statistically significant. Take the area under the curve between pixels 15 and 18, where the difference is greatest, as a representative "vertical" variable image by image.

We now have two discriminators of group difference: one horizontal (the landmark separation, suggested in Figure 4), the other vertical (the sum of four normalized pixels suggested in Figure 6). The scatter in Figure 7 combines them in a single scatterplot. Clearly we can do better by a projection upon the long axis of this plot than along either horizontal or vertical axis separately. This projection corresponds to the appropriately weighted average of the two partial predictors along the axes; our task is to construct that weighted average as a new composite feature in one or the other domain alone. It will prove easiest to combine them by an additional horizontal distortion prior to a vertical re-averaging.

Attend again to Figure 6, and abstract the region of interesting group dif-

189

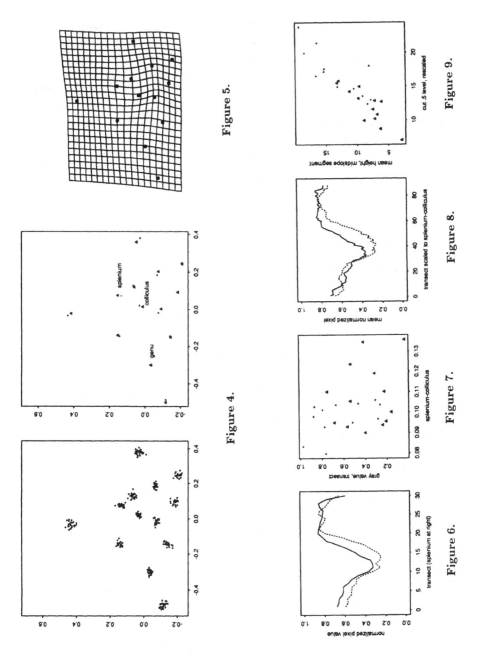

Figure 5.

Figure 4.

Figure 9.

Figure 8.

Figure 7.

Figure 6.

ference (positions 15 – 18 on the horizontal axis) as a parallelogram. The confounded discriminator we seek will, in effect, increase the area of this parallelogram. As the pixel values averaged here are already normalized to range 0–1, it is more reasonable to execute the expansion horizontally. We need to manipulate the *horizontal* discriminator from Figure 4, the distance from splenium to colliculus, in order to introduce intentional crosstalk—a *horizontal* adjustment of about two pixels—in the feature here. As the mean distances differ by about 10%, a division by that difference corresponds to a change of about 1.5 pixels at a distance of 15 pixels from splenium, just about the "adjustment" we seek. To achieve this intentionally confounded predictor, then, the transects of callosal diameter ought to be rescaled to the distance splenium-*colliculus* rather than the distance splenium-*genu*.

Figure 8 displays the averages of these variously stretched transects under the fiction that their re-indexed pixels remain vertically aligned. *These averages have no longer arisen from any unwarping.* The difference between them over the interesting region is now more substantial, corresponding to a statistical signal along the diagonal of Figure 7 rather than one or the other axis. The corresponding group separation is shown in the vertical axis of Figure 9. (Again, dots signify normal cases, and triangles, schizophrenics.)

There is a rhetorical difficulty, however, in expressing exactly what this discriminator is: "averaged pixel value along a transect from splenium to genu indexed according to distance from splenium to colliculus" makes rather little sense as it stands. But there is another choice still available: we can interpret this new discriminator horizontally instead. The point at which the renormalized transect cuts the .50 level can be taken as the location of the new "edge landmark" shown in the inset here. There is already a (horizontal) language available for this oddly mixed construction, in which

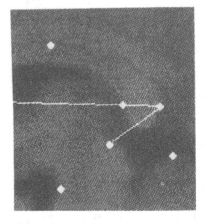

one point is pushed around with respect to a baseline of two others both held fixed: what we have produced is one *shape coordinate* for the triangle formed by splenium, colliculus, and this new landmark. Operationally the discriminator (plotted horizontally in Figure 9) is the ratio of this splenium width to the distance from splenium to colliculus—a very simple measure, although unfamiliar. As Figure 9 shows, the discrimination it affords is just a little better than that using the area under the renormalized curve. Bookstein (1995) demonstrates how a return to the original image data produces this landmark much more accurately by a new round of digitizing. (In reality, the transect shown in Figure 3 sometimes cuts across the fornix. A human operator can interpolate the intended point a great deal more accurately in these cases by considering pixels upon adjacent lines.)

3 Concluding remark

From the somewhat unpromising materials in Figure 2 we have arrived at a quite serviceable discriminator, Figure 9, expressible as a single novel shape variable (along the horizontal axis). To achieve this insight we exploited the interplay between vertical and horizontal descriptors in many different ways. First, each landmark set was transformed by a similarity atop the Procrustes average in Figure 4. Still horizontally, each image was unwarped to those group averages, while a purely horizontal feature of that comparison (divergence of the splenium-colliculus segment) was duly noted. The unwarped images were averaged vertically, and the averages compared by a vertical subtraction, Figure 3. A new vertical feature, Figure 6, was generated by horizontal subsetting of Figure 3, vertically renormalized (to unit range), then re-averaged. Figure 7 suggested combining these two separate discriminators; we chose to do so by a horizontal modification of Figure 6 that could be interpreted either vertically (Figure 8) or horizontally (Figure 9 and preceding inset).

The midsagittal plane in schizophrenia is likely not the only scientific context to which these intertwined maneuvers might be turned. Biometric methods have been crafted over a century of studies of natural variability. Medical image analysts could take better advantage of this well-understood toolkit to enormously simplify the decisions implied by these remarkably rich but exceedingly redundant records of form.

Acknowledgement. Preparation of this contribution was supported in part by NIH grants DA–09009 and GM–37251 to Fred L. Bookstein. The former grant is jointly supported by the National Institute on Drug Abuse, the National Institute of Mental Health, and the National Institute on Aging as part of the Human Brain Project. The Edgewarp program package was developed by William D. K. Green; it can be accessed by anonymous FTP from the **pub/edgewarp** directory on **brainmap.med.umich.edu**. All statistical graphics in this paper were produced in the Splus package available from MathSoft, Inc., Seattle.

References

Bookstein, F.: *Morphometric Tools for Landmark Data.* New York: Cambridge University Press, 1991.

Bookstein, F.: Landmarks, averaging, and the scientific uses of medical images. Submitted to Y. Bizais et al., eds., *Information Processing in Medical Imaging 1995.*

Bookstein, F., Green, W.: Edgewarp: A flexible program package for biometric image warping in two dimensions. In R. Robb, ed., *Visualization in Biomedical Computing 1994.* SPIE *Proceedings*, volume 2359, 1994, pp. 135–147.

Thatcher, R., Hallett, M., Zeffiro, T., John, E., Huerta, M., eds.: *Functional Neuroimaging: Technical Foundations.* Academic Press, 1994.

Registration

3D Multi-Modality Medical Image Registration Using Feature Space Clustering

André Collignon, Dirk Vandermeulen, Paul Suetens, Guy Marchal

Laboratory for Medical Imaging Research*
Katholieke Universiteit Leuven, Belgium.
Department of Electrical Engineering, ESAT,
Kardinaal Mercierlaan 94, B-3001 Heverlee.
Department of Radiology, University Hospital Gasthuisberg,
Herestraat 49, B-3000 Leuven.

Abstract. In this paper, 3D voxel-similarity-based (VB) registration algorithms that optimize a feature-space clustering measure are proposed to combine the segmentation and registration process. We present a unifying definition and a classification scheme for existing VB matching criteria and propose a new matching criterion: the entropy of the grey-level scatter-plot. This criterion requires no segmentation or feature extraction and no a priori knowledge of photometric model parameters. The effects of practical implementation issues concerning grey-level resampling, scatter-plot binning, parzen-windowing and resampling frequencies are discussed in detail and evaluated using real world data (CT and MRI).

1 Introduction

3D multi-modality image registration is a prerequisite for optimal planning of complex radiotherapeutical and neurosurgical procedures. For instance, in radiotherapy planning, the anatomy of the target lesion, usually a soft tissue structure, can best be delineated on magnetic resonance (MR) images, while the electron density map of a CT is needed to calculate the isodose distribution. The specificity of diagnosis can be improved by combining the anatomical information depicted in CT or MR with functional information extracted from emission tomography.

In the past many 3D registration algorithms have been proposed (see [1], [11], [14] for reviews). They can be categorized into: 1) stereotactic [18] or external-marker-based, 2) anatomical-point-landmark-based, 3) surface-based, and 4) VB registration.

Since our work focusses on automatic registration algorithms that can be applied retrospectively, we have excluded algorithms of the first and the second type from our research scope.

Our experience with surface-based registration algorithms ([6] - [4]) leads us to the following conclusions:

---

* Directors: André Oosterlinck & Albert L. Baert

1. Comparison with stereotactic registration has shown that the registration accuracy for real world data, especially when MRI is involved, may be worse than subvoxel due to inaccurate scanner calibration, image distortions and segmentation differences.

2. Completely automatic surface-based registration algorithms require robust surface segmentation algorithms, which are highly data and application dependent. This problem has been tackled by Neiw [12] for CT/MRI/PET, by Mangin [10] for MRI/PET and by van Herk [17] for CT/CT, CT/MRI and CT/SPECT. However, the reliable estimation of the registration error remains an unsolved problem because the "ground truth" is unknown or the "golden standard" is in error itself whenever real world data are involved.

In our work we look for a fully automatic solution and therefore it is an absolute requirement that the accuracy is such that it is impossible to detect the registration error by visual inspection. This can not be guaranteed by a straightforward application of surface-based registration without increasing the robustness of the surface-based matching criterion against errors that will inevitably be introduced by violation of the rigid body assumption (due to image distortion and inaccurate scanner calibration) and by violation of the surface correspondence assumption (due to the different structural image content of different modalities and due to segmentation errors). The robustness of surface-based matching algorithms can be increased by including corresponding pairs of anatomical landmark points, which increases interactivity. Alternatively, one can design outlier treatment methods to eliminate conjectured outliers from the matching evaluation. However, they have not proven to be successful yet [4].

A conceptually different approach to increasing the robustness of automatic registration algorithms is to re-engineer the matching criterion and combine the segmentation and registration process by using VB matching criteria. Voxel-similarity-based matching criteria are measures of misregistration that are functions of the attributes (e.g. grey-level, gradient, texture) of all pairs of corresponding voxels from the images to be registered at a given misregistered position.

Using all voxels is much more constraining than using surface voxels alone, and therefore we expect VB matching criteria to be more robust than surface based criteria. These considerations leave us with the problem of selecting appropriate features and designing a corresponding matching criterion.

Therefore, in the next section we present a brief review and classification of existing VB matching criteria. In Sect. 3 we propose a new matching criterion: the entropy of the multi-modal grey-level scatter-plot. In Sect. 4 we analyse the new matching criterion by looking at its behaviour in function of the registration parameters in the neighbourhood of a stereotactic registration solution for CT and MR images. In [5] we observed that such analyses reveal the influence of the choice of interpolation method used for grey-level resampling. In this paper we also analyse the effects of binning and Parzen-windowing of the grey-level scatter-plot. In Sect. 5 these measurements are interpreted, and in the final chapter some conclusions are formulated.

2 Voxel Similarity Based Registration Algorithms

3D multi-modality medical image registration involves two types of sensor transformations: 1) geometrical (rotation, translation, and scale), and 2) grey-level (CT-to-MR, MR-to-PET, etc.) transformations. While in surface-based registration algorithms grey-level transformations are used only implicitly during segmentation of the surfaces, in VB matching criteria geometric correspondence is modeled implicitly by the rigid body registration assumption.

Let α be an n-tuple of registration parameters - six due to the rigid body assumption and three more to allow for scaling corrections. Let s be the coordinates of the elements of the image grid of one image (the reference image), and let s' be the coordinates of the other image (called the floating image because it will be transformed to resample the reference image for all registration parameter values at which the matching criterion is evaluated during the registration process). Then, if T_α is the geometric transformation relating the image voxel coordinates and (V, V') are the grey-level transformations relating voxel grey-levels $g_R(s)$ and $g_F(s')$, a VB matching criterion optimizes the following:

$$m(\alpha) = f\left(\ \{(a,b) \mid a = V(g_R(s')) \wedge b = V'(g_F(s)) \wedge \forall s, \exists s' = T_\alpha(s)\}\ \right). \quad (1)$$

This general definition of *voxel-similarity* covers a broad collection of matching criteria. This definition also highlights the design problems of VB *matching criteria*: 1) some form of interpolation of voxel grey-levels will be needed to obtain corresponding voxel grey-levels (g_R, g_F) by resampling the reference image, 2) a consistent procedure is needed to account for changes in non-overlapping parts in the images due to changes in the registration parameters α, 3) an appropriate selection of features (V, V') needs to be made, and 4) a global similarity function $f(\{(a,b)\})$ needs to be designed.

The design of a complete VB *registration algorithm* also requires the selection of an appropriate optimisation algorithm in function of the selected matching criterion. Ideally, the optimisation strategy should not affect the registration accuracy. Therefore, in this paper we will focus on the comparison of VB *matching criteria* only.

We have classified existing VB matching criteria into two classes in terms of the complexity of the features used.

1. **0-th Order Image Intensity Based:** V and V' are simple one-dimensional grey-level transformations. The grey-level transformations V and V' relating grey-levels of corresponding voxels of images from different modalities are non-linear and not one-to-one, and thus cross-correlation and its Fourier versions fail when applied to the untransformed grey-levels.

   (a) Gerlot-Chiron and Bizais [8] assume that the histogram $H(T_\alpha, d)$ of the difference image d contains a peak corresponding to registered pixels. Their "Region Overlap" (RO) criterion aims at maximizing the number of registered pixels in d, which it achieves by maximizing the peak area in the difference histogram using a gaussian matched filter.

(b) The algorithm proposed by Woods [19] is based on the idealised assumption that if two images are accurately aligned, then the value of any voxel in one image is related to the value of the corresponding voxel in the other image by a multiplicative factor R. There is a single value of R for all intensity values. In practice, he minimises the "variance of intensity ratios" (VIR) to guarantee optimal uniformness for R. He applied it symmetrically for PET/PET, and non-symmetrically for PET/MRI matching.

(c) Hill et al [9] have investigated several measurements of features space dispersion, the most successful of which they found to be the VIR between voxels of selected tissues. So, they re-implemented Woods's work, but introduced additional flexibility by allowing the calculation of the variance over any combination of groupings (or bins) of denominator image intensity values. They applied the generalized algorithm to the matching of CT and MR. Hill also presents results he obtained minimising a 1D third order moment of the feature space scatter-plot on MR/MR and MR/CT data sets.

(d) Van den Elsen [16] has recently proposed to minimize or to maximize cross-correlation between an MR image and the corresponding CT after the application of a delayed ramp mapping and a triangular intensity mapping respectively.

2. **Higher Order Image Intensity Based:** $V(g)$ represents differential image intensity information, or more general $V(g)$ is a feature characterizing voxel neighbourhoods instead of single voxels. Van den Elsen et al [15] performed cross-correlation of "ridgeness" images using a scale-space based definition of image ridges and applied it to CT/MR matching.

Hill et al [9] describe the dispersing character of the feature space scatter-plot during misregistration. The VB matching criteria reviewed above can all be compared by looking at the driving or "clustering" forces that they generate to counteract the dispersion phenomenon. The analogy with mechanical forces can be made by considering the matching criteria to be potential functions from which the forces can be derived by taking the gradient. The clustering forces in the RO criterion are restricted in direction to minus unit slope lines in the scatter-plot. The VIR criterion apply vertical (and in the symmetric case also horizontal) clustering forces only. In the generalized VIR criterion proposed by Hill the clustering forces can be restricted to a subset of the scatter-plot. Using cross-correlation for $f(\{(a,b)\})$ both van den Elsen's grey-level and ridgeness matching criteria generate clustering forces that are directed toward one of the diagonals of the scatter-plot of the transformed grey-levels and the ridgeness feature respectively.

We believe that all of the above mentioned restrictions on the directions of the clustering forces are heuristics which we prefer to eliminate. Instead we propose to have the clustering forces depend on the data alone. In a first attempt to do so we tried statistically modeling the normalized scatter-plot. We performed a case study [5] in which we interactively outlined parts of distinct regions t of the brain (skull, soft tissue, background, skin and fat) in CT and MR images from which we determined their grey-level statistics (vector mean $\mu(t)$ and variance $\sum(t)$) in the 2D multi-modality grey-level scatter-plot. Using these statistics to define Gaussian feature space probability distributions $N\left(\mathbf{G}(s); \mu(t), \sum(t)\right)$ we traced two new candidate matching criteria: 1) the "number of unlabeled voxels" according to a set of labeling thresholds applied to the Mahalanobis distance, and 2) the "geometric mean maximum likelihood labeling probability" based on the same Gaussian distributions. The advantage of both criteria is that the clustering forces that they invoke are pointed to the $\mu(t)$ which are determined by the data. The disadvantage is that a "photometric model" ($\mu(t)$ and $\sum(t)$) needs to be determined which requires user interaction.

In general, we call "photometric model" any 0-th order image intensity model, and we refer to any higher order model as a "scene model". In the next section we present a new VB matching criterion that does not require any user interaction for the specification of its photometric model and that does not introduce any artificial constraints on the clustering forces.

3 Entropy of Multi-Modal Scatter Plot Histogram

While Hill based his choice of the third order moment of the feature space scatter-plots on a list of detailed observations of such scatter-plots when moving them away from the registration solution (obtained by point landmark based registration), a new 0-th order image intensity based matching criterion is presented here based 1) on the information theoretic consideration that the entropy of a random variable is a measure of the information required on the average to describe it [13], and 2) on the general observation that misregistration diffuses the multi-modal grey-level distribution. Since diffusion of the grey-level scatter-plot corresponds to an increase in the information required to describe it, we propose to use the entropy of the scatter-plot of image intensities as a matching criterion since we expect it to be minimal in the registered position. Formally:

$$\alpha^* = \arg \min_\alpha \left(-\sum_s p(g_R(T_\alpha s), g_F(s)) \log \left[p(g_R(T_\alpha s), g_F(s)) \right] \right) \quad (2)$$

where $p(g_R(\alpha), g_F)$ is obtained by normalizing the scatter-plot into a probability distribution.

Solving (2) requires the calculation of $p(g_R(\alpha), g_F)$. However, since the number of possible pairs of (g_R, g_F) (e.g. 4096*4096 for 12 bit images) is larger than the number of samples that are available in the multi-modal image (e.g. 256*256*128 for full 3D MRI images), robust induction of $p(g_R(\alpha), g_F)$ is not trivial. In principle this can be solved by parzen-windowing [7]. In practice, because it is much faster to implement and to execute, and because it reduces memory consumption, we have chosen to perform simple binning of the image grey-levels in order to reduce the number of possibilities. Binning has been performed uniformly by neglecting the least significant bits, i.e. $p(g_R, g_F) \approx$

$\frac{H(g_R>>n_R, g_F>>n_F)}{N}$ where $H(g_R >> n_R, g_F >> n_F)$ equals the binned version of the scatter-plot $H(g_R, g_F)$, N equals the number of voxels taken into account in the estimation of $p(g_R, g_F)$, n_R and n_F are the number of bits neglected in the respective images.

In principle what needs to be proved for any matching criterion is that: 1) for a wide range of unregistered positions around the true registered position, 2) the matching function is uni-modal, 3) and the optimum of the function should be located at the registered position. In practice, at best, matching criteria can be evaluated by looking at traces of the matching function.

4 Experiments and Results

The data consist of a 12 bit, 39 slice (256 x 256) CT image, a 12 bit, 30 slice (256 x 256) T2-weighted MR image, and the same MR image after gadolinium enhancement (MRE), all having $(1.33 \times 1.33 \times 4)$ mm^3 voxels. The images contain stereotactic localisation marks, and can thus be registered fairly accurately. As a matter of fact, both MR images were registered by acquisition while the CT image is only shifted and not rotated with respect to the MR images. This shift however involves subvoxel translations in all three directions. Note that all measurements shown hereafter have been performed using a 30 slice CT image acquired by trilinearly resampling the original CT image on the image grid of the MR images. Since we will be looking at the effect of resampling algorithms this should be kept in mind. In order to avoid the overlap problem only part of the floating images is considered by deliberately eliminating all voxels within 20 voxels from the image boundaries.

Figures 1, and 2 present traces for rotations of the MRE volume relative to the CT volume about the axis perpendicular to the image slices ranging from -12 to +12°, while Fig. 3 presents traces for medial-lateral translations of MRE relative to MR ranging from -2 to 2 cm. All entropy traces in the figures have been normalized for optimal use of figure space. Figure 1 shows the influence of the type of interpolation used for resampling the reference images (nearest neighbour, trilinear, and cubic convolution). Figure 2 shows the influence of the resolution of the sample s relative to that of the data. These traces were obtained using 'all voxels' (46656 in number), by in-plane 'sub-sampling' (1 sample in 3 voxels in both directions), and by in-plane 'super-sampling' (10 samples in 3 voxels in both directions). Figure 3 demonstrates the problem of image grid interference and shows the effects of parzen-windowing and super-sampling on this problem. It should be remarked that the traces were calculated taking into account voxels from the central slice only, so, essentially 2D. We have chosen to do so after we found out that the behaviour of the 3D and the 2D traces was the same which saves us a lot of computer time.

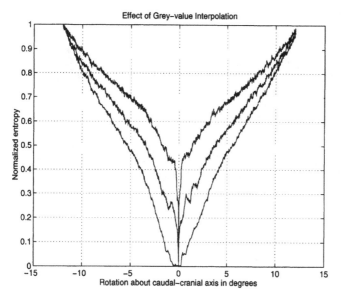

Fig. 1. Normalized entropy traces in axial rotation space for CT/MRE volume pair around the stereotactic reference solution. The traces have been obtained using nearest neighbour (bottom), linear (middle), and cubic convolution interpolation (top) respectively. Nearest neighbour interpolation has a flat minimum. Its size is determined by the sampling resolution. The higher the order of the interpolation, the sharper is the minimum, that precisely coincides with the stereotactic reference, and the 'noisier' the local behaviour. No parzen-windowing, 'all voxels', and $(n_R, n_F) = (2, 2)$ were used. The range of grey-values is 4092 for the CT volume, and 3580 for the MRE volume.

5 Discussion

Figure 1 clearly shows that nearest neighbour interpolation tends to find the best fit of the image grids and is inherently less accurate. The ringing effect in the close neighbourhood of the registration solution that is clearly visible for trilinear interpolation disappears with super-sampling. The opposite happens when combining super-sampling and nearest neighbour interpolation. Currently, we believe trilinear interpolation to offer the best compromise between speed and accuracy.

Figure 2 shows that the trace for super-sampling has its minimum slightly off from the stereotactic reference. There are two possible causes for this deviation. Either the stereotactic ground truth is in error, or one of the assumptions underlying the derivation of our entropy matching criterion is not satisfied, e.g. the rigid body registration assumption is probably in error due to small image distortions.

The translation traces in Fig. 3 are more complex due to large interpolation effects. Trilinear interpolation introduces ripples with a frequency that equals the grid spacing in the direction of the translation. Super-sampling considerably

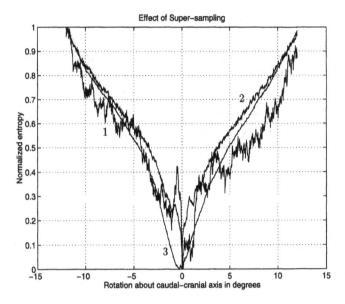

Fig. 2. Normalized entropy traces in axial rotation space for CT/MRE volume pair around the stereotactic reference solution. The traces have been obtained using: 1) sub-sampling (1/3 sample/voxel), 2) all voxels (1/1 s/v), and 3) super-sampling (10/3 s/v) respectively. Both the scale and the amplitude of the 'noise' on the traces decrease with increasing sampling ratio. $(n_R, n_F) = (2, 2)$.

reduces this artefact. Parzen-windowing did not have the effect that was hoped for, i.e. the ripple effect is only slightly reduced.

6 Conclusion

We have classified and reviewed VB matching criteria by looking at the complexity of the features used, and the heuristic constraints used to determine feature space clustering forces. We have shown the entropy of the scatter-plot to be the simplest possible criterion that introduces no such heuristic constraints.

From the experiments we may conclude that if the entropy of the grey-level scatter-plot is calculated using super-sampling on a rectangular grid with trilinear grey-level interpolation then traces of the rigid body rotation and translation parameters are well-behaved minimisation functions for registration of CT and MR. From the experiments we can not determine the critical super-sampling resolution. Super-sampling renders the use of binning and/or parzen-windowing superfluous. Binning can be used though to reduce memory requirements.

Acknowledgements

This work is part of COVIRA (Computer Vision in Radiology), project A2003

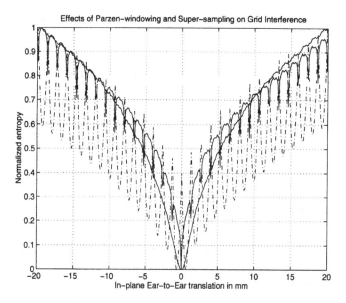

Fig. 3. Normalized entropy traces in medial-lateral translation space for MR/MRE volume pair around the stereotactic reference solution. These traces have been obtained using plain linear interpolation (dashed), linear interpolation combined with parzen-windowing, and linear interpolation combined with super-sampling (10/3 s/v) (ragged). In the abscence of relative rotation, and due to interference of image grids (MR and MRE have identical grids), the entropy matching criterion shows a relatively large periodic ripple, which is reduced by parzen-windowing, but even more by super-sampling. $(n_R, n_F) = (2, 2)$. The range of grey-values is 3357 for the MR volume.

of the AIM (Advanced Informatics in Medicine) programme of the European Commission.

The software was developed on an IBM RS/6000 workstation using xlC C++. Graphics were created with MATLAB 4.2a from The MathWorks, Inc.

We are grateful to Petra van den Elsen and Derek Hill for sending us their work in press.

References

1. Brown L.G.: A Survey of Image Registration Techniques. ACM Computing Surveys 24:4 (1992) 325-376
2. Collignon A., Vandermeulen D., Suetens P., Marchal G.: Surface based registration of 3D medical images. SPIE Int'l Conf. Medical Imaging 1993: Image Processing, 14-19 februari, 1993, Newport Beach, California, USA. SPIE **1898** (1993) 32-42
3. Collignon A., Vandermeulen D., Suetens P., Marchal G.: An Object Oriented Tool for 3D Multimodality Surface-based Image Registration. Computer Assisted Radiology, CAR93, 24-26 juni, 1993, Berlin, 568-573

4. Collignon A., Vandermeulen D., Suetens P., Marchal G.: Registration of 3D Multi-Modality Medical Images Using Surfaces and Point Landmarks. Pattern Recognition Letters **15** (1994) 461-467

5. Collignon A., Vandermeulen D., Suetens P., Marchal G.: Automatic Registration of 3D Images of the Brain Based on Fuzzy Objects. SPIE Int'l Conf. Medical Imaging 1994: Image Processing, 13-18 februari, 1994, Newport Beach, California, USA. SPIE **2167** (1994) 162-175

6. COVIRA, Computer Vision in Radiology: Deliverable 55, D5/2.5 - Demonstration of Final Pilot System for Conformal/Stereotactic Radiotherapy Planning. AIM Programme Project A2003 of The European Commission DG XIII, April 1994

7. Duda R.O., Hart P.E.: Pattern Classification and Scene Analysis. Stanford Research Institute, Menlo Park, CA, USA, A Wiley-Interscience Publication (1973)

8. Gerlot-Chiron P., Bizais Y.: Registration of Multimodality Medical Images Using Region Overlap Criterion. CVGIP: Graphical Models and Image Processing **54**:5 (1992) 396-406

9. Hill D.L.G., Studholme C., Hawkes D.J.: Voxel Similarity Measures for Automated Image Registration. SPIE Int'l Conf. on Visualization in Biomedical Computing, October 4-7, 1994. SPIE **2359** (1994) in press

10. Mangin J.-F., Frouin V., Bloch I., Bendriem B., J. Lopez-Krahe: Fast nonsupervised 3D registration of PET and MR images of the brain. Journal of Cerebral Blood Flow and Metabolism **14** (1994) 749-762

11. Maurer C.R., Fitzpatrick J.M.: A Review of Medical Image Registration. Interactive Image-Guided Neurosurgery, Maciunas R.J. (Ed), Park Ridge, IL, American Association of Neurological Surgeons (1993) 17-44

12. Neiw H.M., Chen C-T., Lin W.C., Pelizzari C.A.: Automated three-dimensional registration of medical images. SPIE Int'l Conf. Medical Imaging V: Image Processing, California, USA. SPIE **1445** (1991) 259-264

13. Shanmugam K.S.: Digital and Analog Communication Systems, University of Kansas, John Wiley & Sons (1979)

14. Van den Elsen P.A., Maintz J.B.A., Pol E.J.D., Viergever M.A.: Image fusion using geometrical features. SPIE Int'l Conf. on Visualization in Biomedical Computing, 1992. SPIE **1808** (1992) 172-186

15. Van den Elsen P.A., Pol E-J.D., Viergever M.A.: Medical Image Matching - A Review with Classification. IEEE Engeneering in Medicine and Biology Magazine **12**:1 (1993) 26-38

16. Van den Elsen P.A., Pol E.J.D., Sumanaweera T.S., Hemler P.F., Napel S., Adler J.R.: Grey value correlation techniques used for automatic matching of CT and MR brain and spine images. SPIE Int'l Conf. on Visualization in Biomedical Computing, October 4-7, 1994. SPIE **2359** (1994) 227-237

17. Van Herk M., Kooy H.M.: Automatic three-dimensional correlation of CT-CT, CT-MRI, and CT-SPECT using chamfer matching. Med. Phys. **21**:7 (1994) 1163-1178

18. Verbeeck R., Vandermeulen D., Michiels J., Suetens P., Marchal G.: Computer Assisted Stereotactic Neurosurgery. Image and Vision Computing **11**:8 (1993) 468-485

19. Woods R.P., Mazziotta J.C., Cherry S.R.: MRI-PET Registration with Automated Algorithm. Journal of Computer Assisted Tomography **17**:4 (1993) 536-546

Registration of Non-Segmented Images Using a Genetic Algorithm

Jean-José Jacq and Christian Roux

Département Images et Traitement de l'Information Télécom Bretagne,
Laboratoire de Traitement de l'Information Médicale
Technopôle de Brest Iroise, B.P. 832 - 29285 Brest-Cédex - France
E-mail JJ.Jacq@enst-bretagne.fr,Christian.Roux@enst-bretagne.fr

Abstract. The proposed method aims at solving the global 3–D automatic non–rigid registration problem of two volume datasets coming from the same modality without any segmentation. The tested algorithm combines a voxel based approach with an optimization procedure carried out by a simple genetic algorithm. The method is based on the search for the polynomial warping model which minimizes a L_1 distance between two volumes datasets. To avoid prohibitive computational cost, the genetic algorithm uses a stochastic fitness function which operates on randomly selected measure sites in neighbourhoods of contours, with an adaptive search space scaling scheme. Application of the method is made to the elastic registration of 3–D CT volumes and gives good results in a reasonable processing time.

1 Introduction

The registration of two different 3–D images defined on a regular lattice is a very general and basic issue in medical imaging. Registration models including non–rigid deformations leads to consider a high dimensional search space which, in turn, involves a high computational cost. Usual approaches are based on a geometric description of the information. They involve complex and sophisticated 3–D segmentation procedures, which quality strongly influences the registration accuracy. Nevertheless, if the datasets come from the same modality, a simple voxel based approach can be carried out without any segmentation; it consists in finding a global polynomial warping that minimizes a distance between the two 3–D datasets. The high number of parameters involved in such a model prevents us from an exhaustive search for the solutions. In order to reach the global solution in the search space, this approach requires a very efficient optimization algorithm. Such an approach based on a genetic algorithm has been proposed in 1984 for the 2–D case and applied to angiographic images [1]. An improvement can be achieved by considering only a stochastic subsampling of the dataset while evaluating the distance associated with one point of the search space [2]. In [3] such a method is presented in the case of the registration of two consecutive DSA images, where stochastic subsampling operates on a map describing the neighbourhoods of the major contours. This paper presents an extension of the previous approach to the case of 3–D images. In addition, we propose to perform a reduction of the search space after each global iteration, which leads to a succesive refinement of the location of the optimal solution.

The used genetic algorithm is restricted to a simple one, containing only the basic operators and based on a simple use of them. Such an algorithm reduced to essentials allows us a simpler way to evaluate the overall performance of the method.

2 Warping model

We will assume that the registration transform between the two images can be modeled by a polynomial warping. In the 3–D case, such a model can be expressed as:

$$\begin{cases} x_1 = \sum_{p=0}^{n} \sum_{q=0}^{m} \sum_{r=0}^{l} a_{p,q,r} x_0^p y_0^q z_0^r \\ y_1 = \sum_{p=0}^{n} \sum_{q=0}^{m} \sum_{r=0}^{l} b_{p,q,r} x_0^p y_0^q z_0^r \text{ with } \quad p+q+r \leq J \\ z_1 = \sum_{p=0}^{n} \sum_{q=0}^{m} \sum_{r=0}^{l} c_{p,q,r} x_0^p y_0^q z_0^r \end{cases} \quad (1)$$

where $(x_1, y_1, z_1) = T(x_0, y_0, z_0)$ denotes the transformed positions of site (x_0, y_0, z_0) of the reference image. Since we aim at implementing the registration of two 3–D structures showing noticeable morphological variations, the linear case $(J = n = m = l = 1)$ must be extended at least to the trilinear one $(J = 3; n = m = l = 1)$. The corresponding search space has 24 dimensions. With such a direct equation (1), it is not easy to express the bounds of each of the 24 dimensions of the search space. The transformed locations of eight reference points enable an indirect description of the involved transformation. A bound associated with each of the reference points permits to describe easily the sub–space in which the search procedure operates. Let $X_0(x_0(i), y_0(i), z_0(i)), i = 1, , 8$ be the coordinates of the eight reference points and $X_1(x_1(i), y_1(i), z_1(i))$ be their transformed coordinates. Denoting by M the transformation matrix deduced from X_0, Y_0, Z_0, the tranformed vectors X_1, Y_1, Z_1 are given by:

$$\begin{cases} X_1 = M(X_0, Y_0, Z_0)A \\ Y_1 = M(X_0, Y_0, Z_0)B \\ Z_1 = M(X_0, Y_0, Z_0)C \end{cases} \quad (2)$$

Such a geometric model is simple and general. However, higher order polynomials can produce numerical instability due to truncation of higher order coefficient. The estimated model can also exhibit spurious oscillations in informationless areas. It is straightforward to obtain a 2–D model from the 3–D case, by simplifying the former equations.

3 Basic principles of the genetic algorithm

A genetic algorithm (GA) is a global stochastic optimization procedure which uses the properties of the evolution of natural systems. The algorithm acts on an iterative way by allowing parallel evolution in a population of N individuals. Each individual represents a point of the search space. It is represented by a string or chromosome, which is composed of a list of L features or genes. The list of the features represents a coding of the characteristics of a string. The appropriateness of the various individuals (the tentative solutions) to the environment (the criterion) is reached through a fitness function, which gives a performance value to the string. The choice of the coding scheme, as well as the definition of the evaluation function are the only issues to be addressed when dealing with a specific optimization problem. The basic principle of a GA (figure 1) is to let the population evolve by recombining on a random way chromosomes two by two (it is the crossing–over operator), and by modifying, still on a random way, the features of a chromosome (it is the well–known mutation). At each step, the selection of the N individuals is carried out by emphasizing the survival of the most fitted individuals resulting from the previous iteration. Three kinds of operators are involved in a genetic algorithm: selection, crossover and mutation. Successive applications of these operators let evolve the population with a constant number of individuals for one generation to another. Hence the major topics of the used genetic algorithm are generics, we will describe briefly the basics operators. An extensive study can be found in [4].

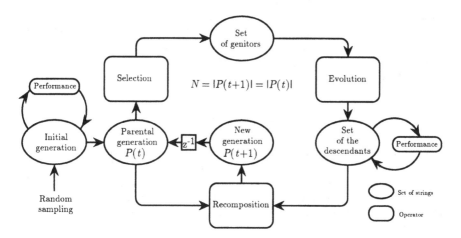

Fig. 1. Basic Genetic Algorithm

The goal of selection is to build the set of genitors, in such a way that the most fitted chromosomes are most likely to survive through reproduction. The fundamental rule consists, for a chromosome which performance is equal to the mean of the fitness value of parental generation, of selecting, on the average, one sample among the reproduction step. The set of the genitors is formed on a stochastic way by a serie of N successive samples in the parental set. The basic principle of the selection operator assumes that the fitness is an increasing positive function. Thus, a rescaling has to be applied that transforms the raw performance given by the fitness function into a corrected performance actually used in the selection process. But it is also necessary to limit the deviation between the offsprings of respectively the most fitted and the less fitted chromosomes. These constraints can be included in a linear rescaling transformation [5], applied to the raw performance and parameterized by a dynamic range α. This dynamic range can be seen as the competition rate between individuals of the parental generation for the selection. As a consequence, a too fast domination of the most fitted individuals, and in the same time, a premature convergence on a local extremum, is avoided.

In a classical genetic algorithm, the two evolution operators are used sequentially (crossing-over and then mutation). By recombining schemes, the crossing-over operator emphasizes the emergence of better solutions. A random permutation of the N selected chromosomes permits to form a series of $\frac{N}{2}$ couples of progenitors. Each of the $\frac{N}{2}$ couples are considered successively: they undergo a crossing-over according to a probability related to the crossing-over rate pc.The crossing point is randomly selected according to a uniform law ($L - 1$ opportunities).

The mutation operator is applied uniformly to the complete population. The genes of all the chromosomes are considered consecutively: for each of the $N.L$ genes, the current value is modified according to a probability defined by the mutation rate pm.

Once the former step has been performed, the parental generation and the new generation are recomposed in order to form the population of individuals for the next iteration of the genetic algorithm. In the simplest case, this operation is reduced to the substitution of the parental generation by all the offsprings.

4 Adaptive search space scaling

Each parameter is quantified on b bits, which results in a length of 24.b bits for the overall string. The parameter encoding is obtained by a random permutation of the 2^b states of the binary code. In our implementation the bottleneck of the genetic algorithm is the fitness function, thus, only a fraction of the reference VOI (Volume of Interest) is considered: M measures sites are used to determine the L_1 distance. These sites are chosen randomly in a map of discriminant sites, obtained from a rough segmentation of the reference VOI. To offset subsampling, the M sites are replaced before each iteration of the genetic algorithm. Therefore, the performance function will have a stochastic behaviour; the solution estimated from the last iteration cannot be issued from the most fitted string since it has only a high performance value with respect to a sole set of M sites. The retained solution is the vectorial mean of the N solutions described by the last genetic iteration. Table 1 summarizes the application procedure.

At a higher hierarchical level, an iterative implementation of the registration procedure is used in order to reduce the search space by a progressive refinement of the solution. The heuristic rule we propose, is based on the comparison of the first two moments of the actual distribution of the estimated solution at the last

Table 1. One global iteration of the application procedure

Data
• distortion model (trilinear)
• boundaries of the search space
• parameters of the genetic algorithm, further parameters
• number of trials t_m , number of considered points in the search space N
Initialization
• description sites $(x_0(i), y_0(i), z_0(i)), i = 0, ..., 7$
• $t = 0$
• compute $M^{-1}(x_0, y_0, z_0)$
• extraction of the discriminant sites in the reference image
• random sampling of K measure sites
• random sampling of N chromosomes (strings) - first generation
• compute the raw performance of each string using the measure sites
While $t \le t_m$, Do
• Compute the corrected performance of the parental generation
• Selection of N strings in the parental generation
• Evolution (crossing-over, mutation)
• Estimation of the raw performance of the new generation:
• Random sampling of the K measure sites
• Compute the raw performance: (elementary L_1 distance to each pair of matched points,corresponding performance) of each string using the measure sites (decoding of the string $\rightarrow$ translation to apply to $(x_0(i), y_0(i), z_0(i)) \rightarrow T(t)$).
• Recomposition
Final Solution
• average of the solutions pertaining to the last generation.

iteration to those corresponding to a uniform distribution on the same interval [6].When the standard deviation of the estimated solution is close to the one of the uniforma law, the interval remains practically unchanged.

5 Application to the registration of non-segmented images

Parameters setting used are : $\alpha = 0.75$, $N = 500$, $pc = 0.8$, $pm = 0.001$, $b = 8$, $K = 500$, recomposition mode is set to full replacement. First experiments show that the tuning of the parameters is not that critical. Stability of the method is experimentally demonstrated in the 2–D case [6]. For each global iteration, the genetic algorithm produces 100 generations, which ensures, in the tested applications, the convergence of the algorithm. A study of the influence of the parameters, specially N,K and the number of generations, would certainly lead to a more efficient use of the genetic algorithm [2]. The proposed method was applied, first to pair of artificially distorted images according to a predefined transform. Such simulations allowed us to evaluate the behavior of the method and to assess the accuracy of the results. The registration (figure 2) is applied to a volume data $(V1)$ set containing one extremity of a humerus bone. A 3–D elastic distortion is applied to $V1$. The corresponding volume $V1$ is considered as the reference volume with respect to the registration procedure. The simulated transform corresponds to a spiral (helicoidal deformation with a compression along the axis of the helix), with major distortions on the side of the humeral head. The registered volume is obtained after 5 global iterations and displayed with maximization and minimization over the reference volume. It shows a similar shape in both cases, which leads to conclude that the estimated solution is close to the global optimum. Further iterations would however give more information regarding the accuracy of the registration. Since the proposed registration algorithm does not require any segmentation, the visual assessment must make use of a direct volume rendering algorithm; such a rendering technique works without explicit segmentation. In order to obtain a simultaneous projection of two or more 3D–functions defined on different regular grids, a specific tool has been developped [7]. This tool is an extension of a standard direct volume rendering technique; such an approach models the data through a density emitters cloud; the computation of the overall contribution of the emitters relies on the radiative transport theory. The major step of the rendering process involves material mapping on 3D–functions values basis; the fundamental parameter is the optical depth (or optical density) per unit length for each material. Simultaneous rendering of 3D–functions requires some ad hoc rules; the simplest ones are maximization or minimization; these can be applied before material mapping (on physical density) or after material mapping (on optical density). Applicability of the algorithm in the case of two different datasets showing an unknown transformation has been demonstrated in [8]. With the used parameters, 100 generations of the genetic algorithms used in the 3–D registration process are performed in 130 sec on a DEC Station 3000–500 (ALPHA) under OpenVMS.

6   Conclusion

A registration approach based on polynomial warping and taking into account non-rigid deformations (24 degrees of freedom) has been developped and applied at voxel level to volume datasets. One of the main features is that the method operates on non–segmented volume data. The results obtained in different experiments lead us to conclude to the accuracy, the stability and the efficiency of the method. Although the basic problem of estimating higher order geometrical tranforms in 2 and 3–D space is highly complex, the stochastic use of a simple genetic algorithm enables us to obtain acceptable results within reasonable computer time on a sequential workstation. At the geometric level, a different approach can be followed, in which the registration is decomposed into several local registration problems performed locally on a mosaïc of patches. A careful evaluation of the results in terms of accuracy and complexity of both strategies (global and local) should conclude to an appropriate compromize.

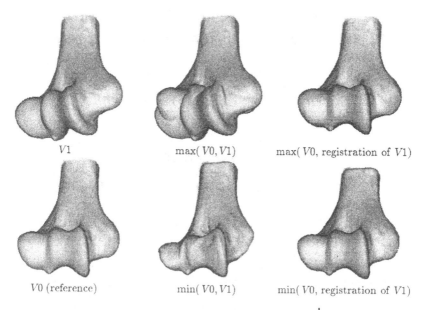

$V1$ max($V0, V1$)   max($V0$, registration of $V1$)

$V0$ (reference)   min($V0, V1$)   min($V0$, registration of $V1$)

Fig. 2. Elastic 3–D registration of humerus bones [†]

References

1. Fitzpatrick, J.M., Grefenstette, J.J.: Image registration by genetic search. Proceeding of IEEE Southeast conference (1984) 460–464.
2. Fitzpatrick, J.M., Grefenstette, J.J.: Genetic algorithms in noisy environments. Machine learning **3** (1988) 101–120
3. Jacq, J.J., Roux, C.R.: Registration of successive DSA images using a simple genetic algorithm with a stochastic performance function. Proceeding of 19th IEEE Northeast Bioengineering Conf., Newark. NJ (1993) 223–224
4. Goldberg, D.E.: Genetic algorithms in search, optimization, and machine learning. Addison–Wesley. (1989)
5. Bramlette M.F.: Initialization, mutation and selection methods in genetic algorithms for function optimization. Proceeding of the fourth international conference on genetic algorithm, San Diego. (1991)
6. Jacq, J.J., C. Roux: Recalage mono–modalité automatique en imagerie médicale 2D et 3D l'aide d'un algorithme génétique traditionnel. Actes du 9ième congrès Reconnaissance des Formes et Intelligence Artificielle. (1994) 109–120
7. Jacq, J.J.: Rendu volumique direct multi–objets. Implantation et application en imagerie médicale. Internal Report. ITI department. Telecom Bretagne. (1994)
8. Jacq, J.J., C. Roux: Automatic registration of 3D images using a simple genetic algorithm with a stochastic performance function Proceeding of EMBS'93 (1993) 90–91

[†] CT scan data were provided by the University Hospital of Brest, France. Thanks to the help of Drs. Ch. Lefévre, D. Colin and E. Stindel.

Anatomy-based Registration
for Computer-integrated Surgery

Ali Hamadeh[1], Stéphane Lavallée[1], Richard Szeliski[2],
Philippe Cinquin[1], Olivier Péria[1]

[1] TIMC - IMAG
IAB, Faculté de Médecine de Grenoble, 38 706 La Tronche, France
e-mail : Stephane.Lavallee@imag.fr
[2] Digital Equipment Corporation, Cambridge Research Lab
One Kendall Square, Bldg. 700, Cambridge, MA 02139

Abstract. In Computed-integrated Surgery (CIS), the registration between pre- or intra-operative images, anatomical models and guiding systems such as robots or passive systems is a crucial step. In our methodology, rigid or elastic transformations are estimated using non-linear least-squares minimization of euclidean distances computed on data that can be 3D surfaces or 2D projections. This paper shows the variety of results that is achieved with this framework on several clinical applications.

1 Introduction

In Computer-integrated Surgery (CIS) , the registration of the whole information available for a given patient is an essential step [TLBM95]. See [Lav95] for a review of standard methods. Several kinds of data may have to be registered :

- *Pre-operative data:* medical images such as CT, MRI, TEP, SPECT, ... or models, such as brain atlases (usually the basis for the surgical planning).
- *Intra-operative data:* medical images provided by low-cost systems (X-rays, echography, microscopes or endoscopes), or positioning information provided by various sensors (optical, ultrasonic, mechanical, or electro-magnetic 3D localizers, range imaging systems). Guiding systems that can be passive 3D localizers or active robots have also to be registered with the images on which the surgical planning has been defined and updated. For that purpose, the guiding systems have often to be calibrated with intra-operative sensors, which are in turn registered with the whole information.
- *Post-operative data:* similar to pre-operative data. They have to be registered to measure the efficiency of an intervention and to update the models.

A typical application will have to register pre-operative CT images with a 3D passive or active manipulator during surgery [LST+94]. In most of standard registration techniques used in CIS, material structures such as reference pins or balls have to be fixed to the patient. For several years, our group has been working on the concept of anatomy-based registration, according to which some reference anatomical structures of the patient provide sufficient features for registration. See [Lav95, LSB95] for a description of our methodology.

2 Registration method

In this section, we briefly present the algorithms that enable us to register a 3D surface model S with various sensor data. For all these algorithms, it is necessary to precompute and store a 3D distance map associated with the 3D surface model S. This distance map is a function that gives an approximation of the minimum signed euclidean distance $\tilde{d}$ to the 3D surface model S from any point q inside a bounding volume V that encloses S. This signed distance function is positive for a point located outside the surface S and negative for a point located inside it. Therefore, the zero of the 3D distance function gives a unique implicit representation of S. The distance map that we use is built from just a collection of 3-D points lying on the surface S and it is represented by an octree-spline which is a 3D adaptive and continuous distance map whose resolution increases near the surface, see [LSB91] for more details.

Rigid 3D-3D registration algorithm

In most of applications, the 3D model is the result of a segmentation procedure applied to MRI or CT images of a reference structure and sensor data can be represented by a collection of 3D points obtained through segmentation of a second series of 3D images (CT, MRI,...), through manual digitization of surface points (e.g., using an optical pointer), through 2.5D ultrasound image segmentation, or through range image acquisition.

In this case we look for the rigid transformation $\mathbf{T}(\mathbf{p})$, that depends on a 6-components vector $\mathbf{p}$ (3 translation components and 3 Euler angles), between the surface S known in Ref_{3D} and a set of M_P points $\mathbf{q}_i$ known in Ref_{sensor} (we make the assumption that most of the points $\mathbf{q}_i$ match to the surface). We look for the parameters p that minimize an error function given by the sum of squares of distances between the surface S and the 3D sensor points transformed by $\mathbf{T}(\mathbf{p})$ in the 3D reference system. The criterion to minimize is:

$$E(\mathbf{p}) = \sum_{i=1}^{M_P} \frac{1}{\sigma_i^2} [e_i(\mathbf{p})]^2 = \sum_{i=1}^{M_P} \frac{1}{\sigma_i^2} [\tilde{d}(\mathbf{T}(\mathbf{p})\,\mathbf{q}_i, S)]^2. \tag{1}$$

where $\tilde{d}(\mathbf{T}(\mathbf{p})\,\mathbf{q}_i, S)$ is the minimum signed distance between the surface S and the data point $\mathbf{q}_i$ transformed by $\mathbf{T}(\mathbf{p})$ in the 3D reference system. σ_i^2 is the variance of the noise of the measurement $e_i(\mathbf{p})$. The minimization of the error function is performed using the Levenberg-Marquardt algorithm [PFTV92]. Robust estimation is also performed by simply removing the outliers exceeding a given threshold and starting again new series of iterations.

Rigid 3D-2D registration algorithm

Sensor data may be also 2D X-ray or video projection images that have to be registered with a 3D surface model [LS95]. To perform such 3D-2D registration, the first step is to use the result of sensor calibration to calculate in Ref_{sensor} the projection lines L_i associated with some pixels P_i that lie on the external contour of the projections of the reference structure. We then use a least-squares formulation similar to the previous one, except that the criterion (1) is now replaced by:

$$E(\mathbf{p}) = \sum_{i=1}^{M_P} \frac{1}{\sigma_i^2} [\tilde{d}_l(l_i(\mathbf{p}), S)]^2, \tag{2}$$

where $\tilde{d}_l(l_i(\mathbf{p}), S)$ is the minimum, along the projection line $l_i(\mathbf{p})$, of the distance, computed in the octree-spline distance map, to the surface S. $l_i(\mathbf{p})$ is the result of transformation $\mathbf{T}(\mathbf{p})$ applied to the projection line L_i.

Non-rigid 3D-3D registration algorithm

The data can also correspond to a structure slightly different from the model (e.g., registration of a patient's brain with an Atlas, or tracking of deformations). For such non-rigid registration, we extend the rigid 3d-3d registration algorithm by a significant modification of the transformation $\mathbf{T}$. Instead of 6 parameters, we have now hundreds of parameters $\mathbf{p}$ that describe the transformation between Ref$_{3D}$ and Ref$_{sensor}$. Although we match surfaces, we represent the deformation as a volumetric transformation, that is represented by a second octree-spline. The coarsest level of the deformation encodes the global (e.g., affine) transformation between the two surfaces, while finer levels encode smooth local displacements which bring the two surfaces into closer registration. A 3D displacement vector is associated with each corner of each cube of the octree-spline built on the 3-D data points. The xyz coordinates of all these vectors constitute the parameters we are looking for. For any point $\mathbf{q}_i$ in Ref$_{sensor}$, the transformed point $\mathbf{r}_i = \mathbf{T}(\mathbf{q}_i; \mathbf{p})$ is computed in Ref$_{3D}$ by interpolating the displacement vectors located at the corners neighboring the point $\mathbf{q}_i$. Therefore, the parameters $\mathbf{p}$ can be seen as the coefficients of an adaptive 3-D spline. The energy that we minimize in this problem is given by :

$$E(\mathbf{p}) = \sum_{i=1}^{N} \frac{1}{\sigma_i^2} [d(\mathbf{r}_i, S)]^2 + \mathcal{R}_m(\mathbf{p}), \tag{3}$$

where $d(\mathbf{r}_i, S) = d(\mathbf{T}(\mathbf{q}_i; \mathbf{p}), S)$ is the minimum Euclidean distance from the point $\mathbf{r}_i$ to the model surface S. Compared to equation (1), we have added a regularization term $\mathcal{R}_m(\mathbf{p})$ that makes the problem well posed (the solution is unique). This term is a combination of 0th and 1st order stabilizers that tend to minimize and smooth the amount of deformations. The minimization of this energy is much more complex than the previous one, and the use of the Levenberg-Marquardt algorithm now requires to solve a very large sparse system. Therefore, we have chosen to use a single step of preconditioned conjugate gradient descent using also hierarchical basis preconditioning techniques to make this process converge faster [SL94].

3 Results of registration algorithms in various clinical cases

MRI-CT registration using 3D scalp surface

In this application the scalp surface of a patient has been segmented on both MRI and CT images . The 3D-3D registration algorithm is applied on these two surfaces. The convergence takes only one second on a DEC-alpha workstation. Once this registration has been performed, for each MR image, the corresponding resliced CT image is computed and superimposed as we can see on Fig. 1.

The application of the same algorithm for SPECT/MRI registration using an intermediary Range Imaging Sensor is also presented in [PLC$^+$93].

Registration using a manual digitization of surface points.

Using an optical 3D localizer makes it possible and easy to collect a set of surface points manually. For example, during an operation on spine, a surgeon can acquire some surface points lying on the posterior part of the vertebra. These points are registered with a CT surface model of the same vertebra. The overall accuracy is better than 1mm. This technique helps the surgeon drill a trajectory which has been defined on pre-operative CT images. Fig 2 shows the algorithm convergence between 3D surface points of a vertebra and the 3D surface model of this vertebra. This technique has been applied for open spine surgery on 6 patients [LST$^+$94].

Registration using an ultrasound probe (2.5D ultrasound pointer)

It is also possible to replace a simple 3D digitizing probe by an ultrasound probe to acquire 3D data points during an operation. The idea is to measure the position of the ultrasound probe in space by adding a sensor on top of a standard ultrasound probe. On each image, some points that lie on the edge of a reference structure such as a bone are segmented, and this process is repeated for several images. The result is a set of 3D points in Ref$_{sensor}$, arranged in pieces of planar curves. The whole system that encompasses the ultrasound image digitization and segmentation is named *2.5D ultrasound pointer*. Such data can be registered with a 3D surface model as in previous examples. This technique has been successfully used for percutaneous spine surgery [BTML93] and for patient positionning in external radiotherapy [TMB$^+$94] (see Fig. 3).

Registration of a 3D Surface with 2D projections.

The technique of 3D/2D registration has been tested on vertebra and skull surfaces interactively segmented on a pair of calibrated X-rays and semi-automatically segmented on CT data. Independant error measurements were obtained for both cases: less than 1mm for the vertebra, 2mm for the skull. This method has been technically validated for percutaneous spine surgery [SCLT92]. Fig. 4 shows the results obtained on a skull.

3D-3D elastic registration between two faces

To demonstrate the local non-rigid matching, we use two different sets of range data acquired with a Cyberware laser range scanner. In their initial positions, the data sets overlap by about 50% and differ in orientation by about 10° (Fig. 5a). Here, the octree spline distance map is computed on the larger of the two data sets (**george1**), and the smaller of the two data sets is deformed (**heidi**). After 8 iterations of rigid matching and 8 iterations of non-rigid affine matching, the registered data sets appear as in Fig. 5b. We then perform 8 iterations at each level of the local displacement spline for 1 through 5 levels. The octree spline has a total of 5728 cubes for a total of about 17000 degrees of freedom. Even with our large number of parameters, the algorithm converges very quickly, because it is always in the vicinity of a good solution (a typical iteration at the finest level takes about 2 seconds). From Fig. 5c, we see that the two data sets are registered well, except for the eyebrows.

4 Conclusions

In this paper, we have presented the application of quite simple registration techniques that we developed in the past five years for the domain of Computer-integrated Surgery. We have shown on real examples that a methodology based on distance minimization between anatomical reference structures can be used efficiently with many different types of data (3D images, range images, 3D points digitized manually, 3D points extracted on 2.5D ultrasound images, X-ray projections, models). All the results presented in this paper were obtained in a few seconds on DEC-Alpha workstations. The accuracy required for the specific applications was obtained in all cases.

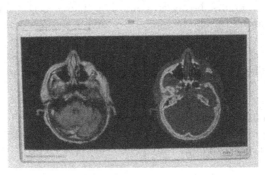

Fig. 1. superimposition of MRI and resliced CT images after rigid 3D-3D registration using the scalp surface. The result is visually perfect.

References

[BTML93] C. Barbe, J. Troccaz, B. Mazier, and S. Lavallee. Using 2.5D echography in computer assisted spine surgery. In *IEEE*, pp 160–161, San Diego, 1993. IEEE Engineering in Medicine and Biology Society Proceedings.

[Lav95] S. Lavallee. Registration for Computer Integrated Surgery : methodology, state of the art. In R. Taylor, S. Lavallee, G. Burdea, and R. Mosges, editors, *Computer Integrated Surgery (to appear)*. MIT Press, 1995.

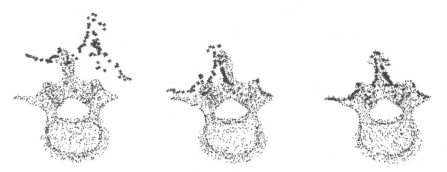

Fig. 2. Rigid 3-D / 3-D registration: during spine surgery, a set of surface points acquired manually with an optical 3D localizer converges towards the 3-D model of the vertebra segmented on pre-operative CT images.

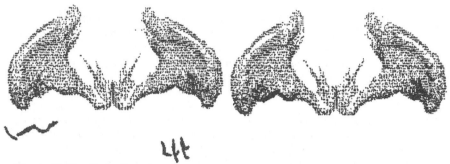

Fig. 3. Rigid 3-D / 3-D registration : during an operation, 3D data points are acquired with a 2.5D ultrasound pointer and they are registered with a 3D model of the pelvis bone segmented on CT images. This method gives a millimetric accuracy.

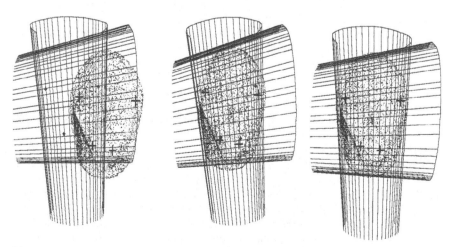

Fig. 4. Convergence of 3-D / 2-D algorithm : A set of projection lines issued from a pair of X-rays of the skull converges towards the skull surface segmented on CT images.

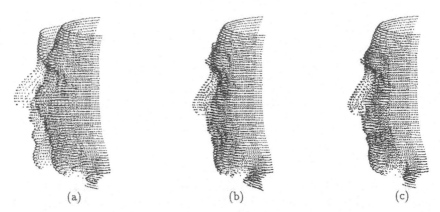

Fig. 5. Elastic registration : (a) initial position (b) affine registration (c) final result

[LS95]   S. Lavallee and R. Szeliski. Recovering the position and orientation of free-
           form objects from image contours using 3-D distance maps. *IEEE PAMI
           (Pattern Analysis and Machine Intelligence)*, to appear, 1995.

[LSB91]   S. Lavallée, R. Szeliski, and L. Brunie. Matching 3-D smooth surfaces with
           their 2-D projections using 3-D distance maps. In *SPIE Vol. 1570 Geomet-
           ric Methods in Computer Vision*, pp 322–336, San Diego, CA, 1991.

[LSB95]   S. Lavallee, R. Szeliski, and L. Brunie. Anatomy-based registration of 3-D
           medical images, range images, X-ray projections, 3-D models using octree-
           splines. In R. Taylor, S. Lavallee, G. Burdea, and R. Moges, editors, *Com-
           puter Integrated Surgery (to appear)*. MIT Press, Cambridge, 1995.

[LST+94]   S. Lavallee, P. Sautot, J. Troccaz, P. Cinquin, and P. Merloz. Computer
           Assisted Spine Surgery : a technique for accurate transpedicular screw fixa-
           tion using CT data and a 3D optical localizer. In *First International Sym-
           posium on Medical Robotics and Computer Assisted Surgery (MRCAS94)*,
           pp 315–322, Pittsburgh, Pennsylvania, USA, september 1994.

[PFTV92]   W. H. Press, B. P. Flannery, S. A. Teukolsky, and W. T. Vetterling. *Nu-
           merical Recipes in C : The Art of Scientific Computing*. Cambridge Uni-
           versity Press, Cambridge, England, second edition, 1992.

[PLC+93]   O. Peria, S. Lavallee, G. Champleboux, A.F. Joubert, J.F. Lebas, and
           P. Cinquin. Millimetric registration of SPECT and MR images of the brain
           without headholders. In *IEEE EMBS Conf.*, pp 14–15, San Diego, 1993.

[SCLT92]   P. Sautot, P. Cinquin, S. Lavallée, and J. Troccaz. Computer assisted spine
           surgery : a first step towards clinical application in orthopaedics. In *14th
           IEEE RMBS Conf.*, pp 1071–1072, Paris, November 1992.

[SL94]   R. Szeliski and S. Lavallée. Matching 3-D anatomical surfaces with non-
           rigid deformations using octree-splines. In *IEEE Workshop on Biomedical
           Image Analysis*, Seattle, June 1994. IEEE Computer Society.

[TLBM95]   R.H. Taylor, S. Lavallee, G.C. Burdea, and R.W. Mosges. *Computer inte-
           grated surgery (to be published)*. MIT PRESS, 1995.

[TMB+94]   J. Troccaz, Y. Menguy, M. Bolla, P. Cinquin, P. Vassal, N. Laieb, and S.D.
           Soglio. Patient set-up optimization for external conformal radiotherapy.
           In A. DiGioia, T. Kanade, and R. Taylor, editors, *MRCAS 94, Medical
           Robotics and Computer Assisted Surgery*, pp 306–313, Pittsburgh, PA,
           september 1994.

Comparison of Feature-Based Matching of CT and MR Brain Images

J.B. Antoine Maintz[†], Petra A. van den Elsen[††], and Max A. Viergever[†]

[†]Computer Vision Research Group, University Hospital
Utrecht, Utrecht, The Netherlands. email: twan@cv.ruu.nl
[‡] Radiological Sciences Laboratory,
Stanford University School of Medicine, Stanford, CA, USA.

Abstract. Geometrical image features like edges and ridges in digital images may be extracted by convolving the images with appropriate derivatives of Gaussians. The choice of the convolution operator and of the parameters of the Gaussian involved defines a specific feature image. In this paper, various feature images derived from CT and MR brain images are defined and tested for usability and robustness in a correlation-based two and three dimensional matching algorithm. A number of these feature images is shown to furnish accurate matching results. The best results are obtained using gradient magnitude edgeness images.

Keywords: multi-modality registration/matching, CT, MRI, differential geometry, edge & ridge features, scale space.

1 Introduction

Modern medicine frequently employs several imaging techniques within a single patient's case. In many cases, proper integration of the different modalities information greatly facilitates clinical diagnosis or treatment. In this paper we focus on the matching of CT and MR brain images. This type of matching is useful, for example, in radiation therapy planning [3], or skull base surgery [18].

Medical image matching can be divided into methods based on artificial marking devices, and methods using patient related image properties, both of which have distinct advantages [26]. The method described here falls into the latter category.

Matching algorithms using patient related image properties maximize a similarity measure between two images. This similarity may apply to the original grey value images [25], to feature images derived from the original images, or to objects defined in the initial or the derived feature images. Features used in image matching are, for example, edges [2] and ridges [16, 7, 22, 21, 20, 13]. Object based matching may, e.g., be based on surface definitions [17, 8]. Object based image matching has the disadvantage that the objects must be defined first, which is a high-level image processing task which might prove difficult, and not without error for complex images. The use of low-level differential geometric features for image matching is attractive, but requires the careful choice of feature measuring operators that produce sufficiently similar feature images when applied to multi-modal images.

When CT and MR brain images are depicted as intensity landscapes, the skull forms a ridge in the CT image, and a negative ridge (trough) in the MR image. If a 'ridgeness' extracting operator is applied to these images, the resultant feature images show remarkable similarity when compared visually. Moreover, since the skull is a virtually undeformable structure, its ridge/trough is ideally suited for matching purposes. Edgeness images of CT and MRI brain scans often have less visual similarity than ridgeness images. Enough similarity, however, is present to furnish a good match, as we will show later on. It is the aim of this paper to compare the quality of registration using ridgeness, edgeness and other geometrical operators, using grey value cross-correlation of the feature images for matching.

Feature images can be extracted by means of differential operators. Conventional differentiation, however, is ill-posed in the sense of Hadamard since we are dealing with digital, sampled images instead of smooth mathematical functions. Section two deals with this problem. In section three we define ridgeness and edgeness measuring differential operators, as well as some other feature operators. A matching algorithm is proposed in section four. In section five, the operators are applied to CT/MRI matching and the results are reviewed.

2 Differentiation of images

2.1 Invariants

Image features obtained by means of differential operators should be independent of the choice of coordinate system. Hence invariance under the group of orthogonal transformations (translations, rotations, reflections) is demanded. An operator that conforms to this restriction is called an (orthogonal) *invariant*. All operators presented in this paper satisfy this requirement.

In our expressions, L denotes the image luminance as a function of spatial coordinates. Subscripts denote derivation with respect to some spatial variable, and the Einstein summation convention is employed where subscripts are concerned.

2.2 Scale space

The differentiation of any sampled signal (e.g., an image) is ill-posed as opposed to the well-posed differentiation of smooth mathematical functions. Well-posed differentiation is possible by convolving the image with derivatives of a Gaussian [6]. The width of the Gaussian used introduces a new parameter, the *image scale*, σ, extending the image dimensionality by one. The extended image is usually referred to as the *scale space* of an image [28, 10]. By convolving an image with derivatives of Gaussians, we can compute image derivatives that are coupled to the scale (i.e., the locality or globality) of structures.

The scale space can be computed using
$$L(x, \sigma) = (L_0 * G)(x, \sigma), \qquad (1)$$
where G is the Gaussian kernel, x is the coordinate vector, σ is the smoothing factor, i.e., the scale. Computing a derivative of L is equivalent to replacing the Gaussian G with its appropriate derivative in the convolution operation:
$$(L_{i_1 \ldots i_n})(x, \sigma) = (L_0 * G_{i_1 \ldots i_n})(x, \sigma), \qquad (2)$$
where subscripts i_j denote the order of derivation with respect to the spatial variables $i_j \in \{x, y, z\}$, $n \in \mathbf{N}^+$, $j = 1 \ldots n$.

The numerical complexity of the computation of a derived image at a certain scale is vastly reduced when all computations are done in the frequency domain, were the convolution operation collapses to a series of simple multiplications.

3 Feature measures

3.1 Ridgeness measures

For the differential-geometrical detection of ridge-like structures, many different schemes and mathematical ridge definitions have been proposed, some dating back for well over a century [15]. Koenderink showed that for some popular definitions based on the water drainage pattern of a landscape, a local ridge detector does not exist [11]. However, there are a number of geometrical invariants that approximate ridges well in a wide variety of images [4]. We have selected the so-called L_{vv} and closely related operators [22, 23]. A comparison with other ridge operators can be found in [14], which also illustrates known shortcomings of this local operator.

L_{vv}: For two-dimensional images, the ridgeness operators used in this paper are derived from the L_{vv} ridgeness operator. In this formula v is defined in a local gradient based coordinate system (v, w): $w_i = L_i$, and $v_i = \varepsilon_{ij} L_j$ in tensor notation. Therefore L_{vv} represents the second order derivative in the direction perpendicular to the local gradient. The value of L_{vv} can be computed using (Cartesian) local derivatives:

$$L_{vv} = \frac{1}{||v||^2}(v \cdot \nabla)^2 L = (L_y^2 L_{xx} - 2L_x L_y L_{xy} + L_x^2 L_{yy})(L_x^2 + L_y^2)^{-1}. \quad (3)$$

In 3D the v direction as being perpendicular to the local gradient, is as yet undefined. The generalization to 3D can be found in [14].

L_{vv}/L_w: L_{vv}/L_w Can also be considered a ridgeness measuring operator. This formula derives from the observation that in two dimensional images, the local gradient changes direction when crossing a ridge. Consequently, an alternative definition of ridgeness is the rate by which the gradient direction changes when moving along the v direction. Let the two-dimensional gradient orientation be denoted by $\theta = \arctan(\frac{L_y}{L_x})$. The new ridge measure then is

$$\frac{\partial \theta}{\partial v} = \frac{1}{||v||}(v \cdot \nabla)\theta = \frac{1}{||v||}(L_y \frac{\partial \theta}{\partial x} - L_x \frac{\partial \theta}{\partial y}) = \frac{2L_x L_y L_{xy} - L_y^2 L_{xx} - L_x^2 L_{yy}}{(L_x^2 + L_y^2)^{\frac{3}{2}}}, \quad (4)$$

Notice that $\frac{\partial \theta}{\partial v} \equiv -\frac{L_{vv}}{L_w}$, so in fact the only difference with L_{vv} is a negation and a normalization with respect to the gradient magnitude. $-\frac{L_{vv}}{L_w}$ Often appears in literature as the *isophote curvature*, frequently denoted by κ. The normalization of L_{vv} with respect to the gradient magnitude ($\frac{L_{vv}}{L_w}$) causes it to react stronger than L_{vv} in areas of the image where the variation in image intensity is relatively small, i.e., relatively flat areas in the intensity landscape.

$L_{vv}L_w^\alpha$: Both L_{vv} and $L_{vv}L_w^{-1}$ have been identified as ridgeness measures. The notion of L_{vv} and L_{vv}/L_w as ridgeness measures can be readily expanded towards the more general formula $L_{vv}L_w^\alpha$, where α is bounded. The ridgeness operators used in this paper can be written in this form, with $\alpha \in \{-1, -0.5, 0, 0.5\}$, although other values for α could be considered as well.

3.2 Edgeness measures

Well known edge measures are the gradient magnitude (L_w), and the Laplacean (L_{ii}). L_w measures the local 'steepness' of the intensity landscape, which presumably has a local maximum at an edge. It is a good detector for step edges. When edges get less steep, use of the Laplacean often gives better results. For example, in the 1D case of an edge, the Laplacean has a positive response in the convex part of the edge flank, and a negative response in the concave part. The edge locus is presumed to be at the zero crossing between these two parts.

3.3 Miscellaneous measures

Besides edge and ridge measures, we employed some other invariant measures, which are briefly mentioned here. Cartesian expressions are given in their 2D form.

$L_{vv}L_w^2$: $L_{vv}L_w^2$ is a cornerness measure based on the work of Kitchen and Rosenfeld [9] and Blom [1]. Note that it equals the (negated) isophote curvature times the gradient magnitude cubed: $L_{vv}L_w^2 = \frac{L_{vv}}{L_w}L_w^3$. The idea behind this detector is that the isophote curvature is extremely high at corners. As the isophote curvature reacts equally strong at 'background' structures and 'real' objects, and has a response at ridges, it is multiplied by a power of the gradient magnitude, to avoid phantom responses. This also solves the faulty detection of corners at local extrema (where $L_w = 0$). In the strictest sense, $L_{vv}L_w^2$ is categorized in our class of ridge detectors $L_{vv}L_w^\alpha$. However, valid values for α are bounded, and —although the exact bounds are subjective— 'cornerness measure' is a better description of $L_{vv}L_w^2$ than 'ridgeness measure': the strong response at corners relatively suppresses the response at ridges. Some ridgeness information can be extracted from $L_{vv}L_w^2$ images by windowed display, or by enhancing the response at ridges by re-mapping the operator as $(L_{vv}L_w^2)^{(1/n)}$, where $n > 1$. Experiments have shown $n = 3$ to be a satisfying choice. In Cartesian notation, $L_{vv}L_w^2$ equals the numerator of the Cartesian expression of L_{vv}: $L_{vv}L_w^2 = L_y^2 L_{xx} - 2L_x L_y L_{xy} + L_x^2 L_{yy}$.

$\boldsymbol{L_{vw}}$: As $-\frac{L_{vv}}{L_w}$ equals the isophote curvature, $\frac{L_{vw}}{L_w}$ equals the flowline curvature, where the flowline is defined as the integral curve of the gradient. In each point of an image, the local flowline and isophote are perpendicular by definition. We employ L_{vw}, obtained by multiplying the flowline curvature with the gradient magnitude, thus diminishing its response in uninteresting areas. The Cartesian expression of L_{vw} equals $(L_x L_y (L_{yy} - L_{xx}) + L_{xy}(L_x^2 - L_y^2))/(L_x^2 + L_y^2)$.

$\boldsymbol{L_{ww}}$: $\frac{L_{ww}}{L_w}$ is a measure for isophote density. As with the previous expressions, we use the expression L_{ww} to reduce uninteresting responses. L_{ww} is closely connected to the Laplacean and L_{vv} ridgeness by the relation $L_{ww} = L_{ii} - L_{vv}$. The Cartesian expression of L_{ww} equals $(L_{xx}L_x^2 + 2L_{xy}L_x L_y + L_{yy}L_y^2)/(L_x^2 + L_y^2))$.

umbilicity, $\boldsymbol{L_{ij}L_{ji}}$: The umbilicity of a point can be determined by computing $\varepsilon_{ij}\varepsilon_{kl}\frac{L_{ik}L_{jl}}{L_{mn}L_{nm}} = \frac{L_{ii}L_{jj} - L_{ij}L_{ji}}{L_{kl}L_{lk}}$. The numerator equals twice the determinant of the Hessian det L_{ij}, which is a measure for local ellipticity (positive value) or hyperbolicity (negative value) of a surface patch. A zero value of this determinant indicates a parabolic or planar patch. The denominator normalizes the umbilicity measure so as to be bounded by -1 and 1, which is most obvious when examining the form containing the ε tensors. The denominator can therefore be regarded as an 'unflatness'-measure. The Cartesian expression of umbilicity equals $2(L_{xx}L_{yy} - L_{xy}^2)/(L_{xx}^2 + 2L_{xy}^2 + L_{yy}^2)$.

checkerboard detector, Y-junction detector: The third and fourth order binary forms L_3 and L_4 of an image L at coordinates $\mathbf{x}$ are $\frac{1}{3!}L_{ijk}x_i x_j x_k$ and $\frac{1}{4!}L_{ijkl}x_i x_j x_k x_l$ respectively. The discriminants D_3 and D_4 of these forms can serve to detect Y-junctions and 'checkerboard' patterns respectively. The reader interested in a theoretical expansion of these expressions is referred to [5, 19]. The Cartesian expressions are: $D_3 = 6L_{xyy}^2 L_{xxy}^2 - 2L_{xxx}^2 L_{yyy}^2 - 8L_{yyy}L_{xxy}^3 - 8L_{xyy}^3 L_{xxx} + 12L_{yyy}L_{xyy}L_{xxy}L_{xxx}$ and $D_4 = (L_{xxxx}L_{yyyy} - 4L_{xxxy}L_{xyyy} + 3L_{xxyy}L_{xxyy})^3 - 27(L_{xxxy}(L_{xxxy}L_{yyyy} - L_{xyyy}L_{xxyy}) + L_{xxyy}(L_{xxxy}L_{xyyy} - L_{xxyy}L_{xxyy}))^2$.

4 Matching method

The method we use to match CT (L_1) and MR (L_2) feature volumes or slices is based on cross-correlation of grey values. By using the grey values directly we avoid segmentation of our feature images. We try to find the global optimum of the correlation value $c(t)$ over all rigid transformations t, where $c(t)$ is defined

$$c(t) = \sum_{(x,y,z)\in L_1} L_1(x, y, z)L_2(t(x, y, z)).$$

Since a brute force approach by trying all possible values of t is computationally infeasible, we resort to a multi-resolution method and a number of assumptions on the behavior of $c(t)$ with respect to t to find the optimal t within an acceptable number of computational operations. In our method, a multi-resolution pyramid is created, with the original image at its bottom. The next level is formed by maximizing, or minimizing each group of up to eight neighboring voxels into one voxel. The choice between maximizing and minimizing is based on the sign of interesting responses. New pyramid levels are formed as long as the largest image structures are clearly discernible. Between the (very low resolution) top levels of the feature pyramids the optimal match is found by optimizing the correlation value over an extensive range of t. Local extrema within a certain percentage of the best extremum found are passed on as search seeds to the next pyramid level, where new searches are started. As we progress further down in the pyramid, the absolute search range of t (i.e., the actual range in parameter space in terms of millimeters and degrees around a certain origin) diminishes, as do the step sizes. By keeping the search range small, the number of values for t to test remain computationally feasible. To avoid the risk of a search range around a seed being too small, and a correlation optimum being missed, a hill-climbing operation may be performed after the search for a local optimum. Details on the procedure are furnished in [23, 21]. These references also explain in more detail the advantages of the correlation method over, e.g., surface based methods [12, 17], which are computationally more attractive. These advantages include the absence of a segmentation step and low sensitivity to differences in the structures used for matching.

5 Application of feature measures to CT/MRI matching

5.1 2D matching experiments

To test all of the operators for matching performance, five representative matched pairs of CT and MRI transverse slices were chosen. These slices were chosen from volumes matched using skin markers [27]. An initial run of 1820 experiments was carried out to select promising features: each of the 13 operators was tested by matching the 5 slice pairs, at scales ranging from 1 to 7 mm, using 4 different artificially induced initial transformations of one of the images of the matching pair (ranging from no transformation to 15 mm translations and 15 degrees rotation). After applying the initial transformation, the operator in question was applied to both the images of the pair, and the resultant feature images were matched. Ideally, the found matching transformation equals the inverse of the applied initial transformation, since the images were taken from sets registered beforehand. We must be careful to accept this transformation as a golden standard however, since the original registration will inevitably have a (small) error. Moreover, the original registration was based on 3D information, while we now match using the 2D slice information only. To make sure the original registration is an acceptable standard, it was re-assessed visually within the 2D slice, and compared visually to typical transformations found in the experiments. The original registration was visually found to be an excellent standard.

Based on this run of experiments, the checkerboard, Y-junction, umbilicity, L_{vw}, L_{ww}, and $L_{ij}L_{ji}$ operators were discarded: in none or only very few cases a correlation optimum was found at the ideal matching transformation. The $L_{vv}L_w^2$ operator was replaced by the re-mapped version $L_{vv}^{1/3}L_w^{2/3}$ which performed notably better. The L_{vv}/L_w operator showed merit, but often there are many local optima near the value of the optimum obtained at the correct matching transformation. Since all of these optima had to be investigated by the matching program, the runtime increased dramatically. Because the $L_{vv}/\sqrt{(L_w)}$ and L_{vv} operator had no such problems, the L_{vv}/L_w operator was discarded too.

This leaves only the edgeness and ridgeness measuring operators as good candidates for correlation matching. The remaining five operators (L_{vv}, $L_{vv}/\sqrt{(L_w)}$), $L_{vv}^{1/3} L_w^{2/3}$, L_{ii}, and L_w) were tested further in three experiment runs, comprising 2100 experiments. Each run is similar to the initial run of experiments, except we now 'maim' the CT image before the start of the experiments, increasing the difficulty of matching considerably. (The maimings used induced an image power loss of 16%, 56%, and 64% respectively.)

To interpret the large amount of experimental results, each matching result was categorized as belonging to one of six classes of increasing matching accuracy. These classes were subsequently indexed, where the index ranged from '0' for the class of failed matches (more than 10 pixels or degrees deviation, or no matching transformation found at all), to '1' for the class of sub pixel-accurate matches.

For each operator, the average experimental index was computed. Note that specific values of this index have no quantitative interpretation. Within one slice pair it can be used to compare operators though, because a higher index can be interpreted as a better matching performance. The overall performance index for each operator as a function of scale can be seen in figure 1.

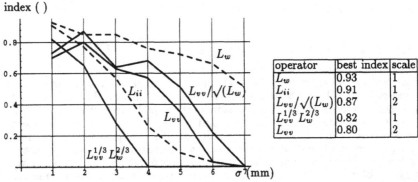

Fig. 1. *The performance index of five operators, accumulated over all experiments, as a function of scale (left), and the value of the best index that occured for each operator (right). In the graph, edge operators are represented by dashed lines, and ridge operators as solid lines.*

The best performance index and the scale at which this index occured of each operator are also included in this figure.

Evidently, L_w has the best overall performance. The edgeness measuring operators (L_w, L_{ii}) perform slightly better than the ridgeness measuring ones on their respective optimal scales. L_w is the least sensitive to changes in scale, as the graph shows. The optimum of the edge operators is a boundary optimum, which suggests the actual optimum may occur at a lower scale than 1 mm. As computing derivatives at such low scales is infeasible on most image volumes, scales lower than 1 mm have not been examined.

5.2 3D matching experiments

The 3D experiments comprised correlation matchings of the L_{vv}, $L_{vv}/\sqrt{(L_w)}$, $L_{vv}^{1/3} L_w^{2/3}$, L_{ii}, and L_w feature images of high resolution 3D CT and MR brain images[1]. The optimal scale was derived from the 2D experiments. The matching transformation found was compared to a previously established match based on a marker method [27]. Additionally, the same experiments were carried out on volumes of lower transverse resolution (3 mm), which were simulated from the high resolution sets by averaging slices. We use simulated sets instead of directly acquired sets, because an accurate matching reference standard is needed, which is difficult to check visually for low-resolution sets. Finally, we repeated all of the above described experiments on maimed sets. Both the CT and MR volumes were maimed. The power loss induced by the maiming is 27.1% in the case of the MR volume, and 56.9% in case of the CT volume.

The results are summarized in table 1. We increased the edge operator scale

operator	σ	high res	maim	result						miss	#
				translation			rotation				
				x	y	z	x	y	z		
L_w	1	•		-0.02	0.04	0.44	0.45	-0.62	2.04		1
L_w	2			0.22	-0.20	-0.39	0.68	-0.17	1.37		1
L_w	1	•	•	0.22	0.98	0.44	0.00	0.28	1.37		6
L_w	2		•	0.45	0.27	-3.61	-0.22	1.17	2.04		0
L_{ii}	1	•		-0.02	0.04	1.22	0.45	-0.39	2.04		11
L_{ii}	2			0.22	0.04	1.16	0.68	0.05	2.94		0
L_{ii}	1	•	•	0.22	0.74	0.84	0.00	0.05	2.04		15
L_{ii}	2		•	0.45	0.98	-1.19	-0.44	0.05	2.04		1
L_{vv}	2	•		-0.25	0.04	1.60	0.45	-0.39	2.27		0
L_{vv}	2			-0.25	0.04	1.20	0.45	-0.17	2.04		0
L_{vv}	2	•	•	-0.25	0.04	1.60	0.45	-0.39	2.27		0
L_{vv}	2		•	∞	∞	∞	∞	∞	∞	•	(97)
$L_{vv}/\sqrt{(L_w)}$	2	•		-0.48	0.98	1.60	0.68	-0.17	2.04		0
$L_{vv}/\sqrt{(L_w)}$	2			0.45	-0.66	-1.20	1.35	0.73	4.28		1
$L_{vv}/\sqrt{(L_w)}$	2	•	•	0.22	0.98	0.83	0.23	0.05	1.82		4
$L_{vv}/\sqrt{(L_w)}$	2		•	0.22	1.21	-4.34	-0.44	0.50	0.92		16
$L_{vv}^{1/3} L_w^{2/3}$	2	•		-0.25	-0.27	-1.23	-0.45	0.93	-1.82		(21)
$L_{vv}^{1/3} L_w^{2/3}$	2			-1.19	-4.18	-15.40	2.69	2.74	11.89	•	14
$L_{vv}^{1/3} L_w^{2/3}$	2	•	•	0.22	0.98	0.46	0.23	-0.17	1.82		(21)
$L_{vv}^{1/3} L_w^{2/3}$	2		•	-1.19	12.93	-18.67	2.69	2.74	-5.57	•	32

Table 1. *The results of the 3D matching experiments. The 'result' column shows the difference between the found transformation and the reference transformation obtained by marker matching. The parameters indicate the translation and rotation of the center CT volume voxel. All values mentioned are in millimeters or degrees. The obvious mismatches have a mark in the 'miss' column. The last column shows the number of extra local minima examined. If this number is bracketed, convergence of the particular correlation was too slow, and the number of minima to be examined was reduced manually.*

when using the low resolution sets, to maintain an appropriate scale relative

---

[1] The MR data set is a transverse T1 weighted 3D/FFE set, TR=30 msec, TE=9 msec, containing 180 slices, no gap, with cubic voxels of approx. $1mm^3$, obtained on a 1.5 Tesla Philips Gyroscan S15/ACS. The CT data set is a contiguous 100 slice set, pixel size approx. 0.9 mm, slice thickness 1.5 mm, obtained on a Philips Tomoscan 350, set to 120 kV and 120 mA.

to the slice thickness. If the scale were not increased, the operator is asked to supply information on an under-sampled level of detail.

Of the high resolution experiments, we applied the found transformation furthest from the reference match and compared the obtained match visually with the reference match. This comparison was done by segmenting the bone contours –by grey value thresholding– from various transversal and sagitally and coronally reformatted slices from the matched CT volume, and overlaying these contours onto the corresponding MR slices [14, 24, 23]. Two independent observers concluded the reference match inferior to the newly found L_{vv} correlation match. When visually comparing the high resolution/no maiming matches in the table in the same manner –excluding the $L_{vv}^{1/3} L_w^{2/3}$ match– no conclusion could be drawn regarding the best match. Owing to the inevitable intrinsic distortion of the MR image, *the* perfect rigid match does not exist, but these four matches are clearly good approximations, and were judged to be equally accurate.

From the table it is clear that when either the low resolution sets are employed, or the sets are maimed, the performance of all operators except $L_{vv}^{1/3} L_w^{2/3}$ is still accurate. All $L_{vv}^{1/3} L_w^{2/3}$ experiments were troublesome, since the algorithm did not converge to a single optimum. In the table, the last column shows the number of extra found local minima examined (i.e., besides the best minimum found on each pyramid level) by the algorithm. This number is bracketed when the algorithm showed no or too slow convergence, e.g., too many incorrect minima remained to be examined on the high resolution pyramid levels. In these cases, after the algorithm had run for a certain amount of time, all results but the best one were removed from the list of minima to be examined, and the algorithm was continued. The final result is shown in the table.

When maimed low resolution sets are used, performance diminishes with almost all operators. With the L_{vv} operator, the matching algorithm fails to converge on a single minimum. The L_w and L_{ii} operators furnish matches with a less accurate z-translation. Considering the low z-resolution and severe maiming of the CT volume, these cannot be called poor results.

6 Conclusion and discussion

In this paper, we have tested and compared the matching of CT and MR brain images by correlation of image features, most notably edge and ridge features. In 2D experiments, the matching merit of 13 different feature operators was established using brute force experiments. The edge and ridge operators used showed the best performance, with the edge operators having a slight advantage. Five operators and their optimal scale were selected for 3D matching experiments, the edge operators L_w (the gradient magnitude), and L_{ii} (the Laplacean), and the ridge operators L_{vv}, $L_{vv}/\sqrt{(L_w)}$, and $L_{vv}^{1/3} L_w^{2/3}$. The 3D matching results were accurate, visually even more accurate than the marker based results used as a reference. All operators showed proper convergence, except for the $L_{vv}^{1/3} L_w^{2/3}$ operator. This last operator seems therefore unsuitable for matching purposes. Regarding the remaining four operators: only when severely maimed low resolution images were employed, the L_{vv} matching failed, and the L_w and L_{ii} matchings were less accurate. The maiming of the volumes used exceeds the limits of normal protocol scope, however. Based on both the 2D and 3D experiments, the gradient magnitude L_w seems to be the best choice of the original 13 proposed operators. In the 2D experiments, it produced accurate matching results, and appeared robust under changes in scale, initial transformation and maiming of the original CT and MR images. In the 3D experiments, it led to accurate results when realistic initial CT and MR images were used. Moreover, of all 13 operators, L_w is the fastest to compute, since only the three first order derivatives are needed.

Our findings regarding the use of the differentio-geometrical operators tested were based on their performance in a multi-resolution cross-correlation algorithm. It is plausible that features we deemed unsuitable for matching purposes may very well be used adequately in a different matching algorithm. Moreover, considering the limited number of data sets employed, repeated execution of our test-suite on other data sets is needed to confirm the results obtained.

For the matching of 3D CT and MR brain images, we propose a matching scheme using scaled L_w feature images in a multi-resolution correlation algorithm. This scheme requires no interactive actions, and is therefore devoid of human subjectivity. Only patient-related geometrical features are used for the matching, so matching can be performed even if pre-acquisition matching accommodations have not been made. The use of patient-related features is also more patient friendly than the use of external features, since no marking devices are required to be attached to the patient's head.

References

1. J. Blom. *Topological and Geometrical Aspects of Image Structure*. PhD thesis, Utrecht University, the Netherlands, 1992.
2. G. Borgefors. Hierarchical chamfer matching: a parametric edge matching algorithm. *IEEE Transactions on Pattern Analysis and Machine Intelligence*, 10:849–865, 1988.
3. George T. Y. Chen and Charles A. Pelizzari. Image Correlation Techniques in Radiation Therapy Planning. *Computerized Medical Imaging and Graphics*, 13(3):235–240, 1989.
4. D. Eberly, R. Gardner, B. Morse, S. Pizer, and C. Scharlach. Ridges for image analysis. Technical report, dep. of Computer science, University of NC, Chapel Hill, Chapel Hill, NC, USA, 1993. submitted for publication.
5. L. M. J. Florack, B. M. ter Haar Romeny, J. J. Koenderink, and M. A. Viergever. Differential invariants in scale-space. Technical report 91-20, 1991.
6. L. M. J. Florack, B. M. ter Haar Romeny, J. J. Koenderink, and M. A. Viergever. On scale and the differential structure of images. *Image & Vision Computing*, 10:376–388, 1992.
7. A. Guéziec and N. Ayache. Smoothing and matching of 3-D space curves. In R.A. Robb, editor, *Visualization in biomedical computing*, volume 1808 of *Proc. SPIE*, pages 259–273. SPIE Press, Bellingham, WA, 1992.
8. P. F. Hemler, T. Sumanaweera, R. Pichumani, P. A. van den Elsen, S. Napel, and J. Adler. A system for multimodality image fusion. In *IEEE symposium on computer-based medical systems*, pages 335–340, Los Alamitos, CA, 1994. IEEE Computer Society Press.
9. L. Kitchen and A. Rosenfeld. Gray-level corner detection. *Pattern Recognition Letters*, 1:95–102, 1982.
10. J. J. Koenderink. The structure of images. *Biological Cybernetics*, (50):363–370, 1984.
11. J. J. Koenderink and A. J. van Doorn. Two-plus-one dimensional differential geometry. *Pattern Recognition Letters*, (15):439–443, 1994.
12. D. N. Levin, C. A. Pelizzari, G. T. Y. Chen, C.T. Chen, and M. D. Cooper. Retrospective geometric correlation of MR, CT, and PET images. *Radiology*, 169(3):817–823, 1988.
13. A. Liu, S. M. Pizer, D. Eberly, B. Morse, J. Rosenman, and V. Carrasco. Volume registration using the 3D core. In *Proc. SPIE Medical Imaging VIII*, Newport Beach, CA, February 1994. In press.
14. J. B. A. Maintz, P. A. van den Elsen, and M. A Viergever. Evaluation of ridge seeking operators for multimodality medical image matching. 1994. submitted for publication.

15. J. C. Maxwell. On hills and dales. *The London, Edinburgh and Dublin Philosophical Magazine and Journal of Science*, 40(269):421–425, 1859.
16. O. Monga, S. Benayoun, and O. D. Faugeras. From partial derivatives of 3D density images to ridge lines. In R. A. Robb, editor, *Visualization in biomedical computing*, volume 1808 of *Proc. SPIE*, pages 118–127. SPIE Press, Bellingham, WA, 1992.
17. C. A. Pelizzari, G. T. Y. Chen, D. R. Spelbring, R. R. Weichselbaum, and C. T. Chen. Accurate three-dimensional registration of CT, PET, and/or MR images of the brain. *Computer Assisted Tomography*, 13(1):20–26, 1989.
18. C. F. Ruff, D. L. G. Hill, G. P. Robinson, and D. J. Hawkes. Volume Rendering of Multimodal Images for the Planning of Skull Base Surgery. In H. U. Lemke et al, editor, *Computer Assisted Radiology '93*, pages 574 – 579. Springer-Verlag, 1993.
19. B. M. ter Haar Romeny, L. M. J. Florack, J. J. Koenderink, and M. A. Viergever. Scale-space: its natural operators and differential invariants. In Colchester and Hawkes, editors, *Information Processing in Medical Imaging, Proceedings of the 12th International Conference*, Springer-Verlag, Berlin, 1991.
20. J. Thirion. Extremal points: definition and application to 3D image registration. In *Proc. CVPR*, pages 587–592, Los alamitos, CA, 1994. IEEE Computer Society press.
21. P. A. van den Elsen. *Multimodality matching of brain images*. PhD thesis, Utrecht University, the Netherlands, 1993.
22. P. A. van den Elsen, J. B. A. Maintz, E. J. D. Pol, and M. A. Viergever. Image fusion using geometrical features. In R. A. Robb, editor, *Visualization in biomedical computing*, volume 1808 of *Proc. SPIE*, pages 172–186. SPIE Press, Bellingham, WA, 1992.
23. P. A. van den Elsen, J. B. A. Maintz, and M. A. Viergever. Automated CT and MR brain image matching using correlation of geometrical "ridgeness" features. Technical Report 3DCV 93-07, Utrecht University, 1993. submitted for publication.
24. P. A. van den Elsen, J. B. A. Maintz, and M. A. Viergever. Geometry driven multimodality matching of brain images. *Brain Topography*, 5:153–158, 1993.
25. P. A. van den Elsen, E. J. D. Pol, T. S. Sumanaweera, P.F. Hemler, S. Napel, and J. Adler. Grey value correlation techniques used for automatic matching of CT and MR brain and spine images. In *Visualization in Biomedical Computing*, volume 2359 of *Proc. SPIE*, pages 227–237. SPIE Press, Bellingham, WA, 1994.
26. P. A. van den Elsen, E.D. Pol, and M. A. Viergever. Medical image matching- a review with classification. *IEEE Engineering in medicine and biology*, 12(1):26–39, 1993.
27. P. A. van den Elsen and M. A. Viergever. Marker guided multimodality matching of the brain. *European Radiology*, 4:45–51, 1994.
28. A. Witkin. Scale space filtering. In *Proceedings of the 7th International Confernece on Artificial Intelligence*, pages 1019–1021, Karlsruhe, 1983.

7 Acknowledgments

This research was supported in part by the industrial companies Philips Medical Systems, KEMA, and Shell Research, as well as by the Netherlands ministries of Education & Science and Economic Affairs through a SPIN grant, by the Murray Foundation, and by the Netherlands Organization for Scientific Research (NWO), through a TALENT fellowship. We wish to thank Dr. G. Wilts, L.M. Ramos, Dr. P.F.G.M. van Waes and Dr. F.W. Zonneveld for their efforts to supply the images. The help of Karel Zuiderveld and Dr. Bart ter Haar Romeny in the course of this work are also greatly appreciated. Carolien Bouma, Wiro Niessen, Rik Stokking, and Dr. Evert-Jan D. Pol are thanked for reading early manuscript versions.

Posters I

Automatical Adaption of Anatomical Masks to the Neocortex

F. Kruggel

Neurologische Klinik, Klinikum Rechts der Isar
Möhlstraße 28, 81675 München

Abstract: We describe an image processing chain that is capable of identifying sulci and gyri in MRI brain slices. Contrary to current interactive map fitting schemes it tries to simulate a radiologist's way of image analysis - a process we call *image understanding by landmark detection*. In a nutshell, we detect the entry points of the neocortical sulci by an automated procedure. These entry points are identified as belonging to a specific sulcus by comparison with an anatomical database. From these landmarks a further analysis of the surrounding region can be performed. This algorithm is used for an anatomical mapping facility in a multimodal image editor for medical volume datasets.

1 Introduction

The brain is the most complex organ in the human body. The current available magnetic resonance (MR) imaging techniques give an excellent pictorial description of a patient's brain morphology and pathology. In a normal brain are in the order of 500 locations of interest which are big enough to be detectable by MR techniques. A precise anatomical analysis of a brain MR tomogram requires a working anatomical knowledge and a good understanding of the spatial relationships of the brain locations which is usually only found with a trained neuroradiologist. This process can be eased by fitting an anatomical map to an image slice.

Current approaches of map fitting take a MR slice and adapt it by transformation to a model map [1, 2]. This map is represented as a *geometrical model* which is based on a model brain or a stereotactical atlas [7]. We call this method *example-based map fitting*. This approach works sufficiently in parts of the brain where the anatomy has low individual differences, like in the brainstem and midbrain areas. The neocortical gyri and sulci however display an individual variability so this approach of map adaptation can reach only a moderate degree of accuracy. Pathologic cases with space-consuming properties like tumors or edemas are even harder to handle.

Our approach tries to simulate a radiologist's way of analyzing an image series. One of the first steps in this process is finding any landmarks. Landmarks are well-defined anatomical points that are easily detectable in MR tomograms, f.ex. the eyes, the ventricles and the primary sulci. Once a set of orientation points has been established, a finer analysis of the area „in between" can be performed. In pathologic cases either the landmarks are simply displaced or only a subset can be successfully detected. Since our approach uses an algorithm to detect and assign structures (i.e a *symbolic model*) we call this approach in derivation of similar problems in computer vision *map fitting by image understanding*. Another important difference between these two approaches lies in the fact that example-based map fitting is usually an interactive process - i.e. (expert) user-based and thus time-consuming - whereas our approach can be automated.

2 Description of the algorithm

We show how the position of the neocortical sulci can be detected by an automated image processing sequence. In short, we compute the brain contour and its *Voronoi segmentation* figure [5]. The entry point of a sulcus is found at the crossing of the brain's convex hull with the outer segmentation figure. The purpose of the core algorithm in this sequence can be explained for a u-shaped test contour (Fig. 1a). Nonstrictly spoken, the outer Voronoi segmentation figure consists of a „crown" around the test contour and a „finger" exploring the sulcus. An outline of the complete sequence is given as follows:

1. Take an MR brain slice with good contrast between liquor and tissue as input
   Comment: Since we want to detect sulci, a good contrast between liquor and brain tissue is necessary. The usual T1-weighted images produced in clinical routine are sufficient. This slice belongs to a volume dataset that has been registered with the stereotactical coordinate system [4]. Note that the current formulation of our algorithm requires a „skull-removed" brain image (Fig. 1b).
2. Compute a polygonal approximation of the brain contour
   Comment: This step approximates the brain contour (preferrably) as a *closed* polygon. We detect the edges in the brain slice by a Canny operator and convert the edge image into a set of line segments by pixel chaining (Fig. 1c).
3. Perform a Voronoi segmentation [5] of the vector image
   Comment: We increase the resolution of the segmentation figure by subdividing long line segments in the input figure. A maximum segment length of 4 pixels yields an optimum between resolution and computation time. The set of Voronoi edges between the bounding rectangle and the brain contour (the exoskeleton) „explores" the sulci (Fig. 1c).
4. Clean out the branches of the segmentation figure („pruning")
   Comment: To include only prominent „fingers" in subsequent steps, a cleaning of the segmentation figure is performed. We determine the adjacency [5] of the Voronoi edges and discard those with an adjacency lower than a predetermined threshold. Usually we prune by a level of 2.
5. Compute the crosspoints of the outer segmentation figure with the hull
   Comment: First we construct a convex hull from the polygon approximation of the brain contour. The cutpoints of the exoskeleton with the convex hull are collected as probable entry points of the sulci. Note that the endoskeleton is disregarded since it lies completely within the hull. Usually 4 to 8 crosspoints per hemisphere are found (Fig. 1d).

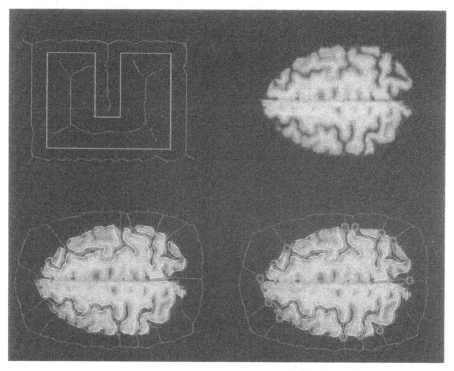

Fig. 1. Top left (a): Test figure „U" and its corresponding Voronoi segmentation. Top right (b): T1-weighted input MR slice 40mm above CA-CP. Bottom left (c): Polygonal approximation of the brain contour and its Voronoi segmentation. Bottom right (d): Crosspoints (shown as rings) with the convex hull are denoted as suspected sulcus entry points.

6. Compare the crosspoints with sulcus locations in the anatomical database (i.e. assign identification probabilities)

   Comment: The z position (slice position) is added to each of the computed crosspoints. The point list is handed to an anatomical database, which contains „usual" positions of the sulci and their variation. These positions were determined initially be manually tracing the sulci in 20 randomly chosen brain MRI datasets. We include sulcus positions successfully assigned by this algorithm (and confirmed by an expert) in a „bootstrap fashion". For all crosspoints we assign probabilities p for belonging to a specific sulcus by comparison with reference locations and their variance using a bivariate normal distribution statistic.

7. Repeat this process for other slices

   Comment: To further enhance the identification process, we perform steps 1-6 for neighbor slices.

8. Define sulci by concatenation of identified crosspoints

   Comment: We collect the crosspoints of all slices including their probabilities for belonging to a specific sulcus and construct a weighted graph (using 1/p) of these points. The path with the lowest cost is accepted as the series of points defining a specific sulcus. The cost can be used as a quality measurement of the adaptation process. Output is a series of points defining an identified sulcus.

9. Define gyri as structures surrounded by identified sulci

Comment: The area between two sulci can be identified as a specific gyrus if both limiting sulci are known. Sulci and gyri are shown by name in the dataset currently under investigation by a user of this system (Fig. 2).

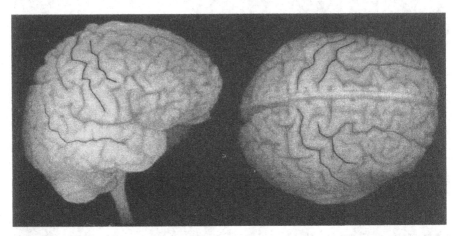

Fig 2. Example of automatically detected sulci in a 3D MR dataset. On the left (L to R): S. temporalis sup., F. Sylvii, S. postcentralis, S. centralis, S. praecentralis. On the right (L to R): S. postcentralis., S. centralis, S. praecentralis, S. frontalis sup.

This algorithm has been implemented as a part of a medical documentation system [3]. It was implemented in about 2000 lines of C++ code. It needs about 10 s per slice on a SGI Indy workstation. Time-consuming steps are the contour formation and the Voronoi segmentation.

Although the details of this algorithm appear complex the whole processing chain can be handled as a black box since the only parameters needed are in the initial edge detection step. Values for these parameters can be supplied by a knowledge database or estimated by histogram analyzation of the slices.

3 Discussion

Several approaches of fitting anatomical maps to MR tomograms have been proposed in the last five years. These approaches use model brains as the base of an anatomical atlas. Former proposals applying rigid matching show adaption problems especially in neocortical structures like sulci and gyri due to their individual variances. Second generation schemes were build on various methods of non-rigid matching [1, 2]. These methods can adapt masks with an accuracy of about 2-3 mm which is sufficient for a physician's orientation but barely acceptable for quantitative volumetric purposes. Furthermore, these adaption schemes work barely in the presence of space-consuming pathologic changes.

In this paper we have outlined a new way of map adaption by feature detection. Our basic idea is to follow a radiologist's way of orientation by finding any landmarks. In our first attempt we identify the primary sulci as landmarks, which are formed first during ontogenesis and develop relatively regular among subjects. By detecting these landmarks, a considerable amount of the interpersonal variability of the neocortical structures can be ruled out. We use a Voronoi segmentation to detect sulci and identify them by comparison with a probabilistic database of their „usual" locations. This distinguishes our approach from static atlases like the one recently introduced by Tiede et al. [7]. Furthermore, by working completely in the „patient space", our scheme does not depend on problems in the adaption of a geometric model as it is the case with non-rigid matching schemes mentioned above.

Our work is related to the study of the neocortical surface topology introduced recently by Mangin et al. [4]. They segment a MR volume dataset to yield a union of gray-matter and cerebro-spinal fluid, which undergoes a skeletonization to form an attributed relational graph that contains a 3D description of the brain's surface topology. This description can be labeled by a neuroanatomist.

While our processing chain appears as a promising approach of map fitting to us, several open problems exist which have to be addressed before this procedure can be applied in an automated system:

1. This algorithm needs a „skull-removed" MR image set. This is currently done by hand editing the original dataset. An automatical algorithm for removing the non-brain parts is under construction in our workgroup.
2. The detection of sulci is depended on a successful edge detection. Most edge detection schemes yield open brain contours, so that the exoskeleton „leaks" into the endoskeleton.
3. Quality measurements of the detection process are not yet available. In a short series using routine MRI slices (20 patients) the primary sulci we correctly assigned in 93%. No incorrect assignments were found.
4. The performance of this algorithm has not been tested with severe distortions of the brain (i.e. large cortical infarcts, malformations).

A possible 3D implementation of this algorithm seems to offer no advantage for us. 3D Voronoi segmentation schemes require high computational efforts, especially due to the amount of boundary planes involved. The resulting topological structures are hard to analyze and to compare. A parallel formulation of this algorithm would be desirable to speed up the computation. In spite of the serial nature of this processing chain, a simple parallelization can be performed by computing several slices in parallel. Candidates for a true parallel formulation are the time-consuming steps 2 and 3.

In the future, we will extend this map adaption scheme to include landmark information of different origin. Through a combination of a region-based growing and a watershed segmentation algorithm [6] we were able to segment deep white-matter structures like the basal ganglia (caudate nucleus, pallidum, putamen and thalamus). This leaves maximum distances of 3 cm to be bridged by patches of conventional model maps, which are still necessary to locate structures that are (currently) undetectable by MRI in terms of their shape or intensity characteristics.

The use of the inner segmentation figure for analyzation of white matter structures appears interesting. The idea of using a Voronoi skeletonization to represent and analyze shapes has recently been published by Mayya and Rajan [5]. The endoskeletons are reminiscent of the course of the white-matter tracts and thus may reveal valuable informations about these not directly traceable structures. It seems necessary to include the segmentation of the basal ganglia (as „holes" in the white matter) to restrict the formation of the endoskeleton to the natural compartment of tracts in the brain.

Our map adaption scheme currently undergoes a test phase in the clinical routine. We need to collect experiences when applying this algorithm in the presence of brain pathologies. During the next months we will analyze the performance, accuracy and failures of our approach under routine conditions. The „gold standard" of an automated analysis is still the approval by an expert. However, we can add successfully matched sulcus locations to our growing anatomical database and thus yield a more robust assignment.

The implementation enhances a multimodal image editor for the neurologic sciences which is currently under development in our clinic.

References

1. Dann R, Hoford J, Kovacic S, Reivich M, Bajcsy R: Evaluation of elastic matching system for anatomic (CT, MR) and functional (PET) cerebral images. Journal of Computer Assisted Tomography 13(4), 603-611 (1989).

2. Davatzikos C, Prince JL: Brain image registration based on curve mapping. IEEE Workshop on Biomedical Image Analysis. Seattle June 1994, 245-249 (1994).

3. Kruggel F, Horsch A, Mittelhäußer G, Schnabel G: Image processing in the neurologic sciences. IEEE Workshop on Biomedical Image Analysis. Seattle June 1994, 214-224 (1994).

4. Mangin JF, Frouin V, Bloch I, Regis J, Lopez-Krahe J: Automatic construction of an attributed relational graph representing the cortex topography using homotopic transformations. Mathematical Methods in Medical Imaging III, Proceedings SPIE Vol. 2299, San Diego July 1994.

5. Mayya N, Rajan VT: Voronoi diagrams of polygons: a framework for shape representation. IEEE Conference on Computer Vision and Pattern Recognition. Seattle June 1994, 638-643.

6. Mittelhäußer G, Kruggel F: Region-based watershed segmentation. See this volume (1994)

7. Tiede U, Bomans M, Höhne KH, Pommert A, Riemer M, Schiemann T, Schubert R, Lierse W: A computerized three-dimensional atlas of the human skull and brain. American Journal of Neuroradiology 14, 551-559 (1993).

Fast Segmentation of Brain Magnetic Resonance Tomograms

Gangolf Mittelhäußer[1] and Frithjof Kruggel[2]

[1] University of Kaiserslautern, 67663 Kaiserslautern, Germany
e-mail: gangolf@informatik.uni-kl.de

[2] Technical University Munich, 81675 Munich, Germany
e-mail: kru@upc.muc.de

Abstract. We describe a combination of a region growing and a watershed algorithm optimized for the detection of homogeneous structures in magnetic resonance (MR) volume datasets. No prior knowledge is used except a segment model. The adaptation to different data sets is controlled by parameters which can be determined interactively due to the high speed of the algorithm. Results are shown for the segmentation of the basal ganglia and the white matter of the brain.

1 Introduction

The basic idea of the segmentation method described in this paper is to combine a region based approach using homogeneity and connectivity to yield segments with an morphological approach using watersheds on gradients to achieve a good localisation of the segment borders. The segmentation method is based on a simple but very general segment model which is defined in section 2. An extremly efficient implementation of this algorithms is given in section 3. Except the segment model no other a priori knowledge is used. The algorithm is adapted to different data sets by parameters, whose values can be determined automatically or interactively. The results shown in section 4 are generated with the second method, which is favored because of the short computing times even for large datasets. An approach for the knowledge based automatic determination of the parameters for a similar algorithm can be found in [1].

As a testbed for our algorithm we have selected the detection of the white matter and the basal ganglia in brain MR tomograms. A special property of the algorithm needed to segment these structures is its ability to differentiate very similar neighboring structures that are seperated only by a very slight inhomogenity.

2 The Algorithm

To segment the structures of the brain mentioned above a segment model is defined:

A segment is a connected, homogeneous region surrounded by inhomogeneous regions (edges) or by other segments (with different mean gray values).

Homogeneity refers to a suitable predicate. If a segment is not enclosed totally by edges it must have neighboring segments with a smooth intensity transition between them. These smooth transitions appear frequently in MR brain images but can hardly be detected by a purely gradient oriented segmentation approach. Nevertheless for both types of neighbors the segment borders should be located at the local extreme values of the gradient between the structures. To achieve these goals the following region growing algorithm is proposed:

The growing starts at the most homogeneous regions, found due to their small gradient magnitude and continues to the less homogeneous regions. Therefore the voxels are sorted by their gradient magnitude and are processed in that order. This avoids expensive neighbor search during the segmentation and makes the algorithm orders of magnitude faster than classical approaches [3]. Interestingly, this procedure is comparable to the implementation of the watershed algorithm based on immersion simulation [2].

During the region growing process the assignment of voxels to segments is controlled by a voxel-segment homogenity predicate. To avoid the creation of one segment for each local minimum, what happens if the watershed transformation is applied, a segment-segment merging step is introduced. It is controlled by a segment-segment homogeneity predicate. This algorithm yields stable results since the segments grow at first as large as possible in the homogenous regions. Additionally, the algorithm needs no seed points and the shape of the segments is purly data driven. However, with increasing gradient magnitude during the segmentation process an increasing fragmentation would occur. To prevent this, two methods are proposed:

a) "Relaxed region growing": the voxel-segment and the segment-segment homogeneity predicate are relaxed with increasing gradient magnitude.

b) "Region growing plus watershed": the region growing with fixed homogenity predicates is stopped at a certain gradient magnitude and the segmentation is completed with a modified watershed transformation.

"Relaxed region growing" has the advantage to form large segments even in less homogeneous areas. But regions may be connected if they are separated only by a slight edge. Hence this method is suitable to segment regions with neighbors of different intensity values for example the white matter of the brain (Fig. 2).

"Region growing plus watershed" stops the region growing process as soon as the gradient magnitude reaches the parameter value h_{stop}. This value should be chosen small enough to avoid the formation of many small segments. The result would be an incomplete segmentation. The idea is to extend the existing segments up to the surfaces of maximum gradient magnitude of the neighboring edges. We achieve this by a modified watershed transformation, which let the segments grow up to the next neighboring edge. Consequently all edges with magnitude > h_{stop} lead to segment borders. Hence the separation of distinct structures can be forced if an edge lies between them.

The difference between the modified and the morphological watershed transformation is that the assignment of a voxel with several segmented neighbors is still controlled by the voxel-segment homogeneity predicate, i.e. the voxel is assigned to the most suitable segment. Problems with deviated watershed lines [2] does not occur.

3 Implementation

The voxels are segmented from the minimal gradient magnitude up to $h\_max = h_{stop}$ ("Region growing plus watershed") or to $h_max = $ maximum gradient magnitude ("Relaxed region growing") (see Fig. 1).

```
for ( h = 0; h < h_max; h = h + 1) {
    while there are unsegmented voxels v with gradient magnitude h {
        while there are voxels g of v have neighboring segments {
            put voxels g in queue Q;
            for all voxel x in Q {
                if x can be merged with best matching neighboring segment then { (**)
                    voxel-segment merge;
                    if segments have become new neighbors then try seg.-seg. merge; }
                else create new segment; }}
    /* Treat local minima now: */
    for all unsegmented voxels v create new segment; } }
if "Region growing plus watershed" then perform modified watershed transformation;
```

Fig. 1. Segmentation algorithm

The final modified watershed transformation ("Region growing plus watershed") is equivalent to the region growing algorithm except that the segment-segment merge is omitted and the statement in line (**) is unconditional.

Both the region growing and the subsequent watershed algorithm use the same data structures and exploit the excellent performance $O(n)$ (without sorting, n number of voxels) of this implementation. Furthermore they are independent of the underlying coordinate grid and can be extended to graphs and m dimensional images.

4 Results and Discussion

We have applied the algorithm to segment the white matter and the basal ganglia of the brain. Fig. 2.a) shows the segment border of the single segment containing the white matter superimposed on the initial volume (slice 110 from 256 slices, size 256 x 109 voxel). The 3D visualization in Fig. 2.b) is computed with the V-Buffer algorithm [4] using the volume with the segment labels. For this segmentation the "Relaxed region growing" has been used. In spite of considerable intensity changes in the white matter a single segment is formed.

Next, results of the segmentations of the basal ganglia are presented:

Fig. 3 shows a computed segmentation of the caudatum. The used volume consists of 154 slices with 127 x 154 voxel. Here and in the following all computations were made using the "Region growing plus watershed" algorithm. The segmentation compares well to hand segmentations although the border lines are more jagged. All segmentations are computed without smoothing the data to avoid suppression of small structures (Canny operator: $\sigma = 0.7$).

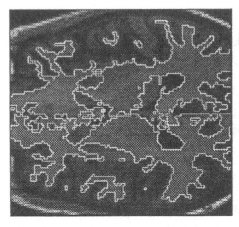 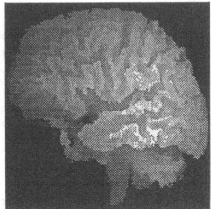

Fig. 2. a) Segmentation of the white matter   **Fig. 2. b)** Visualization of the white matter

The segmentation in slice 55 (Fig. 3.b) shows that the caudatum splits into two segments. The reason are different gray values in the area of the tail of the caudatum. As can be seen in Fig. 4 the gray values of the caudatum and the putamen are very similar where they are close together. So an increased homogenity threshold parameter would

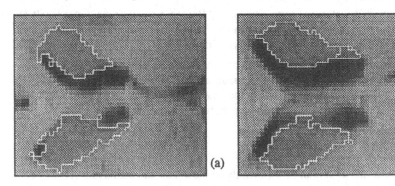

Fig. 3. Segmentation of the caudate nuclei. a) Slice 59, b) Slice 55

yield an incorrect segment merge. For the same reason the putamen and the thalamus (Fig. 4) also split into two main segments. This splitting is a principle property of this segmentation approach when segmenting structures of a high inhomogeneity relative to their vicinity. The complexity of the named brain structures can not be modelled perfectly with our simple segment model. Rather, the complex objects decompose into their homogeneous substructures. Because of its high speed the algorithm seems to be well suited to serve as a tool for higher level systems to achieve a first decomposition of an image into a small number of homogeneous regions highly correlated with the anatomical strucure.

The computing time including the sort on a SUN Sparc 10/40 for the first data volume (14 MBytes) is 142 seconds, for the second data volume (6 MBytes) 69 seconds. For repeated segmentations of the same volume the algorithm may be speeded up by storing the array of sorted voxels once it is computed.

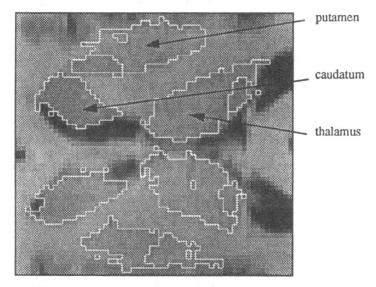

Fig. 4. Segmentation of thalamus and putamen

5 Conclusions

We have presented a 3D segmentation algorithm optimized to segment homogeneous structures in MR data volumes at a very high speed. The algorithm is based on a segment model exploiting homogenity as well as inhomogenity. The implementation is a very efficient immersion simulation [2]. Results are shown for the segmentation of the basal ganglia and the white matter of the brain. Two different variants of the algorithm are given. One is optimized for the segmentation of inhomogenous regions well seperated from similar structures, the other for the segmentation of adjacent structures with very alike properties. It shows that complex objects decompose into their homogenoeus substructures that may be reassambled later by an expert (system). This seems to be a good result since the number of substructures is small and depends only on the complexity of the object.

References

1   Kruggel F, Horsch A, Mittelhäußer G, Schnabel M: "Image Processing in the Neurologic Sciences", Proc. IEEE Workshop on Biomed. Image Analysis, Seattle, June 1994, pp. 214-223

2   Vincent L, Soille P: "Watersheds in Digital Spaces: An Efficient Algorithm Based on Immersion Simulations", IEEE PAMI, Vol. 13, No. 6, June 1991, pp. 583-598

3   Gambotto J P, Monga O: "A Parallel and Hierarchical Algorithm for Region Growing", Proc. IEEE Conf. on Comp. Vision Pattern Recognition, 1985, pp. 649-652

4   Upson C, Keeler M: "V-Buffer: Visible Volume Rendering", Computer Graphics, Vol. 22, No. 4, Aug. 1988, pp. 59-64

Comparison of Two Multi-Scale Approaches to Edge Detection in Medical Images

Wolfgang Beil and H.Siegfried Stiehl

Universität Hamburg, FB Informatik, AB KOGS,
Vogt-Kölln-Str. 30, D-22527 Hamburg, Germany

Abstract. Based on an image model of smooth regions separated by scaled discontinuities we compare two multi-scale approaches to the problem of edge detection and characterization in two-dimensional images from X-ray (CT) and magnetic resonance tomography (MR). Both approaches have been evaluated and compared on both synthetic images reassembling characteristic properties of tomograms and real MR images from the human brain.

1 Image Structure in Computed Tomograms

A computed tomogram is considered a discrete noisy 2-d intensity function representing measurements of physical phenomena in a continuous spatiotemporal domain (e.g a human body). The anisotropic spatial sampling, which we assume to be common to clinical routine examinations, induces the well known partial volume effect resulting in contrast edges with varying slope, e.g. ranging from a step edge to arbitrary scaled intensity transitions. Furthermore assuming homogeneous material within an (idealized) organ bounded by its surface, the 2-d region within a contour exhibits constant intensity. As a consequence, the resulting *image structure* is mainly defined by homogeneous, i.e. piecewise constant, regions and locally scaled intensity transitions (see also [1]).

To a first-order approximation, such scaled transitions can be treated as sigmoidal or ramp-shaped structures with arbitrary transition width. The robust detection of these scaled intensity transitions, along with estimation of local attributes for a token-based image description, necessitates a *scale-space* approach. The set of attributes we set up for this particular class of discontinuities is:

(a) Location,
(b) spatial width (scale),
(c) local contrast between the connected intensity plateaus,
(d) and local orientation (in 2-d).

Our two approaches utilize different analytical models of discontinuity of image structure and both result in multi-scale discontinuity detection, localization, and description schemes extracting the above set of attributes. These attributes, encoded in a set of token elements, may then serve as constraints for subsequent computational processes, e.g. relaxation-based smooth contour grouping and region definition (see [2].

The goal of this comparison is to evaluate which of the two approaches is best suited to extract this token set description accurately and robustly. The fidelity of subsequently computed results heavily relies on the reliability of this first processing step.

2 Scale-Space Edge Detection and Attribute Estimation

The two different models of discontinuity of image structure discussed here are both 1-d analytical functions of the contour cross section.

The discontinuity model of the first multi-scale approach is a sigmoidal intensity transition which exhibits inherent smoothness, the degree of which is controlled by the space constant λ, being the standard deviation of the generating Gaussian kernel (see [1]). The *generalized error integral curve* with arbitrary level a and contrast c is defined in 1-d by

$$\Phi_{sig}(x, \lambda) = (a + c \cdot \mathcal{H}(x)) \otimes G(x, \lambda) \quad \text{with} \quad G(x, \lambda) = \frac{1}{\sqrt{2\pi}\lambda} \exp(-\frac{x^2}{2\lambda^2})$$

being the generating Gaussian and $\mathcal{H}(x)$ the Heaviside function.

The second approach to detect scaled intensity variations in tomographic images is based on a *ramp-shaped transition* (see [3]). A 1-d representation of this transition is given by convolution of a bar $\Pi_R(x) = \mathcal{H}(x+R) - \mathcal{H}(x-R)$ with the Heaviside function $\mathcal{H}(x)$, yielding for a ramp with offset a, local contrast c, and transition width $w = 2R$

$$\Phi_{ramp}(x, c, R) = a + \frac{c}{2R} \Pi_R(x) \otimes \mathcal{H}(x).$$

To detect these scaled intensity transitions a scale-space is generated by discrete convolution with sampled Gaussian kernels of increasing width. For both of these discontinuity models specific derivative operators have been derived which are applied on every scale level. For 2-d images this means to compute directional derivatives along the gradient direction which is in line with the contour cross section.

For every scale proceeding from fine to coarse the following steps are performed:

(a) Convolution of the image with the first-order partial derivatives of a Gaussian and calculation of gradient amplitude and orientation,

(b) localization of candidate edges by non-maximum suppression of the gradient amplitude in gradient direction and thresholding (edge locations are determined with sub-pixel accuracy by utilizing a parabolic fit to the gradient magnitudes),

(c) comparison of the operator responses for all candidate edges in the current scale with those in the last scales to test a termination criterion (location of candidate edges may differ by one pixel in adjacent scales), and

(d) computation of the edge attributes from the last operator responses if the criterion is met.

The approach based on the sigmoidal transition will in the following be abbreviated with BNS-scheme, whereas the approach for the detection of ramp-shaped transitions will be denoted NO-scheme.

3   Evaluation and Comparison

Both segmentation schemes have been evaluated and compared regarding the accuracy of the estimated edge attributes and the dependency of these attributes on noise, curvature, transition width and type. The results of the evaluation on noise-free synthetic images can be comprised as follows:

(a) Both schemes estimate the local orientation very accurately.
(b) Both schemes yield inaccurate results for step edges. (Fig. 1 a,b)
(c) The NO-scheme underestimates the transition width of sigmoidal transitions. (Fig. 1b)
(d) The BNS-scheme estimates the contrast more accurately than the NO-scheme. (Fig. 2 a,b)
(e) The subpixel localization of the NO-scheme is more accurate than that of the BNS-scheme. (Fig. 3)
(f) The localization accuracy decreases with increasing curvature. (Fig. 3)

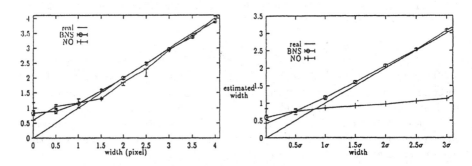

Fig. 1. estimated transition width vs. true width (linear contour with orientation 15 degree) ramp-shaped (a) and sigmoidal (b) transition

Additionally both approaches were tested on the same synthetic images with added Gaussian or signal dependent (Rice distributed) noise. These tests revealed that noise results in an underestimation of the contrast. The BNS-scheme is generally more robust against noise than the NO-scheme. Signal dependent noise has a greater effect than Gaussian noise with the same signal-to-noise ratio. (Fig. 4 a,b)

Test were also performed on MR images of the human brain. An example visualizing the subpixel location and orientation of the detected edge elements is shown in Fig. 5.

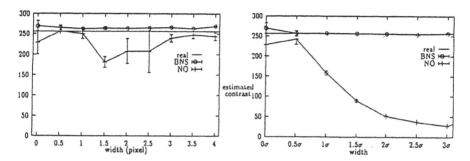

Fig. 2. estimated contrast vs. true width (linear contour with orientation 15 degree) ramp-shaped (a) and sigmoidal (b) transition

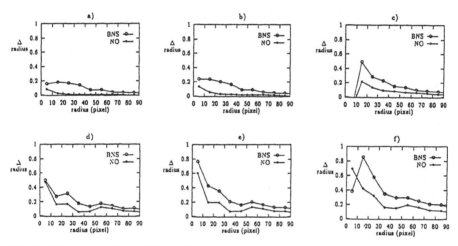

Fig. 3. Mean deviation of the estimated location vs. contour radius: step edge (a), ramp-shaped transition of width 2 (b), ramp-shaped transition of width 4 (c), sigmoidal transition with $\sigma = 0.7$ (d), sigmoidal transition with $\sigma = 1.4$ (e) and sigmoidal transition with $\sigma = 2.8$ (f)

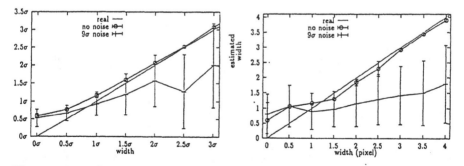

Fig. 4. estimated transition width vs. true width with and without noise (sigmoidal transition, linear contour with orientation 15 degree) BNS-scheme (a) and NO-scheme (b)

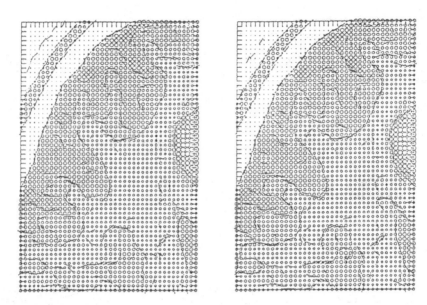

Fig. 5. oriented edge elements found in a MR image of the human brain (circles encode image intensities) BNS-scheme (a) and NO-scheme (b)

The conclusion of this comparison is that the NO-scheme based on a ramp-shaped discontinuity model has serious shortcomings and should be discarded in favor of the BNS-scheme.

4 Acknowledgement

This work was funded by COVIRA (Computer Vision in Radiology), project A2003 of the AIM (Advanced Informatics in Medicine) programme of the European Commission.

References

1. Back, S., Neumann, H., Stiehl, H.S.: On Segmenting Computed Tomograms. in: H.U. Lemke, M.L. Rhodes, C.C. Jaffee, R. Felix (Eds.) Proc. 3rd International Symposium on Computer Assisted Radiology CAR'89, Springer Berlin (1989) 691–696
2. Beil, W., Ottenberg, K., Stiehl, H.S.: Towards Automatic Segmentation of Two-Dimensional Brain Tomograms. in: L. Beolchi, M.H. Kuhn (Eds.) Medical Imaging - Analysis of Multimodality 2D/3D Images, Studies in Health Technology and Informatics, IOS Press 19 (1994) 158–174
3. Neumann, H., Ottenberg, K.: Estimating attributes of smooth signal transitions from scale-space. Proc. 11th IAPR Int. Conf. on Pattern Recognition (ICPR-92), Le Hague III (1992) 754–758

Computer Aided Surgery (CAS) System for Stereotactic Neurosurgery

Yoshitaka Masutani[1], Ken Masamune[1], Makoto Suzuki[1], Takeyoshi Dohi[1], Hiroshi Iseki[2] and Kintomo Takakura[2]

[1] University of Tokyo. 7-3-1 Hongo, Bunkyo-ku, Tokyo 113 Japan
[2] Tokyo Women's Medical College, 8 Kawada-cho, Shinjuku-ku. Tokyo 162 Japan

Abstract. Computer Aided Surgery (CAS) system for stereotactic neurosurgery has been developed by means of robotics and software technology. In this paper, we describe design concepts and features of our system which consists of a needle insertion manipulator, a navigation system and a software system for visualization, surgical planning and manipulator control. And a phantom study for the estimation of manipulator control accuracy and a clinical application of the navigation system are also reported.

1 Introduction

Since the establishment of fundamental techniques for stereotactics by Clarke [1] early in this century, various technologies such as robotics, softwares, etc., have been employed in this area to improve the quality of surgical operation. The most serious problem in neurosurgery for surgeons was the difficulty to recognize and perceive the precise position under their manipulation. To overcome this problem, various navigation systems have been developed using various sensors, frames and image processing softwares, to point out the accurate position under operation on the sliced images in monitor display [2] [3] [4]. Medical software technologies for surgical support [5] [6] had been applied mainly to the plastic surgery in its early phase. One of the problems in these software development was that the surgical plannings were based on just a visualization or interactive trials and errors of surgical simulation. To use the maximum ability of computers, a surgical support software should propose some suggestive ways of operation based on quantitative analysis and evaluation. Early in the medical application of robotics, industrial robots were applied directly to the stereotactic neurosurgery. Recent reports warned against the application of industrial robots to medical use for its questionable safety in surgical operation. Davies [7] analyzed the safety problems of clinical applications of robotics, and gave some suggestions for system design. Taking such safety problems into consideration, several sophisticated systems have been developed [8] [9].

We have been developing Computer Aided Surgery(CAS) system [10] [11] [12] for abdominal surgery and neurosurgery since the middle of 80's. Its main concepts are quantitativeness and optimization of surgery by using computers and robots. Especially in stereotactic neurosurgery, quantitative spatial information of lesions or tumors and quantitative control of surgical equipments are important. The meaning of optimization here is both in surgical planning process and in surgical operation itself. The former process automatically leads to the optimized way of operation instead of interactive trials and errors. In the latter, from the view of low invasiveness, positioning accuracy and rapidity of the operation, it can be realized due to the technologies of mechanics and electronics. In this paper, we describe our surgical planning system, our intra-operative navigation system and our needle insertion manipulator system for quantitative and optimized stereotactic neurosurgery.

2   System Description

2.1   Software system for surgical planning

In this system, organ objects are expressed by surface model. They are reconstructed from 3D medical images like MRI and X-ray CT by 3D image processing techniques including the marching cube algorithm [13]. The surgical optimization is based on the computation of the degree of invasion in all possible cases of approaches by the needle insertion manipulator. In each orientation of the needle to the target, the degree of invasion is estimated by the minimum distance between the needle and objects which must be prevented from puncturing. They are blood vessels and functional area on the surface of brain like auditory area. The optimized insertion point can be obtained from the case of the minimum invasion. The system was implemented in UNIX based SUN workstation and XView environment. The user-interface of software was designed and developed in consideration of its use in a notebook-styled workstation. This information of the optimized way of needle insertion is utilized for manipulator control.

2.2   Navigation system

Figure 1-a shows the scheme of the navigation system. The main unit(Figure 1-b) attached to a stereotactic frame, consists of a pair of CCD cameras and a pair of laser pointers of which focus is located 120 mm from the arc. The focus of laser pointers is displayed with surface objects in the software system describe above. The three linear encoders are detachable and the main unit is compact enough for whole body sterilization. The CCD cameras were equipped to obtain a stereoscopic image of the field of operation. Its additional purpose is the image fusion with surface shaded organs of computer graphics. The most important consideration is that the structure of movements do never interfere with the patient's head in any cases. Though they are driven manually, the theoretical errors were estimated as under 0.1 mm, excepting errors caused by mis-installation of stereotactic frame, brain deformation, etc..

2.3   Needle insertion manipulator system

A needle insertion manipulator for X-ray CT guided stereotactic neurosurgery equipped with six degrees of freedom(Figure 2) was designed for the purpose

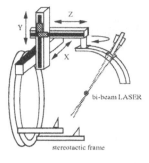
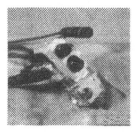

Fig. 1. Laser navigation system: a) scheme(left), b)main unit with CCD cameras and aser pointers(right)

such as biopsy, hyperthermia, etc.. These kinds of equipments can optimize a surgery from the view of not only accuracy and rapidity of operation but also safety of surgeons. In the case surgeon may be exposed to a radio-active source for radiotherapy, the manipulator displays its real worth. The movements were constrained as well as our navigation system. And the closest element to a patient, which is an arc for the latitudinal movement. was designed so that any sliced images of the patient never contain it to avoid the imaging artifact. The whole body of the manipulator was designed to be compact enough for whole sterilization and to be smaller than 600mm in diameter, which is a standard gantry size of X-ray CT scanner. The all movements are driven by step motors.

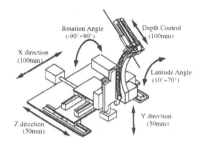
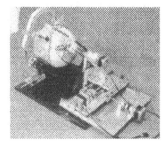

Fig. 2. The needle insertion manipulator with six degrees of freedom

3 Experimental Results and Clinical Application

3.1 Surgical planning

Brain surface and functional areas were reconstructed from a MRI data of normal volunteer excepting the virtual target. A needle insertion optimization was carried out for this case. The result is shown in Figure 3. Each color of the area indicates the degree of invasion, and the catheter shows the approach direction and position in the minimum invasion. As the computation time to obtain the solution, 4-9 minutes were required with Sparc 10 ZX SUN workstation.

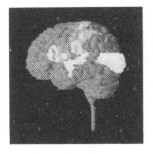 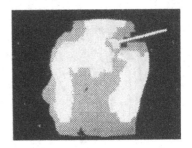

Fig. 3. Surface shaded brain with functional areas(left), result of invasion minimization in needle insertion(right)

3.2 Clinical experience of the laser navigation system

Our navigation system was employed in a surgery for removal of the tumor located above the left ventricle. Through the whole process of operation, the surgeon could confirm the operating position on the reconstructed brain models of brain and tumor visualized in the notebook-styled workstation (SPARCbook 2, Tadpole Technology Inc.) beside him (Figure 4-a). In this case, the main unit of navigation system including laser pointers was covered by a sterilized sheet, instead of whole sterilization. The error in the clinical use was estimated as about 1.0-2.0 mm mainly caused by the resolution limit of source MR images.

3.3 Phantom study of the needle insertion manipulator

Experiments for the motion accuracy test were carried out in the laboratory. As the results, the error in positioning was estimated as 0.1 mm, and the error in orientation was 1.0 degree. A phantom study was also carried out to the evaluation of the needle insertion accuracy under the guidance of X-ray CT images (Figure 4-b). A water melon was used as a phantom, and one of its seeds was regarded as an imaginary target for puncturing. By monitoring in CT images, the positioning error was estimated as under 1.0 mm which equals the size of image pixel as the limitation of measurement. Through these experiments, it was clarified that our manipulator can be controlled in enough accuracy for clinical use.

4 Conclusions

(1) We have developed Computer Aided Surgery (CAS) system for stereotactic neurosurgery which provides the optimized way of surgery. (2) By the surgical planning system, the optimized needle insertion position and direction were computed based on the minimum invasion evaluation. (3) The error of navigation system was estimated as about 1.0-2.0 mm in clinic use. (4) Through phantom studies, the needle insertion manipulator was controlled in accuracy, under 1.0 mm of positioning error, and under 1.0 degree of orientation error.

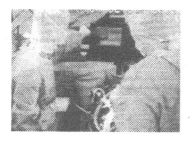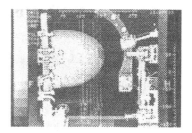

Fig. 4. a) Surgeons with the navigation system in clinical use. b) phantom study of the manipulator system (X-ray CT's scout view)

References

1. R. H. Clarke et al. On the intrinsic fibers of the cerebellum. its nuclei and its efferent tracts. Brain. **28** (1905) 12–29

2. P. J. Kelly Future perspectives in stereotactic neurosurgery: stereotactic microsurgical removal of deep brain tumors. J. of Neurosurgical Sciences **33** (1989) 149–154

3. E. M. Friets et al. A Frameless Stereotaxic Operating Microscope for Neurosurgery. IEEE Trans. on biomedical Eng. **36** (1989) 608–617

4. E. Watanabe, et al. Open surgery assisted by the neuronavigator, a stereotactic articulated, sensitive arm. Neurosurgery **28** (1991) 792–800

5. R. A. Robb, et al. Interactive display and analysis of 3-D medical images. IEEE Trans. on Medical Imaging **8** (1989) 217–226

6. S. Yokoi, et al. A craniofacial surgical planning system. Proc. of the 8th Ann. Conf. and Expo. of NCGA **3** (1987) 152–161

7. B. Davies Safety of Medical Robotics Proc. of Int. Conf. on Advanced Robotics(ICAR) (1993) 311–317

8. D. Glauser, et al. Neuro Surgical Operation with the Dedicated Robot Minerva. Proc. of ICAR (1993) 347–351

9. W. S. Ng, et al. Robotic Surgery A First-Hand Experience In Transurethral Resection of the Prostate. IEEE Engineering in med. and biol. March (1993) 120–125

10. T. Dohi, et al. Computer aided surgery system(CAS):development of surgical simulation and planning system with three dimensional graphic reconstruction. Proc. of the 1st Conf. on Visualization on Biomedical Computing (1990) 458–462

11. D. Hashimoto, et al. Development of computer aided surgery system: Three-dimensional reconstruction for treatment of liver cancer. Surgery (1991) 589–596

12. 18) T. Dohi, et al. A Needle Insertion Manipulator For Stereotactic Neurosurgery. Proc. of 2nd World congress of Biomechanics (1994) 99

13. W. E. Lorensen, et al. Marching Cubes: A High resolution 3D surface Construction Algorithm. Computer Graphics **21** (1987) 163–169

Registration of 3D Objects Using Linear Algebra

Gilles BUREL, Hugues HENOCQ, Jean-Yves CATROS

Thomson Broadband Systems, Av. Belle Fontaine, 35510 Cesson-Sévigné, France

Abstract. A method for estimating the orientation of 3D objects without point correspondence information is described. It is based on the decomposition of the object onto a basis of spherical harmonics. Tensors are obtained, and their normalization provides the orientation.

1 Introduction

Methods for estimating the orientation of 3D objects have largely focused on polyhedral models [5], and numerous methods need point correspondence information [6]. Another kind of approach is based on the minimization of a distance between the objects to register, with respect to a set of parameters modelizing the 3D transformation. Such approaches avoid the need of correspondence information, and may modelize non-rigid transformations, but they are computationally intensive. The use of genetic algorithms has been proposed recently to speed up the algorithm [3].

In this paper, a method which is not restricted to polyhedral objects, and which does not need point correspondence information is proposed. The method is fast because the 3D transformation is computed directly, without iterative search. The basic idea is to take profit of linear algebra theory. The 3D object is decomposed onto a basis of spherical harmonics, wherefrom tensors are obtained. The normalization of these tensors determines the orientation of the object with respect to a standard position. The input of the method is a 3D representation of the surface of the object. For instance, in the medical domain, such information can be easily derived from scanner data.

The paper is organized as follows. In the next section, the principle and the interest of the representation of a 3D object in the basis of spherical harmonics are presented. Then, the determination of the 3D transformation is explained. Finally, experimental results on a problem of registration of vertebrae are shown.

2 Decomposition onto the basis of spherical harmonics

Let us note $\mathcal{F}_S$ the space of differentiable functions from $[0, \pi] \times [0, 2\pi]$ to $\mathcal{C}$, with finite energy. To each 3D object, we associate a function $|\Psi\rangle$ such that $\Psi(\theta, \phi)$ is the distance between the center of gravity of the object and the farthest point still belonging to the object in the direction given by the spherical coordinates (θ, ϕ). This kind of representation is usual for 3D medical data [1] [2].

The spherical harmonics are functions of $\mathcal{F}_S$ which can be computed using Legendre polynomials [4]. In the medical domain, they have been used to represent cranial surfaces [1]. The set of spherical harmonics $\{|Y_{lm}\rangle;\ l = 0, ..., \infty;\ m = -l, ..., l\}$ is an orthonormal basis of $\mathcal{F}_S$. Hence, any function $\Psi(\theta, \phi)$ can be described by its coordinates in this basis:

$$c_l^m = \langle Y_{lm}|\Psi\rangle = \int_0^{2\pi} d\phi \int_0^\pi \sin\theta\ d\theta\ Y_{lm}^*(\theta, \phi)\ \Psi(\theta, \phi) \tag{1}$$

The effect of a rotation of the object on these coordinates is given by:

$$
\begin{pmatrix} \varepsilon_0^0 \\ \varepsilon_1^{-1} \\ \varepsilon_1^0 \\ \varepsilon_1^1 \\ \varepsilon_2^{-2} \\ \varepsilon_2^{-1} \\ \varepsilon_2^0 \\ \varepsilon_2^1 \\ \varepsilon_2^2 \\ \cdot \end{pmatrix}
=
\begin{pmatrix} D_0 & & & \\ & \begin{pmatrix} & & \\ & D_1 & \\ & & \end{pmatrix} & & \\ & & \begin{pmatrix} & & \\ & D_2 & \\ & & \end{pmatrix} & \\ & & & \cdot \end{pmatrix}
\begin{pmatrix} c_0^0 \\ c_1^{-1} \\ c_1^0 \\ c_1^1 \\ c_2^{-2} \\ c_2^{-1} \\ c_2^0 \\ c_2^1 \\ c_2^2 \\ \cdot \end{pmatrix}
\tag{2}
$$

This equation shows the interest of reasoning in the basis of spherical harmonics: $\mathcal{F}_S$ is decomposed into a direct sum of orthogonal subspaces globally invariant by rotation, such as $\mathcal{E}_2$ whose basis is $\{|Y_{2,-2}\rangle, |Y_{2,-1}\rangle, |Y_{20}\rangle, |Y_{21}\rangle, |Y_{22}\rangle\}$. Using group theory [7], one can prove that is is impossible to find a basis in which the rotation operator takes a simpler form.

Let us define a rotation by Euler angles. A rotation of the coordinates system (x,y,z) is decomposed into 3 elementary rotations: a rotation α around z, which transforms y into u, followed by a rotation β ($0 \leq \beta < \pi$) around u, which transforms z into Z, and finally a rotation γ around Z. The effect of the rotation on c_l^m is [7]:

$$c_l^m(\alpha, \beta, \gamma) = \sum_n D_{nm}^l(\alpha, \beta, \gamma)c_l^n \tag{3}$$

$$D_{nm}^l(\alpha, \beta, \gamma) = e^{-i\alpha n}.d_{nm}^l(\beta).e^{-i\gamma m} \tag{4}$$

Let us note $c = \cos\beta$ and $s = \sin\beta$. In $\mathcal{E}_2$ we have:

$$d^2(\beta) = \begin{pmatrix}
(\frac{1+c}{2})^2 & -\frac{(1+c)}{2}s & \frac{\sqrt{6}}{4}s^2 & -\frac{(1-c)}{2}s & (\frac{1-c}{2})^2 \\
\frac{(1+c)}{2}s & \frac{(1+c)}{2}(2c-1) & -\sqrt{\frac{3}{2}}sc & \frac{(1-c)}{2}(2c+1) & -\frac{(1-c)}{2}s \\
\frac{\sqrt{6}}{4}s^2 & \sqrt{\frac{3}{2}}sc & \frac{3}{2}c^2 - \frac{1}{2} & -\sqrt{\frac{3}{2}}sc & \frac{\sqrt{6}}{4}s^2 \\
\frac{(1-c)}{2}s & \frac{(1-c)}{2}(2c+1) & \sqrt{\frac{3}{2}}sc & \frac{(1+c)}{2}(2c-1) & -\frac{(1+c)}{2}s \\
(\frac{1-c}{2})^2 & \frac{(1-c)}{2}s & \frac{\sqrt{6}}{4}s^2 & \frac{(1+c)}{2}s & (\frac{1+c}{2})^2
\end{pmatrix} \tag{5}$$

3 Determination of the orientation

3.1 Principle of the method

The method determines the Euler angles that rotate the object to a standard orientation characterized by constraints on the tensor c_l^m. Using basic properties of the spherical harmonics, one can prove that $c_l^{-m} = (-1)^m (c_l^m)^*$. Hence, we consider only coefficients with $m \leq 0$. Since we have 3 degrees of freedom, we can, for instance, cancel one complex coefficient, plus one imaginary part. We will try to determine the rotation which yields to:

$$
\begin{cases}
c_2^{-1}(\alpha, \beta, \gamma) = 0 \\
c_2^{-2}(\alpha, \beta, \gamma) \text{ real, positive and maximal} \\
Re\{c_1^{-1}(\alpha, \beta, \gamma)\} \geq 0 \text{ and } Im\{c_1^{-1}(\alpha, \beta, \gamma)\} \geq 0
\end{cases}
\tag{6}
$$

We have $c_1^{-1}(\alpha, \beta) = \cos\beta\, Re\left\{c_1^{-1}(\alpha)\right\} + i\, Im\left\{c_1^{-1}(\alpha)\right\} - \frac{\sin\beta}{\sqrt{2}} c_1^0(\alpha)$. The interest of positivity and maximality constraints is to avoid residual ambiguities.

3.2   Determination of α and β

In $\mathcal{E}_2$, the effect of a rotation α is given by $c_2^m(\alpha) = e^{-im\alpha} c_2^m$. Let us note:

$$
c_2^0(\alpha) = a_0 \qquad c_2^{-1}(\alpha) = -a_1 + ib_1 \qquad c_2^{-2}(\alpha) = a_2 - ib_2
\tag{7}
$$

Then, according to equation (5) the effect of a rotation β is given by:

$$
c_2^{-1}(\alpha, \beta) = A \sin(2\beta) - a_1\cos(2\beta) + i(b_1\cos\beta - b_2\sin\beta)
\tag{8}
$$

where $A = (\frac{a_2}{2} - \frac{1}{2}\sqrt{\frac{3}{2}}a_0)$. To cancel $c_2^{-1}(\alpha, \beta)$, we must have:

$$
\frac{2\tan\beta}{1 - \tan^2\beta} = \frac{a_1}{A} \quad \text{and} \quad \tan(\beta) = \frac{b_1}{b_2}
\tag{9}
$$

By replacing the second equation in the first one, and assuming $Ab_2 \neq 0$ and $b_1^2 \neq b_2^2$, we get $\mathcal{F}(\alpha) = 0$, where:

$$
\mathcal{F}(\alpha) = a_1(b_2^2 - b_1^2) - b_1 b_2 (a_2 - \sqrt{\frac{3}{2}} a_0)
\tag{10}
$$

Then, α must be a solution of $\mathcal{F}(\alpha) = 0$. One can prove that the number of solutions in the interval $[0, \pi[$ is always comprised between 1 and 3. These solutions can be found by any zero-finding method. Once α is determined, β is given by the second equation of (9). Finally, (α, β) which produces the largest value of $|c_2^{-2}(\alpha, \beta)|$ is kept.

3.3   Determination of γ

A rotation $\gamma \in [0, \pi[$ produces: $c_2^{-2}(\alpha, \beta, \gamma) = e^{2i\gamma} c_2^{-2}(\alpha, \beta)$. We obtain $c_2^{-2}(\alpha, \beta, \gamma)$ real and positive if:

$$
\gamma = -\frac{1}{2} Arg(c_2^{-2}(\alpha, \beta))
\tag{11}
$$

Until now, we restricted α and γ to $[0, \pi[$. One can prove that, when this restriction is cancelled, we get 3 new candidates. Hence, the possible solutions are $\{(\alpha, \beta, \gamma), (\alpha, \beta, \gamma + \pi), (\alpha + \pi, \pi - \beta, \gamma), (\alpha + \pi, \pi - \beta, \gamma + \pi)\}$. The constraint on the sign of the real and imaginary parts of $c_1^{-1}(\alpha, \beta, \gamma)$ determines the solution to keep. In fact, the sign of the real and imaginary parts of any $c_l^{-1}(\alpha, \beta, \gamma)$ with $l \neq 2$ could be used for this determination.

4 Experimental results: registration of vertebrae

Let us note R_{std1}, R_{std2} the rotations which bring objects 1 and 2 to their standard position. Then the rotation between the two objects is given by: $R_{12} = R_{std1}^{-1} \cdot R_{std2}$.

Figure 1 illustrates the result obtained for a medical imaging application. We have two 3D images of a vertebra provided by a scanner. The acquisitions took place at different times. Using the method described above, the second acquisition has been registered with respect to the first one. The residual angular errors are usually less than a degree. This registration helps the specialist to compare the 3D images.

The method does not need the determination of specific points for correspon-

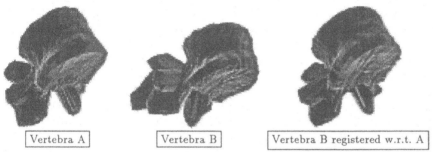

| Vertebra A | Vertebra B | Vertebra B registered w.r.t. A |

Fig. 1. *Medical imaging application: registration of a vertebra*

dence. Such points could be hard (and computationally expensive) to reliably determine on this kind of shape. Furthermore, because the vertebrae above have similar variances on two principal axes, methods based on the moments of inertia as in [2] do not apply.

The vertebra to register is originally represented by a 3D voxel matrix of size 100x120x150. Figure 2 shows the error on the estimation of angle β with respect to the error on the estimation of the barycenter position. An error on the estimation of the barycenter could be due to incomplete scanning, for instance. The effect on the estimation of β becomes noticeable when the translation estimation error is about 15 pixels (that is more than 20% of the including sphere radius).

The experimentations above have been done with a discretization step of 5° for the computation of the c_l^m. Since the spherical harmonics can be precomputed, equation (1) shows that the number of multiplications is $(360/5)(180/5) = 2592$ for each of c_2^0, c_1^0, and $2 \times 2592 = 5184$ for each of $c_2^{-2}, c_2^{-1}, c_1^{-1}$ (because in that case the spherical harmonic is complex). Hence, the total number of multiplications is 20736. On a standard PC machine realizing more than 1 multiplication per μs, this represents a computation time of $20ms$ only.

5 Conclusion

A method for determining the orientation of 3D objects has been proposed. It is not restricted to polyhedral objects, it does not need point matching, and it

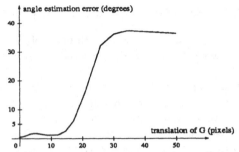

Fig. 2. *Evaluation of the robustness of the method*

is fast because it is not iterative. Since it needs 3D information on input, it can be applied to any domain in which such an information is available, but it is not appropriate for domains in which only 2D information is available, unless 3D reconstruction by computer tomography can be performed. On the theoretical point of view, this work opens new directions of investigation: approaches based on linear algebra and tensor theory instead of structural methods.

Determination of the orientation of 3D objects is a problem of practical interest in medical applications. It allows the registration of 3D data taken at different times or in different conditions. It might also be useful in future medical robotics applications. Since the method is fast and simple it does not require expensive hardware or software.

Acknowledgements: The scanner images of vertebrae have been provided by the LTSI Laboratory, University of Rennes.

References

1. E.J. Holupka & H.M. Kooy, "Spherical harmonic expansion of cranial surfaces", Medical Physics, **18** (4), pp 765-768, Jul/Aug 1991
2. E.J. Holupka & H.M. Kooy, "A geometric algorithm for medical image correlations", Medical Physics, **19** (2), pp 433-438, Mar/Apr 1992
3. J.J. Jacq & C. Roux, "Recalage Monomodalité Automatique en Imagerie Médicale 2D et 3D à l'aide d'un Algorithme Génétique Traditionnel", 9e congrès RFIA, Paris, 11-14 janvier 1994, pp 109-120
4. R. Lenz, "Group theoretical methods in image processing", Lecture notes in computer science, n° 413, 1987
5. S. Linnainman et al., "Pose Determination of a three Dimensionnal Object Using Triangle Pairs", IEEE-PAMI, vol. 10, n° 5, Sept. 1988
6. K.D. Toennies et al., "Registration of 3D Objects and Surfaces", IEEE Computer Graphics and Applications, vol. 10, n° 3, pp 52-62, May 1990
7. E. Wigner, "Group Theory and its application to Quantum Mechanics of Atomic Spectra", New-York: Academic, 1959

Talairach-Tournoux/Schaltenbrand-Wahren Based Electronic Brain Atlas System

Wieslaw L. Nowinski[1], Anthony Fang[1], Bonnie T. Nguyen[1], Raghu Raghavan[1]
R. Nick Bryan[2], Jerry Miller[2]

[1] JHU–ISS Center for Information-enhanced Medicine, CI$_E$Med
Institute of Systems Science, National University of Singapore
Heng Mui Keng Terrace, Kent Ridge, Singapore 0511
[2] Department of Radiology, Johns Hopkins University, Baltimore, MD, USA

Abstract. The paper addresses design and development of an interactive, fully labeled Talairach-Tournoux/Schaltenbrand-Wahren based electronic brain atlas system. The primary goal of our atlas is to allow the user to choose any name from the anatomical index, find the corresponding object in the MRI/CT data, and visualize, manipulate in real-time and quantify it in 2–D/3–D. The atlas system provides several tools for registration, visualization, image processing and analysis, reformatting, anatomical index operations, object extraction/editing, quantification, and file handling. The atlas system is implemented in C++ and uses texture mapping. The work is a precursor to a fully computational 3–D brain model and atlases supporting function, vasculature, pathology, and brain connections.

1 Introduction

The 1990s have been declared to be the Decade of the Brain, and research in all aspects of the brain is receiving widespread attention throughout the world. One of our contributions is in constructing electronic brain atlases. There is a number of paper brain atlases, e.g. [1-5]. Electronic brain atlases, e.g. [6-10], are more convenient and flexible to use than paper atlases. Moreover, they can provide additional and powerful features not available in paper atlases.

The CI$_E$Med electronic brain atlas system contains digitized, enhanced, and labeled: *Co-Planar Stereotactic Atlas of the Human Brain* by Talairach and Tournoux [1]; *Atlas of Stereotaxy of the Human Brain* by Schaltenbrand and Wahren [2]; *Referentially Oriented Cerebral MRI Anatomy. Atlas of Stereotaxic Anatomical Correlations for Gray and White Matter* by Talairach and Tournoux [3]; and *Atlas of the Cerebral Sulci* by Ono, Kubic and Abernathey [4]. Combined anatomical indexes have about 1000 items.

The primary goal of our atlas is to allow the user to choose any name from the anatomical indexes, find the corresponding object in the MRI/CT data, and visualize, manipulate in real-time and quantify it in 2–D/3–D. The primary applications of this atlas system are in neurosurgery, neuroradiology, and neuroeducation. The novel features of our system include: it is based on standard anatomical atlases, commonly used in day-to-day clinical practice; the system is able to extract, edit, visualize, manipulate and quantify 3–D anatomical structures; any new data can be added to the system and labeled; the Schaltenbrand-Wahren and Talairach-Tournoux atlases are combined together and preregistered; electronic versions of the Referentially Oriented Talairach-Tournoux and the Cerebral Sulci atlases are available; rich set of operations; atlas and patient data navigation is simple and powerful; and low cost.

2 Atlas system design

The general philosophy of the atlas system design is illustrated in Fig. 1.

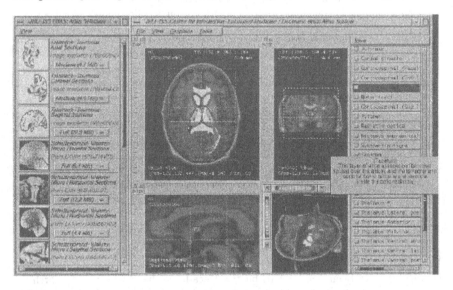

Fig. 1. Brain Atlas Interface. (left) Atlas selection panel: a scrollable and expandable list of atlases. (center) The main work area with the axial, coronal, and sagittal 2–D views and a 2-1/2–D triplanar view. The most common operators on the views, such as resize, magnify, position, blend, etc., are mapped to the mouse buttons while the less frequent operators are accessible via pulldown menus. (right) Anatomical index: names may be displayed in full or abbreviations. Functional descriptions of structures are displayed via a popup menu. Entries are highlighted as image parts are selected, and vice versa.

Three of the graphic windows depict the 2–D orthogonal views of the data and atlases. Each window is smoothly and continuously resizable to allow directing attention to a particular view. A fourth window shows a 2-1/2–D display of a triplanar intersection, or alternatively a 3–D image. Intuitive operations are provided to transform (rotate, scale, etc.) the triplaner or 3–D image in real-time using texture mapping. The atlas data is overlayed onto the patient data with a variable degree of blending. The user can probe into any region on the image to query the anatomical details, or to click on the anatomical listing to find the corresponding structure on the image display.

3 Atlas data

The Talairach-Tournoux atlas describes cerebral structures through series of frontal, sagittal, and horizontal cross-sections of a single brain specimen. Atlas image data are digitized with high resolution, aligned, and organized into volumes. The digitized images are preprocessed and enhanced, see Fig. 2: left.

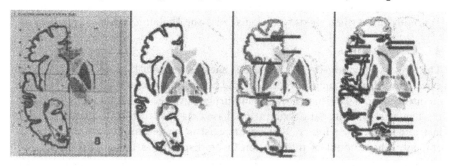

Fig. 2. Talairach-Tournoux atlas. (left) Digitized original image. (center-left) Processed and enhanced image: grid, rulers, and annotations are removed; a unique color is assigned to each structure; the left hemisphere structures which are only outlined in the paper atlas are displayed as labeled (colored) regions along with their substructures. (center-right) Gyri labeling; (right) Brodmann areas labeling.

Talairach-Tournoux atlas image data are organized in five fully labeled volumes: horizontal (908 x 768 points); verticoronal (768 x 664 points); sagittal (both hemispheres); Brodmann areas (Fig. 2: center-right); gyri (Fig. 2: right). Note that the last two volumes are not available in the paper atlas. In addition, three indexes (about 170 items) are provided: anatomical; Brodmann areas; and gyri.

The Schaltenbrand-Wahren atlas contains photographic plates based on several brains, Fig. 3: left.

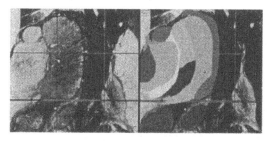

Fig. 3. Schaltenbrand-Wahren atlas: (left) digitized and (right) color-coded.

Atlas image data are organized in 18 volumes: macroseries (frontal/ sagittal/ horizontal); microseries (frontal/sagittal/horizontal); electroanatomical microseries (motor function and sensation for coronal/sagittal/axial sections, vegetative effects for coronal/sagittal/axial sections). The microseries sections are fully labeled, Fig. 3: right. Full Schaltenbrand-Wahren anatomical index containing about 500 items is available.

Both Talairach-Tournoux and Schaltenbrand-Wahren atlases are combined together and preregistered [11]. This way any data registered with the Talairach-Tournoux atlas is automatically registered with the Schaltenbrand-Wahren atlas. Because the Schaltenbrand-Wahren atlas focuses on the deep structures, we chose to blend in the atlas only when the deep structures are amplified. In effect, we gradually "switch" from the Schaltenbrand-Wahren atlas to the Talairach-Tournoux atlas when the user "zooms" into the thalamic region.

4 Operations

The system provides several operations such as reformatting, registration, navigation and display, image processing and analysis, structure extraction/editing, quantification, 3-D visualization (contouring, surface, and volume rendering).

The atlas-patient data registration, based on Talairach transformation [1], is fast and simple, see Fig. 1. Non-linear registration techniques are under development. The amount of information to be displayed is huge: MRI axial/coronal/sagittal slices; the Talairach-Tournoux axial/coronal/sagittal sections; the Schaltenbrand-Wahren axial/coronal/sagittal microseries sections; the Referentially Oriented Talairach-Tournoux coronal/sagittal sections; triplanar; 3–D image; anatomical index, etc. In order to trace anatomical structures, we propose a new way of navigation. The user is provided with all these data on the screen, and is able to continuously navigate through the data such as that any structure from the anatomical index can be traced continuously in space both for the patient and the atlas data. Continuous navigation (see Fig. 1) includes continuous resizing of axial, coronal, sagittal, and triplanar views; continuous atlas - MRI blending; continuous (blended) switching between the Talairach-Tournoux and the Schaltenbrand-Wahren atlases; continuous (blended) switching between the Referentially Oriented Talairach-Tournoux atlas and the Talairach-Tournoux atlas; unified triplanar for the Talairach-Tournoux and the Schaltenbrand-Wahren brain atlases (Fig. 4); continuous triplanar - 3–D image blending.

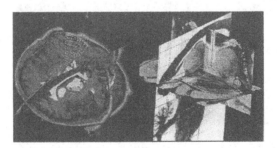

Fig. 4. Unified triplanar display. (left) Talairach-Tournoux atlas overlayed onto MRI data. (right) Schaltenbrand-Wahren atlas (3 different hemispheres are registered).

The registered patient data are fully labeled. In addition, any structure in the anatomical indexes can be extracted from the patient data, edited, and displayed in 3–D. For example, Fig. 5: left shows the extraction and 3–D reconstruction of the putamen. The atlas system also allows to extract structures not visible on

MRI data, see Fig. 5: right-top. 3–D display of the thalamic nuclei extracted from the Talairach-Tournoux atlas is shown in Fig. 5: right-bottom.

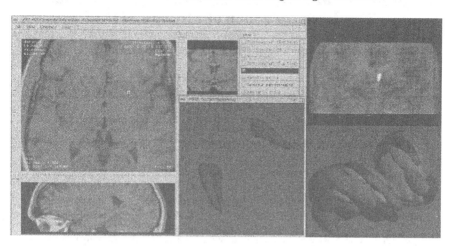

Fig. 5. Extraction and 3–D reconstruction. (left) The putamen. (right-bottom) The thalamic nuclei. (right-top) Volume rendered image of the antero-principalis nucleus.

References

1. Talairach J. and Tournoux P.: *Co-Planar Stereotactic Atlas of the Human Brain.* Georg Thieme Verlag, Stuttgart 1988
2. Schaltenbrand G. and Wahren W.: *Atlas of Stereotaxy of the Human Brain.* Thieme Verlag, Stuttgart 1977
3. Talairach J. and Tournoux P.: *Referentially Oriented Cerebral MRI Anatomy. Atlas of Stereotaxic Anatomical Correlations for Gray and White Matter.* Georg Thieme Verlag, Stuttgart 1993
4. Ono M., Kubic S. and Abernathey C. D.: *Atlas of the Cerebral Sulci.* Georg Thieme Verlag, Stuttgart 1991
5. Andrew J. and Watkins E. S.: *A Stereotaxic Atlas of the Human Thalamus and Adjacent Structures. A Variability Study.* Williams and Wilkins, Baltimore 1969
6. Sundsten J. W. and Kastella K. G.: *The Digital Anatomist - Human Brain Animations.* Videodisc Series, University of Washington, 1991
7. Hoehne K. H., Bomans M., Riemer M., Schubert R., Tiede U., Lierse W.: *A volume-based anatomical atlas.* IEEE Comp. Graphics and Applications, July 1992, 72-78
8. Dann R., Hoford J., Kovacic S., Reivich M. and Bajcsy R.: *Evaluation of elastic matching system for anatomic (CT, MR) and functional (PET) cerebral images.* Journal of Computer Assisted Tomography, 13(4), 1989, 603-611
9. Greitz T., Bohm C. Holte S. and Eriksson L.: *A computerized brain atlas: construction, anatomical content, and some applications.* Journal of Computer Assisted Tomography, 15(1), 1991, 26-38
10. Evans A. C., Collins L. and Milner B.: *An MRI-based stereotactic atlas from 250 young normal subjects.* Soc. Neurosci. Abstr., 18, 1992, 408
11. Nowinski W. L., Fang A. and Nguyen B. T.: *Schaltenbrand-Wahren Talairach-Tournoux brain atlas registration.* SPIE Med. Imaging '95: Image Display (accepted)

Co-Registration of MRI and Autoradiography of Rat Brain in Three-Dimensions Following Automatic Reconstruction of 2D Data Set

Boklye Kim[1], Kirk A. Frey[2], Sunil Mukhopadhyay,[2] Brian D. Ross [1], Charles R. Meyer[1]

[1] Department of Radiology, University of Michigan Medical Center, Ann Arbor, Michigan 48109-0553, U.S.A
[2] Department of Internal Medicine, University of Michigan Medical Center

This work supported in part by DHHS PHS NIH 1RO1 CA59412

Abstract. Brain images obtained in 2DG-autoradiography have been reconstructed into 3D volumes for the purpose of accurate three dimensional registration with MRI data to obtain spatially registered, histologic "truth" data. Modalities were chosen to closely model the current clinical interest in correlation of MRI and FDG-PET imaging. An automatic 2D-registration algorithm that takes into account variations in sample orientation and shearing has been developed for accurate alignment of brain slices. It uses a multivariate optimization algorithm on the peak correlation between the gradient filtered autoradiograph image and the corresponding video image of the specimen's block face. Registration of the reconstructed 2DG-autoradiography volume data with 3D reconstructed *in vivo* multislice MRI of rat brains was accomplished with a 3D registration algorithm utilizing user identified homologous feature pairs consisting of points, line segments, and planar patches.

1 Introduction

Co-registration of three dimensional (3D) data sets of low spatial resolution, functional imaging such as positron emission tomography (PET) with high spatial resolution, anatomical imaging modalities such as magnetic resonance imaging (MRI) or x-ray computed tomography (CT) is used as a means of quantitatively assessing regional function. Our study has applied a 3D registration technique to fuse *in vivo* MRI and high resolution volume data reconstructed from digitized 2DG autoradiography images of rat brains with transplanted intracerebral tumors. Accurate registration of 2DG data set with 3D MRI requires proper reconstruction of the 2DG images. The 2DG autoradiography images are developed by exposing thin tissue slices containing long half-lived radioactive isotopes to a film for extended period of time. As many as 60 to 100 slices constitute an 2DG data set and, after digitization, volume reconstruction may involve tedious and time consuming alignment procedures for proper orientation of slices with respect to one another. Investigators have employed several approaches with varying degrees of success[1-4]. In our study an automatic 2D registration method which finds in-plane transformation parameters with respect to reference image data using a multivariate function minimization algorithm has been developed. After video digitization in an orientation visually matched to a reference image (block face image), the 2DG images are reconstructed into a 3D data set by the automatic 2D registration with respect to the video digitized images of the remaining specimen block face acquired during sectioning. The 2D registration routine uses negative peak of the cross correlation function between gray scale edges of the block face and 2DG images as a cost function for minimization. The technique avoids problems with partial correlations due to gray scale differences between the two modalities by operating on the magnitude of edge-enhanced images for both sets. After reconstruction, the 3D autoradiography data is registered with the corresponding *in vivo* MRI volume using an affine 3D algorithm that simultaneously uses homologous feature pairs consisting of points, lines and plane segments [6]. The modalities are chosen to closely model the current clinical setting of MRI and FDG-PET imaging with much smaller partial volume effect and higher in-plane resolution.

Our goal is to provide unbiased "truth" bases which can be used to compare the results of segmentation algorithms operating on MRI multivariate data sets. Many investigators develop algorithms, but, unfortunately, have no access to realistic test sets for validation. Human "expert" readings are often too subjective and variable to provide such truth bases. This study demonstrates the feasibility of obtaining spatially registered, histologic "truth" data without need for external markers for pixel level comparisons with MRI and can be utilized for validation of automatic segmentation algorithm.

2 Materials and Methods

2.1 Image Acquisition and Digitization

Rat brain Images Intracerebral brain tumors (9L or SF767 cell line) were induced in anesthetized (ketamine/xylazine, 87/13mg/kg, i.p.) adult male Fischer 344 or nude rat weighing between 125 and 150g. Images of rat brains with either normal or harboring intracranial glioma models were acquired.

Magnetic Resonance Imaging In vivo MR images were acquired with a 7 Tesla horizontal bore magnet system (SISCO) using a multislice spin echo sequence. Rats were anesthetized and, using a 40 mm diameter "birdcage" rf coil, 25 contiguous slices of horizontal T_1-, T_2- and proton density weighted brain images were acquired with TR/TE=1000/22, 3300/60, 3000/22, respectively. Parameters were FOV= 30x30 mm in 128x128 matrix, slice thickness=500 μm and separation =500 μm.

Autoradiography Immediately following the MR imaging, a venous catheter was introduced into one of the femoral veins and the rat was allowed to become fully conscious before [^{14}C]-deoxy-D-glucose (2DG), 125 μCi/kg, was injected bolus, through the cannula. After 45 minutes, the rat was sacrificed, brain was resected and frozen in embedding media in dry ice. For autoradiography, 20 μm thick frozen sections were cut in an automated microtome and video images of the block face were recorded with a fixed magnification in 512X480 matrix at an interval of 16 sections. The sections along with isotope standards were exposed to Kodak photographic film (MRM-1) at room temperature for five to six weeks and the films were developed with Kodak D-19 developer.

Digitization Autoradiography images were digitized manually from the developed film by visual approximation of the orientation used for the block face images.

2.2 Volume Reconstruction and Registration

Image reconstruction and registration were performed using Application Visualization System software from Advanced Visual Systems on DEC 3000/500x OSF1/Alpha.

2D Registration   Automatic sequential optimization routine extracts an individual 2DG image and finds in-plane transformation parameters with respect to the selected corresponding video block face image.

Reference Image   Video digitized block face images were aligned by vertical translation determined by cross correlation of grid lines of the specimen's mounting block to correct for the vertical movement of the microtome in the halted horizontal position. Images of the specimen were selected by applying ROI after the alignment.

Edge enhancement   Different gray scale ranges from the two modalities were chosen by window-leveling followed by gradient amplitude operation. Edge images of the main features were obtained by applying Gaussian low pass filter and threshold to control the weighting of selective edges for matching between two images.

Rotation/Translation and 1D scaling: An up-stream feedback loop to maximize correlation peak amplitude, computed using FFT/IFFT of gray scale edge images, employing a multivariate optimizer, that implements the "amoeba" simplex method [5], was used to estimate the in-plane rotation (Θ) and 1D-scaling(Y-coeff) of gray scale edge images. Translation parameters for selected Θ and Y-coeff were estimated from the peak location in the cross correlation image. Problems with local minima are resolved by using two optimization loops. The first optimization performs a broad initial search based primarily on outer edge obtained using a large scale Gaussian followed by the second optimizer, which uses the output of the first as initial conditions and small scale edges of internal features for fine adjustment of Θ.

3D Registration   User identified homologous feature pairs typically consisting of points along midline structures and scaling tangent planes (infrequently lines from vascular and tract segments) were used to register the reconstructed 3D autoradiography with the MRI volume [4]. Depending on the availability of identified homologous feature pairs typically a rotate-anisotropic scale affine transformation was computed. From the computed geometric transformation a trilinearly interpolated autoradiograph volume data set was computed to match the MRI volume data set. Partial volume artifact in the autoradiography data set ranges between 20-100 μ depending on the geometric mapping.

3 Results

Figure 1(a) depicts the result of the large scale optimization by displaying a block face overlaid with the gray scale frame of a 2DG image after automatic in-plane transformation. The block face is shown in green with blue enhanced edges while the red represents filtered edge from a 2DG image; mixing of the three colors represents matched edges. The small scale edges of the internal features selected for the 2nd optimization and the final result are displayed in Fig. 1(b) and 1(c), respectively. The alignment accuracy as a result of the 2D registration of 2DG images in reference to the aligned block face images was evaluated by standard deviation calculated in comparison with the "*Human Expert*" using a hole drilled, by a #76 bit, through the rat brain prior to sectioning for assessment of optimization performance. The average deviations as results of automatic 2D registration show Δx=2, Δy=2 pixels and

$\Delta\Theta=2°$. The in-plane resolution of autoradiography slice was 93 x 93 μm.

Reconstructed MRI and 2DG volume of the same rat brain in three dimension are displayed in Fig. 2 with the user defined feature pairs. The blue spheres designate points used in longitudinal and vertical scaling as well as features to match. Red spheres belong to two sets of tangential planes used for lateral scaling. Figure 3 displays the results of 3D-registration (a) and reconstructed MRI (b) and 2DG (c) volume. The gray scale in MRI and 2DG data represents the T_2-weighting and the activity level measured by 2DG count from the exposed autoradiogram, respectively. Intensity of the blue hue in Fig.3(a) was derived from the MRI data set, and the red hue was driven by negative intensity of the specimen autoradiography exposures and is a function of the isotope 2DG uptake in the brain. Misregistration is identified by the sole appearance of each color, e.g. visible in part of cerebellum due to the localized shearing artifact, while accurate alignment results in equal mixing, as depicted by well matched internal features as well as the lesion in the frontal lobe.

3 Conclusions and Discussions

A homologous feature pair registration technique has been used to provide "fused" volumetric metabolic map for pixel level comparison with MRI imaging data. The unique application of 3D registration of autoradiography and MRI to obtain spatially registered data without need for external markers for pixel-for-pixel comparison demonstrates its feasibility for fusion of functional and anatomical images. The sequential pairwise registration with block face image is ideal for automatic reconstruction scheme implementing multivariate function minimization algorithm using the cross correlation peak to obtain 3D metabolic data set to be correlated with anatomical image. Deformation coming from the microtome procedure includes shearing and skewing of each slice and needs to be considered carefully for accurate volume registration. The current optimization loop needs to include warping algorithm for better correction of the non-linear shearing effect. This initial study using images of rat brain images with experimental gliomas, which represent characteristic metabolic activities, as exhibited in our autoradiogram, enhances the application of the 2D and 3D registration techniques to assess localized metabolism or functionality across definable neuroanatomy in joint with segmentation algorithms.

References

[1] Hibbard, LS, Hawkins, RA: Three-dimensional reconstruction of metabolic data from quantitative autoradiography of rat brain. *Am.J.Physiol.*, **247** (1984)E412
[2] Hibbard, LS, Hawkins, RA: Objective image alignment for three-dimensional reconstruction of digital autoradiograms. *J. Neurosci. Meth.*, **26** (1988) 55
[3] Toga AW, Banerjee PK: Registration revisited. *J.Neurosci.Meth,* **48** (1993) 1.
[4] Zhao W, Young TY, Ginsberg MD: Registration and three dimensional reconstruction of autoradiographic images by disparity analysis method, *IEEE Trans.Med.Img,* **12** (1993) 782
[5] Press WH, Flannery BP, Teukolsky SA, Vetterling WT: Numerical Recipies in C: The art of Scientific Computing, Cambridge University Press, Cambridge (1988)
[6] Meyer CR, Leichtman GS, Brunberg JA, Wahl RL, and Quint LE: Simultaneous usage of homologous points, lines and planes for optimal, 3D, linear registration of multimodality imaging data. Accepted *IEEE Trans. Med. Imag.* (1995)

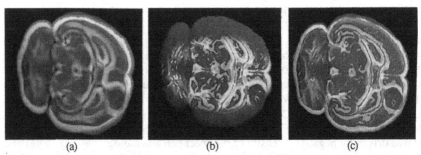

Fig. 1. Results of (a) the 1st optimization, (b) selected edges of internal features and (c) the 2nd optimization. A block face(green) with the edge outline (blue) is overlaied with the gray scale edge of 2DG image(red).

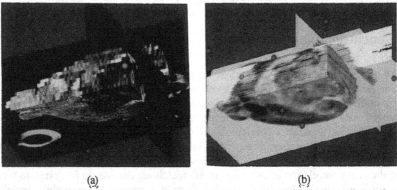

Fig. 2. Sagital view of reconstructed gray scale MRI (a) and 2DG autoradiography (b) displayed along with the user-defined feature pairs.

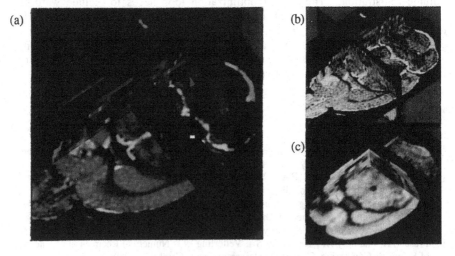

Fig. 3. (a) Co-registered MRI (blue) and 2DG (red) volume data. Red hue intensity is a function of isotope 2DG uptake in the brain. Reconstructed gray scale MRI (b) and 2DG autoradiography (c) of the rat brain used in the 3D registration shown in (a)

Computer Assisted Analysis of Echocardiographic Image Sequences

Andrea Giachetti[1], Guido Gigli[2] and Vincent Torre[1]

[1] Dip. Fisica Università di Genova, Via Dodecaneso 33, 16146 Genova
Tel: 39-10-3536311 Fax: 39-10-314218
[2] Servizio di Cardiologia, Ospedale di Rapallo, Piazza Molfino 10, 16035 Rapallo(GE)
Tel: 39-185-683231 Fax: 39-185-683277

Abstract. In this paper we present a semi-automatic system for the analysis of echocardiographic image sequences, able to provide useful information to cardiologists. The proposed approach combines well known techniques for the detection of left ventricular boundaries with the computation of optical flow. The initial detection of the cavity contour is based on an improved balloon model, the computation of optical flow is performed with a correlation technique and the contour tracking is obtained combining motion information provided by the optical flow with a snake-based regularization. The system is able to follow precisely the cavities motion, to provide several quantitative features of the heart beat and a dynamic representation of systolic and diastolic motion. Preliminary experimental results are presented and commented.

Introduction

Echocardiography is the commonest technique for cardiac imaging and provides a large quantity of clinical information on cardiac structures and functions in an incruent manner. The evaluation of left ventricle is one of the most valuable clinical application of echocardiography [1]; its volume and its ejection fraction have an extraordinary diagnostic and prognostic value [2]. In ischemic heart disease, echocardiography is useful in the diagnosis of myocardial infarction and transient ischemic episodes [3]. The analysis of echocardiographic image sequences is usually performed by visual inspection. However, some systems are able to produce image processing helpful to enhance the definition of the heart cavities and to provide some other useful parameters [4]. Computer Vision tools have been used in pilot studies to perform heart cavity detection: interpolations of calculated edges [5, 9], snakes [7, 9] and segmentation techniques based on Markov Random Fields [10] have already been exploited, while optical flow has been used to study heart motion [12, 13]. In this paper we describe some preliminary results of a system for the automatic analysis of echocardiographic images, based on the use of snakes [6, 7] and the computation of optical flow [11]. This system detects the left ventricular contour on final echocardiographic images (i.e. without any intervention in the processing cascade of ultrasonic signal), computes its area, tracks it and analyses its motion.

1 The detection of ventricular cavities.

The analysis of the image sequence starts with the detection of the left ventricular cavity in the first image. This function is performed by an active contour model, inspired by the recent work on snakes [6] and balloons [7]. The contour is represented by a closed curve, parametrized by the arc length s: $p(s) = (x(s), y(s))$. In our model, similar to the balloon model of Cohen & Cohen [7], the initial shape of the contour is taken as an ellipse, centered inside the cavity. The curve undergoes an evolution driven by an internal force $F_{int} = \alpha p_{ss}$ tending to minimize the contour length, an inflating force $F_g = f_g \gamma$ (where $\gamma(s)$ is the unit normal vector of the curve) tending to enlarge it, and a deflating force that stops the contour expansion near the cardiac boundaries. This force has been introduced because due to noisiness and low contrast of echocardiographic images, the use of the usual edge force $F_{edge}(p) = -\nabla |\nabla E(p)|$. (where $E(p)$ is the grey level at the point p) was not convenient. The new force is defined as follows:

$$F_d = -f_d \left(1 - \left(exp\left(\frac{E(p) - k}{T}\right) - 1\right)^{-1}\right) \gamma \qquad (1)$$

This is a smooth step function where T controls the smoothing, k is the center of the small region where its value changes from zero to f_d. When the grey level is low (inside the cavity), the deflating force is approximately zero. When the grey level is above the threshold k, the force quickly reaches the maximum value f_d and if the bright region is sufficiently large, the contour is stopped at its border. The implementation of the active contour is made substituting the curve $p(s)$ with a closed chain $p(i)$ of N points, replacing the derivatives of the internal force with finite differences and approximating the other forces with vectors applied to the points. Finally the points are simultaneously shifted of the quantity obtained giving unitary masses to the points and computing their approximated dynamics for a unitary time step. The procedure is then iterated until the growth of the contour is stopped.

2 Cardiac walls motion and contour tracking.

The analysis of the motion of the ventricular contour can be useful to build a model of the complex motion of the heart and to detect the presence of ischemic regions from irregular motions during the contraction. Given the chain representing the initial ventricular boundaries, we simply compute the *optical flow* at each point of the chain. The procedure used for our system is the following: after a simple smoothing of the images with a gaussian filter $exp(-(x^2 + y^2)/2\sigma^2)$ with a value of 1.5 pixels for σ, the point (x', y') at time $t + 1$ corresponding to point (x, y) at time t is the one with the lowest value of the quantity:

$$\sum_{i=-n}^{n} \sum_{j=-n}^{n} (E(i + x', j + y', t + 1) - E(i + x, j + y, t))^2 \qquad (2)$$

where $E(x, y, t)$ is the grey level of pixel (x, y) of the frame labelled by the integer variable t. Usually the value of n was set equal to 15. The displacements computed at the chain points can be used to compute the new contour for the next image, by simply shifting the points according to their values. This procedure, however, is not accurate enough to produce a reliable detection of the new ventricular contour: the existence of erroneous displacements and the presence of the quantization noise can generate some problems. If the wrong matches are not eliminated, after a few frames the contour becomes irregular, with many points far from the cardiac walls. To overcome this problem, after shifting the contour points with the computed displacements, we applied a regularization procedure consisting in a few iterations of the forces described in Section 1. In this way, there is a good and fast convergence towards the true cardiac walls. An improvement of the tracking accuracy could be obtained with an appropriate filtering of the point evolution as proposed by Blake et al. [8] exploiting, in this case, the periodicity of the motion and will be studied in the future.

Area evolution of the ventricular cross section. A useful parameter for the analysis of heart functionality is the area S of the computed ventricular section. For each computed contour $p(i)$, an application of Gauss-Green's theorem gives the following formula for the area:

$$S = \frac{1}{2} \sum_{1}^{N} \mathbf{p}(i) \cdot \boldsymbol{\gamma}(i) |\mathbf{p}(i) - \mathbf{p}(i-1)| \tag{3}$$

The evolution of the area of the cavity section can also be used for the estimate of ventricular volumes and functional parameters like the ejection fraction [2].

3 Experimental results

The proposed approach was tested on ten image sequences of healthy and anomalously beating hearts acquired from a video used for cardiologists training. The aim of this experimentation was to establish whether the proposed approach was able to track the left ventricle reliably and to evaluate whether the description of cavity motion with the optical flow was useful. The performance of the

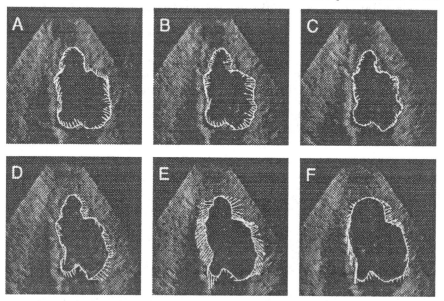

Fig. 1. A, B, C: Contour detection, tracking and optical flow computation for three consecutive frames of systolic motion of the left ventricle. D,E,F: The same for diastolic motion. Flow vectors are magnificated by a factor 2.

system depended rather critically, as it might be expected, on the numerical values of the different parameters used. Contours chains were usually formed by 100 points. In order to have a strong but a short range deflating force and an equilibrium position near the true boundaries of the cavity the values of the parameters T and f_r were both set equal to 1. The range of the inflating and internal forces was rather short, approximately of the order of 0.1 pixels and their ratio was tuned for each sequence to have the better results. The computation of optical flow of points lying on the cavity walls provided correct vector displacements for most of the points. Displacements were rather large because of the low acquisition rate (25 frame/s.). Fig. 1 shows the initial contour detection (A) and during a whole beat, where the computed boundaries of the ventricular cavity are superimposed to the corresponding images together with the optical flow vectors. The tracking of the contour was obtained shifting the chain points with the described technique. After an entire beat (in this case 14 frames), the contour was approximately in the original position.

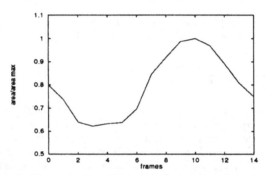

Fig. 2. A: The evolution of the area during the whole heart beat of Fig.1.

The computed area of the cross section had a correct periodic behaviour (Fig. 2). The proposed approach may also provide new useful insights for evaluating the wall motion. Fig 3 shows the comparison between two sequences relative to another patient, the first sequence was acquired when the heart was in good conditions, the second one during an ischemic episode in which significant motion abnormalities were present in the lower right part of the cavity. The optical flow in the lower right part of the images, within the circles, indicates a larger motion in the case of the healthy heart.

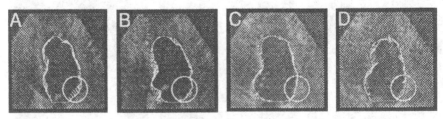

Fig. 3. Comparison of systolic and diastolic optical flows for a normal beat and the correspondent one after the induction of an ischemic episode. A,B: Diastolic (A) and systolic (B) frames of normal beat. C,D: Diastolic (C) and systolic (D) frames during ischemia. The white circles indicate the region of mechanical impairment due to myocardial ischemia.

4 Discussion

The proposed approach for the analysis of echocardiographic image sequences is based on the use of optical flow, that is used for three reasons: to improve the accuracy of the tracking of the cavity walls, to show the complex sequence of ventricular contractions, and as an independent test for contraction abnormalities, as shown in Fig. 3. Indeed, the computation of optical flow restricted on the points on the cavity walls, provides a good description of the dynamics of the heart and therefore of its functional state. In previous studies the computation of the optical flow on echocardiographic image sequences was impaired by several problems because of noise [12]. The computation of the flow over the entire image requires also a long computing time, which is not suitable for real-time clinical application. We solved these problems by computing motion only in the contour points and by using a robust correlation-based technique able to provide good results even in the presence of noise and even in the case of large shifts of the contour in successive frames. The preliminary results obtained with our system are promising: with good quality images the system identified wall motion abnormalities and the left ventricle area changes occurring through the cardiac cycle. The method is also sufficiently fast for clinical applications: the computation of flow vectors and the regularization of the contour are performed in about one second for each frame on a Sun 10 workstation.

References

1. S.J. Mason and N.J. Fortuin, "The use of echocardiography for quantitative evaluation of left ventricle function" Prog. Cardiovasc. Dis. **21**: 119 (1978)
2. M.A. Quinones et al. "A new simplified method for determining ejection fraction with two-dimensional echocardiography" Circulation **64**:744 (1981).
3. R. E. Kreber, M. L. Marcus, "Evaluation of regional miocardial function in ischemic heart disease by echocardiography". Prog. Cardiovasc. Dis. **20**:41 (1978).
4. V. F. Vanderberg et al. " Estimation of left ventricular cavity area with an on line, semiautomated echocardiographic edge detection system" Circulation **86**:159 (1992).
5. C. H. Chu, E.J. Delp and A.J. Buda, "Detecting Left Ventricular Endocardial and Epicardial Boundaries by Digital Two-Dimensional Echocardiography" IEEE Trans. on Medical Imaging 7:2 266 (1988)
6. A. Kass, A. Witkin and D. Terzopoulos, "Snakes: Active contour models," Int. J. of Comp. Vision **1**, 321–331 (1988).
7. L.D. Cohen and Isaac Cohen, "A finite element method applied to new active contour models and 3D reconstructions from cross-sections" Proc. of 3rd Int. Conf. on Comp. Vision, pp. 587–591 (1990).
8. A. Blake et al. "Affine-invariant contour tracking with automatic control of spatiotemporal scale" Proc. 4th I.C.C.V. pp. 66–75 (1993).
9. I. L. Herlin and N. Ayache, "Features Extraction and Analysis Methods for sequences of Ultrasound Images" Proc. 2nd E.C.C.V., pp. 43–55 (1992).
10. I. L. Herlin, D. Breziat, G. Giraudin, C. Nguyen and C. Graffigne, "Segmentation of echocardiographic images with Markov random fields" Proc. 3rd E.C.C.V., **2** pp. 201-206 (1994).
11. B.K.P. Horn and B.G. Schunck, "Determining optical flow," Artificial Intelligence **17**, 185–203 (1981).
12. G. E. Mailloux, A. Bleau et al., "Computer Analysis of Heart Motion from Two-Dimensional Echocardiograms" IEEE Trans. Biom. Eng. **34**:5 356 (1987).
13. S. C. Armatur and H. J. Vesselle, "A New Approach to Study Cardiac Motion: The Optical Flow of Cine MR Images". Nuclear M. R. in Medicine **12**, 59–67.

Computer Tracking of Tagged ^{1}H MR Images for Motion Analysis

Dave Reynard[1], Andrew Blake[1], Ali Azzawi[2], Peter Styles[2] and George K Radda[2]

[1] Department of Engineering Science, University of Oxford, Oxford OX1 3PJ, UK
[2] Department of Biochemistry, University of Oxford, Oxford OX1 3QU, UK

Abstract. Magnetic Resonance Imaging has become popular over the last few years as a technique for non-invasively imaging the internal structures of live subjects. In this paper we describe a technique to assist in the analysis of this type of data. We use quadratic B-splines and dynamic contours to track tagged regions of an infused rat heart, and analyse the motion of the tagged regions in terms of various predefined characteristic motions.

1 Introduction

Non invasive techniques for assessing the condition of soft tissue have become increasingly common over the last few years. In particular tagged MR images have been used to study the heart's dynamic behaviour. Tags are produced by altering the magnetisation of small regions of the heart tissue which then show up in the MR images as dark bands whose motion characterises the movement of the heart. Zerhouni et al (1988) utilised a star burst array of tags on a short axis view of the heart. Axel et al (1992) implemented a grid pattern. However the motion in all of these techniques appears to have been analysed qualitatively, or by hand. More recently Amini (1994) presented a system that would track the cardiac motion automatically using B-spline snakes. Their technique could be used to produce a stress strain analysis of the motion. Our approach utilises the dynamic contours of Blake et al (1993) which has the advantage that the allowable motion of the contour can be tightly controlled. Additionally it is also possible to run our system on a standard SGI Indy. At the moment we can analyse images at 25 Hz. Although most MR images are produced at very low rates the most recent echo planar techniques can produce images in real time.

In our experiments tags were overlaid on images of the cardiac tissue of an isolated perfused rat heart using a DANTE tagging sequence [7] combined with a standard spin echo ^{1}H imaging sequence. Nine images were obtained over a single cardiac cycle at an interval of 100 ms. The tags show up in the images as dark lines which form valleys in the pixel intensity. A closed quadratic B-spline contour was constructed to produce a rectangle lying over a small region of the heart as shown in Figure 1 (a). This was tracked using dynamic contours. These consist of a prediction and measurement stage where the prediction step uses an a priori model of the system dynamics. It is straightforward to analyse the tracked data in terms of a number of basic motions. Section 2 studies the dynamic contour approach used here and Section 3 presents the results from a single application.

2 The Dynamic Contour

The tracker described in this section consists of a Kalman filter used to follow the motion of a dynamic contour. The contour, a quadratic, closed B-spline can be described in terms of a number of control points. Measurements are made at points along the spline which relate the contour to the tracked feature. The estimate of the current position of the spline is then calculated from the measurements and a prediction based on the spline's history. A more detailed discussion of the method can be found in Blake et al (1994).

To improve the stability and performance of the tracker the contour can be restricted to lie in a small subspace. One possible option is the affine subspace. However, we used a larger seven dimensional space that allows the contour to "pin cushion" as well as to move in an affine manner. This type of motion is thought to be appropriate for the heart. One of the advantages of our approach is that specific types of motion may be designated as allowable and any other type of motion in the image will be ignored. It is then possible to study each type of allowable motion qualitatively.

The seven dimensional space is designed in the following way. First define the six dimensional affine space Q_6. This is related to the control point space by the following equations:

$$Q_6 = M_6 \begin{pmatrix} X \\ Y \end{pmatrix} \quad \text{and} \quad \begin{pmatrix} X \\ Y \end{pmatrix} = W_6 Q_6$$

where W_6 is related to the original 'template' position $(\bar{X}, \bar{Y})^T$ of the contour in the following way:

$$W_6 = \begin{pmatrix} 1 & 0 & \bar{X} & 0 & 0 & \bar{Y} \\ 0 & 1 & 0 & \bar{Y} & \bar{X} & 0 \end{pmatrix}$$

and $M_6 = (W_6^T \mathcal{H} W_6)^{-1} W_6^T \mathcal{H}$ where $\mathcal{H}$ is the L_2 metric norm defined in Blake et al (1993).

The seventh element of the subspace is constructed by defining a second 'keyframe' template that is similar to the original template but has been deformed under the particular non affine transformation required — in this case pin cushioning. If the key frame is represented as $(X_k, Y_k)^T$ then the seventh element W_7 is defined as:

$$W_7 = (I - W_6.M_6) \begin{pmatrix} X_k \\ Y_k \end{pmatrix}$$

and the matrix W is defined by appending W_7 to the end of the matrix W_6. Similarly, the matrix M can be calculated and Q defined as a 7-vector.

Motion is defined in terms of a second order differential equation so that, given $\mathcal{X} = (Q, \dot{Q})^T$ then:

$$\mathcal{X}_{n+1} - \bar{\mathcal{X}} = A(\mathcal{X}_n - \bar{\mathcal{X}}) + \begin{pmatrix} 0 \\ \omega_n \end{pmatrix}$$

Where the noise term ω_n is Gaussian and the parameters for A were chosen to allow significant amounts of movement in each of the seven dimensions.

Measurements are made at a number of points along the contour. To reduce the data processing overhead each measurement is made along a line normal to the spline. The length of the normal is restricted by a range gate mechanism [3]. Each measurement $\rho(s, t)$ is related to the state vector through the following relationship:

$$\rho(s, t) = \hat{n}^T(s, t)[H(s)\mathcal{X}(t) + \mu(s, t)]$$

Where μ is a one dimensional Gaussian noise process and $\hat{n}(s, t)$ is the unit normal to the spline. $H(s)$ is the B-spline matrix defined in Blake et al (1993).

Since the measurement process is very strong, the covariance of the measurement process was chosen to reflect this. The covariance of the process dynamics were chosen to ensure that the range gate mechanism behaved sensibly.

3 Robust Tracking

Figure 1 presents the results of tracking the heart's motion. It should be noted that there were only nine images in the sequence because it takes a considerable amount of time to produce each image and the function of the heart begins to deteriorate after a relatively short period of time. Each image was sampled at 10Hz and the heart was paced electronically. Reynard et al (1994) demonstrated that tracking the heart in the affine space can be reasonably successful. However Figure 2 shows that the amount of pin cushioning is significant, and that therefore non-affine motions are important.

The data was analysed in terms of several different basic types of motion. So far we have analysed the area of the B-spline, its rotation, translation and the amount of pin-cushioning. These are plotted in Figure 2. The data is plotted over two heart beats, produced by running through the same data twice. The data is not particularly smooth because only nine frames were used to capture an entire cardiac cycle. Additionally the lack of data means that it is difficult to produce any idea of the repeatability of the results. Since the absolute position of the hearts is not important, the translational information has been omitted from the results presented here.

4 Conclusions

The work carried out here has demonstrated the effectiveness of using a Kalman filter approach to analyse tagged MR images of the heart. The advantage of our technique is that it is very adaptable. The subspace mechanism allows us to

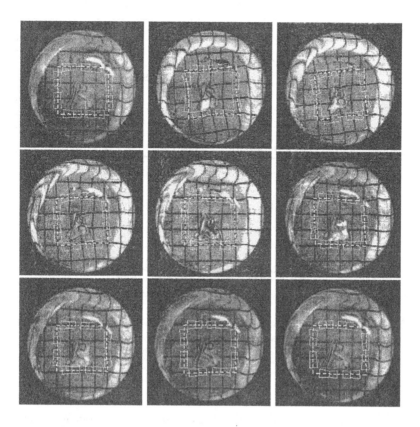

Fig. 1. Tracking using a seven dimensional space across a single heartbeat of an infused rats heart. The sequence runs from left to right, top to bottom. Note that the tracking is good at every time step, and that a significant amount of pin cushioning occurs, demonstrating its importance.

design specialist spaces to study particular types of motion, and to plot their effects over time. At present only a few images are available for each image set. This is caused by the speed of the imaging process. With better imaging techniques, perhaps echo planar MRI or ultrasound, our system will be able to analyse the motion at 25 Hz with modest hardware. Additionally, when longer image sequences become available the dynamics of the heart can be learnt [5]. Initially this would be for improved tracking only. However, ultimately, it might be possible to classify heart disease be comparing a heart's motion with the dynamics caused by known heart conditions.

The use of a rectangular grid pattern also means that in future we will be able to study several smaller regions of the heart simultaneously and compare them in parallel. This should allow biochemists to study the effects of cardiac disease on different regions of the heart.

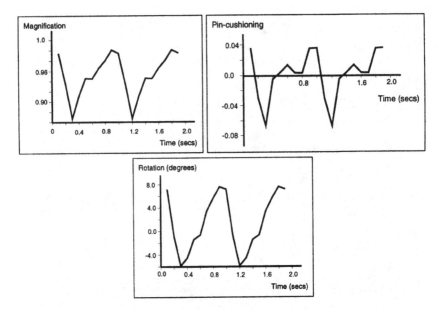

Fig. 2. The results of analysing the tracking data in terms of some basic types of motion. Two cardiac cycles are shown.

References

1. A. A. Amini, R. W. Curwen, R. T. Constable, and J. C. Gore. Automated motion tracking and dense deformations from tagged mr images. In *Proceedings of the Society of Magnetic Resonance*, 1994.
2. L. Axel, R. Goncalves, and D. Bloomgarden. Regional heart wall motion: Two dimensional analysis and functional imaging with mr imaging. *Radiology*, 183:745–750, 1992.
3. Y. Bar-Shalom and T. Fortmann. *Tracking and Data Association.* Academic Press, 1988.
4. A. Blake, R. Curwen, and A. Zisserman. A framework for spatio-temporal control in the tracking of visual contours. *Int. J. Computer Vision*, 11:127–145, 1993.
5. A. Blake, M. Isard, and D. Reynard. Learning to track curves in motion. In *Proc. IEEE Int. Conf. Decision Theory and Control, in press.*, 1994.
6. D.Reynard, A. Azzawi, P. Styles, G. Radda, and A. Blake. Cardiac motion analysis using computer tracking of tagged ^{1}h images. In *Cardiovascular MRI, Present and Future*, New Mexico, USA, 1994.
7. E. A. Zerhouni et al. Human heart tagging with mr imaging — a method for noninvasive assessment of myocardial motion. *Radiology*, 169:59–63, 1988.

Simulation of Endoscopy*

Bernhard Geiger[1] and Ron Kikinis[2]

[1] Institut National de Recherche en Informatique et Automatique
BP 93 – 06902 Sophia Antipolis Cedex, (France)
[2] Dept. of Radiology, Harvard Medical School and Brigham and Women's Hospital
Boston MA

Abstract. We present a simulation for endoscopic procedures. The anatomy of the patient is represented by 3D polyhedral models, computed from tomographic images. The simulation program can be used as a training system, or for prior simulation of complicated individual cases to reduce the error rate and to decide on the feasibility of biopsies. Additionally, we show how the system could be used as an online monitor during the intervention without the use of external tracking devices. The parameters used are the inserted length and the axis-orientation of the endoscope. An example of a bronchoscopy is shown.

1 Introduction

Minimally invasive procedures like endoscopy and laparascopy play an increasing role in interventional treatment. Modern endoscopic devices are flexible tubes that are inserted into body cavities and the interior of hollow organs. They are equipped with an optical channel that transmits an image to a video display. One typical task is to reach a tumor and perform a biopsy. This implies:

- *a navigation problem*: The exact position and orientation of the device is not easily determinable from the local view, especially in a branching organ.
- *a visual problem*: The tumor may be visible on CT or MRI, but not on the endoscopic surface view, if the wall is not directly affected.
- *a verification problem*: We want to know if the whole surface of the organ has been inspected.

Therefore it is desirable to provide a global view of the region showing the hollow organ, the exact position of the endoscope and the target (tumor). While the final goal is to have this information available in real time during the intervention, we propose as a first step an offline simulation on a computerized 3D model. This permits the procedure to be conducted beforehand, determining parameters like the choice of branches and the length of the trajectory. Such a simulation may also reveal whether the endoscope can reach the target or not, due to an incompatibility between the diameters of the endoscope and the conduit. Furthermore, we show that in a tree structure like the respiratory system, it is possible to determine the position of the endoscope if the inserted length and

---

* This work was supported in part by ESPRIT III Bra Project (PROmotion 6546)

the axis orientation are provided in addition to the video image. This paper is organized as follows:

- We show how to calculate a 3D model of the organs of interest from spiral CT images,
- We define a simple physical and optical model of the endoscope
- We show a method to automatically calculate the camera trajectory.
- We propose a method to detect the endoscope's position online.

2 Geometric modeling

The Delaunay reconstruction can be used to obtain both a volume and a surface representation from contours distributed on parallel cross-sections [2, 1]. This method is based on geometric closeness. It is a simple heuristic method, similar to that of the voxel technique. However, the volume elements are not equally shaped, but consist of tetrahedra that are adapted to the object shape. The advantages of this method are as follows:

- It gets directly to a 3D polyhedral representation composed of tetrahedra. The surface is a subset of the tetrahedra faces.
- The property of connecting contours on adjacent planes by triangles avoids the need for anti-aliasing or interpolation steps, especially for large cross-section distances (anisotropic sampling).
- Complex contours with multiple branchings, birth and death of holes, and complicated splitting lines, are all handled correctly.
- We get a considerable reduction in data compared to other volume oriented methods. Real time display of reconstructed human organs is therefore possible on standard graphics workstations.
- The tetrahedral structure is appropriate for applications like simulation of motion or finite element methods.

3 Physical model of the endoscope

We use a very simple model of an endoscope. The camera is represented by a cylindrical object. The viewing direction is the longitudinal axis (z-axis). The camera has three functions simulating the properties of a real endoscope:

- go forwards/backwards in the direction of the z-axis
- turn around its z-axis by -180—180 deg
- pivot around the x-axis by -90—90 deg

If the camera hits the wall, we calculate the force and moment and then produce small corrective motions to reduce the forces to zero[3]. The allowed motions are rotations around the x- and y- axes and translations orthogonal to the z-axis of the camera (see Fig. 1). Due to the geometry of the camera, it usually turns

---

[3] Details on the intersection test and force calculation can be found in [2]

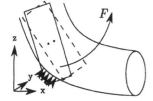

Fig. 1. Avoiding a penetration of the wall

its z-axis parallel to the conduit. If the camera size is chosen according to the actual diameter of the endoscope, the force minimization loop gives a response as to whether the endoscopy can pass or whether it would get stuck in a small branch. In this first approach, we did not try to define a more complex model, and in particular we did dot build a complete flexible chain. However our simple model turns out to be a good approximation.

4 Trajectory calculation

Besides the possibility of reaching a target by using the above functions repeatedly, we also provide a method of calculating a trajectory automatically. The user can specify the target point interactively. We can rapidly find the tetrahedron C containing the current camera position and the tetrahedron T containing the target point. Then we search for a set of tetrahedra S connected face to face and linking C with T. We then connect C with T by a straight line segment s, and verify that it lies completely inside the trachea tetrahedra. If not, we choose M a tetrahedron from the middle of S and replace s by two segments s_1 connecting C and M and s_2 connecting M and T. This procedure is repeated recursively until all segments are inside the trachea. When the camera finally follows this trajectory, we detect an eventual penetration of the wall and modify the trajectory. At this stage, we can also detect if the diameter of the conduit is adequate for the endoscope. This procedure does not necessarily provide the closest path.

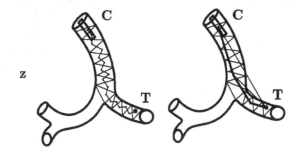

Fig. 2. Automatic calculation of the endoscope trajectory

5 Experimental Results

We implemented this system on a Silicon Graphics workstation (Indy) using the SGI graphics library gl. Three windows are displayed: The *global view*, the *local view* and the nearest CT slice with the camera position indicated. The global view shows the model of the organ, the target and the endoscope. The scene can be viewed from any angle, and details can be zoomed in. The local

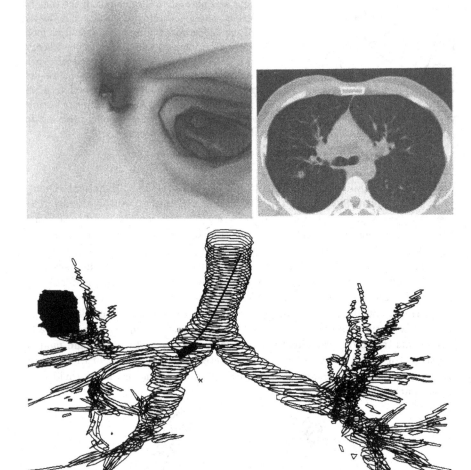

Fig. 3. A biopsy of a lung tumor. The local view (top left) the closest CT image (top right) and the global view (below).

view is the endoscopic surface view. We use the same model as for the global view, but place the viewpoint in the tip of the endoscope (see Fig. 3).

We run the simulation with several datasets: lungs, sinus, brain ventricles and colon, all obtained from spiral CT acquisitions. While the sinus data was successfully segmented by simple thresholding (air), we used statistical segmentation and interactive editing in the other cases. The example in Fig. 3 has been manually segmented to add the smaller bronchi. A typical model consists of about 60000 tetrahedra and 5000 surface triangles. The time for calculating the contact between surface and camera is clearly inferior to the display time. On a Silicon Graphics Indy with an MIPS R4400 processor chip (no hardware rendering) we obtained a rate of about one frame per second.

This model can be improved by mapping texture onto the walls, using advanced lighting models, and adding gravitational forces to the camera model.

6 Online tracking of the endoscope position

Given a path-length in a tree-like structure, there is only a discrete set of points where the camera may be found. If the endoscope could be equipped with a device measuring both the inserted length and the endoscope's rotation around its axis, we might be able to calculate its exact position in the model [4]. The inserted length and rotational values could be obtained for example by measuring the remaining part and the orientation relatively to the patients teeth. The crucial points would then be the branchings, and we must provide a way of automatically deciding which branch the endoscope took. We can think of two complementary ways: Firstly, if the endoscope approaches a branching, we can generate two series of synthetic images inside the model, one showing the local image when taking one branch, and the other showing the local image taking the other. By correlating the synthetic images with the real video images, we may then find out the correct branch.

Secondly, a path in a tree may be represented by the sum of the distances between the nodes. A node may be represented by a vector $l = (l_1, l_2, \ldots l_i)$ where l_1 to l_i are the distances between the i nodes that have been passed. If we are able to automatically detect branchings on the real video image, we can, by comparing this vector to all possible vectors, determine the closest match and therefore the exact position, given that the tree is sufficiently asymmetrical. This second method may be employed complementarily to the first one.

Since the range of a CT acquisition never shows the teeth, the endoscope length has to be initialized to 0 at a characteristic position, like the branching of the trachea into the two main bronchi (carina).

Acknowledgement

We are grateful to Olivier Dourthe for providing the CT images of the lung.

References

1. J-D. Boissonnat and B. Geiger. Three dimensional reconstruction of complex shapes based on the Delaunay triangulation. In R. S. Acharya and D. B. Goldgof, editors, *Biomedical Image Processing and Biomedical Visualization*, volume 1905, pages 964–975. SPIE, 1993.
2. B. Geiger. Three-dimensional modeling of human organs and its application to diagnosis and surgical planning. Report 2105, INRIA Sophia-Antipolis, Valbonne, France, 1993.
3. B. Geiger and R. Kikinis. Simulation of endoscopy. In *AAAI Spring Symposium Series: Applications of Computer Vision in Medical Images Processing*, pages 138–140, Stanford University, 1994.
4. W.M. Wells III. Personal communication.
5. J Toriwaki. Study of computer diagnosis of X-ray and CT images in Japan - a brief survey. In *IEEE Workshop on Biomedical Image Analysis*, pages 155–164. IEEE Computer Society Press, 1994.

A Virtual Reality Medical Training System

Rolf Ziegler, Wolfgang Mueller, Georg Fischer and Dr. Martin Goebel

Fraunhofer Institute for Computer Graphics,
Department Visualization and Simulation,
Wilhelminenstr. 7, D-64283 Darmstadt

Abstract. This paper presents the result of the interdisciplinary cooperation of traumatologists of the Berufsgenossenschaftliche Unfallklinik
(BGU) in Frankfurt am Main and a team of computer graphics scien-
tists of the Fraunhofer Institute for Computer Graphics in Darmstadt.
We have developed a highly interactive medical training simulator system
for arthroscopy by means of computer graphics and Virtual Reality techniques. This system offers an effective alternative to conventional training
systems for training and establishing of arthroscopic techniques. The two
main development tasks will be discussed: the 3D reconstruction process
and the 3D interaction.

1 Motivation

Virtual Environments provide a new dimension of graphical simulation [1]. The
human computer interaction meets now the intuitive perception of the user. This
paper looks into the field of training of arthroscopic skills, which we have simulated by means of Virtual Reality techniques. Since minimally invasive surgery,
especially arthroscopical diagnosis, is increasingly applied in operating theatre,
training is becoming an important issue [2]. Arthroscopy is a special endosco-
pical diagnosis method to recognize pathological changes and diseases of joints
(e.g., knee, hip, shoulder, etc.). So far, the skills required for an arthroscopy
have been taught the learning-by-doing way. In addition, the various orthopedic
operations have been practised using a plastic replica of the knee joint. However,
with training on synthetic knees only, the first surgical operation on the human
knee is very critical.

Against this background, the Fraunhofer Institute for Computer Graphics, in
cooperation with the "Berufsgenossenschaftliche Unfallklinik (BGU)" in Frankfurt am Main, developed a prototype based on the idea of using computer simulation applying Virtual Reality (VR) techniques for training and establishing of
arthroscopic techniques.

The main intention of the project was to develop a training simulator as
an enhanced alternative to conventional training systems (i.e. plastic replica of
the knee joint). The surgeons are criticizing the insensitiveness of the plastic
replica with regard to incorrect handling of the instruments. Furthermore, the
conventional training system does not provide any mechanism to verify (and
protocol) the training progress.

2   The Virtual Environment

To provide the Virtual Environment a realistic three-dimensional representation of the knee joint with all relevant anatomical parts is necessary. The interaction with the system is realized by means of Virtual Reality techniques. Thus, intuitive handling of the instruments is guaranteed. At least an appropriate hardware and software platform has to be configured to achieve a real-time simulation with seamless image generation.

2.1   Generation of the 3D representation

For the generation of a realistic three-dimensional representation of any knee joint a concept for creating it semi-automatically was developed. This concept, based upon data of tomographic imaging modalities, is not limited to the generation of a specific virtual knee joint.

The goal of the reconstruction process was to obtain a representation of the knee joint, which had to be suitable for computer simulation, while preserving as accurately as possible important anatomic features. Our representation of the knee joint has been derived from a MRI (magnetic resonance imaging) data set. The reconstruction process was divided into seven principal steps, starting with the data acquisition and ending with the integration of the 3D representation in the VR arthroscopy simulator [3]. This process or parts of it are adaptable to other applications, i.e. for simulation and visualization of respiratial airflow in the human nose.

The original knee joint MR data consisted of 64 contiguous slices with sagittal orientation. By using segmentation algorithms the contours of anatomic structures within the knee joint were extracted from the preprocessed images. This step needed manual intervention. Even after performing of contrast enhancement methods the edges between various tissues were not well defined in the available MRI data sequence. The sagittal resolution of the original MR image sequence was poorer than the in-slice resolution. Therefore, the individual segmented slices were interpolated to obtain an isotropic data set using an interpolation technique similar to the shape-based interpolation [4].

Next, surfaces of each object were constructed by applying the Marching Cubes algorithm to the segmented data [5]. This surface polygonization method creates triangles which approximate the isosurface of an object within a volume. A shortcoming of this triangulation step is, that due to the high resolution of medical data sets a huge amount (300.000) of small triangles were generated. Therefore, in an additional processing step the total number of triangles had to be reduced, while forming a good geometric approximation. Moreover, a distance to plane criterion, which was under user control, was applied evaluating the importance of a vertex according to its contribution to the detail [6]. Finally, this decimation algorithm has been successfully applied to isosurface representations derived from volume data. We have achieved acceptable performance for the virtual knee joint consisting of nearly 20.000 polygons.

2.2   Virtual Reality interface

The training simulator has to provide a realistic environment for arthroscopy simulation. In a real arthroscopy the surgeon is piloting the instruments, under the guidance of the arthroscopic image projected on a video monitor.

The trainee interacts with the system via a 2D user interface (see Figure 1) [7]. In addition to the display area a functional range has been integrated in order to specify parameters and read status information while rehearsing arthroscopic procedures. For instance the angle of the arthroscope optic can be selected (0° or 30°). Moreover, by choosing left or right knee the simulator enables the training of piloting the instruments in both hands. One advantage in comparison to conventional training systems is the possibility to verify the training progress by recording the session. Applying VR techniques the training

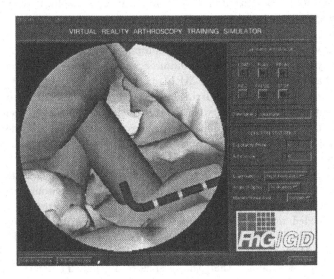

Fig. 1. User interface

simulator can provide the necessary interactive realism. The 3D interaction of the system simulates a real arthroscopy. An original exploratory probe and a replica of an arthroscope are inserted into a synthetic model of the knee through two small incisions located underneath the patella. As in common Virtual Reality applications, the simulator uses the tracking technique. Tracking means to monitor the sensors in a 3D electro-magnetic field, in order to get the position and orientation. Three sensors are used in the arthroscopy simulator. One sensor is fixed on the arthroscope in order to simulate a virtual camera, optics and lightsource located on the tip of the arthoscope. The sensor on the exploratory probe enables the integration of this instrument in the virtual environment. The third sensor is located on the lower leg of the synthetic knee. According to the current position of this sensor the attitude of the knee joint is computed and rendered in the scenery. Now the trainee is able to bend the knee joint similar to a real arthroscopy. One fundamental topic in virtual environments is the problem of interference detection or contact determination between any pair of objects. During an arthroscopic procedure we have checked for collisions between exploratory probe/arthroscope and the anatomical structures of the knee joint. These potential collisions are continuously checked in the VR arthroscopy training simulator. In addition an acoustic response is implemented as an effect of collision. A collision statistics gives information about the training progress of the necessary skills for arthroscopic techniques.

3 Conclusions

The prototype was presented at the "Frankfurt sports medicine weekend" on the 4th and 5th of December 1993 [8]. During the weekend an arthroscopy course for surgeons was included (see Figure 2). The course comprised talks and practices on conventional training systems and the training simulator. We had very

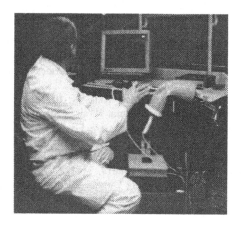

Fig. 2. Presentation in Frankfurt

positive assessments of the training simulator. The simulator is well suited for the training of the 2-axis-coordination. Furthermore, with the protocol option it is possible to have a "documentation" of the training.

The Silicon Graphics Indigo Extreme workstation is an appropriate platform with a high frame rate (6-10 images per second) for the prototype. Actually we are working on the enhancement of the reconstruction pipeline. An important aspect of the system is the capability to adapt it to additional joints, e.g., the hip joint (surgical planning).

At least the main drawback of the simulator is the missing of resistance, which we call force feedback. In cooperation with the Department of Electro-Mechanical Construction at the Darmstadt Technical University we have finished a conceptual study. Based upon the results of this study we are working on the realization. Besides the development of a force feedback system we are working on the simulation of arthroscopical surgical techniques (e.g. resection of a patch at the meniscus). Then, the trainee will be able to select several training scenarios referring to different pathological findings.

4 Acknowledgements

We wish to thank Prof. Dr. h.c. Dr.-Ing. José L. Encarnação for providing the environment in which this work was possible. We also thank all our colleagues and students at our lab, especially Jens Schmidt and Lutz-Otto Batroff. Without their work we would not have been able to achieve the results presented in this paper. Furthermore, we wish to thank the team from the BGU, Dr. Bauer and Dr. Soldner for the successful cooperation.

References

1. M. Goebel (Ed.): Virtual Reality, Computers and Graphics, Special Issue. Vol. 17, 6, Nov. 1993.
2. M. R. Satava: Virtual Reality Surgical Simulator. Surgical Endoscopy, pp. 203–205, Springer-Verlag, 1993.
3. W. Mueller: 3D Reconstruction of MRI Data for the Generation of a 3D Model for a Medical Training Simulator. Diploma thesis, Darmstadt Technical University, Department of Computer Science Interactive Graphics Systems Group, 1994. In german language.
4. G. T. Herman, J. Zheng, C. A. Bucholtz: Shape-based Interpolation. IEEE Computer Graphics and Applications, pp. 69–79, Vol. 12, No. 3, 1992.
5. W. E. Lorensen, H. E. Cline: Marching Cubes: A High Resolution 3D Surface Construction Algorithm. Computer Graphics (Proc. SIGGRAPH), pp. 163–169, Vol. 21, No. 4, 1987.
6. F. Schroeder, P. Rossbach: Managing the Complexity of Digital Terrain Models, Computers and Graphics, Special Issue on Modelling and Visualization of Spatial Data in GIS, 1994.
7. G. Fischer: Design of a 3D User Interface for a Medical Training Simulator. Diploma thesis, Darmstadt Technical University, Department of Computer Science Interactive Graphics Systems Group, 1994. In german language.
8. R. Ziegler, G. Fischer, W. Mueller, M. Goebel: Virtual Reality Arthroscopy Training Simulator. Computers in Biology and Medicine, Special Issue on Virtual Reality for Medicine, December 1994.

Virtual Simulation in Radiotherapy Planning

Rolf Bendl, Angelika Hoess, Wolfgang Schlegel

German Cancer Research Centre, Im Neuenheimer Feld 280, D 69120 Heidelberg
e-mail: r.bendl@DKFZ-Heidelberg.de

Abstract: We present a new system for 3D radiotherapy planning, which allows the interactive definition of treatment parameters, the simulation of the "visible" part of the treatment and the evaluation of the precalculated dose distributions. The system makes extensive use of advanced 3D visualisation and simulation techniques, introduces a new visualisation technique called Spherical View and a universal description scheme for irradiation techniques.

1. Introduction

With the aid of three dimensional treatment planning in combination with precision radiotherapy it is possible to fit the dose distribution very precisely to the shape of the target volume. The clinician will be able to apply a higher dose and in this way, the tumor control probability can be improved and negative side effects decreased. Because of the large number of treatment alternatives in each individual case, three dimensional treatment planning is a complex and time consuming task, and therefore it has not been widely used in clinical routine up to now. In order to support that complicated task appropriately, we have developed and collected different visualisation tools in a graphical user interface which allows the complete virtual simulation and evaluation of radiation therapy [Fig. 1]. The program is called VIRTUOS (VIRTUal radiOtherapy Simulation) and is part of the VOXELPLAN system of the German Cancer Research Centre, Heidelberg.

2. Methods

3D radiotherapy planning is based on a stack of CT-slices and a set of predefined contours of all clinically relevant volumes like the target volume and the organs at risk.

During the planning phase the most time consuming tasks for the therapist are the definition of the directions of the irradiation fields, which are determined by the angle of gantry and couch, and the orientations, sizes and shapes of the irradiation fields, which are determined by the angle and size of the collimator. During therapy, the shape of the fields can be adjusted exactly to the shape of the tumor by means of a multi leaf collimator which consists of two rows of thin moveable tungsten leaves, so the therapist must also be able to define the position of the leaves.

In order to define all these parameters appropriately it is necessary that the therapist get a precise conception of the patient's anatomy, the whole irradiated volume and the resulting dose distribution. Therefore the user interface presents simultaneous 3D models of the patient's anatomy from different points of view.

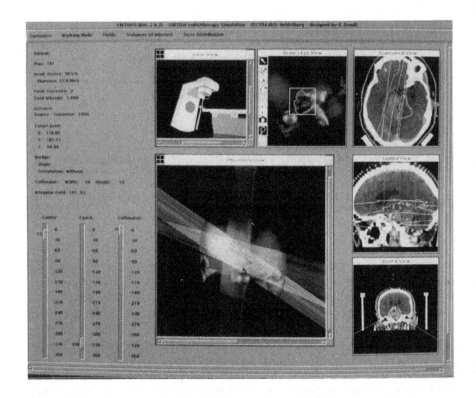

Fig. 1: VIRTUOS: The user interface

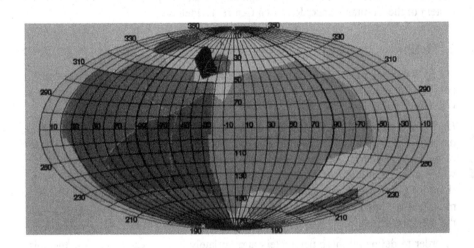

Fig. 2: Spherical View
Solid areas: The central ray first crosses an organ at risk and then the target point.
Hatched areas: The central ray first meets the target point and then an organ at risk.
Crosses: Positions of the fields of the current plan

Beam's Eye View and Observer's View

The most difficult task is to determine and combine appropriate irradiation directions. The most useful tool for this is a Beam's Eye View, where the therapist looks from the position of the radiation source through the collimator's aperture on the 3D model of the patient. Thus he can decide immediately if any organs at risk are enclosed by the field and adjust the shape of the beam exactly to the shape of the target volume. According to the defined shape the leaves of the multi leaf collimator will be adjusted during therapy. The Beam's Eye View is the best tool to check if the target is situated completely within the radiation field, but still it is rather difficult to get a realistic 3D impression of the whole irradiated volume and it is impossible to imagine the spatial relation of the different fields of a plan. The visual impression of the relations of all beams of one plan is a very important prerequisite for the definition of complex irradiation techniques. This information is provided by the Observer's View. There, the patient's model is presented together with all defined beams.

Spherical View

Even with an interactive Beam's Eye View and an Observer's View it is still difficult to determine which combination of gantry and couch angles should be selected, so the search for appropriate irradiation directions is still a trial-and-error process. Since it would be helpful to provide information about good combinations of gantry and couch angles, we have developed a new tool called Spherical View which shows all promising irradiation directions in parallel.

The radiation source moves around the target point on a spherical orbit. On that sphere we visualize all points with the same gantry angles and with the same couch angles. The connected positions of the gantry angles look like the meridians and those of the couch angles look like the parallels of latitude on a globe. For the next step we project the contours of the organs at risk on that sphere. The projections of the organs at risk look like continents on a globe. Each point inside such a "continent" (where a projection of an organ is visible) indicates that the central ray will cross that organ on its way from the source to the target point. At those points where no organ is visible (in the "ocean") the central ray will not run through an organ at risk. So it be a good direction for irradiation. The regions where a beam runs through an organ at risk after having passed the target point are of course visualized as well. When we look at the globe in 3D we can only examine half of its surface. In order to show all irradiation directions in parallel 2D maps of that globe, presenting the whole surface in one plane, are created [Fig. 2].

Now we are able to select very quickly combinations of gantry and couch angles where the central ray does not run through an organ at risk. But, depending on the necessary field size and shape, it might is possible, that the field includes some organs at risk which are near to the central ray. Therefore our Spherical View is input sensitive. One single mouse click on the map selects and displays the corresponding Beam's Eye View thus, showing the answer to this question very easily.

Other applications where it is only neccessary to find an appropriate direction, and field sizes need not be considered (e.g. a planning system for stereotactic neuro-surgery), will also show the power of this new visualization technique.

Schweikard et. al. [3] have proposed an similiar approach for the automatic optimization of gantry arcs of a special Convergent Beam technique.

Linac View and Collision Control

During the planning phase a programm should automatically avoid collisions between the gantry and the patient or the treatment table [1]. The numerical detection of collisions between gantry and couch is possible, but not the detection of collisions between the gantry and the patient, because the program does not know the exact dimensions of the patient, only the dimensions of the part which was previously scanned by the CT (e.g. only the head or the abdomen). Therefore we have added an exact 3D model of the irradiation device, which is moved synchronously according to the definitions of the irradiation direction. The therapist, knowing his patient quite well and being able to keep his size in mind, can estimate quite well if the sequence of the desired fields will cause a collision.

Beamgroup Concept and Simulation of Complex Irradiation Techniques

Other treatment planning systems which are currently available [4] support a few simple irradiation techniques only (e.g. Isocentric Fields and Gantry Rotations, sometimes Convergent Beams). In order to support the definition, and to simulate the application, of complex and dynamic treatment techniques we have developed a universal description scheme of radiation techniques by grouping the single beams of a certain technique hierarchically according to different dynamic parameters. The hierarchical structure is built up by introducing parent-child relations between the different beamgroups. Beamgroups will inherit the parameter settings of their parents, so settings which are identical for all children have to be determined only once. Of course all irradiation parameters can be defined individually on each level of the hierarchical beamgroup structure. For example, a Convergent Beams technique consisting of a number of gantry rotations with different couch angles (described by 100 - 200 beams) can be defined very quickly by delivering just one gantry and one couch interval, but it is also possible to move the couch angle of a gantry rotation slightly, or to define a specific irregular field shape for each single beam. New irradiation techniques can be described and added easily by creating simple template files. The program interpretes these templates at run-time, and provides support in the definition of the particular parameters.

Dose calculation

The previously described features simulate the visible part of the treatment. Another significant task is to predict the effects of the irradiation on the patient's tissue. In the recent years our group has put a lot of effort in developing different algorithms that calculate and optimize dose distributions. A description of that work is beyond the scope of this paper which concentrates on the "visible" parts of the simulation.

Evaluation and Comparision of Dose Distributions

After the visual and physical simulation of the treatment, the therapist has to evaluate and compare the calculated dose distributions. The process of redefining treatment parameters, calculating and checking the dose distribution will then be repeated until a sufficient result is achieved.

VIRTUOS provides different methods for the qualitative and quantitative evaluation of dose distributions. They can be visualized either in 2D or in 3D. In 2D the dose can be overlayed on the CT images either as isodose lines or colorwash, or by displaying the dose matrix without the underlying patient data (e.g. for visual comparison with dosimetric films). The 2D display has the advantage of an exact location of the dose with respect to relevant anatomical structures in the original patient data, but it is difficult to get an impression of the spatial extensions of the dose distribution. In 3D this information can be retrieved easily, therefore isodose ribbons can be integrated in the Observer's View. The 3D display of the surface dose distribution supports the detection of hot spots in organs at risk and cold spots in the target volume.

In Compare Mode, dose distributions of different plans can be loaded and then the therapist can page simultaneously through corresponding slices of different dose cubes. During the iterative refinement of plans, the dose distributions become more and more similiar to each other and it is often difficult to perceive small differences. A difference display mode enhances the perception of small deviations in dose.

Besides those qualitative evaluation tools, quantitative evaluation of the dose distribution is provided by dose volume histograms and by calculating some statistical parameters. A dose volume histogram shows which portion of each relevant structure will be exposed to a specific dose. Because the effects of radiation are different for different types of tissue, these biological effects are considered by calculating TCP (Tumor Control Probability) and NTCP (Normal Tissue Complication Probability) values for the target volume and the different organs at risk.

3. Conclusions and Results

A visual simulation of radiotherapy has to display and support the definition of the "visible" part of the therapy, the irradiation directions, field sizes and shapes, the movement of the gantry and the couch, as well as the results of the "invisible" part of the therapy, the irradiation itself. So in large areas, a radiotherapy planning system can benefit from the latest developments in 3D visualisation and virtual simulation, but it has to calculate and supply a lot of additional information. With the aid of three dimensional representation and visualization of patient data, the therapist gets an excellent impression of the patient's anatomy which allows a fast and intuitive definition of all relevant treatment parameters. But beyond this, a therapist needs further information which cannot be retrieved directly out of 3D scenes (e.g. dose volume histograms), and sometimes visualisation tools which do not need such advanced graphic techniques (e.g. the Spherical View) can show possible solutions more easily. Therefore a treatment planning system should provide all the different types of information in parallel, so that the user can retrieve any information at any time.

Beside the implementation of advanced visualisation techniques, the issue of how the user may interact with the system should be properly considered. Windows on a workstation screen should never be designed as output only devices, but should allow direct interaction with the system and the manipulation of the presented data.

It must be emphasized that an immediate response of the system to changes in the parameter settings is much more important than the visual quality of the 3D scene, so in former planning systems only line graphics were used for rendering the patient's model. Due to the development of graphic accelerators and new powerful workstations it is now possible to use advanced surface rendering algorithms with transparency and other sophisticated features in real time, but volume rendering algorithms [2] are still too slow.

4. Summary

We have presented a new comprehensive system for 3D radiotherapy planning which was designed to give an optimal support to the therapist during the planning and evaluation process of radiotherapy. Special attention was paid to tools which support the design and application of new complex and dynamic treatment techniques. The system makes use of advanced 3D visualisation and simulation techniques, and has introduced a new technique called Spherical View which shows all promising irradiation directions in parallel, information which cannot be retrieved from a 3D scene directly. The system not only visualizes the therapy relevant data, but it also provides many mechanisms for the interactive and intuitive definition of the treatment parameters. A prototype of this system has been used in clinical routine for more about three years, and it has been shown that with new tools and increased experience, the planning time can be markedly reduced. Our therapists suppose that the new tools presented in this paper but not included in the initial prototype, (e. g. the Spherical View), the possible design of new treatment techniques via template files and the graphical simulation of the complete treatment will again reduce planning time significantly.

Acknowledgement
The work was supported by the EC in the frame of the AIM COVIRA project. We triangulate our patient data with the NUAGES software from Bernhard Geiger, INRIA, France.

References

1. Kessler ML et. al. (1994). A Graphical Simulator for Design and Verification of Computer Controlled Treatment Delivery. In: Hounsell AR et. al. (eds.),
   Proc. of the XI. ICCR, Manchester: pp 80 - 81

2. Schiemann T et. al. (1993). 3D Visualisation for Radiotherapy Treatment Planning; In Lemke HU et. al. (eds.),
   Proc. of the Int. Symp. CAR 93, Berlin: pp 669 - 675

3. Schweikard A et. al. (1992). Motion Planning in Stereotaxic Radiosurgery Depart. of Comp. Science, Stanford University, Report No. STAN-CS-92-1441

4. Sontag M, Purdy JA, Photon Treatment Planning Collaborative Working Group (1991). State-Of-The-Art of External Photon Beam Radiation Treatment Planning. Int. J. Radiation, Oncology Biol. Phys. 21: pp 9 - 23

Motion

2D and 3D Motion Analysis
in Digital Subtraction Angiography

J.L. COATRIEUX, F. MAO, C. TOUMOULIN, R. COLLOREC

Laboratoire Traitement du Signal et de l'Image, INSERM, Campus de Beaulieu,
Université de Rennes I 35042 RENNES Cédex FRANCE

Abstract. A very active research is conducted on motion analysis. Most of the concepts, methods and assumptions are well established and lead to additional improvements in computer vision applications. Even in medicine where we have to deal with noisy data, low contrast structures and deformable objects, they bring new cues at all the processing stages. This paper emphasizes the specificities of this area and also the potential difficulties to face. A compilation of results is given aimed at the quantification of heart kinetics in Digital Subtraction Angiography (DSA). They illustrate the benefits of cooperative schemes such as motion based segmentation, moving object identification, three dimensional reconstruction and interpretation.

1 INTRODUCTION

These last ten years, an important evolution has been observed in imaging research. Motion analysis has been one of these components. It allows to have at our disposal elaborated formalisms and methods which efficiency has been demonstrated in a variety of areas: television (image coding), satellite imagery (cloud motion and winds), mobile robotics (inspection task, automatic picking, trajectography), military domain (target tracking), telemonitoring (traffic control and intrusion detection), human motion analysis. Applied works have, in turn, emphasized the roles of visual motion in detection, segmentation, pattern recognition, depth perception, placement prediction etc... In all cases, the observations consist of one or more time sequence images, acquired through a static or moving viewing system.

These general issues are also of concern in medical imaging [Mongrain et al, 1994]. The impressive growth of imaging sources, depicting the distribution in space and time of different physical parameters, provides new ways to noninvasively explore the human body. Morphological and functional informations are available today that allow to quantify, to follow up and to better understand the pathological processes. However, it must be said that most of the researches have been focussed on time-invariant, multimodal characterization of tissues or lesions. Less attention has been paid to structure dynamics without objective justifications. In fact, the kinetics informations attached to structures and organs complement the features on the diseases under study and participate as well, to the overall diagnosis statement. Moreover, motion analysis, as it has been pointed out before, can help in solving the low and intermediate tasks involved in image processing.

This paper is organized as follows. Section II discusses the methods for motion estimation Sections III to VI report the works undertaken in X-ray coronarography and ventriculography. They address respectively the segmentation using active contours and motion (Section III), the spatio-temporal perceptual groupings (Section IV), the 3-D reconstruction through motion (Section V), the symbolic interpretation of dynamics (Section VI).

2 METHODS

Three main approaches for velocity field estimation are usually distinguished : (1) differential (or gradient based) techniques operating in the image space domain ; (2) feature-based correspondence methods working on the image or the parameter domain ; (3) spatio-temporal frequency techniques operating in the transform domain. Other classifications can be proposed by emphasizing the nature of the motion (translational or rotational), the local computations or global optimization, the short range or long range motion estimation, and so on. The two first classes are the most widely used and are examined below.

- Differential methods : they involve one or several constraints that the spatial and temporal partial derivatives of the image brightness must follow. The fundamental assumption that the brightness, recorded from a point on the physical object (3-D), does not change as the object moves, leads to the "gradient equation". It allows to determine the component of optical velocity in the direction of the spatial gradient. Regularization is introduced by imposing some continuity of the solution. Such methods are of interest for their low computational complexity and because they provide a dense (pixel based) velocity field.

- Correspondence methods : they consist of identifying a number of image structures, determining which structures correspond over the image sequence and recording there successive positions. These primitives can be singular points (local maxima), landmarks such as corners, lines or regions..... Motion is quantified by position coding and can be seen as a matching problem equivalent to feature pairing in stereovision [Venaille, 1992] [Aggarwal, 1988]. Graph theoretic approach, iterative relaxation labeling algorithms and others methods can be used. Correspondence methods provide sparse motion fields related to structural characteristics of the objects and they allow to face large displacements.

Several combined frames where motion interacts with other major tasks will be now exemplified. All are dealing with kinetics cardiac assessment through digital X-ray techniques, ventriculography and coronarography, where most of the problems enlightened before are found : noise, low contrast, superpositions, inhomogeneities are present. The major interest we see is (1) that it is a good reference to discuss the performances of the methods and (2) that these two examinations are systematically carried out.

3 SEGMENTATION AND ACTIVE MODELS

Early studies of ventricular wall motion and coronary motion using epicardial markers or anatomical landmarks such as bifurcation points, suffer from several limitations : very sparse motion descriptions and interactive selection of point sets. More recently, optical flow methods have been applied, X-ray ventriculograms [Cornelius and Kanade, 1986]. A comparison of effectiveness of some gradient based algorithms was conducted in [Rong, 1989]. Horn and Schunck's algorithm [1981] gives good results and its efficiency is slightly improved with a modified version proposed by Nagel [1988]. The experiments conducted on large image sets show that reliable motion informations are difficult to obtain for small vessels (2-5 pixels width) and in the areas where crossings and bifurcations are present. The same conclusions can be drawn from ventriculography data with, in addition, more accentuated variations in the distribution of contrast medium.

Another approach for the automatic analysis of these images, which combines motion estimation with segmentation, has been proposed. The method consists of three steps : feature detection in the first image, motion estimation along this feature, model-guided frame to frame fitting. It has been successfully applied to the vessel centerlines in coronarography [Coatrieux, 1992]. Starting from a rough detection of the contour, the motion is estimated along this contour. This contour is then projected onto the next frame and serves as an initialization of an active contour model, or snake, proposed by Kass et al [1988]. The shape of the snake is changed iteratively until to lock on a position of minimal energy in the current image. This scheme allows to correct errors in motion estimation due to noise and inhomogeneities. This cooperation between motion and deformable model has several advantages : (1) the estimations are restricted to anatomically relevant structures ; (2) the computational cost in low ; (3) comparison with expertise shows that the performance is high.

4 SPATIO-TEMPORAL PERCEPTUAL GROUPING

The previous paragraph pointed out that one primitive (a contour or a centreline) was sufficient to delimit and to describe the object. This is not enough when we have to deal with complex scenes. In fact, venous or arterial networks, if they are easily interpreted in their original 3-D space, lead to very complicated pictures after projection. A more realistic description must be based on the following remarks :
- the density of branches is very high and so the situations where overlapping, crossing occur,
- the originating points of bifurcations are difficult to locate,
- the backflow of dye product leads to a high contrast region superposed to the vessels,
- the arteries can depict high curvature, loops or siphon-like shapes,
- a number of other objects such as the catheter, surgical sutures or wires are present,

- the lesions are expressed by strong variations of vessel widths or even full discontinuities (stenoses) and contralateral circulation.

All these elements motivate the elaboration of more sophisticated models. Centrelines or ribbon like regions are too poor to describe the vessel network. A complete scene analysis is required to filter and extract the information, to identify, modify and associate segments and branches. One of the major issue that arises is how to distribute the processing over space and time, that is to say, what must be done in one image, in two spatially different views or in the time sequence ? The answers to these questions are beyond the scope of this paper (the reader can refer to [Coatrieux, 1994]). They go through intermediate descriptions where motion and tracking can play a major role. Our preliminary results can be summarized as follows [Mao, 1993].

The detection of centrelines and edges being performed in a first frame, the lines are recorded (with identifiers) and parametrized (positions and directions at endpoints, length, mean intensity and contrast etc...). Perceptual grouping properties are then used to associate contour lines [Beasse, 1993] [Sarkar, 1993] : they are based on spatial proximity, attribute similarity, continuity of directions (colinearity or curvilinearity), symmetry and parallelism. These associations lead to eliminate non coherent regions such as the backflow and subtraction artifacts and they provide more robust entities on which the subsequent processing can rely. Meta structures, called triplets, are then built by integration of centreline information : centrelines not only bring new inputs for the validation of the previous constructs but also important cues to go from vascular segments to branches. This process corresponds to a spatial propagation of groupings. The next stage is aimed at extending and better identifying the arteries along the time sequence. It can be carried out in too ways : (1) by processing each frame independently and by matching the triplets afterward ; (2) by estimating the motion of the triplets, projecting them on the next frame to initialize and further perform the detection and formation of longer entities. The basic idea is that all the ambiguities, due to superpositions for example, or detection errors cannot be solved in one frame but over the sequence. Backward and forward procedures along the image sequence can then be applied to get a full description of the scene. The time horizon on which they operate is not reduced to the previous and next frames because each entity (triplet or set of triplets) can be consistently tracked. These concepts can be generalized to several views with pairing relations : their main inconvenience is related to the volume of data and the number of data structures to store and modify. If unidirectional constraints are introduced over time (e.g one way image sequence traversal), then a few cardiac cycles can be sufficient based on cyclostationnarity behavior.

5   3-D RECONSTRUCTION FROM MOTION

According to the issues reported Section II, the access to 3-D informations in medical imaging is critical in order to provide anatomically correct descriptions. When a few static projections are only available (stereopairs or orthogonal views), it is well known that the quality of the 3-D reconstruction depends, among other factors, on the primitive extraction and matching. A priori knowledge may be used and embedded in geometrical, stochastic and cognitive models to compensate the underdetermination of the problem [Garreau, 1991]. Motion, in a same way, can bring a significant contribution to this purpose. Several schemes can be adopted to combine reconstruction and motion. The last solution we have developped makes use of two (quasi) orthogonal projections and rely on the centrelines tracking. [Ruan, 1994].

The method consists of two steps. The first one operates in a point by point mode. A 3-D centreline being formed by a set of connected points, the motion on a given point can be used to process the next point under the assumption that the 3-D motion is smooth. These centrelines are separated in 3-D and can be easily tracked, the 2-D informations being utilized to refine the reconstruction. Here the pairing relations are known and preserved all over the image sequences. A predicted 3-D point is projected onto the left and right images at time (t+1), with its accompanying search window. A correspondance method (e.g. cross-correlation) is applied to look for the next position of the given point. Only local fitting is performed at this level.

The second stage carries out a global optimization of the reconstruction. It includes multiple 2-D and 3-D constraints. They deal with the control of position of the centrelines with regard to the axis of the vessels and the minimization of the residual error according to the epipolar geometry criterion. A 3-D smoothing of the motion is also done by minimizing a cost function built on the residual motion error and the gradient of the 3-D motion. These two stages are iterated for all centrelines at one time and then applied on all subsequent images within the sequences.

The key problems are similar to those already mentionned : the reliability of the initial feature extraction, their temporal stability, the capability to handle superpositions and large (and inverted) motions. Reconstruction from motion, when stated in 3-D is enough robust to face the latter difficulties. However, it must be emphasized that if the centrelines appear the best suited descriptions to model to dynamic properties of the coronary network, they are far from being sufficient to quantify lesions such as stenoses : local reconstructions with a precise estimation of vascular cross-sections are required.

6   INTERPRETATION OF KINETICS

From a diagnosis point of view, the analysis must cover the entire patterns contained in the image sets. Emphasis has been put recently on quantification of tissue features and objective evaluation even if still visual and subjective assessment is performed. The same rules apply to dynamic properties. Interpretation systems do not provide the temporal evolution of a given measurements but rather qualify this evolution and reason on it using prior knowledge of the structures and the underlying processes. Image sequence understanding in medicine implies that normal and abnormal situations (sometimes very discrete), in a subinterval of time and a very local region, must be labeled. The experience gained up to now, from an in-depth examination of inter-individual variability and the wide spectrum of diseases [Windyga, 1994], points out the complexity of the task. The size of the solution space is moreover highly augmented if only projections are explored. Model and data are strongly dependent of the viewpoint (even when standard views are acquired). A solution is certainly to carry out the analysis in 3-D as it has been shown in [Garreau, 1991]. A reference coordinate system to model the object and to be estimated from the data is needed to perform the matching. Qualitative versus quantitative descriptions are also other choices or compromises to make. Our current research is focussed on the interpretation of the coronary dynamics. Having at our disposal the 3-D vessel centrelines and their velocity vectors, it can be thought that motion understanding can be easily derived. This is not the case because the same difficulties have to be solved with additional ones : (1) the heart kinetics have not been explored in 3-D and only very poor information is available ; (2) the anatomical relations between arterial branches and cardiac muscle territories have no crisp descriptions but rather fuzzy ones. Netherveless, promising results have been obtained for symbolic descriptions such as "inward", "outward" motions with "rotation" or "translation" dominance [Puentes, 1994].

7 CONCLUSION

The aim of this paper was twofold : (1) to provide an overview of motion analysis in medical image sequences by pointing out the common and specific issues to deal with and (2) to show, by means of concrete examples, how resolution approaches can be organized. The former point discussed the methodological schemes at our disposal. The latter issue addressed motion based segmentation, feature grouping, reconstruction and symbolic interpretation. It has been emphasized that dynamic characteristics cannot only provide new cues for diagnosis, but also help in low, intermediate and high levels problem solving. Our last decade experience leads to conclusions and views similar to those reported in other computer vision areas with, however, more critical requirements in terms of accuracy and completeness. New advances can be anticipated in a near future. They range from imaging sources with higher spatial and temporal resolution up to algorithmic improvements for motion estimation. Cooperative schemes, the main corpus of this paper, will include the combination of observables (edges, lines, regions, etc...), robust estimation methods, uncertainty processing. Parallelism will be also of major importance according to the real time constraints involved in active vision and surgical interventions.

8 REFERENCES

Aggarwal J.K., Nandhakumar N. : On the computation of motion from a sequence of images. A review, Proceedings of the IEEE, 76, 8, 1988, pp. 917-935.

Beasse C. : Modèle de connaissance pour l'identification d'objets, Thèse, Université de Rennes I, Juin 1993.

Coatrieux J.L., Garreau M., Collorec R., Roux C. : Computer vision approaches for the three dimensional reconstruction of coronary arteries : review and prospects, Critical Reviews in Biomedical Engineering, 22, 1, 1994, pp. 1-38

Coatrieux J.L., Garreau M., Ruan S., Mao F. : Sur l'analyse de mouvement en imagerie médicale, Innov. Technol. Biol. Med., 15, 3, 1994, pp. 253-267.

Coatrieux J.L., Rong J.H., Collorec R. : A framework for automatic analysis of the dynamic behaviour of coronary angiograms, Intern. J. Cardiac Imaging, 8, 10, 1992, pp. 1-10.

Cornelius N., Kanade T. : Adapting optical flow to measure object motion in reflectance and X-ray image sequences, Proc. ACM Siggraph on motion, Representation and perception, 1986, pp. 145-153.

Garreau M., Coatrieux J.L., Collorec R., Chardenon C. : A knowledge based approach for 3-D reconstruction and labelling of vascular networks from biplane angiographic projections, IEEE Trans. Med. Imaging, 10, 2, 1991, pp. 122-131.

Horn B.K.P., Schunck B.G. : Determining optic flow, Artif. Intel., 17, 1981, pp. 185-203.

Kass M., Witkin A., Terzopoulos D. : Snakes : active contour models, Intern. J. Comput. Vision, 1988, pp. 321-331.

Mao F., Coatrieux J.L. : A triplet-based description of vessels in angiography, Proc. 15th IEEE-EMBS Conf., San Diego, Oct. 1993, pp. 102-103.

Mongrain R., Meunier J., Bertrand M. : Motion analysis in biomedical images, Thematic Issue, Innov. Technol. Biol. Med., 15, 3, 1994.

Nagel H.H. : Image Sequences-Ten (octal) years : from phenomenology towards a theoritical foundation, Intern. J. Pattern Recog. Artif. Intelligence, 2, 3, 1988, pp. 459-483.

Puentes J., Roux C., Garreau M., Coatrieux J.L. : Three-dimensional movement analysis in digital subtraction angiography : symbol generation from 3-D optical flow, Conf. Computers in Cardiology 94, Bethesda, USA, September 1994.

Rong J.H., Collorec R., Coatrieux J.L., Descaves C. : Estimation de mouvement en coronarographie, Innov. Technol. Biol. Med., 10, 2, 1989, pp. 175-186.

Ruan S., Bruno A., Coatrieux J.L. : three-dimensional motion and reconstruction of coronary arteries from biplane cineangiography, Image and Vision Computing, 12, 10, 1994, pp. 683-689.

Sarkar S., Boyer K.L. : Perceptual organization in Computer Vision : a review and a proposal for a classificatory structure, IEEE-Trans. Syst. Man. Cybernetics 23, 2, 1993, pp. 382-399.

Venaille C., Mishler D., Coatrieux J.L. : Un algorithme peu contraint d'appariement de primitives courbes par st r ovision trinoculaire, Revue Technique Thomson CSF, 24, 4, 1992, pp. 1071-1099.

Windyga P. : Evaluation et modélisation de connaissances pour la reconstruction tridimensionnelle du réseau vasculaire cardiaque en angiographie biplan, Thèse, Université de Rennes I, Mars 1994.

Measuring Microcirculation Using Spatiotemporal Image Analysis

Yoshinobu Sato[1], Jian Chen[1], Shuzo Yamamoto[1], Shinichi Tamura[1],
Noboru Harada[2], Takeshi Shiga[3], Seiyo Harino[4], and Yusuke Oshima[4]

[1] Div. of Functional Diagnostic Imaging, Biomedical Research Center,
Osaka University Medical School, Suita, Osaka, 565, Japan
[2] Dept. of Structure Analysis, National Cardiovascular Center Research Institute
[3] Dept. of Physiology, Osaka University Medical School
[4] Dept. of Ophthalmology, Yodogawa Christian Hospital

Abstract. This paper describes a method for recognizing and measuring
the motion of each individual leukocyte in microvessels from a sequence
of images. A spatiotemporal image is generated whose spatial axes are
parallel and vertical to vessel region contours. In order to enhance and extract only leukocyte traces with a tuned velocity range even under noisy
background, we use a combination of a filtering process using Gabor
filters with sharp orientation selectivity and a subsequent 3D spatiotemporal grouping process. The proposed method is shown to be effective
by experiments using image sequences of two kinds of microcirculation,
rat mesentery microvessels and human retinal capillaries.

1 Introduction

There have been considerable improvements on imaging techniques of microcirculation for the last few decades. These imaging techniques have made possible
visualization of the motion of blood cells in microvessels. For the purpose of
both clinical use and physiological investigation, a key problem is to measure
the velocity and flux of blood cells [1, 2, 3, 4, 5]. In spite of the improvements
of the imaging techniques, there are few well-developed techniques for analyzing
a large amount of image sequences obtained using these techniques. Therefore,
the quantitative analysis of microcirculation has been quite limited. Although
several image processing systems have been developed, these systems only deal
with tasks which can be performed using simple image processing techniques
such as the measurement of erythrocyte velocity [6], platelet adhesion [7], and
arteriolar vasomotion [8] using differential operation, frame subtraction, and edge
detection, respectively.

In this study, we deal with the problem of recognizing and measuring the motion of each individual leukocyte in microvessels. In order to measure the velocity
of leukocytes, each leukocyte must be recognized and segmented out because each
of leukocytes is flowing separately. In the previous work, these measurements
have been performed manually, for example, by counting the number of video
frames [1, 2, 3, 4, 5], which places limits on their accuracy, reproducibility and
the amount of data that can be collected. Recently, we have developed a method

for recognizing and measuring the motion of leukocytes based on spatiotemporal image analysis [9]. In our previous paper we dealt with the recognition of leukocyte motion in a restricted situation where background noise is low. Also, it was difficult to adjust a velocity range of detectable leukocytes. In this paper, we extend the method so as to be applicable to the recognition of leukocyte motion with an arbitrary specified velocity range even under noisy background, and show the potential usefulness of the method for different kinds of image sequences of microcirculation.

2 Spatiotemporal Image Analysis for Extracting Moving Leukocytes

2.1 Generating Spatiotemporal Image

Figure 1 shows two frames of a microscopic image sequence of a rat mesentery microvessel with moving leukocytes. The sequence consists of 100 frames. It is difficult to find leukocytes from only one frame, whereas we can observe moving leukocytes that adhere to microvessel walls from continuous video images. Figure 2 shows another example of a microcirculation image which was taken from fluorescein angiography by a laser scanning ophthalmoscope. In this case, it is hard to observe the leukocyte flow (although it is visible) even from continuous video images because a leukocyte is imaged only as a small and noisy fluorescent dot and its velocity is fast relative to the video rate.

The basic approach to measuring such motions is based on the method of spatiotemporal image analysis[10]. We assume that vessel regions are extracted automatically using the method based on the temporal variance of each pixel [9] or manually using pointing devises after the registration of all the frames of the sequence. We generate a 3D spatiotemporal image whose spatial axes are parallel and vertical to the flowing direction of blood cells (Fig.3(a)). Figure 4 shows the spatiotemporal images generated from the image sequence shown in Fig.1. The leukocyte trace in Fig.4(a) is relatively easy to see in the image, whereas the ones shown in Fig.4(b) are difficult to detect because they are obscured by erythrocytes. In our previous paper [9], we dealt with the extraction of only leukocytes moving near the contours of the vessel region, which are not obscured by erythrocytes as shown in Fig.5(a), using 2D spatiotemporal image analysis. The traces of such leukocytes are imaged as shown in Fig.4(a), in which background noise is relatively low. However, the previous method cannot extract the traces as shown in Fig.4(b). Our aim in this paper is to improve our previous method so as to extract all the leukocytes flowing through the vessel in the sequence of images by using more elaborate filtering techniques and analyzing a whole 3D spatiotemporal image whose spatial axes are vertical as well as parallel to a vessel contour (Fig.3(a)).

If a vessel is so narrow that only one leukocyte passes through, we generate a 2D spatiotemporal image whose spatial axis is taken along the extracted vessel(Fig.3(b)). Fig.6 shows the spatiotemporal image obtained from the image sequence of the human ocular fundus. Its spatial axis is the curve which is shown as a white line in Fig.2. The trace of a leukocyte manages to be observed as a sequence of noisy fluorescent dots in the middle of Fig.6[5]. The sequence of fluorescent dots is almost horizontal because the velocity of a leukocyte is high relative to the video rate. The previous method is not suitable for such a case because the enhancement of leukocyte traces is performed only to the diagonal direction in a spatiotemporal image.

2.2 Spatiotemporal Filter for Enhancement of Leukocyte Traces

Given a spatiotemporal image as shown in Fig.4 or Fig.6, we try to enhance components originated only from leukocyte motion and suppress other components. The leukocyte traces are imaged as lines with a limited thickness in the 2D spatiotemporal images whose spatial axis is parallel to vessel contours. Furthermore, the orientation of traces has a limited range of angles dependent on the minimum and maximum velocities of a leukocyte. In Fig.6, the trace of a leukocyte can only be observed as a sequence of very noisy fluorescent dots, but we can assume that the orientation of traces has a limited range of angles dependent on the minimum and maximum velocities of a leukocyte. We use Gabor filters having sharp orientation selectivity in order to deal with noisy background and an arbitrary specified range of velocities. Gabor filters have been utilized for optical flow computation [11] and texture analysis [12]. Here, we use Gabor filters in order to recognize and segment out moving objects, i.e., leukocytes, from a noisy image sequence mainly based on motion information.

The 2D Gabor filter in the frequency domain is represented by

$$H(\omega_x, \omega_t) = \exp\{-2\pi^2\sigma^2[(\omega_x{}' - \omega_{x_0})^2 + (\omega_t{}')^2\lambda^2]\}). \tag{1}$$

where $(\omega_x{}', \omega_t{}') = (\omega_x \cos\phi + \omega_t \sin\phi, -\omega_x \sin\phi + \omega_t \cos\phi)$. We use a Gabor filter with relatively large $\lambda(\lambda > 1)$ so as to make a filter have sharp orientation selectivity. Also, we use only real components of the Gabor filters because our aim is to enhance dark or bright lines. Although we assume that the minimum and maximum velocities of leukocytes are limited, the range of the velocity cannot be covered with only one Gabor filter having sharp orientation selectivity. So, we use multiple Gabor filters at different angles between the minimum and maximum angles dependent on the range of velocities of leukocytes. We use the maximum or minimum values among these filter outputs at multiple angles as the final output of filter. If we enhance bright lines, we use the maximum value. Otherwise, we use the minimum value. When we deal with a 3D spatiotemporal image, we apply the 3D Gabor filters given by

$$H(\omega_x, \omega_y, \omega_t) = \exp\{-2\pi^2\sigma^2[(\omega_x{}' - \omega_{x_0})^2 + (\omega_y{}')^2 + (\omega_t{}')^2\lambda^2]\} \tag{2}$$

where $(\omega_x{}', \omega_y{}', \omega_t{}') = (\omega_x \cos\phi + \omega_t \sin\phi, \omega_y, -\omega_x \sin\phi + \omega_t \cos\phi)$.

---

[5] There is another theory that these fluorescent dots are not leukocytes, platelets themselves, or plasma gap between leukocytes.

2.3 Extracting and Grouping Leukocyte Trace Regions

We perform thresholding operations for the filtered spatiotemporal image. We use two threshold values. We select the first threshold value so as to extract regions originated only from true leukocyte traces even if extracted regions do not cover wide area of true regions. On the other hand, we select the second threshold value so as to cover the regions originated from true leukocyte traces as much as possible even if some false regions are extracted. Among the regions extracted using the second threshold, we select only the regions connected with the regions extracted using the first threshold. These regions are regarded as the candidate regions of leukocyte traces.

In order to grouping and selecting leukocyte trace regions, we use the constrains that the velocity of each leukocyte is almost uniform, and the size of leukocytes is known to some extent. We can assume that the leukocyte traces have elongate shape with almost uniform orientation and known diameter in the 3D spatiotemporal image. So, the candidate regions which originated from the same leukocyte trace can be expected to form an elongate cluster having a restricted extent around its principal axis. We try to find such clusters from 3D candidate regions extracted using the thresholding operations.

Our clustering method is based on region growing. First, we select the largest region as an initial region. We use this region as a seed region to merge the regions which belong to the same leukocyte traces. We approximate the shape of leukocytes by the principal axis of the regions. Next, we select a region to be merged with the seed region. We select a candidate region which satisfies the condition that the maximum distance to the principal axis from the candidate region is the shortest of all the regions. If the maximum distance is smaller than a threshold, we merge the region with the seed region and recompute the new principal axis based on the seed region and the merged region to repeat this region growing process. Otherwise, we stop this region growing process and find a next seed region to start another region growing process. Finally, we can obtain several clusters which have elongate shapes. Each cluster can be regarded as an individual leukocyte trace. The velocity of a leukocyte can be computed from the direction of the principal axis of the cluster.

3 Experimetal Results

Figure 7 shows the output images of the spatiotemporal filter for the spatiotemporal image shown in Fig.4. We applied the set of 3D Gabor filters shown in Eq.(2). The angles of Gabor filters were 30°, 40°, and 50°. The parameters in Eq.(2) were set at $\omega_{x_0} = 0.1$, $\frac{1}{2\pi\sigma} = 0.02$, and $\lambda = \sqrt{2}$. We took the minimum of their outputs as the final output. We performed the thresholding operations described in 2.3 for the output of the spatiotemporal filter. Figure 8 is a stereo display of 3D regions extracted by thresholding. We applied the clustering method to the 3D regions shown in Fig.8. We could obtain five clusters as shown in Fig.9. In the image sequence, there were four moving leukocytes, and four traces shown in the left four clusters in Fig.9 corresponded to these four leukocytes. Although the rightmost cluster shown in Fig.9 was a false region, it can be easily regarded as noise because it was very small compared with other clusters.

Figure 10 shows the results of the spatiotemporal filter for the spatiotemporal image shown in Fig.6. First, we applied the Gaussian filter to the spatiotemporal image, and subsampled along the vertical axis to enlarge it vertically. Next, we applied the set of 2D Gabor filters shown in Eq.(1) to the vertically enlarged spatiotemporal image shown in Fig.10(a). The angles of Gabor filters were $50°$, $55°$, $60°$, and $65°$. The parameters in Eq.(1) were set at $\omega_{x_0} = 0.1$, $\frac{1}{2\pi\sigma} = 0.02$, and $\lambda = \sqrt{2}$. We took the maximum of their outputs as the final output. In Fig.10(b), the output of the spatiotemporal filter effectively enhanced a leukocyte trace in spite of fast motion of a fluorescent dot. After the thresholding operations, we could extract a leukocyte trace as shown in Fig.10(c).

4 Conclusion

We have described a method for automatically extracting leukocytes in a microvessel. We regarded the recognition of moving leukocytes as the problem of extracting leukocyte traces in a spatiotemporal image. We have used a set of Gabor filters having sharp orientation selectivity in order to effectively enhance leukocyte traces under noisy background. Furthermore, the 3D spatiotemporal clustering method have been developed to identify each individual leukocyte motion. We have shown experimentally that the method is effective for image sequences of two different kinds of microcirculation.

References

1. G.W.Schmid-Schonbein, S.Usami, R.Skalak, and S.Chien: The interaction of leukocytes and erythrocytes in capillary and postcapillary vessels, Microvascular Research, Vol.19, pp.45-70 (1980).
2. H.Komatsu, A.Koo, and P.H.Guth: Leukocyte flow dynamics in the rat liver microcirculation, Microvascular Research, Vol.19, pp.45-70 (1980).
3. U.H.von Andrian, J.D.Chambers, L.M.Mcevoy, R.F.Bargatze, K.E.Arfors, and E.C.Butcher: Two-step model of leukocyte-endothelial cell interaction in inflammation: distinct roles for lecam-1 and the leukocyte β_2 integrins in vivo, Proc.Natl.Acad.Sci. USA, Vol.88, pp.7538-7542 (1991).
4. S.Wolf, O.Arend, H.Toonen, B.Bertram, F.Jung, and M.Reim: Retinal capillary blood flow measurement with a scanning laser ophthalmoscope, Ophthalmology, Vol.98, No.6, pp.996-1000 (1991).
5. T.Tanaka, K.Muraoka, and K.Shimizu: Fluorescein fundus angiography with scanning laser ophthalmoscope, Ophthalmology, Vol.98, No.12, pp.1824-1829 (1991).
6. B.P.Fleming, B.Klitzman, and W.O.Johnson: Measurement of erythrocyte velocity by use of a periodic differential detector, American Journal of Physiology, Vol.249, (Heart Circ. Pysiol. 18) H899-H905 (1985).
7. N.Tateishi, M.Okazaki, and T.Shiga: Determination and kinetics of platelet adhesion onto material surfaces, Journal of Membrane Science, Vol.41, pp.315-322 (1989).
8. C.Y.J.Yip, S.Y.Aggarwal, K.R.Diller, and S.C.Bovik: Simultaneous multiple site arteriolar vasomotion measurement using digital image analysis, Microvaslular Research, Vol.41, pp.73-83 (1991).
9. Y.Sato, R.A.Zoroofi, J.Chen, N.Harada, S.Tamura, and T.Shiga: Automatic extraction and measurement of leukocyte motion in microvessels using spatiotemporal image analysis, Proc. IEEE Workshop on Biomedical Image Analysis, pp. 134-143 (1994).
10. R.C.Bolles and H.H.Baker: Epipolar plane image analysis: A technique for analyzing motion sequences, Proc. 3rd Int. Symposium on Robotics Research, pp.41-48 (1986).
11. D.J.Heeger: Optical flow from spatiotemporal filters, Proc. 1st ICCV, pp.181-190 (1987).
12. S.C.Bovik, M.Clark, and W.S.Geisler: Multichannel texture analysis using localized spatial filters, IEEE Trans. on PAMI, Vol.12, No.1, pp.55-73 (1990).

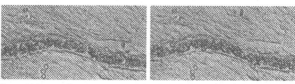

Fig. 1. Two frames in an image sequence of rat mesentery microvessels. (left: 23th frame, right 46th frame.)

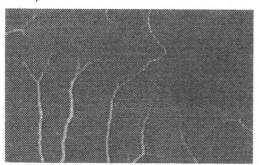

Fig. 2. Fluorescein angiographic image of human ocular fundus taken by a scanning laser ophthalmoscope. The white line is manually traced capillary selected as a spatial axis of the spatiotemporal image.

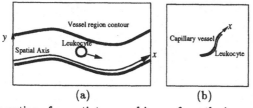

Fig. 3. Generation of a spatiotemporal image from the image sequence.

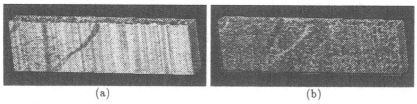

Fig. 4. Generated spatiotemporal images. (a) Spatiotemporal image just along an automatically extracted vessel wall contour. (b) Spatiotemporal image along a curve 10 pixels apart from the vessel wall contour.

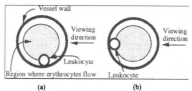

Fig. 5. Axial cross-section of a vessel and viewing direction. (a) Leukocyte whose motion is visualized as motion along contours of a vessel region. (b) Leukocyte obscured by erythrocytes.

Fig. 6. Spatiotemporal image generation from the image sequence of human ocular fundus.

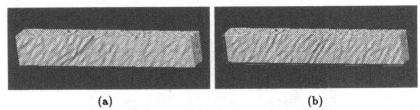

(a)   (b)

Fig. 7. Filtered spatiotemporal images. (a) Filtered result corresponding to Fig.4(a). (b) Filtered result corresponding to Fig.4(b).

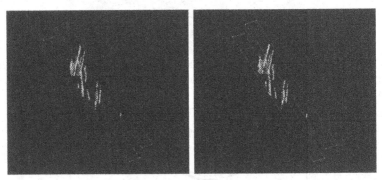

Fig. 8. Candidate regions of leukocyte traces extracted by thresholding the spatiotemporal filtered image.

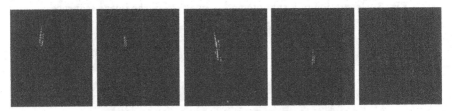

Fig. 9. Results of 3D spatiotemporal clustering method.

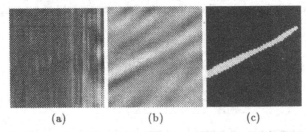

(a)   (b)   (c)

Fig. 10. Results for human ocular fundus angiographic images. (a) Vertically enlarged spatiotemporal image. (b) Spatiotemporal filtered image. (c) Extracted leukocyte trace.

Dense Non-Rigid Motion Estimation in Sequences of 3D Images Using Differential Constraints

Serge Benayoun[1], Chahab Nastar[2] and Nicholas Ayache[1]

[1] Epidaure Project, INRIA, B.P. 93, 06 902 Sophia Antipolis Cedex, France
[2] Perceptual Computing Section, The Media Laboratory, MIT,
20 Ames Street, Cambridge, MA 02139, USA

Abstract. We describe a new method for computing the displacement vector field in time sequences of $3D$ images ($4D$ data). The method is an energy-minimizing method; the energy is splitted into two terms, with one term matching differential singularities in the images, and the other constraining the regularity of the field. In order to reduce the computational time, we introduce an adaptive volume mesh the resolution of which depends on the presence of high gradient. We next perform a modal analysis, which allows a compact representation of the deformation by a reduced number of parameters. We present experimental results on synthetic data and on medical images.

1 Introduction

The problem of the computation of nonrigid motion from $3D$ images is one of the most important challenges of computer vision. There are many applications like model-based image compression [13] or medical diagnosis [2, 5]. Medical imaging produces $3D$ images which describe the complete time evolution of anatomic structures. For example, Magnetic Resonance Imaging (MRI) produces time sequence images of the cardiac cycle. Processing such sequences allows the computation of the motion of the cavities. The analysis of heart deformations can be very useful for cardiologists to detect pathologies or to evaluate effects of a medical treatment.

In this paper we present a method which computes the displacement vector field between two successive frames without any prior segmentation. Furthermore the structures appearing in these images are nonrigid and have some geometric features. In the following we explain how to incorporate such an information.

We pursue the original idea (introduced in a previous paper [7]) of using geometric singularities to anchor the motion field on a few but reliable characterisitic points, and to propagate this sparse motion field to contours first, and then to every image point. The idea of using salient features to guide the components of the nonrigid motion field was also mentioned in different studies reported by [3, 1]. The implementation of our method is based on an energy minimization formulation. This minimization is done with a mathematically rigorous finite element method. This technique allows us to introduce an adaptive mesh whose resolution depends on the presence of high gradient norm points. This allows us to reduce the computational time without decreasing the accuracy of the displacement field (section 2).

Modal Analysis is a very useful tool to reduce and analyze displacement vectors field [12, 8]. We make use of analytical modal analysis [9] as an instantaneous method for analysis and smoothing of the computed displacement field. (section 3).

Finally, we show experimental results on $3D$ synthetic data, and on a time sequence of $3D$ images of canine heart (section 4).

2 Computing Motion Field

2.1 Problem Formulation

Our aim is to compute displacement vector field between two successive frames of a sequence without any prior segmentation. Because it is numerically too expensive to compute the displacement of every voxel, we introduce an adaptive volume mesh. This mesh keeps topological and geometrical properties of the first image. For every node of the mesh we search a correspondent point in the second image. The matching is based on two types of attributes, grey level gradient norm and iso-intensity surface curvature.

We formulate this task as a minimization problem. Consider f the correspondence function which matches nodes in the first frame and points of the second frame, we define an energy $E_e(f)$ which measures quality of the matching. Because this problem has several solutions, we add a second energy $E_i(f)$ which constrains the regularity of function f.

In the following subsections, we present our model of adaptive volume mesh (section 2.2), we define the different energies (section 2.3) and we explain how to obtain numerically a solution of the minimization problem (section 2.4).

2.2 Adaptive Meshes

The use of adaptive meshes is a classical tool in Fluid Dynamics [11]. They have been already used in computer vision, specifically for image reconstruction [14]. The major advantage of this method is to decrease the numerical complexity while preserving the results accuracy.

There are different techniques for building up an adaptive mesh. One makes generally the distinction between *unstructured mesh* and *structured mesh*. For unstructured meshes, the adjacency graph of the nodes is not invariant. For example, the mesh is initialized at the higher resolution (voxel resolution) and non relevant nodes are progressively eliminated. This technique is suited to data compression because no computation follows the adaptation stage. But this is not the case in our application. Thus we prefer to use structured meshes where connectivity between nodes is preserved. We consider first a regular mesh and we move the nodes towards relevant points of the image.

A *mesh* is a set of *nodes* connected by springs. Each spring models the connection between two neighbor nodes by the relationship $S_{ij} = k_{ij}d_{ij}X_{ij}$. The strength S_{ij} exerted by the node j to the node i is directed by the unit vector which relies the two nodes X_{ij}. The intensity of the strength is proportional to the elongation of the spring d_{ij}, and also to the stiffness of the spring k_{ij} which measures the intensity of the link.

Our aim is to increase the density of nodes near the high gradient norm points of the image. We also introduce an image external force. This force pulls the nodes towards high gradient norm points. It is derived from a potential field computed by differentiation of the grey level gradient norm over the whole image.

The adaptation of the mesh is next issued from the resolution of the dynamic equation :

$$m_i \frac{\partial^2 X_i}{\partial t^2} + \gamma_i \frac{\partial X_i}{\partial t} = F_i , i = 1..n \tag{1}$$

where n is the nodes number, $X_i \in I\!\!R^3$ is the location of the node i, m_i its mass, γ_i its damping coefficient, and $F_i \in I\!\!R^3$ the sum of the applied forces.

F_i is composed of two terms. First, a spring term $S_i = \sum_{j \in V_i} S_{ij}$ where V_i is the 18-neighborhood of node i. Then, an image term $G_i = \nabla N_1(i)$ which attracts the node towards high gradient norm points ($N_1(i)$ is the image gradient norm at location of node i).

We use a finite difference scheme to solve this system. In our experiments, we choose to consider a node each four or five voxels. The mesh deforms through the application of the image forces and converges to an equilibrium state.

2.3 Energy Minimization

The correspondences are achieved by minimizing an *external energy* E_e splitted into two terms, a *curvature dependent energy* E_c and a *gradient dependent energy* E_g :

$$E_c(f) = \int_{\Omega_1} (C_1 - C_2(f(x, y, z)))^2 R_c(x, y, z) dx dy dz = \int_{\Omega_1} e_c^2 R_c dx dy dz \tag{2}$$

where C_1 (resp. C_2) is the iso-intensity surface maximal curvature in the first (resp. second) image, Ω_1 is the domain of the first image and R_c is a curvature dependent weighting function.

$$E_g(f) = \int_{\Omega_1} (N_1 - N_2(f(x, y, z)))^2 R_g(x, y, z) dx dy dz = \int_{\Omega_1} e_g^2 R_g dx dy dz \tag{3}$$

where N_1 (resp. N_2) is the gradient norm of the first (resp. second) image, and R_g is a gradient dependent weighting function.

As the minimization of this energy is an ill-posed problem, we add an *internal energy* E_i :

$$E_i(f) = \int_{\Omega_1} \|\nabla f(x, y, z)\|^2 dx dy dz \tag{4}$$

Finally we solve the minimization problem :

$$Min_f E_c(f) + E_g(f) + E_i(f) \tag{5}$$

The internal and external energies are balanced through two *weighting functions* R_g and R_c. R_g (resp. R_c) is a normalized increasing function of the gradient norm (resp. curvature). These weighting functions enforce locally the external energies if relevant points are not well matched. Inversely, they inhibit the external energies when a point has no significant features.

2.4 Finite Element Method

A necessary condition of optimality of $f = (u, v, w)$ is the Euler-Lagrange equation $\nabla E(f) = 0$ which is equivalent to the partial differential equations :

$$\begin{cases} -\Delta u = R_g \dfrac{\partial N_2}{\partial x}(u, v, w)e_g + R_c \dfrac{\partial C_2}{\partial x}(u, v, w)e_c \\[2mm] -\Delta v = R_g \dfrac{\partial N_2}{\partial y}(u, v, w)e_g + R_c \dfrac{\partial C_2}{\partial y}(u, v, w)e_c \\[2mm] -\Delta w = R_g \dfrac{\partial N_2}{\partial z}(u, v, w)e_g + R_c \dfrac{\partial C_2}{\partial z}(u, v, w)e_c \end{cases}$$

with the boundary conditions $f_{/\partial\Omega_1} = f_b$. Consider the first equation ; as its second member also depends on the solution, we study the associated evolution problem :

$$\begin{cases} \dfrac{\partial u}{\partial t} - \Delta u = R_g \dfrac{\partial N_2}{\partial x}(u, v, w)e_g + R_c \dfrac{\partial C_2}{\partial x}(u, v, w)e_c \\[2mm] \text{with } (u_0, v_0, w_0) \text{ initial estimation} \\[2mm] \text{and } f_{/\partial\Omega_1} = f_b \text{ boundary conditions} \end{cases} \tag{6}$$

Solving the variational formulation of equation (6) amounts to search $u \in H^1(\Omega_1)$ with :

$$(\frac{\partial u}{\partial t}, q) + a(u, q) = L_{(u,v,w)}(q) \ , \ \forall q \in H^1(\Omega_1) \tag{7}$$

where (,) represent scalar product in the Sobolev space $H^1(\Omega_1)$; and :

$$a(u, q) = (\nabla u, \nabla q) = \int_{\Omega_1} \nabla u \nabla q \, dx dy dz$$

$$L_{(u,v,w)}(q) = \int_{\partial\Omega_1} (\frac{\partial u}{\partial x} + \frac{\partial u}{\partial y} + \frac{\partial u}{\partial z})q d\sigma + \int_{\Omega_1} R_g \frac{\partial N_2}{\partial x}e_g + R_c \frac{\partial C_2}{\partial x}e_c q \, dx dy dz$$

In order to solve this equation, we make use of a finite difference scheme for the time variable t and the finite element method for spatial variables. We consider the adaptive volume mesh as a tesselation T_h of the domain Ω_1. We use C^0 finite element to approximate $H^1(\Omega_1)$. Thus $H^1(\Omega_1)$ is approximated by the finite-dimensional subspace V_h :

$$V_h = \{v_h \in C^0(\Omega_1)/v_{h/K} \in Q^1(K) \forall K \in T_h\}$$

We decompose u_h, approximation of u, in the functions basis of V_h. Each basis function Φ_i is associated to a node and is defined by :

$$\Phi_i(s) = \begin{cases} 1 \text{ if } s = \text{node } i \\ 0 \text{ if } s = \text{node } j \text{ with } j \neq i \end{cases}$$

Finally the resolution of equation (7) in the space V_h amounts to solve iteratively the linear system $(I + \Delta t A)u_h^{t+1} = \Delta t\, L_{(u_h^t, v_h^t)} + u_h^t$ where Δt is the time step, I the identity matrix, $A = (a(\Phi_i, \Phi_j))_{i,j=1..n}$ and $L = (L(\Phi_j))_{j=1..n}$. We use the conjugate gradient method to solve this system especially because it is efficient for a sparse matrix like A.

3 Modal Analysis

Modal analysis is a standard engineering technique allowing more effective computations and a closed-form solution of the deformation process using low-frequency modes [4]. It was first introduced in computer vision by Pentland's team [12].

Basically, modal analysis consists in changing basis from the standard canonical basis to the vibration basis of our deformable model, defined by its elastic and mass properties. Modes ϕ are the eigenvectors of the n-order eigenproblem :

$$\mathbf{K}\phi = \omega^2 \mathbf{M}\phi \tag{8}$$

where $\mathbf{K}$ is the stiffness matrix and $\mathbf{M}$ the mass matrix of the system, and ω^2 is the mode frequency.

We have recently suggested a novel and powerful approach to modal analysis of deformable surfaces, by computing the analytical expressions of modes for certain surface topologies [9]. We now generalize the results of our analytical modal analysis to deformable volumes, as it is the case of our volume mesh.

We now assume that all mesh points have identical mass ($m_i = m$) and all springs are identical ($k_{ij} = k$). The eigenfrequencies of our volume mesh, derived from equation (1), are obtained by generalizing the analytical expressions for deformable planes described in [9] :

$$\omega_{p,p',p''}^2 = \frac{4k}{m}(\sin^2 \frac{p\pi}{2N} + \sin^2 \frac{p'\pi}{2N'} + \sin^2 \frac{p''\pi}{2N''})$$

where the volume mesh has a size of $N \times N' \times N'' = n$, and mode parameters p, p' and p'' vary respectively in $\{0 \ldots N-1\}$, $\{0 \ldots N'-1\}$ and $\{0 \ldots N''-1\}$.

The modes of vibration of the volume mesh are n-order vectors whose components have the following expression (see the developments in [9] for planes) :

$$\phi_{p,p',p''}(i, i', i'') = \cos \frac{p\pi(2i-1)}{2N} \cos \frac{p'\pi(2i'-1)}{2N'} \cos \frac{p''\pi(2i''-1)}{2N''}$$

where i, i' and i'' give the location of the node in the volume mesh ($i \in \{1, \ldots, N\}$, $i' \in \{1, \ldots, N'\}$, and $i'' \in \{1, \ldots, N''\}$). Note that the modes are orthogonal vectors, and have to be normalized to unity.

We now have a new and complete basis where the displacement field $f = (u, v, w)$ can be accurately written in the following shape :

$$u = \sum_{p=0}^{N-1} \sum_{p'=0}^{N'-1} \sum_{p=0}^{N''-1} \tilde{x}_{p,p',p''} \phi_{p,p',p''} \; ; \; v = \sum_{p=0}^{N-1} \sum_{p'=0}^{N'-1} \sum_{p=0}^{N''-1} \tilde{y}_{p,p',p''} \phi_{p,p',p''}$$

$$w = \sum_{p=0}^{N-1} \sum_{p'=0}^{N'-1} \sum_{p=0}^{N''-1} \tilde{z}_{p,p',p''} \phi_{p,p',p''}$$

In our application, we are mainly interested in the low-frequency smoothing of the computed displacement field $f = (u, v, w)$. Thus, we project the displacement field in a low-frequency modal sub-basis :

$$< u, \phi_{p,p',p''} >= \tilde{x}_{p,p',p''} \; ; \; < v, \phi_{p,p',p''} >= \tilde{y}_{p,p',p''} \; ; \; < w, \phi_{p,p',p''} >= \tilde{z}_{p,p',p''}$$

where $< , >$ represent the scalar product between n-order vectors.

The smoothed displacement field $f_s = (u_s, v_s, w_s)$ is now defined by :

$$u_s = \sum_{p=0}^{P-1} \sum_{p'=0}^{P'-1} \sum_{p=0}^{P''-1} \tilde{x}_{p,p',p''} \phi_{p,p',p''} \; ; \; v_s = \sum_{p=0}^{P-1} \sum_{p'=0}^{P'-1} \sum_{p=0}^{P''-1} \tilde{y}_{p,p',p''} \phi_{p,p',p''}$$

$$w_s = \sum_{p=0}^{P-1} \sum_{p'=0}^{P'-1} \sum_{p=0}^{P''-1} \tilde{z}_{p,p',p''} \phi_{p,p',p''}$$

where P, P' and P'' are three integers defining the total number of low-frequency modes, and $P \times P' \times P'' \ll N \times N' \times N''$.

4 Experimental Results

We first experiment our algorithm on synthetic data. We build a $3D$ image representing a cube. The size of the image is $64 \times 64 \times 64$. By application of an affine transformation, we obtain a second image (the mean displacement issued from this transformation is almost 3.5 voxels). We next consider a $15 \times 15 \times 15$ mesh. After adaptation of the mesh to high gradient points of the cube image, we compute correspondences between the nodes and the points of the deformed cube image. For each node, we then compute the distance between its corresponding point and the exact point. The results are presented on table (1).

We make use of a set of $4D$ ($3D$ Images plus time) nuclear medicine data of a beating canine heart (see an alternative use of the same data in [10]). The size of $3D$ images is $98 \times 100 \times 110$. We use $25 \times 25 \times 25$ meshes. For each pair of successive image (I_1, I_2) we do the following processings :

- Adaptation of the volume mesh to I_1
- Computation of correspondences between nodes in I_1 and points in I_2
- Approximation of the motion field with low frequency modes
- Computation of the displacement for each voxel in I_1 by trilinear interpolation

– Resampling of I_1 from I_2 and the approximated motion field
– Superimposition of the resampled image with real contour points of I_1

Let us detail the algorithm of resampling :

– Consider a voxel v on the first frame I_1
– By application of the motion field obtain a real point on I_2
– Compute its grey level by interpolation
– Affect this value to v.

Figure (1) shows the motion field corresponding to the overall systole. It is computed by addition of all successive motion fields between the two states. We present also several modal approximations of this field by low frequency modes.

Figure (2) shows directional spectra of two deformations from diastole to systole. They represent the modal amplitudes as a function of frequency. The shape of the spectra confirms the low-order approximation of the deformation. They illustrate also the interest of modal analysis to compare different deformations.

In Figure (3) we present several slices of two $3D$ images :

– The first image is the superimposition of the frame corresponding to the systole with contour points of the frame corresponding to diastole. Contour points help to evaluate the intensity of the deformation.
– The second image shows the resampled frame of the diastole. The resampling is computed with several motion fields from systole to diastole. We superimposed again the contour points of the raw frame corresponding to diastole but here to illustrate the accuracy of our algorithm.

Finally we show in figure (4) the overall deformation of the volume mesh from the diastole to the systole. We represent it with the isosurface of the canine heart at the systole.

Distance Error	All	High Gradient	High Curvature
(Voxel)	Nodes	Nodes	Nodes
	(1331 Nodes)	(427 Nodes)	(147 Nodes)
Minimum	0.0321	0.0321	0.0619
Maximum	1.4400	1.4400	0.8510
Mean	0.4720	0.4190	0.4380
Standard Deviation	0.2380	0.1780	0.1540

Table 1. Statistics on the distance error between computed and real correspondences.

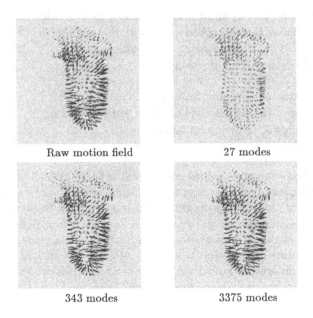

Raw motion field   27 modes

343 modes   3375 modes

Fig. 1. *Modal approximations of this field with low frequency modes.*

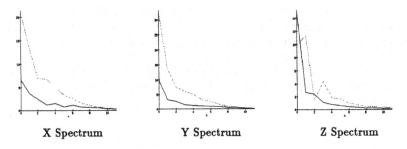

X Spectrum   Y Spectrum   Z Spectrum

Fig. 2. *Directional spectra of the deformation. Black: low deformation (from diastole to intermediate step). Grey: high deformation (from diastole to systole).*

Conclusion

We have described a method which computes displacement fields in a time sequences of $3D$ images. It consists in minimizing an energy which takes into account differential similarities for contour points and imposes a regularity constraint for no salient points. In order to reduce numerical complexity, we have introduced adaptive volume meshes. Smoothing and analysis of the deformation of the volume mesh is performed via a straightforward analytical modal analysis

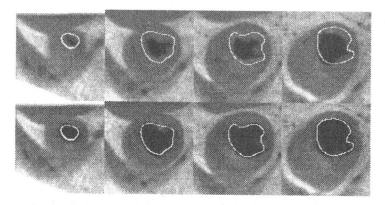

Fig. 3. *Bottom, some slices of the raw systole frame with contour points of the diastole frame. Up, same slices of the resampled diastole frame.*

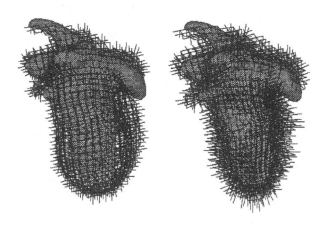

Fig. 4. *On left, iso-surface of the canine heart at the systole with initial volume mesh (at the diastole). On right, same iso-surface with final volume mesh (at the systole).*

on the volume mesh.

Acknowledgments

We wish to thank Eric Bardinet and Alexis Gourdon for helpful discussions. Thanks are also due to Dr. Richard Robb at Biomedical Imaging Resource, Mayo Foundation/Clinic, for providing the DSR heart data. This work was partially supported by Digital Equipment Corporation.

References

1. A.A. Amini, R.L. Owen, P. Anandan, and J.S. Duncan. Non-rigid motion models for tracking the left-ventrical wall. In *Proceedings IPMI '92*, 1992.
2. N. Ayache. *Volume Image Processing, Results and Research Challenges.* September 1993. INRIA Research Report (2050).
3. Ruzena Bajcsy and Stane Kovacic. Multiresolution elastic matching. *Computer Vision Graphics and Image Processing*, 46:1–21, 1989.
4. Klaus-Jurgen Bathe. *Finite Element Procedures in Engineering Analysis.* Prentice-Hall, 1982.
5. S. Benayoun. *Calcul Local du Mouvement, applications l'imagerie médicale multi-dimensionnelle.* PhD thesis, Université Paris Dauphine, Décembre 1994.
6. S. Benayoun, N. Ayache, and I. Cohen. Adaptive meshes and nonrigid motion computation. In *International Conference on Pattern Recognition*, Jerusalem, Israel, October 1994.
7. Isaac Cohen, Nicholas Ayache, and Patrick Sulger. Tracking points on deformable objects using curvature information. In *Proceedings of the Second European Conference on Computer Vision 1992*, pages 458–466, Santa Margherita Ligure, Italy, May 1992. In Lecture Notes in Computer Science: Computer Vision – ECCV92, Vol. 588 Springer-Verlag.
8. C. Nastar and N. Ayache. Classification of nonrigid motion in 3d images using physics-based vibration analysis. In *IEEE Workshop on Biomedical Image Analysis*, Seattle, Washington, June 1994.
9. Chahab Nastar. Vibration modes for nonrigid motion analysis in 3D images. In *Proceedings of the Third European Conference on Computer Vision (ECCV '94)*, Stockholm, May 1994.
10. Chahab Nastar and Nicholas Ayache. Spatio-temporal analysis of nonrigid motion from 4D data. In *Proceedings of the IEEE Workshop on Nonrigid and articulate motion*, Austin, Texas, November 1994.
11. B. Palmério and A. Dervieux. *2D and 3D unstructured mesh adaption relying on physical analogy.* September 1988. Université de Nice Research Report (207).
12. A. Pentland and S. Sclaroff. Closed-form solutions for physically based shape modelling and recognition. *IEEE Transactions on Pattern Analysis and Machine Intelligence*, 13(7):715–729, July 1991.
13. L.A. Tang and T.S. Huang. Quantifying facial expressions : smiles. In *Proceedings of the Workshop Journee INRIA Analyse/Synthèse d'Images*, pages 22–27, Paris, France, Janvier 1994.
14. D. Terzopoulos and M. Vasilescu. Sampling and reconstruction with adaptive meshes. In *Proceedings CVPR '91, Lahaina, Maui, Hawai*, pages 70–75. IEEE, June 1991.

Superquadrics and Free-Form Deformations:
A Global Model to Fit and Track 3D Medical Data

Eric Bardinet, Laurent D. Cohen*
Nicholas Ayache

INRIA Sophia Antipolis
2004, Route des Lucioles BP 93
06902 Sophia Antipolis CEDEX, France.
Email: bard@epidaure.inria.fr

Abstract. *Recovery of 3-D data with simple parametric models has been the subject of many studies over the last ten years. Many have used the notion of superquadrics, introduced for graphics in [4]. It appears, however, that although superquadrics can describe a wide variety of forms, they are too simple to recover and describe complex shapes.*
This paper describes a method to fit to 3-D points and then track a parametric deformable surface. We suppose that a 3-D image has been segmented to get a set of 3-D points. A first estimate consists of our version of a superquadric fit with global tapering. We then apply the technique of free-form deformations, as introduced by [9] in computer graphics to refine the estimate. We present experimental results with real 3-D medical images, where the original points are laid on an iso-surface. This is also applied to give efficient tracking of the deformation of the myocardium

1 Introduction

Over the last ten years, many surface reconstruction problems have been formulated as the minimization of an energy function corresponding to a model of the surface. Using deformable models and templates, the extraction of a shape is obtained through an energy composed of an internal regularization term and an external attraction potential (data term), illustrated for example in [13, 6, 10, 12]. Since the relevant surfaces in medical images are usually smooth, the use of such models is often very efficient for locating surface boundaries of organs and structures, and for the subsequant tracking of these shapes in a time sequence.

The advantage of deformable templates like superquadrics is their small number of parameters to represent a shape. However, if superquadric shapes give a good global approximation to a surface, the set of shapes described by superquadrics is too limited to approximate precisely complex surfaces. Therefore they were coupled with a deformable model in [12] to take into account local deformations.

The contribution of this work is twofold. First, we propose an algorithm for fitting data with a superquadric, based on [10] with some variations. Second, we

---

* CEREMADE, U.R.A. CNRS 749, Université Paris IX- Dauphine, Place du Marechal de Lattre de Tassigny 75775 Paris CEDEX 16, France

improve the shape extraction by introducing the use of free-form deformations (FFD), as introduced by [9] in computer graphics. The idea is to put our previous surface, here a superquadric, in a rubber-like box and then to deform this box by moving its control points. We solve an inverse problem to find the set of control points which minimize the error in the displacement field on the whole object. FFD has also been successfully used by [11] to match anatomical 3-D surfaces.

We show example results for 3-D medical images of the myocardium where the data set is an iso-surface. We also show an efficient tracking of the deformation of the myocardium.

2 Superquadric Fitting

This class of objects was introduced to computer graphics by A. Barr ([4]) and is an extension to 3-D of the superellipse. Their first use in computer graphics and in vision is due to Pentland ([8]), followed by Bajcsy ([10]) and later by Terzopoulos and Metaxas ([12]). A more complete description of Superquadrics and their use in Surface Reconstruction can be found in [3].

2.1 Definition of Superquadrics

Superquadrics form a family of implicit surfaces obtained by extension of the familiar set of quadrics. They are obtained by spherical product (see [4]) of two 2-D curves. The superellipsoid is the spherical product of the superellipse with itself. For a complete definition, see [2].

2.2 Our Superquadric Fitting

In our applications, the original data is a 3-D medical image which represents, for example, the myocardium or the head area. Interesting features can either be edges extracted from the data, corresponding to a potential (gradient), or an iso-surface. We want to approximate this surface by a superellipsoid.

To fit a superquadric to a set of data points, we presented in [2] a revised version of Solina and Bajcsy's Model of a superquadric fit. After initialization of the surface by an ellipsoid defined by the moments of inertia of the data, they made least squares minimization the inside-outside function F for:

$$E(A) = \sum_{i=1}^{N} [(1 - F(a_i, \epsilon_j, \varphi, \theta, \psi, t))]^2 . \tag{1}$$

We improved this approach by modifying the initialization, introducing global tapering and using Conjugate Gradient Descent.

3 Free-Form Deformations

The previous fit gives a first approximation to the surface, but it is not sufficiently close to the data. The superquadric is correctly oriented and the three axes of inertia already have the right size. The problem is that the set of shapes described by superquadrics is too limited to describe complex medical objects, in particular the myocardium or brain. We conclude that we need a more complex model.

In [1], we applied to surface fitting a tool called Free-Form Deformations (FFD) developed in computer graphics (see [9, 7]). This is a 3D-space deformation and consists of including a surface in a box and deforming it as a 3D solid. Our choice was guided by the fact that we wanted to have a simple global model at the end of the process.

3.1 Definition

FFD deforms solid geometric models in a free-form manner. It is independent of the nature of the object to be deformed. An analogy is to consider a rubber box in which the object is situated. Control points are placed on a regular 3D grid in the box. To deform the object, control points are moved, and the object follows accordingly. In graphics and CADs, FFD are used to design complex shapes by successively moving control points of the box to some place and thus retrieving a global deformation of the object.

The forward algorithm used for graphics is based on trivariate Bernstein polynomials, and divided into two steps:

1. Computation of the local coordinates of the object points in the frame defined by the set of control points.
2. Displacement of the control points and estimation of the new position of the object.

See [1] for more details.

3.2 The Inverse Problem : A two-step Iterative Algorithm

To improve the precision of the initial superquadric fit to the data, the superquadric is embedded in a parallelepiped box and a displacement field between the data and the model points is computed.

The FFD algorithm presented in the previous section can be summarised up like this: displacement of the control points permits the computation of a displacement map for any point. Here, we deal with the inverse problem. What we first determine is a displacement field on points of our surface. This displacement field joins a point of the model to the closest data point. The problem is then to find the displacement of the control points which minimizes the error between the displacement field produced by the FFD and the given one.

First Step : Computation of the displacement field. We need to associate with each point on the superquadric a data point M. The distance map is computed using a KD-tree algorithm (see [14] for example). As explained in [2], instead of taking the closest point on the data, we make it the other way :

- First the distance map to the superellipsoid is computed. We thus find for each data point the closest point on the superellipsoid.
- Since some points on the superellipsoid have not been reached, a displacement value is computed by interpolation.

Second Step : Displacement of the control points. We want to find the new position of the control points of our 3D box that best recovers the displacement field obtained in the previous step. For more details, see [1].

Iterative Algorithm: Since after the control points have moved, we have a new position on the surface, the displacement field also changes, and we need to iterate these two steps to improve the quality of the approximation. This makes our algorithm somewhat resemble to the two-steps formulation of the B-splines snakes using auxiliary variables (see [5]), but a difference here is that we have a 3D deformation using 3D Bernstein trivariate polynomials for our 2D surface embedded in the 3D box. We now give a description of the algorithm:

- We begin with P_0 as the regularly spaced control point box; $X_0 = BP_0$ represents the set of points on the parameterization of the initial superellipsoid.
- We then iterate the following steps:

Step 1: Displacement Field Computation: $X_n^a = X_n + \delta X_n$
Step 2: Control Points P_{n+1} Computation by Minimization of $\|BP - X_n^a\|^2$
$X_{n+1} = BP_{n+1}$
Test: computation of the least-square error $\|X_{n+1} - X_n\|$

3.3 Including Regularization in the Inverse Problem

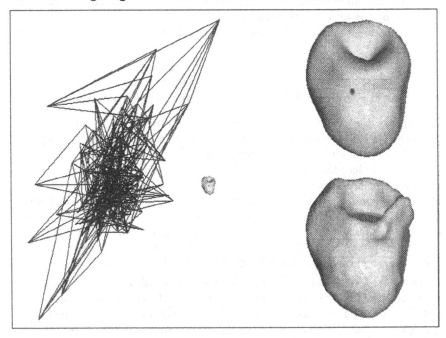

Fig. 1. Left: chaotic 5x5x5 box and the corresponding model. Right: the model compared to the original data.

As shown in figure 1, the control points box may be very irregular. In consequence, it is unstable to study the evolution of these control points in a sequence of images. In [11], the authors deal with a similar problem and introduce m-th order stabilizers. In order to control explicitly the regularity of the box, we add a regularization term into the minimization of the second step. The minimization criterion now becomes :

$$\|BP - X_n^a\|^2 + \alpha \sum_{j=1}^{NP} \sum_{j'} \|P_j - P_{j'}\|^2, \tag{2}$$

where j' corresponds to the neighbours of P. The second term is an internal energy corresponding to the insertion of zero-length springs between control points. This has a regularizing effect on the box to an extent controlled by the weight α. This regularization term can be also written $\|DP\|^2$ where D is a matrix which represents a discretized derivative of the control points position.

We show results of this regularizing effect on the box in figure 2 to compare to the previous figure 1. One drawback of the regularization is that the accuracy of

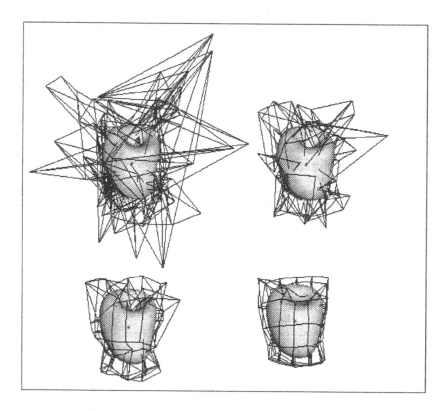

Fig. 2. Regularizing effect. Top left: $\alpha = 0.0001$. Top right: $\alpha = 0.001$. Bottom left: $\alpha = 0.01$. Bottom right: $\alpha = 0.1$.

the approximation decreases when the regularizing effect increases (see table 1).

Regularization weight	Least-square Error
0.0001	0.015065
0.001	0.015935
0.01	0.017489
0.1	0.021123

Table 1. Least-square Error between original data and parametric model as a function of regularization weight.

4 Experimental Results

We present some results obtained from applying the two-step algorithm to iso-surfaces extracted from medical data, followed by tracking results.

4.1 Medical Data: Left Ventricle of the Myocardium

In the following examples, the left ventricle of a myocardium was extracted from a time sequence of 3D SPECT images. Figure 3 was obtained with a $5 \times 5 \times 5$ box, the iterated algorithm and resolution using Singular Value Decomposition. These data are each composed of 6000 points, and the model is defined each time by 11 parameters for the superellipsoid and $5 \times 5 \times 5$ 3D points for the control points box, that is less than 130 3D points. The information is reduced by a factor of 48.

4.2 Tracking and detection of pathology

Figure 4 shows the result of the algorithm on the time sequence of the left ventricle. The model at time t_0 was computed using the corresponding superellipsoid, but the models at time t_n were computed using the previous ones (at time t_{n-1}). One basic application, having a time sequence of 3D data represented by parametric models, is to compute the displacement of each point on the surface during the sequence.For the left ventricle, this modelling can be efficient for the localization of pathological zones: for such zones, surface points have a small displacement, corresponding to necrosed areas on the ventricle.

5 Conclusion

We presented a new approach to shape reconstruction applied to 3-D medical data. It is based on a first approximation giving the best fit with a superquadric model. This is followed by a two-step algorithm for refining the details of the previous shape by making use of free-form deformations. The data is a set of points in a 3-D image, and the closest point to data is used for definition of the displacement field. We also added a regularizing term in the previous algorithm to make the control points box behave better. The interesting aspect of this approach is that it gives a description of a complex shape with only a small number of parameters.

Example results have been shown for a synthetic shape and for iso-surfaces extracted from 3-D medical images of the left ventricle. We also shown application of our method to automatic shape tracking in a time sequence of medical images.

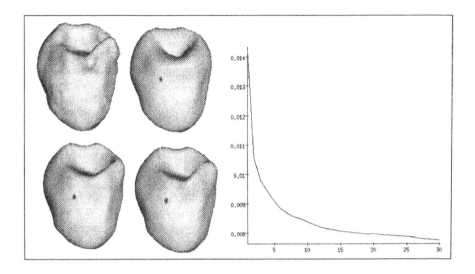

Fig. 3. Left: from top left to bottom right: left ventricle and the final result after 1, 10 and 30 iterations with a 5x5x5 box. Right: Least-square Error between original data and parametric model as a function of the number of iterations.

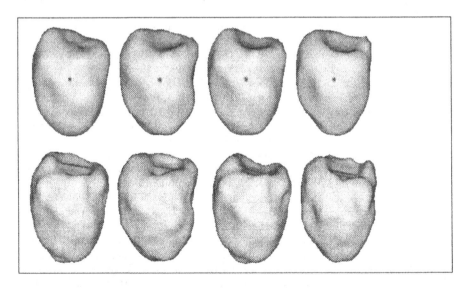

Fig. 4. Tracking the left ventricle with a 5x5x5 box. Top: the models. Bottom: the data.

Acknowledgments

We would like to thank Serge Benayoun and Alexis Gourdon who provided us with substantial help through fruitful discussions and Grégoire Malandain for his judicious remarks. Thanks also to Mike Brady for his careful review of this paper. This work was partially supported by Digital Equipment Corporation.

References

1. E. Bardinet, L.D. Cohen, and N. Ayache. Fitting 3-d data using superquadrics and free-form deformations. In *Proceedings of the IEEE International Conference on Pattern Recognition*, Jerusalem, Israel, October 1994.
2. E. Bardinet, L.D. Cohen, and N. Ayache. Fitting of iso-surfaces using superquadrics and free-form deformations. In *Proceedings of the IEEE Workshop on Biomedical Images Analysis (WBIA '94)*, Seattle, Washington, June 1994.
3. E. Bardinet, L.D. Cohen, and N. Ayache. Representation of surfaces with a global model : Superquadrics and free-form deformations. Technical report, INRIA, October 1994. (in print).
4. A.H. Barr. Superquadrics and angle-preserving deformations. *IEEE Computer Graphics Applications*, 1:11–23, 1981.
5. L.D. Cohen. Use of auxiliary variables in computer vision problems. Technical Report 9409, Ceremade, February 1994. Cahiers de Mathematiques de la Decision.
6. L.D. Cohen and I. Cohen. Finite element methods for active contour models and balloons for 2-D and 3-D images. *IEEE Transactions on Pattern Analysis and Machine Intelligence*, 15, 1993.
7. W.M. Hsu, J.F. Hughes, and H. Kaufman. Direct manipulation of free-form deformations. In *SIGGRAPH'92*, volume 26, pages 177–184, Chicago, 1992.
8. A.P. Pentland. Recognition by parts. In *IEEE Proceedings of the first International Conference on Computer Vision*, pages 612–620, 1987.
9. T.W. Sederberg and S.R. Parry. Free-form deformation of solid geometric models. In *SIGGRAPH'86*, volume 20, pages 151–160, Dallas, 1986.
10. F. Solina and R. Bajcsy. Recovery of parametric models from range images : the case for superquadrics with global deformations. *IEEE Transactions on Pattern Analysis and Machine Intelligence*, 12:131–147, 1990.
11. R. Szeliski and S. Lavallée. Matching 3-d anatomical surfaces with non-rigid deformations using octree-splines. In *Proceedings of the IEEE Workshop on Biomedical Images Analysis (WBIA '94)*, Seattle, Washington, June 1994.
12. D. Terzopoulos and D. Metaxas. Dynamic 3d models with local and global deformations: deformable superquadrics. *IEEE Transactions on Pattern Analysis and Machine Intelligence*, 13(7):703–714, 1991.
13. D. Terzopoulos, A. Witkin, and M. Kass. Constraints on deformable models: recovering 3D shape and nonrigid motion. *AI Journal*, 36:91–123, 1988.
14. Z. Zhang. Iterative point matching for registration of free-form curves and surfaces. *International Journal On Computer Vision*, 13(2):119–152, 1994. Also Research Report No.1658, INRIA Sophia-Antipolis, 1992.

A Unified Framework to Assess Myocardial Function from 4D Images

P. Shi, G. Robinson, A. Chakraborty
L. Staib, R. Constable, A. Sinusas, and J. Duncan

Departments of Diagnostic Radiology, Electrical Engineering, and Medicine
Yale University, New Haven, CT 06520-8042, USA
email: xship@noodle.med.yale.edu

Abstract. This paper describes efforts aimed at developing a unified framework to more accurately quantify the local, regional and global function of the left ventricle (LV) of the heart, under both normal and ischemic conditions, using four–dimensional (4D) imaging data over the entire cardiac cycle. The approach incorporates motion information derived from the shape properties of the endocardial and epicardial surfaces of the LV, as well as mid–wall 3D instantaneous velocity information from phase contrast MR images, and/or mid–wall displacement information from tagged MR images. The integration of the disparate but complementary sources of information overcomes the limitations of previous work which concentrates on motion estimation from a single image–derived source. [1]

1 Introduction

The measurement of regional myocardial injury due to ischemic heart disease is an important clinical problem. It is the goal of many forms of cardiac imaging and image analysis to measure the regional functions of the left ventricle (LV) in an effort to isolate the location, severity and extent of ischemic or infarcted myocardium. The ability to make these measurements has a variety of benefits, including the idea that serial analysis of regional function is helpful in assessing the efficacy of thrombolytic and other therapeutic agents, and angioplasty [5, 8].

In this paper, we describe a unified framework that integrates the two sets (endocardial and epicardial) of shaped–based estimates of the LV surface motion from our previous work [15], along with estimates of mid–wall motion derived from some of the MR physics–based methods, i.e. phase contrast cardiac MR imaging and MR tagging of myocardium, in an attempt to quantify the 3D deformation of the LV. The framework is built upon a continuum mechanical model of the left ventricle, and is embedded in a finite element grid. The integration of the disparate but complementary sources of information provides more accurate and robust measurements of the pointwise motion of the entire LV myocardium. We have reviewed much of the relevant literature on endocardial/epicardial wall motion in our previous work, we will briefly review efforts related to the unified framework we propose here.

---

[1] This work was supported by NIH–NHLBI grant R01–HL44803.

MR Tagging of the Myocardium. While the attractiveness of tracking grid lines that can actually be seen in the underlying image has been noted by many investigators [1, 21], there are difficulties with the use of MR tagging data for the 4D analysis of LV function because: i.) it's difficult to track the tags over the complete LV cycle due to decay of the tag lines and ii.) it's quite difficult to obtain acquisitions and assemble the detected tags into a robust 3D analysis/display. We note, however, the efforts of Young [20] and Prince [7] for assembling MR tagging–derived information into 3D of cardiac motion/function.

Phase Contrast Cardiac MR Imaging. Another approach for motion tracking is the use of phase contrast images to decipher local velocity which in turn can be integrated to estimate trajectories of individual points over time [13]. Several investigators have studied the resolution and accuracy of these techniques for tracking myocardial motion and strain [6]. Currently, phase contrast velocity estimates near the endocardial and epicardial boundaries are extremely noisy since the required size of the regions–of–interest (ROI) due to signal-to-noise limitations is so huge that it includes information from outside the myocardial wall. Thus, as with MR tagging, the most accurate LV motion and function information is obtained from the middle of the myocardial wall, and is least accurate near the endocardial and epicardial wall boundaries.

Computer Vision Approaches to Non–Rigid and Cardiac motion. A body of work has emerged from the computer vision community related to the topic of nonrigid motion and the registration of nonrigid surfaces that is directly relevant to the cardiac motion problem. The efforts in nonrigid surface registration include the use of deformable thin–plate splines [3] and octree–spline based volumetric transformation [18], among others. This research attempts to register entire sets of image data and then quantitatively and statistically look for similarities and differences. The more physical–model motivated work of Pentland [9] and Terzopolous [19] is also aimed at solving this embedding problem. In all of these approaches, any estimates of correspondence between individual points on objects are either specifically assumed to be known to aid in solving the problem, or are not considered at all in the solution. The goal of the nonrigid motion recovery is to find point correspondences between two objects over as dense a spatial field as possible. Goldgof [10] has been pursuing surface shape matching ideas, using Gaussian curvature under conformal stretching models. Recently, Metaxas [12] has utilized the mid–wall point correspondences estimated from MR tagging in conjunction with the deformable superquadrics approach. Ayache [11] has been trying to unify boundary shape landmark approach with physically–based framework to segment and track objects simultaneously.

2 Methods

We are working towards the development of a unified framework which uses the shape properties of the endocardial and epicardial surfaces, as well as incorporates mid–wall 3D instantaneous velocity information of phase contrast MR images and displacement information of tagged MR images if they are available, to track the 4D trajectories of a dense field of points which sample the myocardial wall over the entire cardiac cycle. Furthermore, it is our intent to derive accurate myocardial motion, LV thickening and strain measures from these trajectories, useful (from both a basic research and clinical standpoint) for the study of the location, severity and extent of ischemic injury.

In this section, we first briefly describe the experimental procedures used for our *in vivo* MRI–based validation experiments. Next we describe the MR imaging protocols used in this effort. Finally, we describe the basic ideas of our newly developed unified tracking strategy, earlier versions of which (the shape–based tracking of endocardial and epicardial surfaces) have been described more completely in [15]. [2]

2.1 Experimental Setup for *In Vivo* MRI–based studies

Acute Infarct Animal Model. To date, 12 acute experiments yielding 9 usable datasets have been performed on open chested dogs subjected to permanent coronary artery occlusion, resulting in transmural myocardial infarction. A limb lead of the electrocardiogram was continuously monitored, with non-ferromagnetic electrodes. The femoral vein and both femoral arteries were isolated and cannulated for administration of fluids and medications, pressure monitoring, and arterial sampling. The proximal left anterior descending coronary artery was isolated after the first diagonal branch, for placement of an occluder.

Paired endocardial and epicardial markers were placed in 4 locations on the heart. We implanted a small, bullet–shaped copper plug (1mm x 2.5mm) through the myocardium with a hollow metal insertion tube through an 18 gauge needle track. This *void* marker was loosely tethered to the endocardial surface by an elastic string. The string attached to each endocardial marker passes through the myocardium and is secured to a Gd–DTPA–filled marker sutured onto the epicardial surface. The *bright* epicardial markers are small, plastic encasings (inner volume 73.81mm^3) filled with a solution of saline and Gd–DTPA (200:1). The elastic string attaching the epicardial and endocardial markers keeps the endocardial marker on the endocardial surface during the entire cardiac cycle, without restricting myocardial thickening.

The dogs were positioned in the magnet in the left lateral position for initial 4D imaging under baseline conditions, according to the MR imaging protocols described below. The left anterior descending coronary artery was then occluded, without movement of the animal relative to the imaging planes. 4D images were acquired again after occlusion. After completion of the acute protocol, hearts were rapidly excised for postmortem imaging and histochemical staining. The hearts were then sectioned in 5mm–thick slices perpendicular to the long axis of the heart. 3D *post mortem* injury maps were then reconstructed from digitized photographs of the myocardial slices.

Magnetic Resonance Imaging Protocol. MR imaging was performed on GE Signa 1.5 Tesla scanners with version 4.7 software and hardware using a head coil. Axial images through the LV were obtained with the gradient echo cine technique using the following parameters: section thickness 5 mm, no inter–section

---

[2] We are also testing our approach using high resolution, 4D cine–computed tomographic data, acquired using the Dynamic Spatial Reconstructor (DSR) at the Mayo Clinic in collaboration with Dr. Erik Ritman. The DSR experiments followed roughly the same procedure, but are not described here for brevity.

gap, 42 cm field of view, TE 14 msec, TR 20 msec, flip angle 30 degrees, 256x256 matrix and 2 excitations. Images typically were acquired with 2 locations per acquisition and 16 cardiac phases per location. Each slice location acquisition required approximately an 8 minute acquisition time for 2 excitations. This sequence provides images with an in plane resolution of 1.64 x 1.64 mm for a 128x128 matrix and 5mm resolution perpendicular to the imaging planes. Temporal resolution is 40msec for each location acquisition. Example images at 3 slice levels in a single temporal 3D frame are shown in figure 1, with arrows indicating the locations of the implanted validation markers. For 3 of these studies, phase contrast MR images were also acquired in 3 mid–ventricular slices for the same dog heart, which provide mid–wall velocity information for the imaged regions.

2.2 Image Analysis: A Unified Motion Tracking Framework

Extended from our previous shape–based motion tracking approach [15], we are developing a unified framework using continuum biomechanical model which utilizes both the LV boundary information (which is available from the shape properties of endocardial and epicardial surfaces) and the mid–wall information (which can be provided by the 3D phase contrast MR images and/or the tagged MR images). [3] We construct a complete triangular finite element grid which tessellates not only the LV surface sample points, but also the sample points in the mid-wall. The union of all the tetrahedra forms the solid model of the entire left ventricle (see figure 4). The unified motion tracking algorithm then uses this grid to embed the underlying biomechanical constraints of the LV model, and tracks the motion of points everywhere on the entire LV wall using the known displacement information of the sparse endocardial/epicardial surface sample points and/or the mid–wall tagged points, as well as the velocity information of a sparse set of mid–wall points. From the dense motion trajectory field, other LV function measurements such as 3D LV thickening and strain maps, can be obtained. We note the 3D framework is still in development, but we will report some of the initial ideas and 2D results in this subsection.

Generating the Finite Element LV Model. The first step to construct the finite element LV model is to segment the 4D image data on a slice by slice basis to find the LV boundary. This is currently performed by treating the data as if it is consisted of a sequence of temporal 3D frames where there exists a spatial stack of 2D images in each frame, although we are continuing to investigate complete 3D parametric surface approach as well [17]. We solve the 2D boundary finding problem twice in each slice, once for the epicardial border and once for the endocardial border using a deformable contour approach that we have developed for 2D boundary finding[16, 4]. The boundaries found in this plane are now used as a bias and initial estimate for locating the endocardial and epicardial boundaries in the next plane in the stack. This process repeats until all of the contours that make up the LV surfaces in each frame are completely located. Meanwhile,

---

[3] Although the aim of the unified framework is to utilize multiple complementary sources of constraints to achieve more reliable and robust estimates, it will work if only single source of information is available.

some mid–wall points of the phase contrast MR images (and landmark mid–wall points of the tagged MR images) are also identified. Finally, the contours that form each endocardial and epicardial surface in each 3D frame as well as the mid–wall sample points identified from phase contrast and tagging images will be stacked. A Delaunay triangulation algorithm is then used to tessellate the stacked LV sample points. A solid finite element LV model which consists of many tetrahedra representing all parts of myocardium is thus generated.

Boundary Displacement Information. The movement of a sparse set of LV surface points is performed by following local surface shape [15]. The tessellated dense set of surface points are used to guide shape calculations, and surface curvature maps over the cardiac cycle for both endocardial and epicardial surfaces are computed through multi–level local surface patch fitting. For each time instant, two sparse subsets of the surface points are created by choosing *geometrically significant* shape landmark points, one for endocardial surface and the other for epicardial surface. The best matched point for each shape landmark at the next time frame is located using a 3D bending energy model. In this effort, surface patches on the LV are modeled as thin, flexible plates. The strain energy of the deformation required to bend a curved plate or surface patch to a new deformed state is defined as a function of the changes of two principal curvatures, and is invariant to 3D rotation and translation. Under the assumption that each surface patch deforms only slightly and locally within a small time interval, for each sampled point on the first surface, we construct a search area on the second surface. The point within the search window on the second surface that is best matched (i.e. minimizing the bending energy) is chosen as the corresponding point to the one at the first surface, while the bending energy for all the other points inside the window are also recorded to be used as a indicator of the uniqueness of the match. The result of this matching process yields a set of shape–based, best–matched initial motion vectors $\mathbf{D}_0(u, v)$ for pairs of surfaces derived from 3D image sequence, as well as information from within each search area as to how confident the match is.

A regularization procedure is then adopted to result in a dense displacement vector field that is an optimal compromise between an adherence term and a smoothness term, with the sparse shape landmark points' initial matches being the only matching constraint to find the dense point correspondence between surfaces. The process is embedded in the irregular triangular surface grid generated from the Delaunay tessellation, and is given by the following expression:

$$\mathbf{D}^*(u, v) = \arg\min_{\mathbf{D}} \int_U \int_V \left\{ C_{\mathbf{D}}(u, v)[\mathbf{D}(u, v) - \mathbf{D}_0(u, v)]^2 + (\frac{\partial \mathbf{D}(u, v)}{\partial \mathbf{u}})^2 \right\} \, du \tag{1}$$

In this equation, $[U, V]$ is the domain of the surface at time t in which the grid from the Delaunay triangulation is embedded, $\mathbf{u} = [u, v]^T$ is the surface point at time t, $\mathbf{D}^*(u, v)$ is the optimal smoothed motion vector field between two surfaces at times t and $t + \delta t$, $\mathbf{D}_0(u, v)$ is the initial motion vector estimate, and $C_{\mathbf{D}}(u, v)$ is the confidence measure matrix which weighs both the goodness and uniqueness of the initial match.

In the new unified framework, the displacement vectors between time frames of the shape landmark points will be used only as part of LV deformation constraints, the boundary displacement constraint. In addition, the triangular grid is now a solid volumetric mesh instead of a surface grid.

Mid–Wall Velocity/Displacement Information. The mid–wall region of the 3D phase contrast images can be sampled at a number of points with their instantaneous velocity known at each time frame. This mid–wall information can provide additional constraints to track the LV wall motion. Our group's initial work in this area is documented in [6], in which a stable algorithm that combines forward and reverse integration within a rigorous framework for velocity mapping is presented. Meanwhile, the displacement information from a sparse set of mid–wall MR tagging landmark points can be computed by following trajectories of some MR tag points over time [14]. This will provide yet another set of constraint to track the motion of the dense field LV points.

A Unified Framework to Assess Myocardial Function. We have constructed a 3D finite element LV model which has nodes in the mid–wall region, as well as nodes on endocardial and epicardial surfaces. We also have established the displacement vectors for a sparse set of surface shape landmark nodes and mid–wall tag points, and the velocity information for a sparse set of mid–wall phase contrast nodes. Assuming the boundary and mid–wall nodal points represent the LV reasonably well, a continuum biomechanical LV model based on the theory of finite elasticity and realistic material law is under development. Using the finite element method to solve the deformation of the LV over time, under the known boundary conditions (the displacement and velocity information of some of the nodes) and external forces (i.e. flow pressure, volume change) if available, the equilibrium equations can be established as [2]:

$$\mathbf{M}\ddot{\mathbf{U}} + \mathbf{C}\dot{\mathbf{U}} + \mathbf{K}\mathbf{U} = \mathbf{R} \tag{2}$$

where $\mathbf{M}$ is the mass matrix, $\mathbf{C}$ the damping matrix, $\mathbf{K}$ the stiffness matrix, $\mathbf{R}$ the external load, and $\mathbf{U}$ the nodal displacement vector field. We note that the form in equation (2) describes a very general finite element system, while the known displacement/velocity conditions and the external forces provide more specific constraints for our framework. We want to point out that we intend to use this model to enforce certain real physical constraints related to known cardiac volumes and pressures, as well as realistic biomechanical properties of the myocardium, not just physically analogous ones as described by Pentland [9] and others. Let $\mathbf{U}_a$ be the known displacements, $\mathbf{U}_b$ the displacements of the nodes with known velocity, and $\mathbf{U}_c$ the displacements of the nodes with no prior information, we can rewrite the equilibrium equations in the form[4]:

$$\begin{bmatrix} M_{aa} & M_{ab} & M_{ac} \\ M_{ba} & M_{bb} & M_{bc} \\ M_{ca} & M_{cb} & M_{cc} \end{bmatrix} \begin{bmatrix} \ddot{U}_a \\ \ddot{U}_b \\ \ddot{U}_c \end{bmatrix} + \begin{bmatrix} C_{aa} & C_{ab} & C_{ac} \\ C_{ba} & C_{bb} & C_{bc} \\ C_{ca} & C_{cb} & C_{cc} \end{bmatrix} \begin{bmatrix} \dot{U}_a \\ \dot{U}_b \\ \dot{U}_c \end{bmatrix} + \begin{bmatrix} K_{aa} & K_{ab} & K_{ac} \\ K_{ba} & K_{bb} & K_{bc} \\ K_{ca} & K_{cb} & K_{cc} \end{bmatrix} \begin{bmatrix} U_a \\ U_b \\ U_c \end{bmatrix} = \begin{bmatrix} R_a \\ R_b \\ R_c \end{bmatrix} \tag{3}$$

where $\mathbf{U}_a$ and $\dot{\mathbf{U}}_b$ are prescribed conditions. The iterative solutions of these pre–conditioned equilibrium equations yield displacements for all element nodal points, from which the 3D strain and stress maps can be obtained.

---

[4] For simplicity of the equation, we assume no node has both known displacement and velocity information.

3   Experiments and Results

Using the initial form of our unified framework described above, the initial experimentation with the cardiac motion and function analysis is reported here. As mentioned above, to date we have acquired nine usable sets of 4D MRI data using the acute infarct animal model. The visual results shown here are from two of the MR studies that have been analyzed.

Figure 1 shows three image slices from the same 3D MRI time frame, illustrating the paired markers used for motion tracking validation (white arrows ⇒ epicardial markers, black arrows ⇒ endocardial markers). Implanted markers' centroids are detected over the entire cardiac cycle, and their trajectories are compared to the algorithm–derived points trajectories in order to validate the accuracy of the developed methodology. Figure 2 illustrates the comparison of algorithm–computed (lighter) trajectories with the marker–derived (darker) trajectories of three endocardial points, moving from end–diastole (ED) to end–systole (ES). The paths are shown relative to the endocardial surface rendered at global end–systole (lowest overall chamber volume). The two most right points have almost identical marker- and algorithm- derived trajectories, while the left one is a little bit off after several time intervals (but they are still very close).

Figure 3 and table 1 are presented to illustrate some of the measurements from which useful physiological parameters will be derived. Figure 3 shows an infarcted endocardial surface roughly in its end-systolic state. On the left, the dense motion trajectories are shown in the normal zone of the infarcted left ventricle, while on the right, the dense trajectories locating in the infarct zone of the same LV are shown. Note in this case, the normal zone has far larger motion than the infarct zone does. Table 1 provides the quantitative comparison of normal and infarct zone measurement (path length) before and after the coronary occlusion surgery which causes the myocardial injury. From the table we observe that for both studies, the normal zone points have relatively stable movement pre- and post- infarction while the infarct zone's mobility drops fifty percent or more.

A key additional measurement of interest to us is that of myocardial thickness and strain. By tracking small, related regions of points on both the LV surfaces (endocardium and epicardium) and mid–wall myocardium over time, we can create transmural and non–transmural measures of myocardial strain and use the radial component of strain to infer thickening changes. Non–transmural strain measures are of great value for predicting early myocardial injury and viability. Figure 4 displays of a tessellated 3D LV wall mesh deforming over time from ED to ES, in the order of left, middle, and right. Figure 5 shows the gray scale maps of three 2D principal strain maps, as well as the principal direction associated with the maximum principal normal strain. Here, we denote large positive strain with light white shade, large negative strain with dark shade, and near zero strain with neutral gray. For any given element, the positive principal strain represents the stretching in the associated direction, the negative one represents the compressing effect.

In addition to reporting the above initial results on the motion/function tracking algorithm, we also report here the results of initial steps taken towards comparing the *in vivo* algorithm–based measurements to *post mortem* measures.

	normal zone path length		infarct zone path length	
study	baseline	post − infarction	baseline	post − infarction
1	$17.07 \pm 2.79mm$	$14.50 \pm 2.05mm$	$22.50 \pm 2.13mm$	$8.76 \pm 2.16mm$
2	$13.32 \pm 1.67mm$	$15.79 \pm 2.26mm$	$14.28 \pm 1.81mm$	$7.31 \pm 2.35mm$

Table 1. Table of path lengths of endocardial normal and infarct zones of two canine MR studies, under baseline and post–infarction conditions. These data were average path lengths within each zone (defined by points' closeness to the implanted markers). Note the relative stableness of the normal zone path lengths before and after infarction, and the big drop of the infarct zone path lengths after coronary occlusion.

Ultimately, the image frame in each of the pre- and post- infarction studies whose markers best match the *post mortem* markers by minimizing the overall Euclidean distance between the sets of points will be chosen as the *in vivo* myocardial injury reference frame for that study. Next, color masks representing the infarct zone and normal zone that were found on the *post mortem* surface are mapped onto both the pre- and post- infarction *in vivo* endocardial reference surfaces. Classification of myocardium from *in vivo* image–derived measurement will be compared to the *post mortem* measures. Results from the first step of this process, showing two views of the computer–reconstructed, color coded 3D *post mortem* surface, are shown in figure 6. Note that the right figure shows the non–transmural nature of the myocardial injury in this study.

4 Summary

We have described our ongoing efforts aimed at developing a unified framework to more accurately quantify the local, regional and global function of the left ventricle (LV) of the heart, under both normal and ischemic conditions. Our approach incorporates multiple sources of constraints, including motion information derived from the shape properties of the endocardial and epicardial surfaces, mid–wall 3D instantaneous velocity information from phase contrast MR images, and/or mid–wall displacement information from tagged MR images.

Ongoing and future work includes developing more sophisticated continuum biomechanical model of the myocardium based on viscoelastic material law, incorporating temporal periodic characteristics of the heart motion into the current framework.

References

1. L. Axel and L. Dougherty. MR imaging of motion with spatial modulation of magnetization. *Radiology*, 171:841–845, 1989.
2. K. Bathe and E. Wilson. *Numerical Methods in Finite Element Analysis*. Prentice-Hall, New Jersey, 1976.
3. F. L. Bookstein. Principal warps: Thin-plate splines and the decomposition of deformations. *IEEE Trans. on Patt. Anal. and Mach. Intell.*, pages 567–585, 1989.

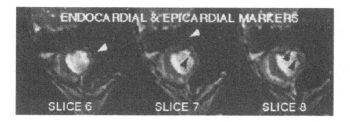

Fig. 1. Three slices from the same 3D MRI time frame, illustrating the paired markers used for motion tracking validation (white arrows ⇒ epicardial markers, black arrow ⇒ endocardial markers).

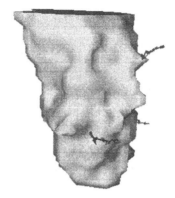

Fig. 2. Comparison of algorithm–computed (lighter) and marker–derived (darker) trajectories of three endocardial points, moving from ED to ES. The paths are shown relative to the endocardial surface rendered at global end–systole. The two right most points have almost overlapping marker- and algorithm- derived trajectories, while the left one is a little bit off after several time intervals.

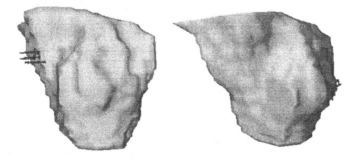

Fig. 3. Display of two sets of dense motion trajectories in the normal and infarct zones of the endocardial surface of an infarcted left ventricle, relative to the surface rendered at global end–systole. The normal zone is shown on the left, the infarct zone is on the right. Note the relatively smaller motion in the infarct zone. (See table 1 for quantitative details).

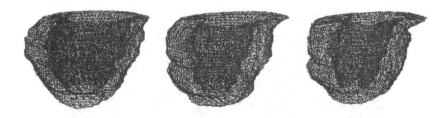

Fig. 4. 3D displays of a tessellated LV wall deforming from ED to ES. Left: end–diastole; Middle: middle of the contraction; Right: end–systole.

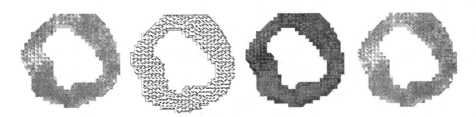

Fig. 5. 2D principal strain maps at ED: maximum principal strain, direction associated with maximum principal strain, minimum principal strain, and shear strain.

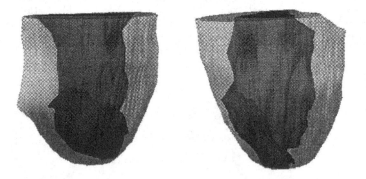

Fig. 6. 3D displays of a reconstructed *post mortem* LV wall from two views: endocardium (inner lighter opaque), epicardium (outer transparent), and injury region (lower darker opaque). Note the right figure shows the non–transmural nature of the myocardial injury.

4. A. Chakraborty, L. H. Staib, and J. S. Duncan. An integrated approach to boundary finding in medical images. In *Proceedings of the IEEE Workshop on Biomedical Image Analysis*, pages 13–22, 1994.

5. J. Chesebro and G. Knatterrud et al. Thrombolysis in myocardial infarction (TIMI) trial phase I: A comparison between intravenous tissue plasminogen activator and intravenous streptokinase. *Circulation*, 76:142–154, 1987.

6. R.T. Constable, K. Rath, A. Sinusas, and J. Gore. Development and evaluation of tracking algorithms for cardiac wall motion analysis using phase velocity MR imaging. *Magnetic Resonance in Medicine*, 32:33–42, 1994.

7. T. S. Denney and J. L. Prince. 3d displacement field reconstruction from planar tagged cardiac MR images. In *Proceedings of the IEEE Workshop on Biomedical Image Analysis*, pages 51–60, 1994.

8. W. Grossman. Assessment of regional myocardial function. *JACC*, 7(2):327–328, 1986.

9. B. Horowitz and S. Pentland. Recovery of non- rigid motion and structure. In *IEEE Conf. on CVPR*, pages 325–330, Maui, June 1991.

10. C. Kambhamettu and D. Goldgof. Point correspondence recovery in non–rigid motion. In *IEEE Conf. on CVPR*, pages 222–227, June 1992.

11. C. Nastar and N. Ayache. Non-rigid motion analysis in medical images: a physically based approach. In *Information Processing in Medical Imaging*. Springer-Verlag, 1993.

12. J. Park, D. Metaxas, and A. Young. Deformable models with parameter functions: Application to heart wall modeling. In *IEEE Conf. on CVPR*, pages 437–442, June 1994.

13. N. J. Pelc, A. Shimakawa, and G. H. Glover. Phase contrast cine MRI. In *Proceedings of the 8th Annual SMRM*, page 101, Amsterdam, 1989.

14. P. Shi, A. Amini, R. T. Constable, and J. Duncan. Tracking tagged MR images with energy–minimizing deformable grids. In *Proceedings of the 18th IEEE Annual Northeast Bioengineering Conference*, pages 133–134, 1992.

15. P. Shi, A. Amini, G. Robinson, A. Sinusas, R. T. Constable, and J. Duncan. Shape-based 4d left ventricular myocardial function analysis. In *Proceedings of the IEEE Workshop on Biomedical Image Analysis*, pages 88–97, 1994.

16. L. H. Staib and J. S. Duncan. Parametrically deformable contour models. *IEEE Trans. on Patt. Anal. and Mach. Intell.*, 14(11):1061–1075, 1992.

17. L. H. Staib and J. S. Duncan. Deformable fourier models for surface finding in 3d images. In *Visualization in Biomedical Computing*, pages 90–104, Oct. 1992. SPIE 1808.

18. R. Szeliski and S. Lavallee. Matching 3d anatomical surfaces with non-rigid deformations using octree-splines. In *Proceedings of the IEEE Workshop on Biomedical Image Analysis*, pages 144–153, 1994.

19. D. Terzopolous and D. Metaxas. Dynamic 3d models with local and global deformation: Deformable superquadrics. *IEEE Trans. on Patt. Anal. and Mach. Intell.*, 13(17), 1991.

20. A. A. Young, D. L. Kraitchman, and L. Axel. Deformable models for tagged MR images: Reconstruction of two- and three-dimensional heart wall motion. In *Proceedings of the IEEE Workshop on Biomedical Image Analysis*, pages 317–323, 1994.

21. E. Zerhouni and et. al. Tagging of the human heart by multiplanar selective RF saturation for the analysis of myocardial contraction. In *Abstracts of the Ann. Meeting of the Soc. of MR in Imaging*, page 10, San Francisco, 1988.

Segmentation II

Detection of Brain Activation
from MRI Data by Likelihood-Ratio Test

S.RUAN(1), C.JAGGI(1), J.M.CONSTANS(2), D.BLOYET(1)

(1) LEI/ISMRA, 6 Bd du Maréchal Juin, F - 14050 Caen Cedex
    e-mail : Su.Ruan@lei.ismra.fr
(2) CHRU de Caen, Unité de Résonance Magnétique, F - 14033 Caen Cedex

Abstract. An image processing strategy for functional magnetic resonance imaging (FMRI) data set, consisting of K sequential images of the same slice of brain tissue, is considered. An algorithm of detection based on the likelihood-ratio test is introduced. The noise model and signal model are established by analysing the FMRI. Due to data having a poor signal-to-noise ratio, and also in order to make more reliable detection, the algorithm is carried out in two stages: coarse detection followed by a fine one. Jumps in mean from non stimulation periods to stimulation ones in the time-course series data are used as decision criteria. The detection method is applied to experimental FMRI data from the motor cortex and compared with the cross-correlation method and Student's t-test.
Key words: FMRI; signal detection; motor cortex; likelihood-ratio test.

I. Introduction

Physiological, anatomical and cognitive psychophysical studies indicate that the brain possesses anatomically distinct processing regions [1] in which neuronal activity causes local changes in cerebral blood flow (CBF), blood volume (CBV), blood oxygenation and metabolism. These changes can be used to map the functional location of component mental operations [2]. Positron emission tomography (PET), which measures the distribution of radioactive tracers within the brain, has provided evidence for localised brain activation during functional tasks. But it suffers from limited spatial resolution and especially from temporal resolution, which is needed for studying the dynamic brain processes. In comparison, functional magnetic resonance imaging (FMRI), developed recently, has higher spatial and temporal resolutions.

MR Imaging is mainly based on contrast derived from tissue-relaxation parameters T_1 and T_2. Several investigators have demonstrated that brain tissue relaxation is influenced by the oxygenation state of hemoglobin (T_2^* effect) [3][4] and intrinsic tissue perfusion (T_1 effect) [5][6]. Local changes produced by neuronal activity can thus be obtained as signal intensity changes by choosing pulse sequences which are sensitive to the variations of T_2^*, T_2 or T_1 [3-7]. The signal observed is usually so small that it is covered by the noise. For example, the percent signal change in activated primary brain regions (motor and visual cortices), at optimised TE for maximum functional contrast, is in a range of 1-5% at 1.5 T [8], 1.5-5% at

2T [9] and 5-20% at 4T [10]. We can repeat the acquisition as often as desired for the same subject (theoretically), thereby yielding improved time resolution to enhance the signal-to-noise ratio (SNR). But, we can't really apply series of images as long as we want to for a human subject; therefore, image processing strategies are used necessarily to deal with functional MRI data.

The basic method for detecting the activation (signal variation induced by stimulation) is to subtract images obtained during a resting state from images obtained during activation [11][12]. This simple subtraction of images is sensitive to noise and to movement artifacts, yielding unprecise localisation of the activated regions. So, this method is usually applied in regions of interest (ROI) determined manually by experts. Statistical methods have been suggested to improve the detection, such as Z-score which tests the difference in signals between the activation and rest states normalised by the standard-deviation [13][14], and the Student's t-test which tests a statistically significant difference between the two conditions according to some known probability density function under the null hypothesis [15][16]. However, these approaches suffer from a lack of robustness. Many spurious areas of activation are present when a low threshold is used and, on the contrary, activated regions are lost in case of a higher threshold. Let us also mention the problem of artifacts which cannot be resolved. For further improvement and also for analysing the dynamic brain process, the time-course data sets are used. The time-series repeat the resting and activated states at a constant frequency. The analysis of these data can be carried out both in the time-domain and in the frequency domain. It also allows differentiation of activation from artifacts. Bandettini et al. [17] have developed a method based on thresholding the correlation coefficient of the data with respect to a reference waveform. They have also used Fourier analysis to deal with the data, which however loses phase information.

A coarse to fine detection method of the brain activation, making use of a time-course MRI data, is proposed in this paper. It is based on the likelihood ratio test (L.R.T). The method proceeds as follows. All regions having significant changes from the stimulated state to the rest state are first noted as regions of interest (ROI). The true activated regions are then selected from these ROI; the obtained regions are finally optimised. This method is described in detail in the next section. The obtained experimental results using FMRI from human motor cortex are presented in section 3 and compared to some other methods. We then conclude in the last section.

II Method

As we mentioned in the previous section, the activation signals are very small in MRI data, which result in low SNR defined as:

$$\text{SNR} = \sqrt{\frac{s^2}{\sigma^2}} = \frac{s}{\sigma} \tag{1}$$

where s denotes the magnitude of signal, and σ the standard deviation of noise. For n signal observations, s^2 is equal to $\sum_{k=1}^{n} s_k^2$ and the SNR becomes $\sqrt{n\dfrac{\overline{s^2}}{\sigma^2}}$, or the initial SNR increased by $\sqrt{n}$ ($\overline{s^2}$ is the average signal power).

To reliably and precisely achieve the localisation of activated regions, the detection should rely on a high SNR. It is obvious that SNR of a pixel is less than one in that region since the SNR is theoretically increased by $\sqrt{n}$ if the region extends over n pixels. Therefore, we surely have more reliability in detecting the time-course of a region than in detecting that of a pixel. Based on this fact, we first only look for the pixels having a significant signal change between the resting state and active state without using the temporal condition, i.e. the time instants of signal changes. This first detection with low constraint allows to merge activated pixels into the regions of interest. From these ROI's, we can then ascertain, with help of the temporal conditions, the regional changes which are of sufficient similarity to the functional signal to be validated as activated regions. Of course, it is possible that, at this step of the processing, some pixels be included in the selected ROIs by error. Therefore, another step is required to further optimisation. This strategy of analysis leads to our algorithm which consists in four main steps. First, coarse detection is performed in all images for each pixel using the likelihood-ratio test (step 1). This step results in some labelled regions defined by merging of pixels, adjacent in eight-connexity (step 2). The pixels, that are not adjacent to at least one other, are eliminated. Based on these regions of interest, we select the activated regions by application of the likelihood ratio test using the same principle as in the first step, but adding this time the temporal conditions (step 3). Finally, each detected region is optimised by examination of every pixel SNR. The low SNR pixels are considered as non activated.

A functional MRI time-series consists in alternately resting images and activated images with several cycles. The time-course of each pixel can be considered, from our point of view, as a signal corrupted by additive noise in the activated region, and as noise in non activated regions. Testing of pixels within the activated region can be modelled as a binary hypothesis:

$$H_0(\text{noise}): \qquad Y_k = N_k \qquad\qquad k = 1,2...n \qquad\qquad (2)$$

versus

$$H_1(\text{signal}): \qquad Y_k = N_k + S_k \qquad\qquad k = 1,2..n$$

where $\underline{Y} = (Y_1.. Y_n)^T$ is an observation vector, $\underline{S} = (S_1..S_n)^T$ is a known signal and $\underline{N} = (N_1..N_n)^T$ is a sampled noise vector. In fact, we wish to derive an optimum detector from a given number of observations. From the theory of hypothesis testing [18][19], optimum procedures for deciding between the hypothesis H_0 and H_1 can be obtained if we know the statistical behaviour of the signal and of the noise. Therefore, the first step is to analyse both behaviours in MRI time series data.

Activation signal modelling : The temporal response of the MR signal to functional brain activity is an incompletely understood process. There is a complex relationship between the activation signal, the neuronal activity and the delayed hemodynamic response. However, we know that there is an increased signal induced by a brain activity on activated pixels during stimulation relative to non stimulation. The change from non stimulation to stimulation is more important than the variation of signal induced by brain activity during stimulation. A simple model of this signal, usually used in FMRI, is shown in figure 1. It implies that the signal jumps occur synchronously with stimulation; the signal is then constant during the interleaved stimulation periods and the interleaved rest periods. This model is an over simplification, but is of considerable practical utility.

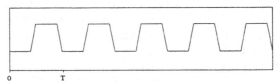

Figure 1 : Signal model: box-car waveform.

Noise distribution modelling : The noise images were generated by subtraction of two successive resting images. We have thus n/2 noise images (n: total resting images). The distribution of the pixel values in a noise image was computed. Figure 2a shows that it is well approximated by a gaussian function. Furthermore, to test if pixel values are statistically independent in noise images, the coefficient of auto-correlation at various distances in a noise image and the coefficients of cross-correlation between noise images were computed. The curves illustrated in Figure 2b show a weak degree of correlation between pixels and between successive images of noise. From these above experimental studies, we can deduce that the noise is white and gaussian. Note that the physiological noise inside the brain has been neglected.

Having established both models for the activation signal and the noise, the time-course of a pixel in one cycle, as depicted in figure3a, can be decomposed as the sum of two or three components : the anatomical MR signal (constant), the noise (white noise) and possibly the activation-induced signal (box-car waveform) in the case of an activated pixel.

Likelihood-ratio test : The noise samples $N_1...N_n$ in (1) can now be considered as independent and as having an identical distribution $p_0(\mu_0, \sigma)$. Given the foregoing assumptions on $\underline{S}$, their effect on the distribution of $\underline{Y}$ is merely to shift the mean from that of $\underline{N}$. Therefore the observation $\underline{Y}$ is a sequence of independent gaussian variables with variance σ^2, piecewise constant mean $\mu_i (i = 0,1)$, and jumps in the mean at known time instants. The problem is actually to detect the jumps appearing at known time instants. Detecting a jump is in fact equivalent to accepting the hypothesis H_1 of change and rejecting the hypothesis H_0 of no change. As the observations are independent of each other, the likelihood ratio test between these two hypothesis takes the following form :

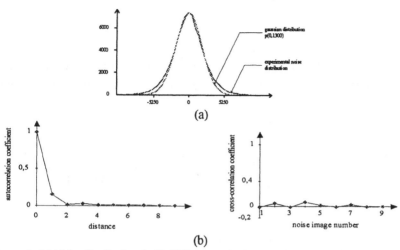

(a)

(b)

Figure 2: (a) Noise distribution for FMRI in one noise image achieved by subtraction of the first and second rest images in the time-course series. This distribution is well approximated by a gaussian function. (b) Coefficients of auto-correlation of the noise image (left) and coefficients of cross-correlation (right) between successive noise images.

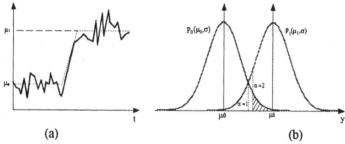

(a)   (b)

Figure 3: (a) Time-course of signal changes in one cycle is supposed to be a Gaussian sequence with a change in mean and constant variance. (b) Illustration of location testing with threshold α.

$$L(\underline{Y}) = \frac{\prod_{k=1}^{r-1} p_0(y_k) \cdot \prod_{k=r}^{n} p_1(y_k)}{\prod_{k=1}^{n} p_0(y_k)} = \prod_{k=r}^{n} \frac{p_1(y_k)}{p_0(y_k)} \qquad (3)$$

where

$$p_i(y) = \frac{1}{\sigma\sqrt{2\pi}} e^{-\frac{(y-\mu_i)^2}{2\sigma^2}} \qquad (i = 0, 1)$$

The test is given by :

$$L(\underline{Y}) \underset{H_0}{\overset{H_1}{\gtrless}} \gamma$$

$$(4)$$

H_1 or H_0 hypothesis are validated depending on whether $L(\underline{Y})$ is higher or lower than γ. The decision threshold γ is established using the following technique. Taking logarithm of (3) gives :

$$\lambda_n = \sum_{k=r}^{n} \ln \frac{p_1(y_k)}{p_0(y_k)} = \frac{1}{\sigma^2} S_r^n(\mu_0, \nu)$$

$$(5)$$

with

$$S_r^n(\mu_0, \nu) = \nu \sum_{k=r}^{n} \left(y_k - \mu_0 - \frac{\nu}{2} \right) \quad , \qquad \nu = \mu_1 - \mu_0$$

The test (4) becomes :

$$\frac{1}{\sigma^2} S_r^n(\mu_0, \nu) \underset{H_0}{\overset{H_1}{\gtrless}} \ln \gamma$$

$$(6)$$

The threshold $\ln\gamma$ is determined by:

$$\ln\gamma = \ln\alpha^{n-r} = (n-r)\ln\alpha$$

$$(7)$$

where α is given by:

$$\frac{p_1(y_k)}{p_0(y_k)} > \alpha$$

$$(8)$$

The overall decision threshold γ for accepting one jump is then based on the α value ($\alpha>1$) which corresponds to the ratio between $p_1(y_k)$ and $p_0(y_k)$. Figure 3b illustrates the basic principle of this test. For a small ν value compared to σ (small magnitude jump), the two gaussian functions will almost be overlaid; the condition (8) will hardly be satisfied (depending on the α value); therefore, no jump will be detected. Conversely, if ν has a high magnitude compared to σ, the curves will be separated, condition (8) is easily satisfied and a jump identified. The α value can, in fact, be considered as a threshold value for deciding whether the magnitude jump is acceptable. However, condition (6) does not identify positive or negative jumps; this is done by adding the conditions: $\nu > 0$ or $\nu < 0$ for a positive jump or a negative jump, respectively.

Optimisation : Activated regions, resulting from the previous steps, may include pixels which were taken into account only on the basis of adjacency with activated ones. The latter must now be rejected. This refinement step is as follows. The SNR of a pixel p_j^i ($SNR_{p_j^i}$) and of a region (SNR_{r^i}) were introduced at the beginning of this section. For each pixel p_j^i of a region r^i, the following test is performed:

$$SNR_{p_j^i} < \frac{1}{\sqrt{n-1}} SNR_{r^i}$$

$$(9)$$

where n is the area of r^i in pixel units. If (9) is satisfied, p_j^i is taken out of the region.

III. Results

Materials and brain activation protocol : MR imaging was performed on a standard GE 1.5 T Signa scanner. A spoiled gradient recalled (SPGR) sequence having an initial 20 degree pulse, a TR of 70 ms and a TE of 60 ms was used. The spatial resolution is: FOV = 22 cm, slice - thickness = 10 mm, matrix = 256×192. The image was coded in 16 bits. To localise the plane of study in the motor cortex, an oblique axial slice was acquired 30 mm above the CA-CP plane.

The motor activation task consisted of tapping each finger of the right hand to the thumb. The subject was instructed to tap continually. Then, five images under stimulation were acquired after five resting images (without finger movement). This stimulus alternation was repeated continually for five cycles. Because of time delay in the activation signal change and steady state equilibrium of the signal, the first resting image and the first activated image in each period were not used for detection. Of course we can adjust the jump instants if we know the delay.

Pixel detection : Three methods of detection of activated regions have been carried out for comparison. The threshold to be applied for each method is chosen in order to build the regions of interest with a priori knowledge (primary motor cortex).

Student's t-test : Figure 4b shows the binary image obtained by Student's t-test [18] thresholding with $p < 0.05$ (p is the probability of detecting an activated pixel by chance). Although we can observe the true activated regions, the result is not satisfactory because of many spurious regions in the background. This is due to lack of accuracy in the estimation of SD (standard-deviation) which directly limits the statistical value of t. Of course, we can reduce some number of spurious regions in the background by lowering the threshold, but at the same time we can lose the activated pixels.

Cross-correlation : As explained in II, we have chosen the reference waveform as shown in Figure 1. The function used to calculate the correlation coefficients was the same as in [17]. A threshold value of 0.35 was applied to the correlation coefficient. The result [Figure 4c] shows that this method is less sensitive to noise than the Student's t-test due to the supplementary temporal condition. But it is not robust enough in the case of low SNR data, because of the lack of tolerance to large noise values. The spurious regions can still be observed in the background. As this method retains only pixels having the same time-course signal as the modeling signal, artifacts are removed directly.

Likelihood ratio test : Due to the weakness of SNR, in a first step, we aim at seeking all the pixels having significant changes from resting to activated states. In this sense, the likelihood-ratio detector tests, for each pixel, the occurrence of a jump between all images on stimulation periods and all images on non stimulation periods, without taking into consideration the temporal constraint. Knowledge of experimental noise allows to reduce spurious pixels as much as possible. The result depicted in Figure 4d ($\alpha = 2$) shows the improvement in detectability : the spurious regions in the background are reduced to a much greater degree than results obtained by the first two methods. At the same time, there is no loss and there is even an increase of ROI's within the head. We can observe that most of the detected pixels are situated approximately along the sulci, which is in agreement with the fact that the signal changes in functional MRI are in relation with signal changes in vessels. We can analyse each region, and understand the origin of any intensity changes. Of course, some of the regions are selected due to artifacts. Here, we are only interested in the activated signals having the same waveform as the signal model. The next steps are carried out to detect them.

Region detection : After labelling the regions obtained and having eliminated isolated pixels, we seek the regions in which time-course signals are similar to the model. As we have mentioned above, the SNR in a region is higher than for an isolated pixel. We apply therefore the temporal condition to detect the regions. Likelihood ratio detector is also used here. Knowing the signal model (5 cycles), we tested in fact 5 positive and 4 negative jumps for time-course series for each region. Choosing the maxima of likelihood ratios, we obtain the activated regions with great reliability and remove the other ones, such as sagittal sinus area which is due to artifacts. It is also possible to generate a color map of all regions with different likelihood-ratios to show the degree of functional changes. For these data series with a motor activation task, six small regions, having maximum likelihood ratios, were detected. These six small regions can be considered as two areas: one occurs in the area of the primary left motor cortex and the other in the supplementary motor area. They correspond to areas that are understood to be involved with finger activity. The SNR of pixel on each region and the SNR of selected regions were then calculated to optimise the results. The final result (optimised six regions), superimposed upon the first image in the time-course series, is illustrated in Figure 5. The averaged percent signal changes for primary left motor area and the supplementary motor area are 5.9% and 3.6%, respectively. The time course signal of these two areas are also depicted in Figure 5. The curves show clearly the signal changes from a non stimulation state to a stimulation state.

IV Discussion and conclusion

We have described a new method for functional MRI, based on the likelihood ratio test. Emphasis has been placed on the detection of jumps in mean by hypothesis testing. This robust method is sensitive to signals, capable of detecting lower-order areas such as the supplementary motor area. The analysis strategy of coarse to refined detection offers means to achieve the functional regions with better reliability due to the increased SNR. The threshold level, which identifies by the likelihood ratio test the interest of pixels in the first step, is less influenced by the stability of final results. The obtained results are further improved by the next steps, which allow to successfully detect the most significant regions among many spurious regions caused by a low threshold or artifacts. Compared to the cross-correlation method, our method is less dependent on the signal model which does not really and truly represent the activated signal, because our method only detects jumps in mean.

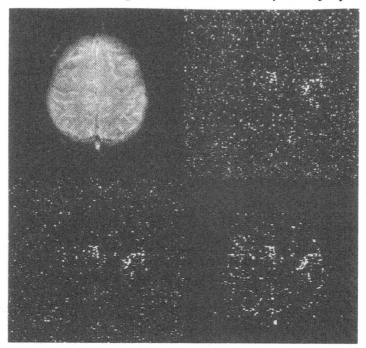

Figure 4: Comparison between three predetection methods: original image (upper left) and binary images resulting from Student's t-test (with p < 0.05) (upper right), cross-correlation (correlation coefficient threshold 0.35) (lower left), likelihood ratio test (α=2)(lower right).

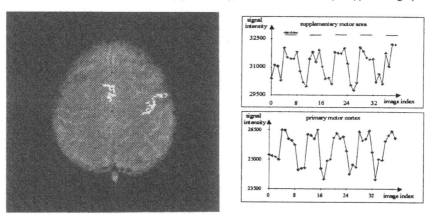

Figure 5: The final regions obtained are superimposed upon the first image in the time-course series. Time courses of signal-intensity changes for supplementary motor area (upper) and left primary motor area (lower) are indicated in two plots.

References

[1] S.Zeki & S.Shipp, Nature 335, 311, 1988.

[2] S.E.Petersen & P.T.Fox, Nature 331, 585, 1988.

[3] S.Ogawa, T.M.Lee, Bertrand Barrere, Magn. Res. Med. 29:205-210, 1993.

[4] S.Ogawa, D.W.Tank, R.Menon, J.M.Ellermann, S.G.Kim, H.Merkle & K.Ugurbil, Proc. Natl. Acad. Sci.USA , Vol. 89, pp. 5951-5955 , 1992 .

[5] S.Ogawa, T.M.Lee, A.S.Nayak & P.Glynn., Magn. Res. Med. 14, pp.68-78,1990.

[6] K.K.Kwong, J.Belliveau, D.A.Chesler, I.E.Goldberg, R.M.Weisskoff, B.P.Poncelet, D.N.Kennedy, B.E.Hoppel, M.S.Cohen, R.Turner, H.M.Cheng, T.J.Brady & B.R.Rosen, Proc. Natl. Acad. Sci. USA, Vol. 89, pp. 5675-5679, 1992.

[7] D.S.Williams, J.A.Detre, J.S.Leigh & A.P.Koretsky, Proc. Natl. Acad. Sci. USA, Vol. 89, pp 212-216, 1992.

[8] A.M.Blamire, S.Ogawa, K.Ugurbil, D.Rothman, G.McCarthy, J.M.Ellermann, F.Hyder, Z.Pattner & R.G.Shulman, Proc. Natl. Acad. Sci. USA, Vol.89, pp. 11069-11073, 1992.

[9] J.Frahm & K.Merboldt, Magn. Res. Med. 29, 1993.

[10] R.Turner, P.Jezzard, H.Wen, K.K.Kwong, D.Le Bihan, T.Zeffiro, R.S.Balaban, Magn. Res. Med. 29, 277, 1993.

[11] J.W.Belliveau, D.N.Kennedy, R.C.Mckinstry, B.R.Buchbinder, R.M.Weisskoff, M.S.Cohen, J.M.Vevea, T.J.Brady & B.R.Rsen, Science, Vol. 254, pp.716-718,1991.

[12] J.R.Zigun, J.A.Frank, F.A.Barrios, D.W.Jone, T.K.F.Foo, C.T.W.Moonen, D.Z.Press, D.R.Weinberger, Radiology , 186: 353-356, 1993.

[13] G.McCarthy, M.A.Blamire, D.L.Rothman, R.Gruetter & R.G.Shulman, Proc. Natl. Acad. Sci. USA, Vol. 90, pp. 4952-4956, 1993.

[14] W.Schneider, D.C.Noll & J.D.Cohen, Nature, Vol. 365, Sept.1993.

[15] D.Le Bihan, P.Jezzard, R.Turner, C.A.Cuenod & A.Prinster, Abstact : Soc. Magn. Res. Med., pp.11, Aug. 1993.

[16] S.M.Rao, J.R.Binder, P.A.Bandettini, T.A.Hammeke,F.Z.Yetkin, A.Jesmanowicz, L.M.Lisk, G.L.Morris, W.M.Mueller, L.D.Estkowski, E.C.Wong, V.M.Haughton & J.S.Hyde, Neurology, Vol. 43, pp. 2311-2318, 1993.

[17] P.A.Bandettini, A.Jesmanowicz, E.C.Wong & J.S.Hyde, Magn. Res. Med. 30: 161-173, 1993.

[18] H.Vincent Poor, *An introduction to signal detection and estimation*, Springer-Verlag, 1994.

[19] M.Basseville, Conf. on Detection of abrupt changes in signals and dynamical systems, Paris,1984.

Probabilistic Hyperstack Segmentation of MR Brain Data

Koen L. Vincken André S.E. Koster Max A. Viergever

Computer Vision Research Group, Utrecht University, AZU E 02.222, Heidelberglaan 100, 3584 CX Utrecht, The Netherlands; e-mail: koen@cv.ruu.nl

Abstract: **A multiscale method (the hyperstack) is proposed to segment multidimensional MR brain data. Hyperstack segmentation is based upon the linking of voxels at adjacent levels in scale space, followed by a root selection to find the voxels that represent the segments in the original image. This paper addresses an advanced linking and root labeling method for the hyperstack. In particular, attention will be paid to an extension of the linking scheme for the detection and classification of partial volume voxels. The result—a list of probabilities for each partial volume voxel—improves the resulting segmentations.**

1   Introduction

Multiscale image processing derives from the idea that a visual system analyses a scene at multiple levels of resolution simultaneously. The scale space, a one-parameter family of blurred replicas of the input image, is based on the diffusion equation and was proposed by Witkin [13] and Koenderink [6] as the image representation for multiscale analysis. Most approaches to multiscale image segmentation involve connecting voxels in adjacent levels of the sampled scale space [1]. A linked set of image replicas has been called a *stack* [9] for 2D images, and a *hyperstack* [10, 2] for 3D images. (Hyper)stack segmentation has—up to now—focused on front-end vision, *i.e.*, automatic analysis of a scene without any prior knowledge. By using this multiscale approach the global image information can effectively be included. In [11] and [12] we have shown that the hyperstack performs well on noisy images and is particularly strong in its ability to segment both small and large objects simultaneously.

The basic idea of the hyperstack is to define relations (*linkages*) between voxels in all pairs of adjacent scale space levels, such that the levels at larger scales—containing the global information—guide the collection of voxels in the original image at the smallest scale (the *ground level*).

In section 2 we briefly discuss the hyperstack process. In section 3 we address the extension of the conventional linking and root labeling scheme to a more robust method. In section 4 we deal with probabilistic linking for proper segmentation of partial volume voxels. Finally, we will show some results in section 5.

2 The hyperstack process

The hyperstack segmentation method consists of four phases (see Fig. 1).

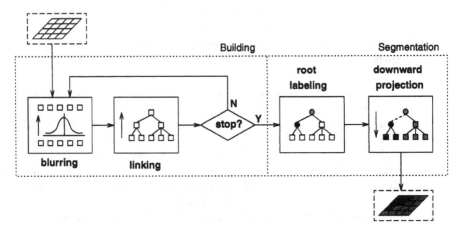

Fig. 1. *Schematic of the hyperstack image segmentation process.*

Blurring. The hyperstack starts by creating a scale space—which is a set of replicas of the original image—blurred by a Gaussian kernel of increasing width. The Gaussian kernel was proposed by Witkin [13] and Koenderink [6] since it is the only solution of the linear diffusion equation that creates no spurious detail in the blurring process (see also Florack *et al.* [5]). According to the property of scale invariance [3] the blurring strategy has to follow an exponential sampling in scale space. Hence, the linear scale parameter $\tau = n \cdot \delta\tau$, $n \in \mathbb{N}$, is related to the absolute scale σ_n at level n by $\sigma_n = \varepsilon \cdot \exp(n \cdot \delta\tau)$, where ε is taken to be the smallest linear grid measure of the imaging device.

Linking. During the linking phase voxels in two adjacent levels are connected by so-called *parent-child* linkages. Linking is a bottom-up process in the sense that we start linking the children of level 0 (the ground level) to parents in level 1, then find parents in level 2 for the children in level 1, and so on. Since only parent voxels that have been linked to before are considered children in the next linking step, convergence of the scale-tree is assured. The area in which a parent is selected for a specific child is defined by a radius $r = k \cdot \sigma$, where k is chosen such that only parents are considered whose intensity has been determined to a significant extent by the child at hand. Typically, $k = 1.5$.

In the conventional hyperstack the parent with the smallest intensity difference compared to the intensity of the child is chosen. Extensions to this basic scheme will be discussed in sections 3 and 4.

Root labeling. The roots—*i.e.*, voxels in the scale-tree that represent segments in the original image—are identified after all levels are connected through the linkages. The children with a large intensity difference with their parents are classified as roots. This is done either by setting a threshold on this difference, or by setting a prescribed number of roots.

To control the size of the resulting segments, a range of levels where roots may be created is defined by setting the *lowest root level* (the lower bound) and the *segmentation level* (the upper bound).

Downward projection. In the actual segmentation phase root values are projected downwards from every root to the connected voxels in the ground level. By using a unique value for each root it is guaranteed that the segments in the original image are distinguishable. This allows for quantitative validation of segmentation results. For visual inspection, the mean intensity of the pixels within each segment is a reasonable alternative.

3 Extended linking and root labeling

A more general framework for child-parent linking is provided by the concept of *linkage strength* or *affection*, which may be based on heuristic features—like intensity proximity, spatial proximity, ground volume [7, 11]—or differential-geometric features [4]. (The ground volume of a voxel is defined as the number of ground voxels with a route to that voxel.)

The affection (denoted by $\heartsuit$) is a weighted linear sum of N normalized components:

$$\heartsuit = \sum_{i=1}^{N} w_i \cdot C_i \ , \quad \text{with } C_i \in [0,1] \, , \text{ and } \sum_{i=1}^{N} w_i = 1 \, .$$

The candidate parent with the highest affection value is selected to become the child's parent.

Research to different statistical and heuristic components has shown that a general and robust linking scheme should use three components [8]: (i) the traditional intensity difference component $C_{\mathcal{I}}$, (ii) the ground volume criterion $C_{\mathcal{G}}$, and (iii) the mean ground volume intensity component $C_{\mathcal{M}}$. They are calculated as follows:

$$C_{\mathcal{I}} = 1 - \frac{|\mathcal{I}_P - \mathcal{I}_C|}{\Delta \mathcal{I}_{max}} \, , \quad C_{\mathcal{G}} = \frac{\mathcal{G}_P}{\mathcal{G}_{max}} \, , \text{ and } C_{\mathcal{M}} = 1 - \frac{|\mathcal{M}_P - \mathcal{M}_C|}{\Delta \mathcal{I}_{max}} \, ,$$

where $\mathcal{I}_P$ and $\mathcal{I}_C$ denote the intensity of the parent and the child, respectively, and $\Delta \mathcal{I}_{max}$ the maximum intensity difference in the original image; $\mathcal{G}_P$ is the ground volume of the parent and $\mathcal{G}_{max}$ the maximum ground volume at the parent's level; $\mathcal{M}_P$ and $\mathcal{M}_C$ are the mean ground volume intensity of the parent and the child, respectively.

For all three components it can be argued that a large value should be preferred for a child to link to that parent. For instance, if the mean ground volume intensity of the child closely resembles the corresponding field of the parent, then it is natural for the child to merge into that parent segment: they both represent (part of) a segment with that intensity value.

Obviously, the linkages formed heavily depend on the local image structure and the relative weights of the affection components. Experiments with different images showed that general, robust weight factors corresponding to the components $C_{\mathcal{I}}$, $C_{\mathcal{G}}$, and $C_{\mathcal{M}}$ typically take the (unnormalized) values of 1, 10^{-7}, and 1000, respectively.

As regards the root labeling, we investigated the applicability of an *adultness* term, similar to the affection formula approach. The two components that turned out to be robust root criteria were: (i) the mean ground volume intensity difference component $C_{\mathcal{I}}'$, and (ii) the ground volume intensity variance component $C_{\mathcal{V}}'$. They are defined as:

$$C_{\mathcal{I}}' = \frac{|\mathcal{M}_P - \mathcal{M}_C|}{\Delta \mathcal{I}_{max}} , \text{ and } C_{\mathcal{V}}' = \frac{\mathcal{V}_P}{\mathcal{V}_{max}} ,$$

with $\mathcal{V}_P$ the intensity variance in the ground volume of the parent, and $\mathcal{V}_{max}$ the maximum variance in the image.

For both components it is plausible that relative large values indicate a *catastrophe* in scale space [6]. At such an event, two different objects merge together. The relative (unnormalized) weight factors turned out to be typically 0.1 and 1, respectively.

4 Probabilistic linking

Despite the robustness of the linking scheme of the previous section, the problem of the partial volume artifact remains—in particular with images of a relative low resolution. Owing to the inherent undersampling of current imaging equipment—at least with respect to the resolution of the visual system—boundary voxels of the different objects and voxels representing relatively thin structures (like blood vessels) belong to more than one object type. These voxels need to be segmented at sub-voxel level in accordance with their partial volumes.

To this end, the hyperstack has been extended from single-parent to *multiparent* (or *probabilistic*) linking [11], where child voxels are allowed to link to more than one parent. The probability value assigned to each link is derived from the corresponding affection values of the multi-parent linkages by straight normalization. Hence, the sum of the probabilities of all parent linkages of one child equals 1.

As a result, there may be multiple roots for each ground voxel as well as multiple routes from a ground voxel to each root. The (root) probability that a ground voxel belongs to the segment defined by a root voxel is determined by multiplication and addition of the probability values between those two voxels. Each partial volume voxel is then assigned a list of probabilities, the entries of which denote the chances that the voxel is part of various candidate objects.

Conventional segmentations can easily be derived from such lists by either focusing on the largest probability of each list, or by focusing on one particular root (that defines one object). In the latter case, for every ground voxel the corresponding root probability (which will be zero for voxels totally outside the object) is represented by an intensity value.

5 Results

In Fig. 2, a histological image of size 256^2, we focused on a simultaneous segmentation of the blood vessel wall (a clustering of several small segments) and of the thrombus in the middle (consisting of a few large segments). The extended root labeling scheme, where the roots are distributed over a relative large range of levels makes this kind of multi-tasking segmentation possible.

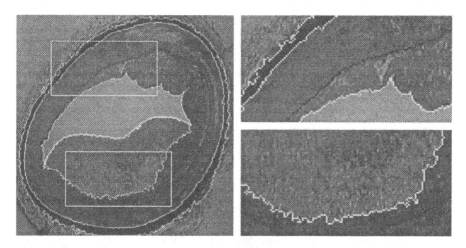

Fig. 2. *Single-parent segmentation of the thrombus and the vessel wall of a histological image. Segment contours have been superimposed in bright white. Enlargements on the right.*

In Fig. 3 we have shown a two-dimensional multi-parent segmentation of a small part of a 2D MR brain image, based on the highest object probability of each list (denoting the probability that each pixel belongs to the cerebellum). Probabilistic linking clearly outperforms its single-parent counterpart in which a voxel can only be part of one object.

In Fig. 4 the surplus value of probabilistic over single-parent segmentations is shown for the ventricle system. The original image is an MR image of the brain containing 32 slices of 128^2 and a grey-level resolution of 12 bits. The single-parent segmentation has several serious shortcomings.

In Fig. 5 a high-resolution 3D MR image has been rendered [14], based on a single-parent segmentation. Because the resolution is significantly higher (128 slices of 256^2) than the ventricle image, we did not compare the result to multi-parent linking. We segmented the image into three segments: brain, skull/skin, and background. The brain has been extracted and separated from the other parts by a simple pixel-connect operation.

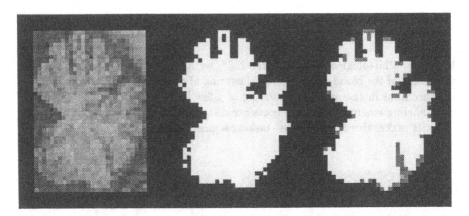

Fig. 3. *Segmentation of the cerebellum of an MR brain image. Original image (left), single-parent segmentation (middle) and a probabilistic result (right).*

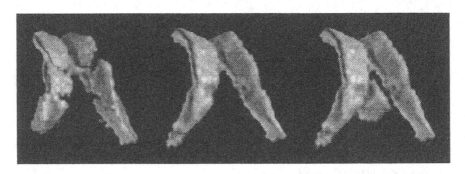

Fig. 4. *Renderings of a single-parent (left) and a multi-parent (middle) segmentation of the ventricle system in a 3D MR image of the brain. Adding objects is very simple (right).*

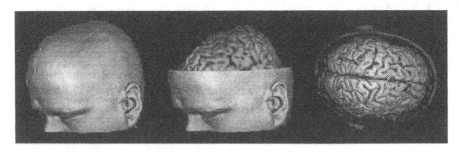

Fig. 5. *Renderings of a high-resolution 3D MR data set, based on single-parent linking.*

Acknowledgements

This work was supported by the Japanese Real World Computing Program through the project Active Perception and Cognition, by the Netherlands Ministries of Economic Affairs and Education & Science through a SPIN grant, by the industrial companies Philips Medical Systems, KEMA and Shell Research, and by the Netherlands Computer Science Research Foundation (SION) with financial support from the Netherlands Organization for Scientific Research (NWO).

References

1. P. J. Burt, T. H. Hong, and A. Rosenfeld. Segmentation and estimation of image region properties through cooperative hierarchical computation. *IEEE Transactions on Systems, Man, and Cybernetics*, 11(12):802–809, 1981.
2. C. N. de Graaf, K. L. Vincken, M. A. Viergever, F. J. R. Appelman, and O Ying Lie. A hyperstack for the segmentation of 3D images. In D. Ortendahl and J. Llacer, editors, *IPMI, Proc. of the 11th conference*, pages 399–413. Wiley-Liss, New York, NY, 1991.
3. L. M. J. Florack, B. M. Ter Haar Romeny, J. J. Koenderink, and M. A. Viergever. Scale-space and the differential structure of images. *Image and Vision Computing*, 10:376–388, 1992.
4. L. M. J. Florack, B. M. Ter Haar Romeny, J. J. Koenderink, and M. A. Viergever. Cartesian differential invariants in scale-space. *Journal of Mathematical Imaging and Vision*, 3(4):327–348, 1993.
5. L. M. J. Florack, B. M. Ter Haar Romeny, J. J. Koenderink, and M. A. Viergever. Linear scale-space. *Journal of Mathematical Imaging and Vision*, 4(4), 1994.
6. J. J. Koenderink. The structure of images. *Biol. Cybernetics*, 50:363–370, 1984.
7. A. S. E. Koster. A linking strategy for multi-scale image segmentation. Report 3DCV 90-05, Utrecht University, 1990.
8. A. S. E. Koster, K. L. Vincken, C. N. de Graaf, O. C. Zander, and M. A. Viergever. Heuristic linking models in multi-scale image segmentation. Submitted for publication.
9. S. M. Pizer, J. J. Koenderink, L. M. Lifshitz, L. Helmink, and A. D. J. Kaasjager. An image description for object definition, based on extremal regions in the stack. In S. L. Bacharach, editor, *IPMI, Proc. of the 9th conference*, pages 24–37. Martinus Nijhoff, Dordrecht/Boston MA, 1986.
10. K. L. Vincken. The hyperstack, a multiresolution technique for the segmentation of 3D images. Report 3DCV 89-04, Delft Univ. of Technology, 1989.
11. K. L. Vincken, A. S. E. Koster, and M. A. Viergever. Probabilistic multiscale image segmentation – set-up and first results. In R. A. Robb, editor, *Visualization in Biomedical Computing 1992*, pages 63–77. Proceedings SPIE 1808, 1992.
12. K. L. Vincken, A. S. E. Koster, and M. A. Viergever. Probabilistic segmentation of partial volume voxels. *Pattern Recognition Letters*, 15(5):477–484, 1994.
13. A. P. Witkin. Scale space filtering. In *Proc. International Joint Conference on Artificial Intelligence*, pages 1019–1023. Karlsruhe, W. Germany, 1983.
14. K. J. Zuiderveld and M. A. Viergever. Multi-modal volume visualization using object-oriented methods. In *1994 Symposium on Volume Visualization*, pages 59–66. ACM SIGGRAPH, 1994.

Multiscale Representation and Analysis of Features from Medical Images

Márta Fidrich, Jean-Philippe Thirion

INRIA, B.P. 93, 2004 route des Lucioles
06902 Sophia-Antipolis FRANCE
Tel: (33) 93 65 76 62

Abstract. We address here the problem of multiscale extraction and representation of characteristic points based on iso-surface techniques. Our main concern is with $2D$ images: we analyze corner points at increasing scales using the Marching Lines algorithm. Since we can exploit the intrinsic nature of intensity of medical images, segmentation of components or parameterization of curves is not needed, in contrast with other methods. Due to the direct use of the coordinates of points, we get a representation of orbits, which is very convenient both for detection at coarse scale and for localization at fine scale. We find that the significance of corner points depends not only on their scale-space lifetime but also on their relationship with curvature inflexion points.

keywords: Scale space, Differential geometry, Singularity theory

1 Introduction

Beginning with Witkin's pioneering paper [18], there have seen many interesting works on *scale space* over the past decade. Research emphasizes several topics: how to construct the best discretized multiscale representation [2, 7, 8, 3, 14, 13]; how the individual features behave [19, 20, 9, 5, 6]; and how to apply this knowledge to various problems, e.g. matching and recognition [1, 11, 12, 5].

If we restrict ourselves to medical image processing, we can exploit the intrinsic nature of intensity using *iso-surface techniques* [10, 16, 17], and we can consider curvature-based features meaningful, such as $2D$ *corner points* and $3D$ *crest lines* [16]. Features which can be defined as zero-crossings of (possibly nonlinear) differential expressions are called *differential singularities*. The singularity set of a differential operator changes with the scale parameter: the orbits of singularity points in the scale-extended space may undergo bifurcations: splitting or merging at catastrophe points. Critical points, a subset of differential singularities, are defined by the zero-crossings of the gradient. They are classified by their Hessian and are called nongeneric if their Hessian matrix is singular; intuitively this means that they are unstable since small perturbations change their nature. Theoretical results about the behavior of singularities have been obtained only in simple cases. Typically, the evolution of 2-3 isolated critical points have been analyzed [5, 9, 6] in generality. Alternatively, a more general singularity, let us say a corner point, has been examined, but only in the case of simple (parameterized) contour models [1, 11, 12]. In practice, the set of configurations can be huge, so instead of depicting all the influences together, we need to exemplify the orbits of some features in scale space, and to do so is the goal of this paper. In the next section we show a natural way to visualize multiscale properties, while in Sect. 3 we analyze the behavior of curvature inflexions and corner points in scale space.

2   Visualization

We have implemented an algorithm that convolves the initial image with the desired combinations of derivatives of a Gaussian kernel as the variance σ logarithmically increases $(\sigma_i = \varepsilon \cdot \tau^i)$. Parameters specify the derivatives to be used and the three smoothing factors: the initial variance (ε), the number of samples at the resolution axis (n) and the ratio of the largest kernel size (corresponding to σ_n) and of the initial image size [4]. We use the ε-smoothed image as the ground level of the *multiresolution extension* image (blurred by the Gaussian itself), thus each of its levels corresponds to a level of the *scaled differential descriptors* image (smoothed by the derivatives of the Gaussian).

We create the $(n+1)D$ multiresolution extension of the nD original image and also the $(n+1)D$ image of a chosen nD differential descriptor at increasing scales. The $(n+1)D$ hyper-iso-surface of the multiresolution extension image can show the development of the nD iso-surface as resolution varies, while the $(n+1)D$ zero-crossings of the scaled differential descriptor image can demonstrate how the number and location of singularities change. Moreover, the intersection of the two hyper-iso-surfaces (one of intensities, the other of zero-crossings) illustrates the orbits of features. This is particularly impressive starting from a planar image. In the sequel, we restrict ourselves to $2D$ images.

The multiresolution extension is a family of gradually blurred images, where annihilation of small structures is not necessarily visible, in contrast for example, to the development of an iso-intensity-contour. The iso-contours become more and more "regular", that is sharp curvatures are attenuated leading to a bowl-like convex shape (see Fig. 1). Note that the sequence of iso-contours extracted independently from the members of a family of blurred images is equivalent to the hyper-iso-contour (i.e. an iso-surface) obtained from the multiresolution extension; assuming, that the same intensity constant I is used. We use this fact: instead of extracting the sequence of iso-contours individually, we extract directly the corresponding iso-surface.

We have already used the intuitive notion of iso-contours $(2D)$ and also of iso-surface $(3D)$, but to define them precisely, the following arbitrary choice (or its opposite) must be made, as pointed out in [16]: *The iso-surface is the interface between the regions of the image f: $f \geq I$ (the inside) and $f < I$ (the outside), where I is a constant.* To extract iso-surfaces and also their intersections (e.g. iso-contours), they implemented a smart algorithm, called "Marching Lines", which insures both sub-voxel accuracy and nice topological properties

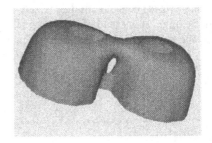

Fig. 1. Original image *(left)* and its multiscale iso-contour *(right)*. The coordinates of points are marked in the (x, y) plane, while resolution is measured logarithmically via the z axis. The delocalization effect can be immediately investigated due to the natural (e.g. not parameterized) coordinate system. We also observe that the connectivity of the iso-contour is not preserved: in the course of blurring, it splits into two, then merges and then splits again.

like connectivity, closeness and no self-intersection. All the pictures of this paper, showing iso-surfaces, are obtained using the Marching Lines algorithm [16].

Now let us examine invariants that are useful to process medical images [15, 16]. Here we specify corner points as the local extrema of the curvature on a $2D$ iso-contour, while ridge lines are their extension to $3D$, corresponding to the successive loci of the iso-surface whose principal curvature is locally extremal.

Definition 1 *Corner points satisfy the extremality criterion $e(x, y) = \nabla c(x, y) \cdot \mathbf{t} = 0$, where $\mathbf{t} = (-f_y, f_x)$ is the iso-line tangent and $\nabla c(x, y) = (c_x, c_y)$ is the gradient of the curvature $c(x, y) = \frac{2 f_x f_y f_{xy} - f_x^2 f_{yy} - f_y^2 f_{xx}}{(f_x^2 + f_y^2)^{3/2}}$. We call the implicit curve $e(x, y) = 0$ the curvature curve, whose intersection with the iso-line $f(x, y) = I$ are the points of extremal curvatures.*

In the same way as iso-intensity-contours extend naturally into hyper-iso-contours in scale space, so do the singularities of the primal image (such as curvature curves). This means that singularities at different scales can be observed with the help of the zero-intensity-surface extracted from the image of scaled differential descriptors.

To be more informative, we can display the sign of the scaled differentials [4], just like curvature extremality, on the iso-intensity-surface; see Fig. 2 *(left)*. Since corner points (ridge lines) are defined as the intersection of two iso-contours (surfaces), their orbits can be explicitly obtained in scale space by intersecting two (hyper-)iso-contours: one of the intensities, other of the zero-crossings. By following the orbits in scale space we can examine how bifurcations occur, that is, how a simple feature can turn into several features when the resolution is increased; see Fig. 3. One important thing to notice is that the orbits of corner points *do not* correspond to the ridge lines of the (hyper-)iso-contour, because the scale is not equivalent to the other dimensions; see Fig. 2 *(right)*.

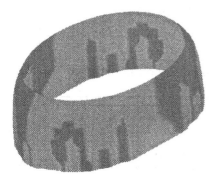 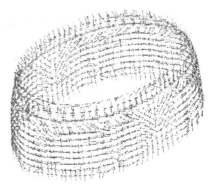

Fig. 2. *left:* The scaled iso-contours of an ellipse are colored due to the sign of curvature extremality (definitely positive, definitely negative and approximately zero). There are two symmetrical zones corresponding to the smaller axis where the curvature is almost zero; here features are very unstable, their spatial positions and even their existences are not well defined. *right:* The principal direction fields of the same image show that the orbits of corner points do not correspond to ridge lines. Since the two principal directions of the surface (i.e. multi-scale iso-contour) generally do not correspond to the tangent of the iso-contours and to the (vertical) resolution axis.

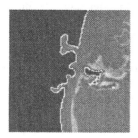 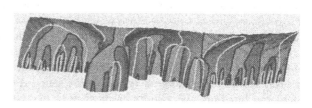

Fig. 3. *left:* CT scan cross section of the ear with the selected iso-contour *right:* The orbits of inflexion (white) and of corner points (black) are marked on the multi-scale contour which is colored according to the sign of the curvature extremality.

3 Analysis of corner points in scale space

First, let us examine various types of characteristic curvature points: corner points (curvature extrema) and inflexion points (zero-crossings of curvature) with the help of Fig. 4 *(top, left)*.

Critical points have already been studied in scale space [19, 9, 5, 6]: their orbits are either lines from small to large scale or bowl-like shapes corresponding to a maximum point (**M**) and a minimum point (**m**) that merge at some catastrophe point. The orbits of corner (resp. inflexion) points have analogous

points	A	B	C	D	E	F	G
curvature	+	+	+ → -	-	-	-	- → +
extremality criterion	- → +	+ → -	- → -	- → +	+ → -	- → +	+ → +
type (value)	m+	M+	infl.	m-	M-	m-	infl.
significance (abs. value)	m	M	m	M	m	M	m

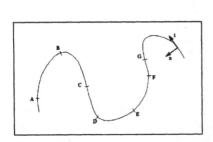 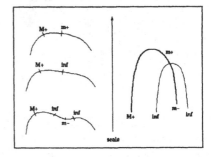

Fig. 4. *top, left:* Description of some characteristic curvature points (m: min., M: max.; +: pos., -: neg.). *right:* The sign of minimum changes due to an inflexion point

structures (see Fig. 3), though closed curves may occur since these points are the extrema of a non-linear expression. The structure of orbits depends only on the transition of the extremality criterion (resp. curvature), which has the consequence that the significant and practically more stable absolute maxima (M+ and m-) form such a sub-structure which makes their orbits difficult to follow. Indeed, because of the influence of a neighboring inflexion point, the sign of a curvature extremum may change as M+ → M- and m- → m+, respectively; see Fig. 4 *(right)*. We call the intersection point of an extremum and an inflexion orbit *second order nongeneric singularity*, since at that point a second order differential function, and also its gradient, a third order differential function, is zero.

We have found that an orbit which is relatively extended along the scale axis, but also has a small "base", indicates the presence of a highly curved feature of limited extent, i.e. a visually significant feature. Also, we can perceive that at some almost-straight contour-parts second order nongeneric singularities occur either at relatively fine scales or at large scales but with great "extent". These observations suggest that stability of corner points should be measured as the ratio of life-time delimited by second order nongeneric singularities and of base in scale space. The usefulness of this measure can be depicted in Fig. 5.

Definition 2 *The effective life-time T_e of a corner point is defined to be:*
- *the scale of intersection, if its orbit is intersected by an inflexion orbit;*
- *the scale of merging, else if its orbit merges with another corner orbit (whereon both annihilates);*
- *else, the largest scale of observation.*

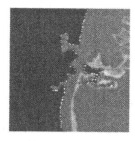 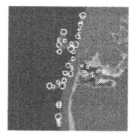 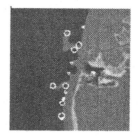

Fig. 5. *left:* All the corner points extracted at $\sigma = 1$. The most significant points measured by scale-space life-time *(middle)* and by the proposed method *(right)*.

Definition 3 *The base B of a corner point is defined to be:*
- *the Euclidean distance between the two branches of the inflexion parabola at the finest scale, if its orbit is intersected by an inflexion orbit;*
- *the Euclidean distance between the two branches of the obtained parabola at the finest scale, else if its orbit merges with another corner orbit (whereon both annihilates);*
- *else, one.*

4 Conclusion

We have presented a natural way to extract and represent multiscale singularity orbits based on iso-surface techniques. We have shown using planar images that the representation is very convenient for observing both bifurcation and delocalization effects. It is also applicable to observe boundary evolution in scale space, assuming that the boundary can be defined as an iso-surface, for example the zero-crossings of the Laplacian. In particular, we have analyzed the behavior of corner and of inflexion points in scale space. Based on our experiments we have proposed a stability measure for corner points in terms of scale-space life-time and base. We believe that this method can help further understanding of the multiresolution properties of differential singularities.

Currently, the marching lines algorithm, which can extract iso-surfaces and their intersections (iso-lines), is implemented in $3D$, so it applies to the multiscale analysis of $2D$ images. In the future we intend to extend this algorithm to higher dimensions, to be able to investigate the multiresolution behavior of features of real $3D$ images.

Acknowledgment
We wish to thank Mike Brady and the members of the Epidaure research team for stimulating discussions about scale space. Part of this study has been supported by the Esprit Basic Research Action VIVA and the French-Hungarian

Cooperation Program BALATON. Thanks also to Digital Equipment who provided us with fast computers.

References

1. Haruo Asada and Michael Brady. The curvature primal sketch. *IEEE PAMI*, 8, 1986.
2. Jean Babaud, Andrew P. Witkin, Michael Baudin, and Richard O. Duda. Uniqueness of the gaussian kernel for scale space filtering. *IEEE PAMI*, 8, Jan 1986.
3. Rachid Deriche. Recursively implementing the gaussian and its derivatives. Technical report, INRIA, 1993.
4. Márta Fidrich and Jean-Philippe Thirion. Multiscale extraction and representation of features from medical images. *Rapport de Recherche INRIA*, (2365), Oct 1994.
5. John M. Gauch and Stephen M. Pizer. Multiresolution analysis of ridges and valleys in grey-scale images. *IEEE PAMI*, 15, 1993.
6. Peter Johansen. On the classification of toppoints in scale space. *Journal of Mathematical Imaging and Vision*, 4:57–67, 1994.
7. Jan J. Koenderink. The structure of images. *Biological Cybernetics*, 50:363–370, 1984.
8. Tony Lindeberg. Scale-space for discrete signals. *IEEE PAMI*, 12, March 1990.
9. Tony Lindeberg. Scale-space behaviour of local extrema and blobs. *Journal of Mathematical Imaging and Vision*, 1:65–99, March 1992.
10. William E. Lorensen and Harvey E. Cline. Marching cubes: A high resolution 3d surface reconstruction algorithm. *Computer Graphics*, 21(4), July 1987.
11. Farzin Mokhtarian and Mackworth Alain K. Scale-based description and recognition of planar curves and two-dimensional shapes. *IEEE PAMI*, 8, Jan 1986.
12. Farzin Mokhtarian and Mackworth Alain K. A theory of multiscale, curvature-based representation for planar curves. *IEEE PAMI*, 14, Aug 1992.
13. Bart M. ter Haar Romeny and Luc M. J. Florack. A multiscale geometric model of human vision. In *Perception of Visual Information*, volume 511, chapter 4, pages 73–114. Springer-Verlag, 1993.
14. Bart M. ter Haar Romeny, Luc M. J. Florack, Jan J. Koenderink, and Max A. Viergever. Scale space: Its natural operators and differential invariants. In *LNCS*, volume 511, pages 239–255. Springer-Verlag, July 1991.
15. Jean-Philippe Thirion. The extremal mesh and the understanding of 3d surfaces. In *IEEE Workshop on Biomedical Imaging*, number 2149, Seattle, June 1994.
16. Jean-Philippe Thirion and Alexis Gourdon. The 3d marching lines algorithm : new results and proofs. *Rapport de Recherche INRIA*, (1881), March 1993.
17. Jayaram K. Udupa. Multidimensional digital boundaries. *CVGIP: Graphical Models and Image Processing*, 56, July 1994.
18. Andrew P. Witkin. Scale space filtering. In *Proc. Int. Conf. Artificial Intelligence*, volume 511, 1993. Karlsruhe.
19. Alan L. Yuille and Tomaso A. Poggio. Fingerprint theorems for zero crossings. *Journal Opt. Soc. Amer.*, pages 683–692, 1985.
20. Alan L. Yuille and Tomaso A. Poggio. Scaling theorems for zero crossings. *IEEE PAMI*, 8, 1986.

A Representation for Mammographic Image Processing

Ralph Highnam, Michael Brady and Basil Shepstone

Departments of Engineering Science and Radiology, Oxford University, U.K.

Abstract. We propose that mammographic image processing should be performed on what we term the h_{int} representation. h_{int} is the thickness of non-fat or "interesting" tissue between each pixel and the x-ray source. This representation allows simulation of any projective x-ray examination and we show simulations of the appearances of anatomical structures within the breast. We follow this with a comparison between the h_{int} representation and conventional representations from the point of view of invariance to imaging conditions and surrounding tissue. Initial results suggest that image analysis will be more robust when specific consideration is taken of the imaging process and the h_{int} representation is used.

1 Introduction

An imaging process creates an image that contains information about certain characteristics of the objects in the scene. Inevitably, the information is confounded by changes in the imaging conditions and scene background and it becomes difficult to judge simply by looking at the image whether the objects have changed or whether the imaging conditions or background has changed. In mammography, we are interested in the former not the latter. In order to overcome this problem for image analysis it is necessary to normalise the image and/or the feature measurements. In this paper we show how mammographic images can be normalised in the form of a representation that makes explicit quantitative measurements of the breast itself and we argue that this is the correct representation to use for mammographic image processing.

The paper starts with the reasoning behind, and a description of, the h_{int} representation - which is a quantitative representation of the breast tissue. The next section demonstrates the power of the h_{int} representation: it allows us to simulate any projective x-ray examination and to simulate the appearance of anatomical structures within the breast. We follow this with a comparison between the h_{int} representation and the conventional representation from the point of view of invariance to imaging conditions and surrounding tissue.

2 The h_{int} representation and its computation

The x-ray attenuation coefficients of many breast tissues (eg. fibrous, glandular, cancerous) are so similar that we can categorize them into three types: "interesting tissue" (ie. non-fat), fat and calcium. For our current purposes we ignore calcium and use as our breast measure the thickness of "interesting" tissue between each pixel and the x-ray source. These thicknesses constitute what we term the h_{int} representation. They are the most fundamental measure that can be obtained from a mammogram due to the projective nature of the imaging process, and similarity of the x-ray attenuation coefficients of the varying tissues.

The key to determining h_{int} is to have full calibration data for the imaging process [1]. Except for the breast thickness, all the calibration data is readily available. To determine h_{int} a practical attenuation measure $\overline{h\mu_P}$ is matched with the theoretical, $\overline{h\mu_T}$, by varying h_{int}, where:

$$\overline{h\mu_P} = \ln\left(\frac{X_c}{X_{ref}E_p^{rel}}\right),$$

where X_{ref} is part of the calibration data, X_c is the time of exposure multiplied by the tube current (mAs), and E_p^{rel} is the primary energy component imparted to the screen relative to the energy imparted in a reference situation (namely when an exposure is taken at X_{ref} mAs with no breast present). The primary component is determined from the total energy imparted by estimating the scatter component, and this process is explained fully in [2].

$$\overline{h\mu_T} = \ln\frac{\int_0^{28} N_0^{rel}(E)\ E\ S(E)\ G(E)\ e^{-\mu_{luc}(E)h_{plate}}\ dE}{\int_0^{28} N_0^{rel}(E)ES(E)G(E)e^{-\mu_{luc}(E)h_{plate}}e^{-h_{int}\mu_{int}(E)-(H-h_{int})\mu_{fat}(E)}dE}$$

where $S(E)$ is the absorption ratio of the screen to primary photons of energy E; $G(E)$ is the transmission ratio of the grid for primary photons of energy E; $N_0^{rel}(E)$ is the number of incident photons at energy E; $\mu_{luc}(E)$ is the linear attenuation coefficient of lucite at energy E and h_{plate} is the thickness of the lucite compression plate.

There are two ways of getting an intial estimate of breast thickness from the calibration data and image. The first way is to use the fact that near the chest wall there is low scatter and the breast tends to be fatty so one can assume $h_{int} = 0$ and $E_s = 0$. The second way is to assume that near the breast edge we have pure fat and a high scatter-to-primary ratio. Bounds on H can also be attained. The lower bound on H is related to the minimum attenuation apparent within the breast image. To achieve such low attenuation requires a certain minimum thickness of breast tissue. The minimum possible H occurs if the breast tissue is entirely interesting tissue (i.e. highly attenuating). An upper bound on H can be determined in exactly the same way except that we now look at the maximum attenuation and consider the breast to be nearly all fat. The estimate of H can be improved by studying the smoothness of the so-called "breast edge", which is where $h_{int} = 0$.

3 Power of the h_{int} representation

Any projective mammographic examination can be simulated from the h_{int} representation. This kind of simulation was the basis for previous work on model-based (or physics-based) image enhancement [1]. Here, we show the results of simulating how different anatomical structures, namely masses, would appear in a mammographic image. Simulation allows comparison between predicted and

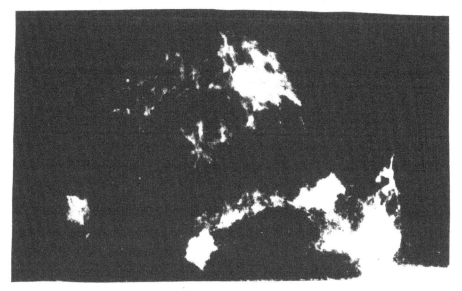

Fig. 1. This fatty breast has had two spherical masses implanted into it, along with two irregular shaped masses. The spherical masses represent simple models of cysts with low interesting tissue to fat proportions. The circular shape in the top right of the image, near the nipple, is a genuine cyst.

actual appearance so that anatomical models can be created and this aids a principled approach for automated detection [3].

To simulate a mass we need to know not only the spatial dimensions of the mass, but also the thicknesses of the relevant tissues at each pixel. The thicknesses can be estimated using a model of the 3D shape of the mass, the spatial dimensions, and the proportion of interesting tissue to fat within the mass (the density). We make several assumptions including that masses develop separately from the breast tissue and do not displace interesting tissue, only fat. Figure (1) shows the result from a simulation of cysts (as spheres) and malignant masses (with the spatial shape taken from a real case). The underlying three-dimensional shapes are assumed to be spherical. This is implemented using binary morphological erosion to define layers within the mass, and then interpolation to find the thickness of the mass at each layer.

4 Invariance to imaging conditions

In this section we consider representations and variance in the imaging conditions. Firstly, we shall demonstrate how conventional image processing is susceptible to changes in the imaging conditions and surrounding tissue. Then we investigate how errors in H propagate into h_{int}. Finally, we use this knowledge to propose appropriate feature measurements on the h_{int} representation that are robust.

4.1   Conventional image processing

To illustrate the susceptibility of conventional features to changes in the imaging conditions consider "contrast" in a image (D) with pixel values linear to film density. One definition of contrast is $C = (D_{max} - D_{min})/(D_{max} + D_{min})$. Figure (2) shows the relative distribution of contrast measures for some normal fibro-glandular tissue when the film gradient changes from 2.0 to 3.0.

Conventional features are also susceptible to changes in surrounding tissue (the background) and this varies from breast-to-breast and with different breast compression. Figure (2) shows the contrast measure on similar tissue in images where the breast was firmly compressed and not so firmly compressed.

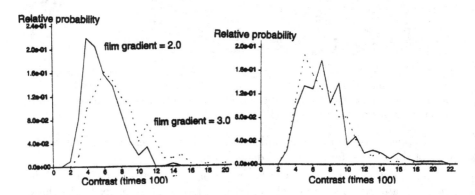

Fig. 2. These show relative distribution of contrast values using a simple contrast measure, 100 samples, and a film density image of a volume of fibro-glandular tissue within the breast. On the left are curves for different film-screen characteristic curves, on the right are curves for different breast compressions.

4.2   Measurement error in H

An error in the estimate of breast thickness results in an error in the estimation of the scatter component and an error in the analysis of the attenuation measure. It can be shown that the error in h_{int} due to an error in the scatter component is small compared to the effect of error in H in the analysis of the attenuation measure. Considering the attenuation at only one energy gives the following equation for h_{int} (from the earlier equations) where ΔH is the error in H:

$$h_{int} = \frac{\overline{h\mu_P} - H\mu_{fat}(E)}{\mu_{int}(E) - \mu_{fat}(E)} - \frac{\Delta H \mu_{fat}(E)}{\mu_{int}(E) - \mu_{fat}(E)}$$

The value of $\frac{\mu_{fat}(E)}{\mu_{int}(E) - \mu_{fat}(E)}$ is always over 1.0 for the energy range that we are interested in. This equation suggests that h_{int} is linearly related with ΔH, and this can be shown in the polyenergetic case by considering specific values or by studying histograms of the h_{int} image. This relationship is of vital importance in choosing features.

4.3 h_{int} image and feature normalisation

Dealing with different breast thicknesses H

The first point to note about normalizing h_{int} images is that there has been little research that considers anatomical structure size relative to breast thickness. In the absence of evidence to the contrary and in the belief that most anatomical structures are from local processes, we assume that feature size is independent of breast thickness H. This means that we should not scale the h_{int} images to a standard breast size and then look for a standard size feature, rather we should take the h_{int} images and look for a standard size feature in them. Another problem with scaling on H is that it can lead to h_{int} values which have little or no relation to the projected spatial size of a feature and we consider this relationship to be of primary importance since it gives an indication of tissue density and this might be useful for diagnosis.

A model of compression is helpful to determine how to deal with different breast thicknesses and there are several plausible alternatives. For this paper, we consider compression to remove a constant value from both h_{int} and h_{fat} across the image. Effectively this assumes that interesting tissue and fat both compress, but that the interesting tissue does not move. With this model the effect on the h_{int} representation is equivalent to changes in the surrounding tissue, and that is the issue we now consider.

Dealing with different tissue surrounds

Breast features might have different tissue surrounds. For example, a mass could be on a fatty surround or a dense surround. In these circumstances features such as the contrast measure defined earlier are exceptionally poor: maximum - minimum remains constant, but maximum + minimum is vastly different.

A problem with the h_{int} representation is that the band of tissues that are classed as interesting is too broad. The breast has much fibrous tissue which helps to support it and which mostly can be ignored although it does give the breast its dense or fatty appearance. We consider large, relatively flat components of h_{int} to be surrounding tissue, and we seek to estimate this component to attain what we term: $h_{feature}(x, y) = h_{int}(x, y) - h_{surround}(x, y)$

Earlier we saw how errors in H lead to translations in the h_{int} values, so that the definition of $h_{feature}$ actually removes the error since it exists in both components. The correct way of estimating $h_{surround}$ depends upon the definition of surrounding tissue that is being used and this in turn depends upon the type of feature required, that is, we have to build in some notion of scale.

Appropriate Features

For this paper we deal with features pertinent to detecting masses, in particular cyst, from fatty tissue. The three example images are meant to be illustrative of our approach; proof of superiority has to be statistical and that is beyond the scope of this paper. The examples we use are at different compressions (FDLC1 and FDLC2) and from an image (also with a cyst) digitized on a different scanner (GCRC1). In all cases the surrounding tissue was relatively fatty.

Cysts often present as being denser than fatty tissue so that the x-ray attenuation and consequently the image brightness is higher. Figure (3) shows the distribution of average pixel value in small windows (1.5mm by 1.5mm) in the film density and $h_{feature}$ images for the cyst and fatty tissue. Clearly, the average pixel values in the film density images for the fatty tissues are not sufficiently clustered to differentiate purely by thresholding. For the $h_{feature}$ measures the value of $h_{surround}$ was taken to be the minimum in the large window over which measurements are performed. In practice one would seek to ensure that the large window covers the feature of interest. The fat values and the cyst values are far better clustered, in particular the fatty tissue and the cysts in the breast at different compressions are giving almost identical responses, which we would expect given the compression model.

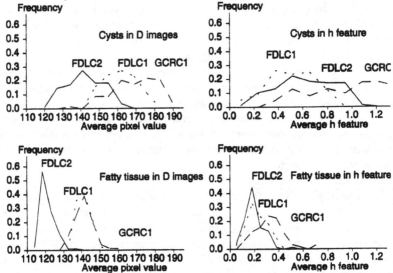

Fig. 3. Distributions of mean values in small windows from film density and $h_{feature}$ images of 3 breasts. Around 100 samples were taken for each example.

Fatty tissue, in particular, has low tissue roughness. There are many possible measures of roughness many of which are based upon the concept of visual contrast so that the feature gives high response for situations where we have a relatively high peak compared to the background. Although such measures might be appropriate for emulating a radiologist, we are more interested in a measure of the tissue roughness that measures the actual tissue property. For this paper we again use a simple measure, this time standard deviation. The simplicity of our features comes in part from the task we are considering but also from not needing to do any further normalisation. Figure (4) shows the standard deviation distribution from the three film density and $h_{feature}$ images for the cysts and surrounding fatty tissue. The distributions show that the average of the standard deviations is lower for the fatty tissue and that the distributions do overlap for the film density images. However, the distributions in the $h_{feature}$ images are closer than those in the film density images: especially in the case of the breasts at different compressions.

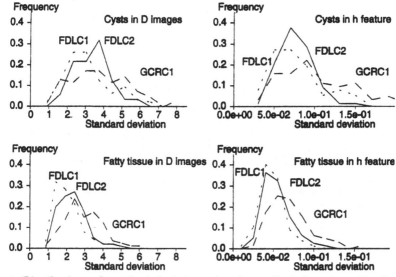

Fig. 4. Distributions of standard deviation values in small windows from film density and $h_{feature}$ images of 3 breasts. Around 100 samples were taken for each example.

5 Conclusions

The mammographic imaging process is prone to variations that make changes in the object hard to detect over changes in the imaging conditions and background. In this paper we have described, and shown how to compute, an image representation devoid of changes due to variations in the imaging conditions. The h_{int} representation has proven to be a powerful and flexible representation allowing simulation of any projective x-ray examination and modelling of anatomical structures such as cysts and malignant masses. Such modelling naturally leads to a principled approach for feature detection. Based upon the h_{int} representation, features were selected that appear to be invariant to changes in the surrounding tissue and degree of breast compression although statistical proof is required.

References

1. R. P. Highnam. *Model-based enhancement of mammographic images.* PhD thesis, Computing Laboratory, Oxford University, 1992.
2. R. P. Highnam, J. M. Brady, and B. J. Shepstone. Computing the scatter component of mammographic images. *IEEE Medical Imaging*, 13:301 – 313, June 1994.
3. N. J. Cerneaz. *Model-based analysis of mammograms.* PhD thesis, Engineering Science, Oxford University, 1994.

Finding Curvilinear Structures in Mammograms

Nick Cerneaz and Michael Brady

University of Oxford
Oxford OX1 3PJ, U.K.

Abstract. We develop a model-based algorithm for the extraction of curvilinear structures in x-ray mammograms, corresponding to milk ducts, blood vessels, fibrous tissue, and spiculations. The diagnostic basis for the problem is sketched. Results of applying the algorithm are shown. The results accord closely with the CLS structures observed by Radiologists, and the algorithm has supported further processing to identify potential lesions and to match left and right breast x-ray pairs. A new perspective is provided on the debate on the relevant merits of film density images versus transmitted light.

1 Introduction

Approximately one woman in twelve develops breast cancer, making it the second biggest cause of death for women (after heart disease) in the West. Early diagnosis greatly improves prognosis, so there are mass screening programs for older women in many countries, including the USA and UK. Currently, and for the foreseeable future, x-ray mammography is the only feasible imaging modality for mass screening: some three million mammograms are taken annually in the UK alone. There is, however, need for improvement in the process: 8–25% of cancers are missed, and 70–80% biopsies turn out to be benign. As is typically the case with medical imagery, there is huge inter- and intra-observer variability, not least because of the lack of quantitative measures. Computer processing of x-ray mammograms is a demanding task: the images have poor signal-to-noise ratio (largely because of scattered photon radiation [6]), are textured, there is only weak control of the imaging process, and abnormalities present as quite subtle, often non-local differences.

The need for image processing that can be trusted by radiologists is plain: one error in 10 000 images corresponds in the UK alone to 300 women per year. The uncritical application of conventional image processing operations can have serious consequences. For example, image smoothing may make lesions easier to locate; but it can remove calcifications and spiculations: as a result a malignancy may be overlooked. Similarly, edge sharpening may appear to reduce the blurred appearance of an image that results from scattered photons; but it can transform a malignant lesion into one that appears to a radiologist to be benign. Our approach has been to develop a model of the mammographic image process [5] and base image enhancement algorithms on that model [6]. This paper continues our model-based approach by first developing a model of curvilinear structures, corresponding to blood vessels, milk ducts, spiculations, and fibrous tissue, then developing an algorithm based on that model to extract the curvilinear structures. At this point, the reader may skip ahead to section 5 to see the only result of applying the algorithm that can be included in a paper of this length.

There are many mammographic signs that typically attract the attention of the diagnostic radiologist during the search for breast abnormality and disease. Two of the main x-ray mammographic signs of breast abnormality are calcifications and densities (indicators of masses, both circumscribed and spiculated). Other indicators such as bi-lateral asymmetry can present in a variety of forms; but almost always these cases can also be classed as being spatially diverse, or of low spatial-frequency.

In the case of calcifications, their shape and arrangement are important in assessing the degree of malignancy. Additionally it is useful to be able to distinguish both the inter-ductal and intra-ductal calcification arrangement, and to differentiate arterial and ductal calcifications. Consequently it would be very useful to have a description of the locations of the ducts and blood vessels in an image, allowing for a comparative analysis of calcifications present in an image.

When assessing a mammographic density, a radiologist routinely checks the border surrounding the density for spiculations or radial fibrous tissue anchored to the density. Spiculations surrounding a mammographic density/mass are a strong indicator of malignancy. Similarly the radial spiculations surrounding a radiolucent centre are possibly indicative of disease as they are the only signs of radial scar. In fact the detection of radial scar is a very difficult problem due to the subtle appearance of these abnormalities in an image. Mammographic densities (spiculated or circumscribed) appear as spatially low frequency patches of higher density. The search for these features is often complicated by the higher-frequency textural variations in image intensity/density due to the fibrous tissue, milk ducts and blood vessels which occur with much smaller spatial extent, but with high incidence (hence high-frequency). A description of these high-frequency features allows compensation for their presence, and thus reduces the complications they cause when searching for mammographic densities.

In both of these cases, it is necessary to construct a high-level description of the milk-ducts, blood vessels, mass spiculations and other higher-frequency fibrous tissues (collectively, for the reason given below, called *curvilinear structures: CLS*) present in an image, and this paper reports an implemented algorithm to produce such a description. As we noted above, the key novelty of the approach presented here is that the algorithm is based upon a model of the expected CLS cross-sectional profile that allows the calculation of the corresponding image pixel intensities. We demonstrate [1] that the predicted intensity profile closely matches those found in images, and we argue that this is a necessary contributing factor to the performance of the CLS detection algorithm. Subsequent use of the CLS structures, for finding masses, interpreting calcifications, and matching left-right breasts [1] depends crucially on the CLS image model.

The mammographic footprint of the vessels that are resolved shows them to be nominally 1-dimensional, with *slightly* increased image brightness compared with its surroundings. The situation is analogous for the case of fibrous tissue, which form part of the breast stroma. They are long, thin and strong, and support the functional material of the parenchymal tissue of the breast. The extra tissue density of the fibrous strands over that of the ducts and vessels attenuates the beam even further; hence they appear often on a film. The net result is that the fibrous tissues, milk ducts and blood vessels of the breast are mammographically detectable from the footprint that they leave on a film in the form of locally linear, nominally 1-dimensional features with lower film density (higher image intensity) than the surrounding tissue.

For the task of describing the milk-duct, blood-vessel and fibrous tissue networks in an image, their respective mammographic features are very similar on a local scale, and subtly different on a more global scale. However for many of the radiological applications to which it is required to apply the feature description, it is not necessary to be able to distinguish between them. Rather, simply being able to identify those areas of an image that are the milk-ducts, blood-vessels and fibrous tissues collectively suffices. The computer vision task to find the regions comprising the milk-ducts, blood-vessels and fibrous tissues can be defined as finding the regions with slightly increased intensity that are nominally 1-dimensional, and locally linear — but may diverge from strictly linear over larger scales, that is they may exist up to some maximum curvature in a continuous sense. For this reason, these features are commonly referred to by the collective term *curvilinear structures* (CLS).

Complicating the issue however is that although these features are generally of higher intensity than the surrounding 'background', the SNR is often very small. Additionally, the features can lie adjacent and closely parallel to each other, yet they are quite distinct and must be resolved individually. Ultimately, this means that the images *cannot* be smoothed prior to analysis. This pre-empts conventional noise suppression techniques which often employ a smoothing step under the assumption that the noise is white-gaussian. Consequently, alternative methods are necessary to suppress noise.

In its most naïve conception, the problem of finding the CLS features is that of ridge finding in digital images, a problem on which considerable effort has been expended (see Haralick and Shapiro [4] for a comprehensive account). We have implemented several published techniques, particularly those by Haralick, and by Sha'ashua & Ullman [1], and find that they perform poorly due to their inappropriate formulation within the context of the present task, re-emphasising the need for a model-based ridge finder such as we propose in this paper.

2 The CLS detector algorithm

The CLS extraction algorithm is presented in this section in its most generic form, stripped of the implementation details which can be found in [1]. Consider a binary image segmented into *foreground* and *background* regions. Without loss of generality, in order to preserve the topology of a feature in the discrete digital representation that is the image, we choose the system of 8-connectivity for the foreground and 4-connectivity for the background. In the description of the algorithm which follows, it is clear which pixels should be considered as foreground at any given time—they are members of the sets N, S, C, B and CLS (see below) when the particular set is under consideration (the background is implicitly defined as the complement of the respective set under consideration)—and accordingly these details are omitted to avoid unnecessary clutter.

Consider an original grey-level mammogram image I. The CLS algorithm for extraction of the curvilinear structures is:

1. Find the set N of all pixels n_i in the image I that are components of the CLS features. This is the key step and is spelt out in much more detail in the remaining sections of the paper.

2. Fill small bounded holes in set N by including the pixels of the holes in set N.

3. Thin the regions of set N, retaining in a new set S the pixels that comprise the simply-connected *skeletons* of N's regions. The algorithm [1] we use for this returns a simply-connected topologically equivalent skeleton lying at most a single pixel from the medial-axis of the region under consideration.

4. Break the skeleton into its segments by scanning the set S collecting into *cantons* c_i those 8-connected pixels that collectively share a common global heading/direction. At each branch (or junction) in the skeleton initiate another canton. Form the set C of all cantons c_i that result from classifying all $s_i \in S$.

5. Scan the set C, merging into *bones* b_i those cantons with both a (nearly) common endpoint and a sufficiently similar heading. Scan the bones b_i searching for merges involving a short intermediate canton joining two dissimilar cantons. Exclude the least convincing of the two merges, returning a junction at this location. At the completion of this phase, those cantons that are not merged with others to form bones are transcribed directly to the set B creating a new bone for each such canton.

6. Search the set B for the known irrelevant branches of the skeleton and reject them.

7. Search the set N in the region surrounding each bone $b_i \in B$, collecting the 8-connected neighbourhood pixels in the new set cls_i associated with b_i.

8. Declare the set CLS of all cls_i (with corresponding bones b_i) to be the curvilinear structures of the original image I.

The algorithm design has evolved through a mix of analysis and extensive experimentation. It is justified on the grounds that it succeeds at the task it was formulated to deal with, since the resulting CLS features accord well with what radiologists perceive, and they support subsequent processing such as the identification and description of potential masses and the matching of a left-right breast pair.

3 Modelling the expected CLS profile

Consider a section of homogeneous breast tissue of thickness H with an x-ray attenuation coefficient μ_1. The incident x-ray beam in a modern mammographic imaging device is poly-energetic. To accurately analyse the attenuation of this beam as it traverses the model tissue sample, it is necessary to integrate analysis over all beam energies. Our numerical simulation does precisely that. However, for simplicity, we assume a mono-energetic incident beam of energy E_o, such that $E_o = \phi X_c \mathcal{E}_p$ where $\mathcal{E}_p$ is the energy per x-ray photon (keV), X_c describes the x-ray tube current and exposure time (in millampere-seconds (mAs)) which effectively is a measure of the *number* of photons in an exposure, and ϕ is a constant of proportionality. The assumption of a mono-energetic beam equates to setting $\mathcal{E}_p$ to a constant value. Given the relative occurrence of photon energies in a typical incident beam we choose $\mathcal{E}_p = 17.4$keV, the value at which the peak occurs.

The energy of the x-ray beam emerging from the sample has two components, the *primary* energy E_p that has traversed a straight path through the material from the x-ray gun to the imaging device (and been absorbed along the way), and the *scattered* energy E_s which has been scattered within the sample. The absorption of the primary beam can be described by $E_p = E_o \exp(-\mu_1 H)$. For analysis, though not for numerical simulation, we assume no scatter. We suppose a CLS feature has an elliptical cross-section, of length b in the principal photon direction and width a, and introduce one into the cross-sectional model of the breast tissue. Suppose it is homogeneous, and that it is composed of a material with an x-ray attenuation coefficient of μ_2.

From the general equation of an ellipse with major and minor radii a and b respectively, and assuming a collimated x-ray beam we can derive the path length the beam traverses through the feature as:

$$h(x) = \frac{2b}{a}\sqrt{a^2 - x^2}, \quad -a \leq x \leq a, \tag{1}$$

and the net beam attenuation for the combined sample to be:

$$E(x) = \begin{cases} E_o e^{-\mu_1(H - h(x))} e^{-\mu_2 h(x)} & -a \leq x \leq a, \\ E_o e^{-\mu_1 H} & \text{otherwise.} \end{cases} \tag{2}$$

Once the beam has been attenuated during its travel through the breast (or in this case, the cross-sectional sample) there are a number of stages before the digitised image is available. Each of these processes must be considered so that the absolute pixel intensities of the image, and thus the image surface, can be estimated.

The film-screen apparatus can be modelled by considering a typical characteristic curve that relates energy imparted to the screen to film density. We can model this as

$$D = \gamma \log_{10}(\beta E). \tag{3}$$

where D is the film density, γ the film gradient, β is related to both the film speed, and within the mono-energetic assumption, the anti-scatter grid and intensifying screen response, and finally E is the x-ray energy imparted to the film-screen system.

To estimate the image intensities resulting from the digitisation of the film, we now consider the digitisation process itself. There are a number of different ways to digitise a film, however they generally can be classed as those that quantise the film density D, and those that quantise the light transmitted through the film T_l for a given back illumination I_l. These representations are related by the following equation

$$D = \log_{10}\left(\frac{I_l}{T_l}\right). \tag{4}$$

The direct digitisation of the film density (for example by a scanning microdensitometer) returns image pixel values $P_d(x, y)$ in an approximately linear relationship with D as

$$P_d(x, y) = mD(x, y) + q \tag{5}$$

whilst the digitisation of the transmitted light (for example using a CCD camera and a film back lit on a light-box) relates the image intensity $P_l(x, y)$ with T_l as

$$P_l(x, y) = \alpha T_l(x, y) + \lambda$$

where m, q, α and λ are digitisation calibration constants. Substituting equation (4) yields

$$P_l(x, y) = \alpha I_l 10^{-D(x,y)} + \lambda. \tag{6}$$

At this point, the analysis of the overall system diverges down the respective paths headed by the choice of image representation. Many people advocate the use of the film density as the domain of choice for analysing mammogram images since it can be equated directly to the raw data of the film. Although clinical practice is to view a mammogram mounted on a light-box, and thus observe the transmitted light T_l, it is believed the human visual system responds logarithmically to light intensities falling on the retina [3, p85]. In effect the human visual system implements the logarithmic transform of equation (4) and thus responds linearly to the film density D. Since the clinical domain of analysis for mammogram images has to date been the human visual interpretation of light-box mounted films, this is often advocated as the domain-of-choice for automated analysis systems. However, since it is possible to form digital images with intensities representing either film-density or transmitted-light (and to convert between them with relative ease by the application of equation (4)). Regarding the selection of which image representation should be used for this analysis, we note that the balance appears marginally to lie in favour of the transmitted-light representation. However, P_l'' is coupled to the imaging parameters $(\beta \phi X_c \mathcal{E}_p)$ whilst P_d'' is not. Due the difficulties this coupling to the imaging parameters can impose (due to the variability of those parameters) it is suggested that the film-density image representation be used when analysing image second-differences, for example when searching for CLS pixels as described in these sections.

Consider initially the direct digitisation of the film-density D given by equation (5). Substitution of equations (1), (2) and (3), and restriction of the domain to the region of interest, ie. $-a \leq x \leq a$, yields:

$$P_d(x) = \frac{m\gamma}{\ln 10} \left(\ln(\beta \phi X_c \mathcal{E}_p) - \mu_1 H - (\mu_2 - \mu_1)\frac{2b}{a}\sqrt{a^2 - x^2} \right) + q \qquad (7)$$

From Fleck's *Spectre* detector [2] it is clear [1] that there is useful information in the second-difference of an image for finding features such as the CLS features [1]. In the continuous sense this equates to the second derivative, or curvature of the image surface. Differentiating equation (7) gives

$$\frac{d^2 P_d}{dx^2} = \frac{2m\gamma}{\ln 10}(\mu_2 - \mu_1)ab(a^2 - x^2)^{-3/2}. \qquad (8)$$

In order to analyse the typical response from these equations, we insert typical values for the constants as given in figure 1. To obtain the best results possible we use the linear attenuation coefficients for various breast tissues reported by Johns and Yaffe [7]. We set the substrate of the model to an attenuation coefficient of 'fat' and the feature to that of 'fibrous' tissues as this reflects the actual composition of the CLS features and the 'background'. The digitisation constants m and q can be measured by solving the set of two simultaneous equations resulting from substitution of known (film-density, digitised-value) data pairs obtained from calibration data into equation (6). Typically, digitisation at 8-bit resolution utilising the linear region of the film-screen characteristic curve, gives two data points at $(0.6, 255)$ and $(3.0, 0)$, yielding $m = -106.25$ and $q = 191.25$. Obtaining a value of ϕ (actually $\beta \phi X_c \mathcal{E}_p$) is harder, since it really is just a scaling factor that accommodates the different imaging parameters. This scaling factor is necessary since it allows similar images to be recorded (ie. remain within the non-saturated regions of the film-screen recording system) for breasts of quite different compressed thickness and density/attenuation (ie. a thicker breast needs a longer exposure to give a similarly satisfactory image). It is set to a value compatible with that chosen during the numerical simulation which follows below, so that the respective intensity profiles have equivalent base-line levels for ease of comparison. Finally, evaluation of equations (7) and (8) for P_d and P_d'' yield curves from which it it is obvious that the image surface corresponding to a CLS feature has a strong second derivative in the continuous domain and this may be useful in detection of the CLS features.

4 From continuous to discrete

For numerical simulations, we use Highnam's [5] suite of implemented models, which analyse the mammogram imaging and digitisation processes, including the x-ray tube/beam characteristics, the anode-heel effect, beam-hardening, scattering, and finally digitisation. Initially this method was applied using a mono-energetic beam, non-scattered radiation and zero noise as specified during the development of the CLS modelling procedures of the previous sections. Thus

Constants	Value
Film density range	$0.6 \leq D \leq 3.0$
Image intensity range (8-bit)	$0 \leq P \leq 255$
Film gradient	$\gamma = 3$
Beam energy (keV)	$\mathcal{E}_p = 17.4$
Attenuation coefficients (cm^{-1})	$\mu_1 = 0.558$, $\mu_2 = 1.028$
Breast thickness (cm)	3.5
Size of feature (cm)	$a = 0.10$, $b = 0.02$

Fig. 1. Parameters for calculation of the CLS model surface equations.

the simulation returns the digital image surface that would be obtained if the sample of the predicted analytical curves were imaged and digitised, allowing a direct comparison between the discrete digital results obtained and the results of the continuous analysis of the previous section. Figure 2 shows the simulated intensity profile for a feature with major and minor radii of $1mm$ and $0.5mm$ respectively, imaging constants of figure 1, and at digitisation resolutions of $50\mu m$, $125\mu m$ and $250\mu m$ square per pixel. The specific digitisation resolutions shown were chosen since $50\mu m$ and $125\mu m$/pixel are commonly available with current digitisation techniques, and $250\mu m$/pixel is a size convenient for analysis of CLS features.

This digital image surface can be directly compared to the continuous surface. To facilitate this comparison, figure 2 includes the respective continuous curve (the dotted curve) for each case.

Figure 2 shows the (simulated) digital image surface resulting from digitisation of both film-density and transmitted-light representations. Note that although there is quite a difference between the continuous image surfaces (dotted lines) of the two representations, the digital surfaces do not reflect the difference in this instance, that is, the digital curves of the film-density representation are *exactly* the same as those of the transmitted-light representation. This inability to resolve the difference between the two digital representations is due mostly to the relatively large intensity quantum. Although the assumptions of the present model (in particular that of no noise) would accommodate a refinement of the intensity quantum (ie. digitise the image to greater depth, say 12-bits) to more faithfully represent the respective image domains in the digital case, in practice this is not possible as any attempt to digitise a film to greater depth simply measures the film-noise with greater accuracy, and therefore does not capture the image surface characteristics as desired. Despite this however, we do find that the second difference responses more closely resemble the continuous case (excepting the positive second difference response in the tails of the discrete case due to the spatial extent of the Δ_N'' kernel) as the pixel size is increased from $50\mu m$ through $125\mu m$ and finally to $250\mu m$/pixel.

380

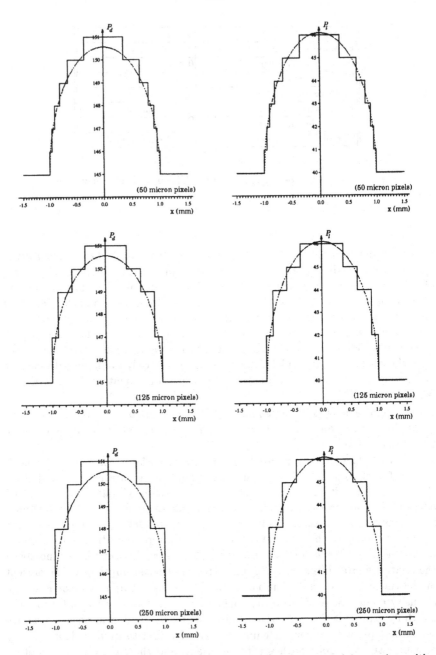

Fig. 2. Comparison between the analytical (continuous) expected image intensities (dotted lines) versus the simulated discrete approximation (solid lines) for an elliptical CLS feature with major and minor radii $1mm$ and $0.5mm$ respectively. The top row shows the simulation at a resolution of 20 pixels/mm ($50\mu m$ pixels), middle at 8 pixels/mm ($125\mu m$ pixels) and bottom at 4 pixels/mm ($250\mu m$ pixels).

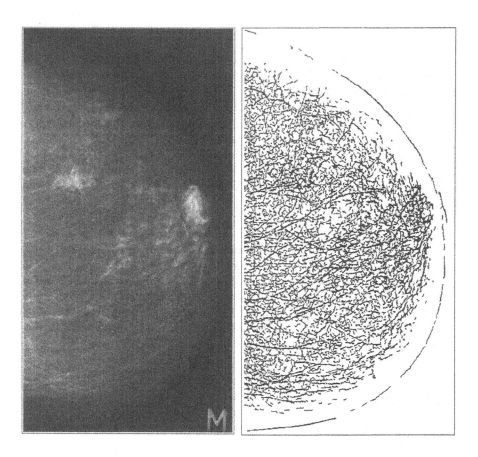

Fig. 3. A cranio-caudal image and the CLS pixels identified.

In conclusion, we find that for a given digitisation resolution and intensity quanta it is possible to tune the second difference kernel size to return second difference responses consistent with the continuous model developed in the previous sections. Therefore if the real CLS features in an image can be adequately represented by the model so developed, then the second difference, or curvature of the image surface can be used to locate the CLS features.

5 Results

An implementation of the algorithm described in section 2 has been developed based explicitly upon the characteristics of the CLS features as described by the model developed in section 3. In this section we report that the implementation has been applied to some 350 mammographic images, and without exception the algorithm has identified the CLS features as expected, from the most salient to the faintest of CLS features in each image.

A typical result of the algorithm is displayed in figures 3, which shows an original mammogram image and a corresponding image displaying the pixels identified as CLS pixels. Note that it is difficult to display the fact that the algorithm has extracted a *single* CLS feature for the longer curvilinear portions of the CLS pixel-trees and thus no attempt has been made to do so, although for completeness it should be noted that such an extraction has been achieved.

Note that as expected from the formulation of the model, the CLS detector algorithm is insensitive to the absolute grey-level in a local region, and is capable of extracting the CLS features at all local image intensities. As mentioned previously these results are typical of the results obtained from extensive application of the algorithm to many mammographic images, and importantly, the CLS feature description thus obtained has allowed a systematic, logical and model-based development of subsequent higher-level mammographic image processing and analysis tools.

References

1. NJ Cerneaz. Model-based analysis of mammograms. D.Phil thesis, Robotics Research Group, Oxford University, 1994.
2. MM Fleck. Spectre: an improved phantom edge finder. In *Proceedings of the 5th Alvey Vision Conference*, pages 127–132, University of Reading, UK, 25–28 September 1989.
3. RL Gregory. *Eye and Brain: the psychology of seeing*. World University Library. McGraw-Hill Book Company, New York, 1973.
4. RM Haralick and LG Shapiro. *Computer & Robot Vision*, volume 1. Addison-Wesley Publishing, Reading, Mass., 1992.
5. R Highnam. Model-based enhancement of mammographic images. D.Phil thesis, Programming Research Group, Oxford University, Trinity 1992.
6. RP Highnam, JM Brady, and BJ Shepstone. Computing the scatter component of mammographic images. *IEEE Transactions on Medical Imaging*, 13(2):301–313, 1994.
7. PC Johns and MJ Yaffe. X-ray characterisation of normal and neoplastic breast tissue. *Physics in Medicine and Biology*, 32:675–695, 1987.

Reconstruction / Vessels

On Reconstructing Curved Object Boundaries from Sparse Sets of X-Ray Images

Steve Sullivan[1], Alison Noble[2], and Jean Ponce[1]

[1] Beckman Institute, University of Illinois, Urbana, IL 61801, USA
[2] GE Corporate Research & Development, Schenectady, NY 12301, USA

Abstract. We propose a hybrid method using both geometric and intensity information to reconstruct multiple curved object boundaries from sparse sets of X-ray images. We have implementated this approach and present several examples on real and synthetic data.

1 Introduction

We propose a hybrid method using both geometric and intensity information to reconstruct multiple curved object boundaries from sparse sets of X-ray (digital radiographic) images. Working in the plane, we reconstruct smooth boundary curves from one-dimensional X-ray images. Our approach has applications in medical imaging (reconstruction of organs and tumors from sparse sets of X-ray images, stereo reconstruction of coronary arteries from angiograms, registration of CT models and X-ray images) and manufacturing (part acquisition and tolerancing, registration, and non-destructive evaluation).

Reconstruction from a sparse or limited-angle set of X-ray images is important for a number of reasons. If a few views are adequate for reconstruction, patient X-ray dosage can be reduced relative to current CT methods. There are also cases (such as cardiac imaging) when a full scan around an object is not possible in the available data acquisition time frame. Finally, from an economic standpoint, stereo X-ray systems are now widely available and generally cheaper than CT machines.

Recent work on geometric boundary reconstruction from X-ray images includes Thirion's method [11], which uses silhouette edges found in a dense set of X-ray images (a sinogram). His approach is related to computer vision research on surface reconstruction from silhouettes [3, 6, 13]. Skiena [10] and Gardner [5] have proposed computational geometry methods for reconstructing polygonal shapes using a small set of X-ray images. In a more general setting, Kergosien [7] has studied the topology of X-ray contours and their relationship to three-dimensional shape. Several authors have also worked on utilizing a priori shape knowledge. Recent examples inlclude the work of Van Tran, Bahn, and Sklansky [12] on reconstructing cross-sections of coronary arteries from biplane angiograms under the assumption that these cross-sections are ellipses, and the work by Bresler, Fessler and Macovski [1] on recovering multiple object boundaries under the assumption that these can be modeled as generalized cylinders. (See also [4, 8] for example.)

Our approach applies in a context where previous approaches do not: we use a sparse set of views to reconstruct object boundaries (rather than material density values), and we assume only that the object regions are uniform with smooth boundaries.

The input to the reconstruction algorithm is a small set of one-dimensional X-ray images, and its output is a set of low-degree spline curves representing the boundaries of the objects present in these images. (These boundaries are assumed to be smooth, as is common in medical images.) The basic idea is to initialize the spline curves using geometric information provided by the silhouette rays detected in each image, then let the intensity information deform the splines while maintaining tangency with the silhouette rays until a good fit is obtained. While shape fitting is the focus of this paper, the feature detection and grouping stages are at least as difficult. We discuss them briefly below.

2 Feature Detection

The features we seek are the discontinuities found in the (one-dimensional) X-ray projection images. Since we restrict our attention to smooth objects, any discontinuities correspond to points where the imaging ray is tangent to the object contour. As shown in Figure 1, there are four possible types of silhouette points in an X-ray image, and they all manifest themselves as tangent discontinuities (with infinite slope): types (a), (b), (c), and (d) correspond respectively to the beginning of a solid region, end of a solid region, beginning of a cavity or a right concavity, and end of a cavity or a left concavity. Note that type (a) and (b) points are convex, with all the matter on the same side of the tangent line, while type (c) and (d) points are concave, with matter on both sides of the tangent line.

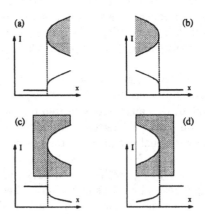

Fig. 1. The four different types of silhouette points in X-ray images.

Tangent discontinuities are usually found as "roofs" in images, but since the slope on one side of the discontinuity is always infinite in our case, these "roofs" are more appropriately detected as "steps". We have used a 1D version of the Canny edge detector [2] to detect the steps with sub-pixel localization. A single scale ($\sigma = 0.4$) and a single threshold (2.0) have been used for all images. Figure 2 shows the steps found in the first X-ray of the blade, overlaid on its CT reconstruction. The intensity profile is shown as a continuous curve, and the detected features are indicated by vertical lines.

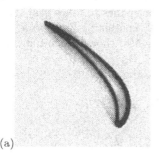 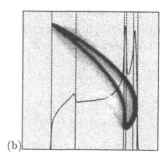

(a)   (b)

Fig. 2. Feature detection: (a) CT reconstruction of the blade. (b) Overlay of the intensity profile of the 0 degree orientation, along with detected step positions.

3   Feature Grouping

Once features have been detected, they must be grouped into subsets associated with the different object boundaries, then ordered along the boundary. Neither of these steps is straightforward, except in the (not too interesting) case of a single convex solid object. We do not yet have a good grouping strategy; in our experiments, we have grouped the features by hand. It should be noted, however, that not every pair of silhouette point types can be neighbors on the curve. From Figure 1, the only legal pairs of neighboring silhouette points are (a)-(d), (a)-(b), (c)-(b), (c)-(d).

Given a set of features, we can reconstruct the corresponding viewing rays, which are tangent to the object contours [3]. And given their ordering, we can compute polygonal approximations to the actual boundaries. Figure 5(a) shows the tangents constructed from the steps found in Figure 2(b), with the polygonal approximation darkened.

4   Shape Fitting

In this section, we describe how a spline approximation to each boundary is first initialized and then refined by minimizing the discrepancy between predicted and observed intensities.

---

[3] In X-ray images, the actual projection is neither orthographic or perspective. Instead, it can be modeled quite accurately by a linear pushbroom model [9]

4.1 Initial Shape

Given an ordered set of n silhouette rays $\Delta_1, .., \Delta_n$, we define the point A_i to be the intersection of the lines Δ_i and Δ_{i+1}. The spline we desire must be tangent to the sides of the polygon $A_1, .., A_n$. Setting P_i to be the point of contact of the spline with side A_i, A_{i+1}, it is natural to define a set of spline curve segments tangent to Δ_i and Δ_{i+1} at endpoints of P_i and P_{i+1}. The sequence of these segments produces an initial closed C^1 shape, parameterized by the position of the tangent points P_i between A_i and A_{i+1} (initially set to be midway; see Figure 3). In our experiments, we used cubic splines to allow easy insertion of new points in the spline while maintaining C^1 continuity. Figure 5(a) shows the Δ_i's for four views of the blade, while Figure 5(b) shows the initial curve.

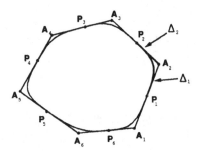

Fig. 3. Silhouette rays Δ_i defining a closed cubic spline curve.

4.2 Shape Refinement

The spline curve defined above has n degrees of freedom corresponding to the position of the contact points along the various tangents. In general, they will not be sufficient to fit the data well, so we propose to subdivide the spline boundary adaptively until a good fit is obtained through non-linear minimization.

In the first stage of our algorithm, we try to improve the match between projections of the object and the given X-ray intensities by moving the points of tangency for each spline segment. A contact point P_i is selected at random and moved a small amount to change the shape. We compute synthetic X-ray images of the new shape (by performing line integrals around the spline boundaries), then sum the L^2 distance between these images and the input intensities. We keep those movements which decrease the total error, and continue making small adjustments to the contact points until the error stabilizes.

Once a fit has been found, we project each segment onto every view, summing the error under all the projections. The segment covering the most error is then split by adding a new point to the middle of the segment. Since this point does not lie on a tangent, it is allowed to move freely in two dimensions, with its slope determined by the adjacent points on the contour.

After splitting, the algorithm again adjusts points at random to decrease the total error in the shape, maintaining the distinction between contact points (which are constrained to slide on silhouette rays) and free points. Once the error stops decreasing, another new point is added, and the process of splitting poorly-fit segments, then minimizing, continues until the errors stabilize across iterations.

4.3 Results

Figure 4(a) shows the reconstruction obtained for a non-convex synthetic object. The ten iterations required for convergence took roughly 30 minutes on a SPARC 10. It should be noted that no geometric information about the boundary concavities was used in this experiment. The objects in Figure 4(b)-(c) were selected to demonstrate the reconstruction of objects with internal structure (holes or smaller objects). In these cases, a single iteration was sufficient for convergence. In all cases, four views (0, 45, 90, and 135 degrees) were used.

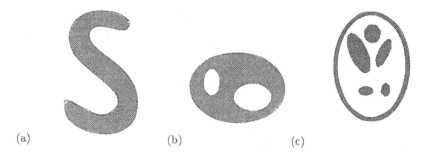

(a) (b) (c)

Fig. 4. Reconstruction from synthetic data: (a) an S figure, (b) an object with interior holes, and (c) an object with interior structure. The grey area shows the actual shape, while the black border indicates the four-view reconstruction.

Figure 5(c) shows our reconstruction of the turbine blade from real data. The input tangents are the projection rays shown in Figure 5(a), and an initial spline approximation is shown in Figure 5(b). Five iterations took approximately fifteen minutes on a SPARC 10. Note that the contour error introduced by feature extraction near the tail and end of the hole were removed by hand for this particular experiment. We are currently investigating approaches to automatically perform such simplification.

Finally, we attempted to reconstruct a blood vessel cross-section from images of a human head. For these images, a nominal set of X-rays were taken of a patient, followed by a set taken after marker fluid had been injected into

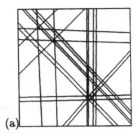 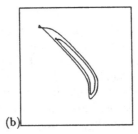 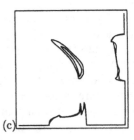

Fig. 5. Linear pushbroom reconstruction of a turbine blade: (a) silhouette rays (b) initial spline approximation (c) recovered shape The dark lines at the bottom and side show input X-ray profiles for the 0 and 90 degree views, while the lighter lines give the thickness of the reconstructed object.

the blood stream. The difference of these sets produced images with highly-contrasted blood vessels. We took four views of one horizontal slice of this data and discarded all low-contrast features to yield the silhouette edges of the veins. Since the attentuation of the veins and marker were unknown to us a-priori, we subtracted the average value of the image from the intensities, then scaled them by the maximum width of the control polygon $(A_1, .., A_n)$. Figure 6(a) shows one of the four images we used, with the slice in question highlighted. Our algorithm required seven iterations (about 45 seconds on a Sparc 10) to produce the reconstruction presented in Figure 6(b). It should be noted that these are only preliminary results on a relatively clean, uncluttered slice, where the silhouette geometry had as much impact on the final shape as the attenuation information. Nevertheless, these preliminary results are encouraging.

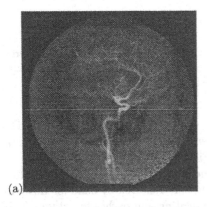 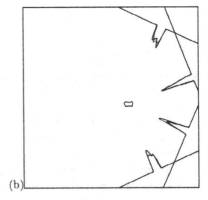

Fig. 6. Reconstruction of a blood vessel cross-section: (a) one of the four images used (reconstruction level indicated in white) (b) reconstruction result and intensity profiles.

5 Discussion

We have proposed and demonstrated a hybrid method for boundary reconstruction from a small set of X-ray images, using both synthetic and real data. Much of this work is preliminary: the next steps will involve improvements to the fitting algorithm, extension to 3D, and a serious attack on the problems of feature detection and grouping. We believe that tools from computational geometry [5, 10] and differential topology [7] will prove useful in this context.

Acknowledgments: This work was supported in part by the Beckman Institute and the Center for Advanced Study of the University of Illinois at Urbana-Champaign, and by NASA grant NAG 1-613. We wish to thank Dr. Yves Trousset from GE Medical Systems S.A. and Dr. Nicholas Ayache and Jacques Feldmar from INRIA for providing medical data to be used in our experiments

References

1. Y. Bresler, J.A. Fessler, and A. Macovski. A Bayesian approach to reconstruction from incomplete projections of a multiple object 3D domain. *IEEE Trans. Patt. Anal. Mach. Intell.*, 11(8):840–858, August 1989.
2. J.F. Canny. A computational approach to edge detection. *IEEE Trans. Patt. Anal. Mach. Intell.*, 8(6):679–698, November 1986.
3. R. Cipolla and A. Blake. Surface shape from the deformation of the apparent contour. *Int. J. of Comp. Vision*, 9(2):83–112, November 1992.
4. J.A. Fessler and A. Makovski. Object-based 3D reconstruction of arterial trees from magnetic resonance angiograms. *IEEE Trans. Medical Imaging*, 10(1):25–39, March 1991.
5. R.J. Gardner. X-rays of polygons. *Discrete and Computational Geometry*, 7:281–293, 1992.
6. P. Giblin and R. Weiss. Reconstruction of surfaces from profiles. In *Proc. Int. Conf. Comp. Vision*, pages 136–144, London, U.K., 1987.
7. Y.L. Kergosien. Generic sign systems in medical imaging. *IEEE Computer Graphics and Applications*, 11(5):46–65, 1991.
8. K. Kitamura, J.M. Tobis, and J. Sklansky. Estimating the 3D skeletons and transverse areas of coronary arteries from biplane angiograms. *IEEE Trans. Medical Imaging*, 7(3):173–187, September 1988.
9. A. Noble, R. Hartley, J. Mundy, and J. Farley. X-ray metrology for quality assurance. In *IEEE Int. Conf. on Robotics and Automation*, pages 1113–1119, May 1994.
10. S.S. Skiena. *Geometric Probing*. PhD thesis, Department of Computer Science, University of Illinois at Urbana-Champaign, 1988.
11. J.-P. Thirion. Segmentation of tomographic data without image reconstruction. *IEEE Trans. Medical Imaging*, 11(1):102–110, March 1992.
12. L. Van Tran, R.C. Bahn, and J. Sklansky. Reconstructing the cross-sections of coronary arteries from biplane angiograms. *IEEE Trans. Medical Imaging*, 11(4):517–529, December 1992.
13. R. Vaillant and O.D. Faugeras. Using extremal boundaries for 3D object modeling. *IEEE Trans. Patt. Anal. Mach. Intell.*, 14(2):157–173, February 1992.

3D Reconstruction of Blood Vessels by Multi-Modality Data Fusion Using Fuzzy and Markovian Modelling

Isabelle Bloch[†], Claire Pellot[‡], Francisco Sureda[†], Alain Herment[‡]

† Télécom Paris, département Images, 46 rue Barrault, 75634 Paris Cedex 13
Tél: 45 81 75 85, Fax: 45 81 37 94, E-mail: bloch@ima.enst.fr

‡ INSERM U256, hôpital Broussais, 96 rue Didot, 75014 Paris

Abstract: We propose an original approach for 3D reconstruction of blood vessels based on fusion of digital angiography and intravascular echography data, without any geometrical a priori vessel model. We aim at better understanding and interpreting vessel morphology and atheromateous vascular lesions. A Markovian and a fuzzy approach are developed, which take into account all information about the problem, including its imprecisions. They both show good and similar results.

1 Introduction

The three-dimensional reconstruction of blood vessels by objective and reproducible methods aims at helping in the interpretation and understanding of pathological vascular structures and at providing quantitative information about vessels and possible lesions. Such a precise and detailed morphological reconstruction (not available from MR images for instance, since they have a too large voxel size w.r.t. vessel size) has several advantages from a medical point of view: for prognosis and diagnosis of atheromateous diseases, for choosing a suitable therapy (including angioplasty and surgery), for controlling surgical gesture, and for a better understanding of restenosis phenomena observed during post-angioplasty examinations.

In order to provide a better 3D description of complex atheromateous lesions, we propose an original approach for reconstructing vascular segments by data fusion, from two different imaging sources: two orthogonal X-ray angiographic projections, and a series of intravascular echographic slices. This approach aims at avoiding the limits inherent to the reconstruction from only one modality: 3D reconstruction from two digital angiographies (DA) leads to imprecise and generally over-regularized results, due to the strong geometrical hypotheses and a priori knowledge on the vascular structures used in the reconstruction; 3D reconstruction from intravascular echography (IE) is limited by physical acquisition factors [5], [8], and the existing methods either ignore the translation and rotation of the catheter inside the vessel [6], [10] or suppose that the catheter follows exactly the vessel axis [7]. Therefore we propose two reconstruction methods

---

* This study has been carried out in the context of GdR CNRS 134 "Traitement du Signal et des Images" and has been partly supported by the French Ministery MESR (DRED founding).

relying on the fusion of both modalities: a Markovian approach and a fuzzy one (more details can be found in [2]).

2 Geometry of angiographic and ultrasonic acquisitions and data, and first reconstruction from IE

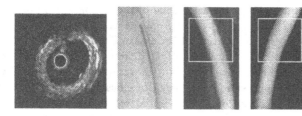

Fig. 1. Images used for the reconstruction. From left to right: echographic slice, control radiography, digital angiographies (the reconstruction will be performed in the surrounded area).

The experience realized in this study was made on a dog aorta, with a well defined acquisition protocole, near from routine acquisition (see Figure 1): two orthogonal contrast injected angiographic projections are first acquired; then the echographic probe is introduced in the vessel and progressively manually withdrawn; at each probe position, an IE slice is acquired, together with a X-ray radiography (with the same incidence than one of the contrasted angiographies), which allows the partial control of position and orientation of the probe through the vessel. The reference frame $(0, x, y, z)$ of the vessel to be reconstructed has been chosen such that the DA coordinates have simple expressions. For the IE images, located in planes which depend on the position and orientation of the probe, we introduced a frame related to the probe, defined by a translation vector (x_t, y_t, z_t) and three rotation angles φ, θ, and ω. This geometrical modelling of the acquisitions leads to the derivation of equations relating polar coordinates (r, α) of an echographic point to its cartesian coordinates (x, y, z) in the reference frame. After a preliminary segmentation step, a geometrical fusion step consists in determining the six parameters. θ, φ, x_t and y_t can be directly determined on the control radiography. The rotation of the probe on its own axis (angle ω) is computed by minimizing the distance between IE points and DA contours. In the same way, the last translation parameter z_t is computed by minimizing the distance between the projection of IE contours onto the right DA and the contours of this angiography. This geometrical fusion step allows to obtain a binary reconstruction by interpolating the IE slices registered in the reference frame, in order to obtain a regularly sampled surface (with the same resolution as the DA data). This reconstruction provides already an improvement over existing techniques, since it takes into account all the geometrical parameters of the acquisitions. However this reconstruction does not yet take into account the imprecision related to the acquisitions and the estimation of parameters, nor the information on vessel thickness provided by the grey levels of the DA images.

3 Reconstruction by Markovian fusion

The first method developed for the fusion of DA and IE data is based on a probabilistic approach which consists in searching the most likely solution amongst the set of possible ones according both to the acquired data and to a priori knowledges on vessel features. The vessel is reconstructed by a stack of parallel binary cross-sections [11] in the referencial of the angiographic projections. The DA cross-sectional data are extracted from the 1D density profiles at the very level of the processed cross-section of the stack. The IE cross-sectional data are given by the echographic contours extracted from the 3D approximated echographic volume obtained previously. For the reconstruction, an initial solution is first obtained by a least squares fitting of ellipsoidal binary sections on the vessel slices from DA data only. This initial solution is then optimized using an algorithm based on Simulated Annealing [4], which leads to the most likely configuration by minimizing an energy function containing the features of the DA and IE images in a Markov random field framework.

Energy model: The reconstructed structure will be consistent with the original data if its projections are close to the acquired angiographies and if its contours are close to the corresponding sections of the 3D echographic volume obtained previously. An additional a priori term is introduced to reduce the ambiguities between the two types of data. This regularization term (derived from Ising model) reflects the contour energy of the cross-section and maintains an anatomic homogeneity of the vessel slice. The energy function is thus composed of three terms (consistency with DA projections, consistency with IE contours, and regularization).

Optimization: Successive configurations of the current solution are then generated by randomly moving preselected candidate pixels (i.e. contour pixels) for transition. This selective scanning prevents unrealistic transitions of intraluminal sites consistent with the fact that pathologic material always deposits on vascular walls, and speeds up the reconstruction. A pixel move is achieved according to the Boltzman probability $P = \exp(-\Delta E/kT)$, which is relative to the variation of energy ΔE induced by the pixel transition and to a parameter T controlling the annealing temperature. A series of moves (a cycle) along all M candidate pixels is performed at a constant temperature level. The algorithm starts with a high temperature T_0, for which most pixel moves are accepted, and then gradually reduces T in order to converge to the global minimum of the energy function. The temperature decrease law $T_k = 0.95T_{k-1}$, where k is the iteration, has heuristically been proved to provide correct results for most vascular structures [9]. The initial temperature [9] is determined as a function of the current morphological features of the slice which are approximated by the initial projection differences of the image. The cycle length (Markov chain length) is proportional to the vessel perimeter. It has been heuristically estimated between 3 and 5 times the perimeter of the initial elliptic configuration. The algorithm stops when the number of agreed transitions remains low compared to the dimension of the image.

Results: The vascular segment has been reconstructed with three different weightings of the energy components. The results are illustrated on Figure 2. The reconstruction based on IE data only leads to an under estimation of the vessel geometry, the reconstructed vessel is too narrow, accounting for the differences located on the borders of the right projection image. The reconstruction based only on DA data gives a lower difference with the original projections, but there is no mean to check up to what precision the reconstructed vascular lumen exactly reflects the shape of the actual cross-section. The quality of reconstruction is improved when the two modalities are taken into account, since the DA longitudinal projections and the IE transversal slices provide complementary information on the general shape and on the cross section of the reconstructed vessel. In addition the difference images indicate no more discrepencies between the projection of the reconstructed vessel and the original ones. We thus believe that the vessel section should be more precise because the high resolution of IE images is integrated while the reprojected structure remains totally consistent with DA acquisition.

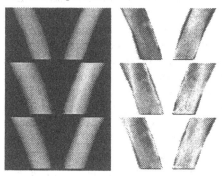

Fig. 2. Left image: left and right projections of the reconstructed vessel using different energy configurations. From top to bottom: IE term only, DA and regularization terms, all three energy terms. Right image: difference between the original projections and the ones of the reconstructed vessel (left and right) using the same energy configurations than on the left image (highest errors in black).

4 Fuzzy fusion

Fuzzy modelization of variables using possibility distributions is well suited for dealing with imprecise information like "the value of parameter θ is approximately equal to the measure θ_0 obtained on a radiography" [12]. For a pixel of the echographies, imprecisions on the geometrical parameters lead to imprecision on the point position in the reference frame. This point may thus have several positions with different possibility grades. We propose to represent the set of these positions by a 3D geometrical imprecise set, called fuzzy structuring element (SE), which will be exploited in the framework of fuzzy mathematical morphology.

Fuzzy structuring element: For representing a fuzzy number, we have chosen a flexible exponential form whose parameters are estimated as function of imprecision on the measured parameters. For instance for θ, it can be considered that the value having possibility 0.5 corresponds to an error of 1 pixel in the detection of each extremity of the probe. According to the geometrical modelization, the coordinates (x, y, z) of an echographic point (r, α) are defined by a function of θ, φ, ω, x_t, y_t and z_t. Each parameter v is modelized by a possibility distribution μ_v. The 3D SE associated with point (r, α) is a function of these imprecise variables, following the extension principle. The SE computation is performed directly in the discrete 3D space by determining, for each point of this space, its associated possibility.

Fuzzy reconstruction: In order to introduce the imprecisions modelized previously, fuzzy mathematical morphology is a well adapted tool, since it allows the propagation of a spatial imprecision around each point used in the reconstruction, in a controlled way, through the structuring element, and has good properties w.r.t. both mathematical morphology and fuzzy sets [1]. For our problem, we have to replace a point, possibly fuzzy, by a fuzzy set ν which represents all possible positions of this point. This is equivalent to dilating this point by the fuzzy structuring element defined by ν. Fuzzy dilation is therefore perfectly adapted for introducing spatial imprecision in the detected contours. Moreover, the compatibility property of the dilation with fuzzy set union allows the direct computation of the dilation of a set of points by the same structuring element. At last, the iteration property of fuzzy dilation allows the dilation of a fuzzy set successively by two fuzzy structuring elements or equivalently by their dilation. These two properties will be used for the fuzzy reconstruction.

In a first step, imprecisions on θ, φ and ω are taken into account for each point $x = (r, \alpha)$ of the interpolated surface V_{bin} under the form of a SE ν_1^x. The possibility degree (or membership degree to the reconstructed vessel) of each point of the 3D space is obtained as the maximum of possibility degrees in this point issued from the different ν_1^x's. A first fuzzy volume V_f' is thus obtained, whose membership function is $\mu_{V_f'}(x) = \sup\{\nu_1^y(x) \mid y \in V_{bin}\}$. In the second step, the final fuzzy reconstruction is obtained by a fuzzy dilation with SE ν_2, which takes into account imprecision on the translation parameters x_t, y_t and z_t. Since ν_2 is constant over the whole volume, the compatibility and iteration properties avoid to dilate each ν_1^x by ν_2 and allow one to perform only one fuzzy dilation, directly on the fuzzy volume V_f': $V_f = \bigcup \{D_{D_{\nu_2}(\nu_1^x)}(\{x\}) \mid x \in V_{bin}\} = D_{\nu_2}(V_f')$.

Fuzzy fusion: Here, the last available information is introduced: the vessel reconstruction provided by the DA data. The binary reconstruction obtained from the two DA projections (see Section 3) has therefore to be combined with the previous fuzzy IE reconstruction. Imprecision is modelized, like for the IE data, by a fuzzy structuring element, which represents membership possibility degrees to the vessel surface of the points situated in a neighbourhood of the reconstructed surface. The variation of vessel surface position corresponding to a possibility degree of 0.5 is estimated to 3 pixels (about 0.5 mm for the DA resolution of 0.1666 mm per pixel) along all 3 axes. The introduction of imprecisions on the binary reconstruction, denoted V_{bin}^{angio}, is then obtained by a fuzzy dilation by ν_2, providing a fuzzy volume V_f^{angio}. The last fusion step consists now in introducing this information in the reconstruction, i.e. in combining both fuzzy volumes V_f and V_f^{angio} by a fusion operator, resulting in a fuzzy volume V_f^F. The introduction of imprecisions in both reconstructions has led to fuzzy volumes V_f and V_f^{angio} which have a large overlapping part (of course with more or less high degrees) and which does not present any more contradiction. So a conjunctive fusion operator (with severe behaviour) can be used, which has the advantage to reduce imprecision in the result. Among the most used T-norms [3], the "min" and "product" have been chosen, which lead to similar results after the decision.

Binary decision: Obtaining a binary volume necessitates a decision step. To overcome the topological problems in the resulting surface inherent to classical decision rules, we prefer to select the points of the "crest surface" of the fuzzy volume. We obtain this way a unit thickness connected surface, going through the maximum membership points, and having thus the required properties. This surface is obtained by a morphological algorithm of 3D watershed. The result is shown on Figure 3, superimposed to the fuzzy fusion. This figure shows the good positioning of the watershed surface w.r.t. to the high membership values. The comparison with DA and IE contours shows that ambiguities are solved in a satisfactory way: in non conflictual areas, the watershed surface coincides with both contours, while in conflicting areas, an intermediary position is found.

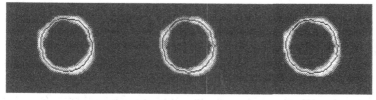

Fig. 3. Superimposition of the fuzzy volume after fusion and of the watershed (in black) on a few slices of the vascular segment.

Comparison between Markovian and fuzzy fusion: Figure 4 presents the result of the watershed on the fuzzy fusion superimposed on the results obtained with the Markovian approach. The remarkable similarity between both results should be noted (only a few slices are shown, but a good 3D coherence is obtained, as it can also be observed from the reconstructed projections).

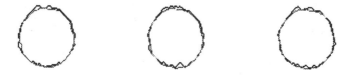

Fig. 4. Superimposition of the reconstruction by tae Markovian approach (in black) and of the reconstruction by fuzzy fusion and watershed (in grey).

5 Conclusion

A complete original approach has been proposed for the reconstruction of vascular segments by DA and IE data fusion. The main advantages of the methods are the following: all geometrical parameters are estimated and their introduction in a geometrical fusion step leads to a first reconstruction which is already an improvement over existing approaches; the Markovian fusion approach provides a reconstruction where radiologic and ultrasonic data fidelity and connexity constraints are all introduced through an energy model of the vessel cross-section; the optimization algorithm used to minimize this energy is based on simulated annealing; fuzzy modelling and fuzzy mathematical morphology allowed to take imprecision into account in an original approach, leading to a reconstruction by fuzzy fusion which takes again all problem data into account and avoids ambiguities; decision by watershed provides a result which is consistent from a topological and geometrical point of view, while going through the maxima of the membership functions. The first results prove the feasibility of the method and the interest of combining several modalities for improving 3D vessel reconstruction, without any a priori geometrical model of the vessels.

References

1. I. Bloch, H. Maître: *Fuzzy Mathematical Morphologies: A Comparative Study*, Technical Report Télécom Paris 94D001, 1994, To appear in Pattern Recognition.
2. I. Bloch, F. Sureda, C. Pellot, A. Herment: *3D Reconstruction of Blood Vessels by Data Fusion from Angiographic and Echographic Images*, Technical Report Télécom Paris 94D026, 1994 (in French).
3. D. Dubois, H. Prade: *A Review of Fuzzy Set Aggregation Connectives*, Information Sciences 36, 85-121, 1985.
4. H. Haneishi, T. Masuda, N. Ohyama, T. Honda, J. Tsujiuchi: *Analysis of the Cost Function used in Simulated Annealing for CT Image Reconstruction*, Applied Optics, Vol. 29, 259-264, 1990.
5. H. Hoff, A. Korbijn, T. H. Smit, J. F. F. Kinkhamer, N. Bom: *Imaging Artifacts in Mechanically Driven Ultrasound Catheters*, Int. Journal of Cardiac Imaging, Vol. 4, No.2-4, 195-199, 1989.
6. R. I. Kitney, L. Moura, K. Straughan: *3D Visualization of Arterial Structures using Ultrasound and voxel Modelling*, Int. Journal of Cardiac Imaging, Vol. 4, No.2-4, 135-143, 1989.
7. H.M. Klein, R.W. Gunther, M. Verlande, W. Schneider et al.: *3D-Surface reconstruction of intravascular ultrasound images using personal computer hardware and a motorized catheter control*, Cardiovascular Interventional Radiology, vol 15, 97-101, 1992.
8. E. Maurincomme, I. Magnin, G. Finet, R. Goutte: *Methodology for three-dimensional reconstruction of intravascular ultrasoung images*, SPIE, vol 1653, Medical Imaging IV: Image Capture, Formatting and Display, 26-34, 1992.
9. C. Pellot, A. Herment, M. Sigelle, P. Horain, H. Maître, P. Peronneau: *A 3D Reconstruction of Vascular Structures from Two X-Ray Angiograms Using an Adapted Simulated Annealing Algorithm*, IEEE Trans. on Medical Imaging, Vol. 13 (1), 48-60, March 1994.
10. K. Rosenfield, D. W. Losordo, K. Ramaswamy, J. O. Pastore, R. E. Langevin, S. Razvi, B. D. Kosowsky, J. M. Isner: *Three-Dimensional Reconstruction of Human Coronary and Peripheral Arteries from Images Recorded During Two-Dimensional Intravascular Ultrasound Examination*, Circulation, Vol. 84, 1938-1956, 1991.
11. L. van Tran, R. C. Bahn, P. W. Serruys: *Reconstructing the cross sections of coronary arteries from biplane angiograms*, IEEE Trans. Med. Imaging, Vol. 11, 517-529, 1992.
12. L. A. Zadeh: *Fuzzy Sets as a Basis for a Theory of Possibility*, Fuzzy Sets and Systems 1, 3-28, 1978.

Three-Dimensional Reconstruction
and Volume Rendering of
Intravascular Ultrasound Slices
Imaged on a Curved Arterial Path

Jed Lengyel[1], Donald P. Greenberg[1], Alan Yeung[2], Edwin Alderman[2], Richard Popp[2]

[1] Program of Computer Graphics, Cornell University, Ithaca, NY 14853
[2] Cardiovascular Medicine Division, Stanford University School of Medicine, Stanford, CA 94305

Abstract. Past techniques for three-dimensional reconstruction of intravascular ultrasound have assumed that the ultrasound slices are parallel and that the vessel being imaged
is straight. These assumptions result in distortions of vessel and lesion geometry. To properly reconstruct the volume data for a curved artery, the position and orientation of the
transducer must be known or calculated. We use angiography to recover the geometry of
the artery centerline, which is then used as a coordinate system to position the ultrasound
slices. To estimate the registration of the slices, several landmark sites are selected by the
physician and imaged over a complete heart cycle. Continuous pullbacks are then used to
sample between the landmark sites, yielding a three-dimensional volume data set. Standard
volume rendering techniques require data on a regular grid. We present new sampling and
rendering techniques that handle the oriented ultrasound slices positioned along the curved
artery.

1 Introduction

Intravascular ultrasound imaging is a relatively new technique for imaging the interior structure
of arteries.[YOCK88] Unlike traditional cardiac ultrasound that uses an exterior probe (limited
to imaging between the patient's ribs) or a transesophageal probe, intravascular ultrasound uses
a miniature ultrasound transducer mounted on the tip of a catheter.

To image the coronary arteries, both intravascular ultrasound and standard contrast angiograms use the same catheter placement technique. The catheter is threaded inside the patient's
arterial system through an artery in the thigh, and then maneuvered through the descending
aorta, around the aortic arch, and into the coronary arteries. For contrast angiograms, radio-
opaque dye is injected at the catheter's tip so that the blood flow in the lumen of the vessel
appears in fluoroscopic x-ray images. For intravascular ultrasound, the transducer at the tip of
the catheter is rotated by a drive shaft that runs the length of the catheter. The rotating transducer can then image cross-sections by emitting pulses of ultrasound (currently in the 20-50 MHz
range) and then receiving time-delayed echos.

The main advantage of intravascular ultrasound over the standard contrast angiogram is that
intravascular ultrasound can make images of the interior structure of the artery wall. The standard
angiogram shows only the lumen of the vessel. Recently it has been shown that intravascular
ultrasound can both reveal disease that does not appear in the standard constrast angiogram
and accurately measure the vessel lumen.[SG92][SG91]

Previous work on three-dimensional reconstruction of two-dimensional ultrasound slices assumed the vessel being imaged was straight, and therefore stacked the slices to form three dimensional cylindrical images. [ROSE91] [KRIS92] [ISNE92] Improvements include cardiac gating
and catheter motion compensation.[DHAW92] Other techniques have been developed for three-
dimensional reconstruction from a forward-viewing intravascular ultrasound catheter [NG94], and
for three-dimensional reconstruction of the geometry of endovascular stents from intravascular

ultrasound data[MINT93]. The images produced by stacking the slices along a linear path show the three-dimensional relations of vessel structures, but distort the geometry.[ROEL94] The work presented here addresses the distortion problem by using the *curved* artery geometry to position the ultrasound slices.

There is a large body of work on the reconstruction of the arterial tree from constrast angiograms. Parker *et al* [PARK87] use an interactive technique where vessel branch points and lines between the branch points are entered on the sequence of frames in both views. O'Brien *et al* [OBRI94] use a seed-fill algorithm. Hyche *et al* [HYCH92] use active contours ("snakes") similar to the technique we describe below.

Section 2 and Section 3 describe our algorithm for recovering the geometry of the artery centerline. Section 4 describes a technique for positioning 2D ultrasound slices on the curved coordinate system calculated above. Section 5 briefly discusses how to reconstruct and render a volume data set from the slices positioned in 3D. Section 6 presents the conclusions and topics for future research.

2 Geometry of the Arterial Tree

Our initial technique for reconstructing a segment of the arterial tree was an interactive one in which the stereo angiograms were presented to the user who then positioned points along the length of the artery segment in both images. Standard stereo inverse techniques were then used to calculate the three-dimensional points. This technique was far too labor intensive to be useful (especially when we consider the eventual goal of capturing the *moving* geometry of the arterial tree.) The goal of automatic tracking motivated the use of the technique described here.

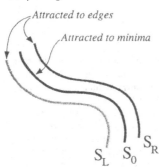

Fig. 1. *Snake — physically-based spline attracted to image features specified in energy functions*

Since arteries are made of elastic material, the model we use to fit to the arteries should capture this behavior. One such model used in computer vision is energy-based splines, or "snakes". Snakes have been used to track edges, to follow moving features, and to do stereo matching—all of which are needed for tracking a moving artery. For a full discussion, please see [KASS88] and [HYCH92]. Our work differs from the previous work by the use of compound snakes with offset energy functions.

Snakes are modeled with an internal energy that gives the snake its elastic character, and external energy functions for getting a desired behavior. For example, if one uses an external energy such as $E_{\text{dark}}(x, y) = I(x, y)$ where I is the image intensity, then the snake seeks dark areas in the image.

Through experimentation, we have found that a compound snake using two types of energies provides good results, and is more effective than the individual energies alone.

Let $s_0(u)$ be the centerline of the snake. Define $s_L(u)$ and $s_R(u)$ to be perpendicularly offset from $s_0(u)$ at each u by a constant r_{width}. Let $s_L(u) = s_0(u) + r_{\text{width}} n(u)$ and $s_R(u) = s_0(u) - r_{\text{width}} n(u)$ where $n(u)$ is the normal to the curve of $s_0(u)$.

The center of the combination snake seeks the center of the artery where the image is most opaque because of the contrast in the vessel lumen, using $E_{\text{dark}} = I(x, y)$. The offset parts of the combination snake seek edges, using $E_{\text{edge}} = -|\nabla I(x, y)|^2$. The combined energy is $E_{\text{total}}(u) = k_{\text{dark}} E_{\text{dark}}(s_0(u)) + k_{\text{edge}}(E_{\text{edge}}(s_L(u)) + E_{\text{edge}}(s_R(u)))$.

There are several free parameters to set, such as the strength of the minima-seeking energy k_{dark}, the strength of the edge-seeking energy k_{edge}, and the radius to seek r_{width}. For the work described here, the constants were set with initial rough estimates and then tuned interactively for good performance. Ideally, these parameters should be assigned from measurements of the physical properties of the actual catheter and actual vessels. This might eliminate the need for a tuning step. Note that r_{width} is an input parameter specifying the desired size of the matching artery. Since we are interested in accurately representing only a portion of the artery containing the catheter, this is a reasonable assumption. To make the combination snake more general, the radius should be made a function of arclength.

3   Stereo Matching

We require at least two views to reconstruct the centerlines of the arteries. We use two of the compound snakes as described above, with an additional energy that tries to minimize the distance between the two snakes in three-dimensions:[KASS88]

$$E_{\text{stereo}}(u) = |M_{\text{left}}^{-1}(S_{0_{\text{left}}}(u)) - M_{\text{right}}^{-1}(S_{0_{\text{right}}}(u))|^2$$

where M^{-1} is the inverse of the viewing transformation. M^{-1} is usually taken as linear, as a 4×4 perspective matrix, but the snake energy based method can also include nonlinear warping corrections. Although we have not yet incorporated this, the warping function can be calculated by imaging a regular grid and calculating the inverse function.

Since the resulting artery is in three dimensions,

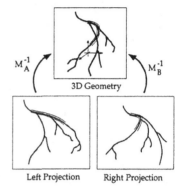

Fig. 2. *Stereo Matching*

we add a third coordinate to our snakes, which is the z-coordinate after the viewing transformation. These coordinates are convenient to express energy functions on the image, and also for the stereo energy. The final output is taken as the average of the two compound snake's centerlines after transforming by M^{-1}.

Since the snakes seek local minima in the energy functions, it is important to start them with the proper initial conditions, or they will find the wrong local minima. The initial placement of the snakes is currently done interactively.

4   Positioning of 2D Ultrasound Slices

Ideally, the catheter would be fitted with a device that would allow external measurement of its position and orientation while the ultrasound transducer is actively gathering data. This would eliminate the need for much of the work described above that locates the catheter in 3D. Since we do not have any method of externally measuring the position of the transducer, we use landmark sites within the arterial tree to estimate the position, twist, and tilt of keyframes. These keyframes are then used as the start and end of continuous pullbacks.

The choice of keyframes is left to the expertise of the doctor performing the intravascular ultrasound study. There are six parameters that need to be estimated for each keyframe

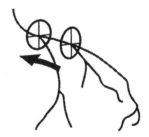

Fig. 3. *Landmark Sites*

site—position in space, tilt along each axis, and axial orientation $(x, y, z, \phi, \psi, \theta)$. A good keyframe requires side branches for axial orientation θ, must be distinct enough to be correlated with the recovered arterial tree for position in space (x, y, z), and the catheter placement must lie fairly close to the center of the artery for a reasonable estimate of the tilt parameters (ϕ, ψ).

Once the keyframes are imaged over a complete cycle, the administering doctor does a continuous pullback of the catheter, attempting to maintain a steady rate, or using a mechanical assist to help make the pullback uniform. The images are currently captured on videotape in slice format. This method of capture introduces many artifacts, such as video noise and errors in the resampling from polar to rectangular coordinates. In the future, we hope to eliminate some of these artifacts by acquiring the raw data digitally. Also included in the captured sequence are motions from the patient's breathing.

Once the catheter coordinate system is estimated, the slices are placed perpendicular to the catheter at intervals according to the distance and time between keyframes. The pullback motion is assumed to be uniform between the keyframes. See Color Plate 1 for an example.

Currently we take the center of the artery to be the position of the catheter. This is not an accurate assumption, and needs to be refined in the future. This technique also assumes that the distortion of the vessel due to the catheter is neglible, which may be a large source of error. Another source of error is the nonuniform rotational velocity of the transducer.[KIMU94]

5 Rendering of Curved Volume Data

To reconstruct a 3D density from 2D slices oriented along a curve in space, we use the curve as our coordinate system. To calculate an echo density value between slices, we assume that the data between the slices is approximated by the slice values. Thus we want to define a smooth coordinate system to move between the slices. Intuitively, we want the coordinates to "match up" neighboring sample points. For resampling in a curved space with variable spacing between sample points, at first it is unclear what size the reconstruction kernels should be.

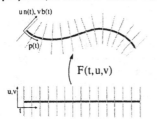

How much weight should be given to each sample point? How much should each sample contribute to the whole function at a point in space? Our solution is to map the data from the slices on the curving path back to rectangular parametric coordinates for sampling, using the inverse of the map F shown in Figure 4. We choose a coordinate system (described briefly in Appendix A) based on the the path of the catheter and a plane perpendicular to the path.

Most of the current volume rendering techniques either require or assume that the input grid of data is on a regular, rectangular grid. We would like to

Fig. 4. *Coordinate Map*

work with the data in curved coordinates for several reasons. One is to reduce memory space requirements. Another reason is to monitor where errors are introduced—and possibly to display the relative reliability of various parts of the data set and algorithms.

The volume data set is sampled at a number of points along each viewing ray and composited. A simple model of emission and absorption is used to provide lighting and occlusion (a good description of emission-absorption models is found in [NOVI93].) The main difference from a standard volume ray-tracing renderer is the handling of the curved geometry. Please see Color Plate 2 for some preliminary examples and Appendix A for more details.

6 Conclusion

By recovering the arterial tree and calculating the position of the ultrasound slices in space, we are able to create 3D ultrasound renderings that are more faithful to the curving geometry of the artery than the previous linear approximations.

Eventually, as machine speeds catch up to our needs, this kind of rendering pipeline might move into the interventional catheter laboratory. Since the ray-traced volume rendering times turned out to be so long (about an hour per frame), other rendering techniques must be pursued. Also for future work, we plan to combine the time-dependent intravascular ultrasound data and the moving geometry of the artery.

Accurate knowledge of the interior anatomy of the diseased vessel permits improved therapy through iterative processes initiated by the physician attempting angioplasty or atherectomy.

A Coordinates and Sampling

Let $p(t)$ be the path of the catheter parametrized so that equal steps in t by Δt map to the location of each slice. Then we can find a function, F, that maps from the rectangular coordinates of the data u, v, t to the spatial coordinates x, y, z.

Let $n(t)$ and $b(t)$ be the normal and binormal of $p(t)$, using the Frenet formulas. This gives us a plane perpendicular to $p(t)$ at each point along its length.

To avoid the sign flips that occur with the Frenet frame and to define the frame on points with zero curvature, associate n_i and b_i with each slice such that $n_i \cdot n_{i+1} > 0$ and $b_i \cdot b_{i+1} > 0$. If the curvature is zero, then use the axes from the previous slice. Then define $\bar{n}$ and $\bar{b}$ to be interpolated linearly between the slices. Let $F(u, v, t) = p(t) + u\bar{b}(t) + v\bar{n}(t)$. With proper constraints on the curvature of $p(t)$, F is a continuous one-to-one map over the entire domain of the input data, and so we can define an inverse function F^{-1} that maps the range of F back to the input data.

Let dF be the jacobian matrix of F. Let $q(s) = q_0 + sQ$ be a ray through the distorted volume. Since we have the starting points that correspond to both the mapped and the unmapped points, we can use the inverse jacobian of F to map the direction of the ray back into the undistorted volume, $\bar{Q}(s) = dF(q(s))^{-1}Q$, and then integrate to obtain the pre-image of the ray, $\bar{q}(s) = \bar{q}_0 + \int_0^s \bar{Q}ds$. Note that the direction of the ray changes as we move forward in s, and so the inverse of the jacobian matrix must be calculated at each integration step, which makes for long rendering times (approximately one hour per frame on a 75MIPS workstation.) More details are available in [LENG95].

B Data Resolution

For the preliminary study, we digitized from videotape to get our digital angiograms, limiting our data to video resolution. Since the theoretical resolution is higher, we are currently seeking digital angiography data. The video data we used covered about 400×400 pixels imaging the heart over an approximately 10cm $\times$ 10cm region. This gives a feature length resolution of about 0.5mm.

The speed of the pullback of the intravascular ultrasound probe is $1 - 2$mm/s and the slices are swept out at 30 frames per second. We select one frame out of every 15-30 frames gated to the heart cycle (which in the case of heart transplant patients is at an elevated rate.) This gives a slice spacing of $0.5 - 1$mm. An alternative is to keep all 30 frames per second, which gives a higher resolution along the catheter axis, but puts together data taken at different times in the heart cycle.

The frequency of the transducer used to obtain our images was 20MHz. Higher frequencies are available, currently up to 50MHz. The higher the frequency, the shorter the penetration depth, but the smaller the feature that can be resolved. According to [BOM92], the current practical axial resolution is about 0.1mm and lateral resolution on the order of $0.3 - 0.5$mm.

References

[BOM92] Bom, Nicolaas, Wenguang Li, Charles T. Lancée, Harm ten Hoff, and Elma J. Gussenhoven. "Basic Principles of Intravascular Ultrasound Imaging," in Tobis, Jonathan M. and Paul G.

Yock, editors, *Intravascular Ultrasound Imaging*, Churchill Livingstone Inc., New York, 1992, chapter 2, pages 7–15.

[DHAW92] Dhawale, Paritosh J., Nobuo Griffin, David L. Wilson, and John McB. Hodgson. "Calibrated 3-D Reconstruction of Intracoronary Ultrasound Images with Cardiac Gating and Catheter Motion Compensation," *Computers in Cardiology*, 1992, pages 31–34.

[HYCH92] Hyche, M., N. Ezquerra, and R. Mullick. "Spatiotemporal Detection of Arterial Structure Using Active Contours," *Proceedings of Visualization in Biomedical Computing*, 1808, 1992, pages 52–62.

[ISNE92] Isner, Jeffrey M., Kenneth Rosenfield, Douglas W. Losordo, and Chandrasekaran Krishnaswamy. "Clinical Experience with Intravascular Ultrasound as an Adjunct to Percutaneous Revascularization," in Tobis, Jonathan M. and Paul G. Yock, editors, *Intravascular Ultrasound Imaging*, Churchill Livingstone Inc., New York, 1992, chapter 16, pages 186–197.

[KASS88] Kass, Michael, Andrew Witkin, and Demetri Terzopoulos. "Snakes: Active Contour Models," *International Journal of Computer Vision*, 1988, pages 321–331.

[KIMU94] Kimura, Bruce J., Valmik Bhargava, Wulf Palinski, Kirk L. Peterson, and Anthony N. DeMaria. "Can Intravascular Ultrasound Yield Accurate Measures of Vascular Anatomy? Documentation of the Critical Importance of Uniform Rotational Velocity," *Journal of the American College of Cardiology*, February 1994, page 173A.

[KRIS92] Krishnaswamy, Chandrasekaran, Arthur J. D'Adamo, and Chandra M. Sehgal. "Three-Dimensional Reconstruction of Intravascular Ultrasound Images," in Tobis, Jonathan M. and Paul G. Yock, editors, *Intravascular Ultrasound Imaging*, Churchill Livingstone Inc., New York, 1992, chapter 13, pages 141–147.

[LENG95] Lengyel, Jed. *Three-Dimensional Reconstruction and Volume Rendering of Moving Coronary Arteries*, PhD dissertation, Program of Computer Graphics, Cornell University, January 1995.

[MINT93] Mintz, Gary S., Augusto D. Pichard, Lowell F. Satler, Jeffrey J. Popma, Kenneth M. Kent, and Martin B. Leon. "Three-Dimensional Intravascular Ultrasonography: Reconstruction of Endovascular Stents In Vitro and In Vivo," *Journal of Clinical Ultrasound*, 21, November/December 1993, pages 609–615.

[NG94] Ng, K.H., J.L. Evans, M.J. Vonesh, S.N. Meyers, T.A. Mills, B.J. Kane, W.N. Aldrich, Y.T. Jang, and P.G. Yock. "Arterial Imaging with a New Forward-Viewing Intravascular Ultrasound Catheter, II: Three-Dimensional Reconstruction and Display of Data," *Circulation*, 89(2), 1994, pages 718–723.

[NOVI93] Novins, Kevin L. *Towards Accurate and Efficient Volume Rendering*, Technical Report TR 93-1395, Department of Computer Science, Cornell University, Ithaca, NY 14853-7501, October 1993.

[OBRI94] O'Brien, James F. and Norberto F. Ezquerra. "Automated Segmentation of Coronary Vessels in Angiographic Image Sequences Utilizing Temporal, Spatial, and Structural Constraints," *Proceedings of Visualization in Biomedical Computing*, 1994.

[PARK87] Parker, Dennis L, David L Pope, Rudy Van Bree, and Hiram W Marshall. "Three-Dimensional Reconstruction of Moving Arterial Beds from Digital Subtraction Angiography," *Computers and Biomedical Research*, 20(2), 1987, pages 166–185.

[ROEL94] Roelandt, Joseph R.T.C., Carlo di Mario, Natesa G. Pandian, Li Wenguang, David Keane, Cornelius J. Slager, Pim J. de Feyter, and Patrick W. Serruys. "Three-dimensional Reconstruction of Intracoronary Ultrasound Images," *Circulation*, 90, 1994, pages 1044–1055.

[ROSE91] Rosenfield, Kenneth, Douglas W. Losordo, K. Ramaswamy, John O. Pastore, Eugene Langevin, Syed Razvi, Bernard D. Kosowsky, and Jeffrey M. Isner. "Three-dimensional Reconstruction of Human Coronary and Peripheral Arteries From Images Recorded During Two-Dimensional Intravascular Ultrasound Examination," *Circulation*, 84, 1991, pages 1938–1956.

[SG91] St. Goar, Frederick, Fausto J. Pinto, Edwin L. Alderman, Peter J. Fitzgerald, Michael L. Stadius, and Richard L. Popp. "Intravascular Ultrasound Imaging of Angiographically Normal Coronary Arteries: An In Vivo Comparison With Quantitative Angiography," *Journal of the American College of Cardiology*, 18, 1991, pages 952–958.

[SG92] St. Goar, Frederick, Fausto J. Pinto, Edwin L. Alderman, Hanna A. Valantine, John S. Schroeder, Shao-Zou Gao, Edward B. Stinson, and Richard L. Popp. "Intracoronary Ultrasound in Cardiac Transplant Recipients—In Vivo Evidence of "Angiographically Silent" Intimal Thickening," *Circulation*, 85, 1992, pages 979–987.

[TOBI92] Tobis, Jonathan M. and Paul G. Yock, editors. *Intravascular Ultrasound Imaging*, Churchill Livingstone Inc., New York, 1992.

[YOCK88] Yock, PG, EL Johnson, and DT David. "Intravascular Ultrasound: Development and Clinical Potential," *American Journal of Cardiac Imaging*, 2, 1988, pages 185–193.

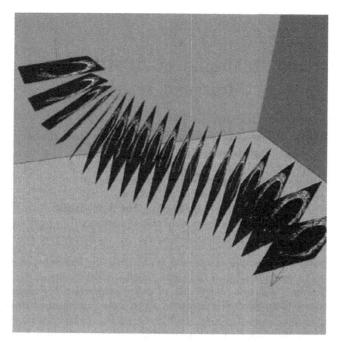

Color Plate 1. Slices positioned along the transducer path

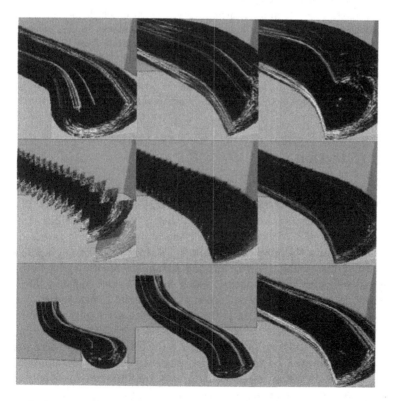

Color Plate 2. Preliminary volume renderings
a,b,c *Coronal split, thin sagittal split, thick sagittal split*
d-f,i *Progression of between-slice opacity from zero to one*
g,h *Two elevation angles*

Analysis and 3D Display of 30 MHz Intravascular Ultrasound Images

Manon Kluytmans[1], Carolien J. Bouma[1], Bart M. ter Haar Romeny[1], Gerard Pasterkamp[2] and Max A.Viergever[1]

[1] Computer Vision Research Group
[2] Heart Lung Institute
University Hospital Utrecht - The Netherlands
e-mail: Manon.Kluytmans@cv.ruu.nl

Abstract. Intravascular ultrasound (IVUS) has the intrinsic potential to visualize and quantify the full three-dimensional structure of the vessel with high resolution. A recently proposed subtraction technique [8] enables automatic contour extraction, a prerequisite for routine clinical use.

This paper presents all image processing steps to come to a feasible procedure for 3D display and quantitative analysis. Segmentation takes place without user-interaction.

An interactive presentation method is suggested in which the obtained information is visualized by using different techniques in one screen, thereby enabling fast extraction of relevant information from IVUS data in clinical routine. Transparent overlay of the segmented images over the original images in real-time mode, allows visual feedback already during the interventional procedure. A volumetric presentation of the lumen is generated, as well as quantitative parameters that characterize the vessel lumen.

1 Introduction

The current standard for guidance of transluminal recanalization techniques is contrast angiography. This technique however has several limitations. The most important impediments arise from the fact that it yields only a silhouette of the lumen. The number of views is restricted and no information is gathered about the vessel wall and the shape of the lumen. Thanks to its tomographic nature intravascular ultrasound (IVUS) has the advantage of displaying both vessel lumen and wall with high resolution, which enables measurement of the luminal cross-sectional area [7] and visualization of the arterial lumen and lesions. This is in particular true for 30 MHz IVUS which provides a higher resolution than the more common 20 MHz version, and is therefore capable of detecting small dissections and irregularities of the vessel wall. Up to now, the acceptance of IVUS has been limited: on the one hand judgement of IVUS data is very time-consuming, mainly owing to the need to view the images sequentially; on the other hand automated analysis is hampered by the high levels of backscatter and noise. Acceptance of IVUS as a routine clinical imaging modality is dependent on the availability of a procedure to preprocess the data automatically. This step notably includes segmentation of the lumen. In several studies segmentation of the lumen from IVUS data was performed automatically [1, 4, 5, 11, 12], but in those studies ultrasound catheters with a frequency of 20 MHz were used, which give little backscatter of the blood. A review of several 3D reconstruction techniques with their advantages and limitations was recently given by Roelandt et al. [10]. With 30 MHz high frequency ultrasound, discrimination between lumen and wall is difficult because of the intense backscattering of the blood [3] (Fig. 1a). This problem can be evaded by flushing the lumen with saline (Fig. 1b). Since flushing is not completely without danger for the patient, and since it is not possible to flush constantly during acquisition of an entire vessel segment, this method is impractical for 3D acquisition. Distinction between wall and lumen can also be enhanced by averaging several images at one location, yielding a texture difference between lumen and plaque (Fig. 1c), but contours are still difficult to detect automatically. In this paper we present a segmentation method based on a recently proposed subtraction technique [8]. This technique consists of subtraction of successive IVUS images at one location, thereby highlighting the lumen (dynamics of the blood) in good apparent contrast with wall and plaque (static)(Fig. 1d). After the preprocessing step the images and parameters derived from them are presented on a display, in which step interaction is admissible and even desirable.

In this paper we will first describe the image acquisition and resume the - slightly adjusted- subtraction and averaging methods. Next the image processing steps that lead to an automatic procedure for analysis and display of IVUS data are discussed. Finally, we will present the design of a workstation feasible for routine clinical use. Features are:

- real-time (red) transparent overlay of the segmented images over the original images thus providing visual feedback already during the interventional procedure,
- a longitudinal view of the total traversed vessel length,
- a 3D presentation of the lumen, real-time growing in length while the catheter is pulled back,
- quantitative data, such as luminal area as a function of vessel length and stenotic index.

2   Image acquisition

In this section the acquisition of IVUS images is described. An electro-optic distance counter built in the catheter shaft yields the position of the catheter. Images are taken by pulling back the catheter stepwise with regular intervals. At each interval (e.g. every mm) the catheter is snapped for several seconds to obtain multiple images at one location, necessary for automatic subtraction and averaging.

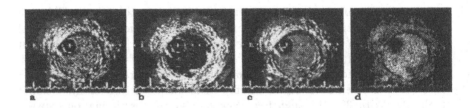

Fig. 1. Intravascular ultrasound images of arteria femoralis (original data, courtesy of dr. H.J. Gussenhoven and dr. H. Pieterman (Dijkzicht University Hospital, Rotterdam)). Frame a. original image, showing adventitia, media, intima and lumen with backscatter caused by the red blood cells; Frame b. image after flushing with saline, the lumen is now clearly visible as a dark hole; Frame c. weighted average image from 12 original images taken at the same location; Frame d. weighted subtraction image from 12 consecutive difference images taken at the same location, highlighting the lumen relative to the static parts of wall and plaque.

2.1 Temporal Subtraction

Two consecutive images taken from the time-series at one location will differ in the lumen because of the changing speckle pattern which results from the flow of blood. Subtraction of those images eliminates the static parts and highlights the dynamic parts of the image. A difference image is generated from two subsequent images and the absolute values of a number of these difference images are averaged (six images are already sufficient to produce an acceptable result), yielding what is referred to in this paper as a 'subtraction image' (Fig. 1d). To make the subtraction method somewhat less sensitive to small movements of the catheter subtraction images were calculated according to the following formula:

$$Sub_n = \frac{\sum_{m=0}^{9}(1 - 0.1m)(I_{n-m} - I_{n-m-1})}{\sum_{m=0}^{9}(1 - 0.1m)} \qquad \text{where } I_x \text{ is the x-th image.}$$

This is weighted subtraction where a difference image closer in time to the last acquired image is given more weight than a previous difference image. (Eleven images are now needed to get an apparent contrast between wall and lumen similar to the contrast obtained with the conventional subtraction method with six images).

2.2 Temporal Averaging

Like the subtraction method, temporal averaging uses the changing scatter of blood with time. Averaging a number of consecutive images gives a texture difference between lumen and wall. The blood scatter variations are smoothed while the relative stable structure of the arterial wall is preserved [6] (Fig. 1c). Weighted average images were calculated from:

$$Av_n = \frac{\sum_{m=0}^{9}(1 - 0.1m)I_{n-m}}{\sum_{m=0}^{9}(1 - 0.1m)} \quad \text{where } I_x \text{is the x-th image.}$$

Although subtraction images are more suitable for automatic segmentation, averaged images can be used for visualization of transversal slides, as will be demonstrated further on in the proposed screen layout for a clinical workstation. Subtraction, average and original images are generated and digitized by a frame-grabber, which is capable of real-time image acquisition.

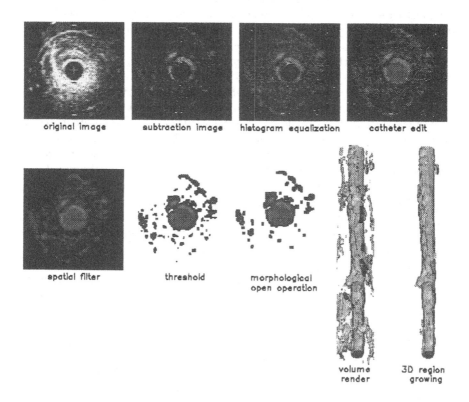

Fig. 2. From upper-left to lower-right: Intermediate steps during 3D reconstruction of the vessel lumen from subtraction images (coronary artery *in vitro*, length=6cm; images were taken every mm).

3 Segmentation

A prerequisite for fast routine clinical use is automatic segmentation. We have designed such a procedure comprising the following processing steps. First, subtraction images are normalized with respect to overall intensity by means of a histogram-preserving stretching of the intensity range of each image. This cancels fluctuations in US power output and overall gain, and allows use of a standard threshold for segmentation. A Gaussian low-pass filter with a standard deviation in the order of the spatial resolution of the IVUS system removes unwanted high frequency speckle. By resampling of the set of IVUS frames, x, y and z dimensions are adjusted to their true proportions, yielding cubic voxels. The contours of the lumen are then found by thresholding. Contours smaller then 3 pixels (0.2 mm) in diameter are removed by morphological erosion and subsequent dilation. 3D images are generated and the lumen is separated from smaller not connected structures by 3D 'region growing' from a seed-point, which may be anywhere in the lumen. By taking the central pixel of the image this step is automated since (in our case) this pixel always represents the center of the catheter. All calculations were carried out with Analyze^{TM} [9].

The segmentation method was capable of detecting very small dissections as small as 0.2 mm, as was validated with agar vessel-phantoms with manually made dissections and deformations. The walls of these phantoms were made by mixing agar with red blood cells, which gives approximately the same backscatter properties as blood. To test the subtraction method and automatic segmentation procedure the phantoms were flushed with blood; as a control the phantoms were flushed with saline followed by manual segmentation. For large dissections the results of the automatic procedure were very much similar to the manual segmentation. One of the phantoms had a very thin dissection, made by light squeezing. The automatic method was better capable of segmenting this thin dissection then an experienced person could do manually.

The calculation time for a stack of 50 images typically is less than 2 minutes on a HP 9000/710 workstation. A summary of the results of the procedures is given in figure 2.

4 Clinical Display

To facilitate quick judgement of the IVUS procedure in routine use, results are displayed in a 'multi-modal' screen in which multiple modes of presentation are combined (Fig. 3). Hardware requirements for such a display are met by current workstation technology.

Already during processing, images appear on the display. The original (or averaged) images are shown in real-time. By transparent projection of the subtraction images in red over the average images, the lumen is colored red and becomes easily visible to the observer, allowing immediate verification of the subtraction procedure. An 'orthogonal' (sagittal/coronal) view is also displayed practically real-time, appearing on the display while the pull-back is proceeding. This 'orthogonal' view is directly comparable with the contrast angiogram, but has the advantage that every arbitrary viewing angle can be chosen. At the same time a graph is drawn, displaying the cross-sectional lumen area against distance. At the end of the procedure the volume rendered lumen is presented to give an

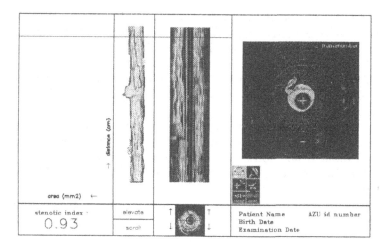

Fig. 3. Multi-modal screen displaying several modes of presentation of IVUS data. Proposed screen layout for presentation of original image, segmented lumen, 3D lumen rendering and quantitative data. From left to right (top): lumen-area as a function of vessel length; 3D reconstruction of the lumen; sagittal cross-section; real-time transparent overlay of subtraction on averaged transversal images. From left to right(bottom): stenotic index; positioning parameters of 3D lumen rendering; viewing angle of sagittal cross-section; patient data.

overview of dissections and other irregularities. A graph with the percentage area obstruction, i.e. the local cross-sectional area divided by (an average value of) the area outside the stenotic region, is also calculated and displayed at the end of the procedure.

After the processing has been completed the information can be manipulated interactively. A marker can be set onto a specific slice or surface location or at an interesting part of the graph. The original or averaged images at that location are then displayed, with the subtraction image transparently projected in red. Also the quantitative figures belonging to that specific location (e.g. cross-sectional area, percentage area obstruction, and the distance traversed by the catheter) are calculated. An important advantage of separately displaying the transversal images is that these provide diagnostic relevant insight into the structure of the vessel wall. Bringing out the characteristics of the wall is an intrinsic property of IVUS which is lost during segmentation and 3D visualization of the vessel lumen.

5 Discussion

A workstation as proposed in this paper might be an important step towards routine clinical use of IVUS. The proposed method to visualize and quantify intravascular ultrasound data appears quite suited. However, introduction into the clinic will require a thorough evaluation of the efficacy of the approach, and a consensus on the clinical 3D viewing protocol. All items displayed on screen should be critically considered with respect to their relevance for a particular intervention. An overload of information will only obscure important details. Maybe some information should be optional, allowing use in complex cases or in validation afterwards.

In our 3D reconstructions no corrections are made for spatial orientation of the vessel [5]. Processing time would be influenced negatively and in most cases it is not expected that assessment of the vessel wall would improve. However, guidance by ultrasound of directed therapeutic catheters (e.g. IVUS combined with laser) is a promising development [2] and when these directional intervention techniques gain importance, knowledge of the spatial structure becomes essential.

References

1. Chandrasekaran, K., et al.: Three-dimensional volumetric ultrasound imaging of arterial pathology from two-dimensional intravascular ultrasound: An in vitro study. Angiology 45(1994)253–264
2. Crowley, R., et al.: Ultrasound guided therapeutic catheters: recent developments and clinical results. Int. J. Cardiac Imaging 6(1991)145–156
3. Kallio, T. and Alanen, A.: A new ultrasonic technique for quantifying blood echogenicity. Invest. Radiol. 23(1988)832–835
4. Kitney, R.I., et al.: 3-D visualization of arterial structures using ultrasound and voxel modelling. Int. J. Cardiac Imaging4(1989)135–143
5. Klein, H.M., et al.: 3D-surface reconstruction of intravascular ultrasound images using personal computer hardware and a motorized catheter control. Cardiovasc. and Inter. Rad. 15 (1992) 97–101
6. Li, W., et al.: Computer-aided intravascular ultrasound diagnostics. 10th Symp. on EchoCardiol. Ed: Roelandt, J. et al. Kluwer Ac. Publ.(1993)79–90
7. Nissen, S.E., et al.: Intravascular Ultrasound assessment of lumen size and wall morphology in normal subjects and patients with coronary artery disease. Circulation 84(1991)1087–1099
8. Pasterkamp, G., et al.: Discrimination of the Intravascular Lumen and Dissections in a Single 30MHz US Image: Use of "Confounding" Blood Backscatter to Advantage. Radiology 187(1993)871–872
9. Robb, R.A., et al.: ANALYZE: A comprehensive, operator-interactive software package for multidimensional medical image display and analysis. Comput. Med. Imag. Grap. 13(1992)433–454
10. Roelandt, J.R.T.C., et al.: Three-dimensional reconstruction of intracoronary ultrasound images. Circulation 90(1994)1044–1055
11. Rosenfield, K., et al.: Human coronary and peripheral arteries: On-line three-dimensional reconstruction from two-dimensional intravascular US scans. Radiology 184(1992)823–832
12. Sonka, M., et al.: Automated detection of wall plaque borders in intravascular ultrasound images. SPIE2168(1994)

Simplification of Irregular Surfaces Meshes in 3D Medical Images

Alexis Gourdon

INRIA, B.P. 93, 06902 Sophia-Antipolis Cedex, France.
Email: alexis.gourdon@sophia.inria.fr

Abstract. Iso surface extraction using the *Marching Cubes* algorithm produces surfaces meshes with often hundreds of thousands of vertices. Even with today's powerful graphic workstations, storage problems can arise and rendering algorithms can be dramatically slow. This paper describes a new method for reducing the number of vertices and facets on orientable surfaces meshes (which may not be triangulations). Vertices or edges are removed using a curvature criterion. When many points are removed, an additional stage is necessary to regularize the relative positions of the vertices on the surface. Experimental results from synthetic data and medical images illustrate the overall process.

1 Introduction

Surface rendering techniques are popular in computer graphics and can generate realistic models of 3D objects. The basic primitive of these techniques is the polygon which can be rendered efficiently with a shading effect on many workstations. Of course, as we deploy more polygons we are able to model more complex shapes ; but as the number of polygons increases so does the necessary disk space and this decreases the rendering speed. For example, typical medical 3D images, such as CT-Scan, can have more than 100 slices at a resolution of 256×256 or 512×512. For such huge data sets iso-surface extraction can produce meshes with more than 250000 vertices. Other computer vision acquisition techniques such as range data or digital elevation models produced by satellite imagery techniques can lead to huge surface meshes. While a number of papers [10, 8, 2, 3] have dealt with the problem of reducing triangular meshes, we propose a new approach which is suitable for any orientable surface mesh. This paper is organized as follows :

- First, we recall some basic topological concepts on surface meshes.
- Next, we present our simplification and regularization algorithms.
- Finally, we show experimental results on synthetic and medical images.

2 Topology on surfaces

From a topological point of view, the notion of surface is intuitive : locally a surface looks like the real plane $\mathbb{R}^2$. More precisely, each point of a topological surface has a neighborhood homeomorphic to the open unit disk in the real plane $\mathbb{R}^2$ [4]. When this topological space is compact, the surface is said to be compact. This definition of a surface tells us about its local aspects. One way to acquire a global understanding of the shape of the surface is to construct a mesh as a partition of points, edges and facets where edges are similar to segments and facets to convex planar polygons [4]. More precisely :

- a **vertex** v is a set reduced to a single point.
- a **closed edge** e is a set diffeomorphic to the closed interval $[0,1]$, the corresponding **open edge** is the mapping by the same diffeomorphism of $]0,1[$. and the points which correspond to 0 or 1 are the **vertices** of the edge.
- under the mapping by a diffeomorphism of the closed unit disk of $\mathbb{R}^2$, n distinct points $(n \geq 1)$ $M_1, ... M_n$ on the unit circle such that two open arcs in $\{M_i M_{i+1}$ with $(i \in \{1, ..., n\})$ $\}^1$ have an empty intersection, is a **closed facet** f. The **open facet** is the mapping by the same diffeomorphism of the open disk. By mapping the n points M_i, we get the **vertices** of the facet, and by mapping the n consecutive open arcs we get the **open edges** of the facet.

A surface mesh is a finite partition of open facets, open edges, and vertices where :

- for each open edge e there exists at least one facet f such that e is an edge of f
- for each vertex v there exists at least one facet f such that v is a vertex of f.

When such a mesh exists on a surface, the surface is compact (the converse statement is also true but harder to prove). If the surface has no boundary, then each edge belongs to exactly two distinct facet edges (the facets may not be distinct). For a mesh on a compact surface with boundaries, each point of the boundary is either a vertex, or on an edge; and each edge on the boundary of the surface belongs to exactly one facet's boundary.

The list of the n consecutive open arcs of the facet define an orientation on the edges and the facet. If we take the points in the reverse order we change the orientation. We say that the mesh is orientable when each edge of the mesh, considered as an edge of two distinct facets has two opposite orientations.If a mesh on a surface has F facets, E edges, and V vertices, the finite number :

$$\chi = F - E + V \qquad (1)$$

is called the Euler characteristic of the mesh. This relation is remarkable in the sense that the Euler characteristic is equal for any mesh on a given surface. Moreover, if two compact connected surfaces have the same number of boundaries, the same Euler number, and are both orientable or non-orientable they are homeomorphic [4].

---

[1] $M_{n+1} = M_1$.

415

3 Simplification of surfaces

In practice we have discrete 3D images and our goal is to obtain an orientable mesh. The standard approach is the Marching cubes algorithm, which partitions the volume into cubic cells. The original algorithm [5] used a look-up table procedure and exploited symmetry between one situation and the situation involving opposite voxels values. Unfortunately, this algorithm can produce holes in the surface, as pointed out by [11]. One way to cope with ambiguous configurations is to make sure that the edges interpolated on each face of a voxel remain the same while going on the adjacent voxel (for more details see [9]). In this case, the mesh which approximates the iso-surface has no holes, and is oriented. It is then possible to compute the principal curvatures of the mesh as expressions of the derivatives of $I(x, y, z)$ computed by a Gaussian convolution filter [6, 9].

Another approach to iso-surface extraction is the Wrapper algorithm [1, 2], which uses a decomposition into 5 tetrahedra of each cubic-cell and yields oriented triangulations with no hole.

The idea of our simplification algorithm is to perform basic operations which remove either vertices, edges or facets and which keep unchanged the topology of the surface. At each stage of a removal procedure we must check the following conditions for any connected component of the mesh :

- the result must be a mesh.
- the Euler characteristic must remain the same.
- the resulting mesh must be orientable.
- the number of connected components of the boundary must not change.

The basic procedure of our simplification algorithm consists of cutting edges. Edges are either interior edges or boundary edges. For the moment, we do not allow the removal of boundary edges. Consider an interior edge e with vertices M_1 and M_2 on an orientable mesh. Then $M_1 M_2$ is an oriented edge of some facet f_1 (with n_1 edges) and $M_2 M_1$ is an oriented edge of a facet f_2 (with n_2 edges). Suppose, for simplicity that $n_1 \geq n_2 > 0$ (if this is not the case, reverse M_1 and M_2). If we want to remove the edge e, several cases can occur :

- $M_1 = M_2$, so that $n_2 = 1$ and $f_1 \neq f_2$
    - if $n_1 = 1$, the mesh is a spherical mesh with one edge, one vertex and two facets : we can't remove the edge e on the mesh without changing its topology.
    - if $n_2 > 1$, we remove f_2 and $e = M_1 M_2$. The number of edges of f_1 becomes $n_1 - 1$, and the Euler number is preserved.
- $M_1 \neq M_2$ then $n_2 > 1$
    - if $f_1 = f_2$, we don't remove the edge.
    - if $f_1 \neq f_2$, and $n_2 = 2$ we can remove safely the edge e and the facet f_2 from the mesh and f_1 remains the same.
    - if $f_1 \neq f_2$ and $n_2 > 2$, let p_1 (respectively p_2) be the number of distinct edges which have M_1 (respectively M_2) in common. Since $f_1 \neq f_2$ we must have $p_1 > 1$ and $p_2 > 1$. Several sub-cases occur :

* p_1 and p_2 are > 2 : if we remove the edge e, we merge f_1 and f_2 into a new facet f with $n_1 + n_2 - 1$ edges. The number of distinct edges shared by M_1 (resp. M_2) becomes $p_1 - 1$ (resp $.p_2 - 1$).

* if $p_1 = 2$ (resp. $p_2 = 2$), let M_3 be the point distinct from M_1 and M_2 on the second edge coming to M_1 (resp. M_2) (because $n_2 > 2$). We can replace the edges $M_1 M_2$ and $M_1 M_3$ (resp $.M_2 M_3$) by a single edge $M_2 M_3$ (resp. $M_1 M_3$) and delete M_1 (resp. M_2) . During this operation the number of edges of f_1 and f_2 decrease by one, and since exactly one vertex and one edge on the mesh are removed, the Euler characteristic is preserved.

These conditions, can lead to strange situations such as meshes with facets reduced to either a single point or many points, or distinct edges shared by the same facet, which can be troublesome. Hence, we have added more conditions on our mesh :

- facets or vertices with one or two edges are not allowed (n_2, p_1 and p_2 are ≥ 3,).
- an edge shared by the same facet is not allowed ($f_1 \neq f_2$).
- facets with more than $N = 12$, and vertices with more than $P = 6$ edges, are not allowed.

More complex operations can be defined : removing a vertex and all the p distinct edges shared by it, can be done with the elementary edge removal procedure. Instead of removing edges on the mesh we could have performed the same operations on the dual mesh. The edge removing procedure on the dual mesh amounts to the same operation as merging the vertices of an edge of the mesh, while the dual operation of vertex removal is a facet deletion.

In practice, we have to find an efficient data structure to perform edge deletion. The doubly-connected-edge-list (DCEL) [7] is well suited to our problem. In each edge e we have the information about its vertices M_1, M_2, a pointer towards the two oriented facets f_1, f_2 that it belongs to, and also a pointer towards the previous edge in the oriented facets f_1, f_2.

4   Regularization stage

When many edges and vertices are removed from the mesh, the facets may become very irregular, elongated or may even have concavities. This is sometimes troublesome when applying a shading effect to the mesh. The basic idea to overcome this problem consists of moving the vertices of the mesh for a given number of iterations in order to minimize an energy function. In our case we use a spring energy [3] (Sum of the squared lengths of the edges of the mesh). When the neighbors of a given point are fixed, this can be achieved by moving the point towards the barycenter of its neighbors. The improvement consists of constraining the displacement of the point parallel to the average plane of its neighbors, and towards their barycenter (see figure 1).

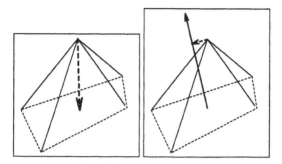

Fig. 1. left : basic regularization method , the point is moved towards the barycenter of its neighbors. right : our regularization method, the resulting point is the projection on the average normal of its neighbors

5 Experimental Results

In the first example, we performed the algorithm of simplification by removing edges and vertices at random on the iso-surface of a torus. The resulting mesh is very irregular. The use of a basic regularization algorithm leads to a dramatic shrinking effect after only 50 iterations. On the contrary, our regularization stage preserves the size and the shape of the object with the same number of iterations (see figures 2).

Finally, we applied our algorithms to a CT-Scan of a skull [2]. The original iso-surface mesh had about 160000 vertices, and more than half of the vertices were removed in flat areas (where maximum absolute value of the principal curvatures is low) (see figure 3).

6 Conclusion

In this paper we have presented a new algorithm for reducing the number of vertices on an irregular surface mesh. On real medical images, half of the vertices can be removed without losing quality. When a greater percentage of points are removed, the facets of the surface become very irregular. This problem is reduced by using a regularization step which consists in moving each point in its associated tangent plane. However the algorithm can still be improved, especially by taking into account the edges of the boundary.

Acknowledgments

The author thanks Serge Benayoun, Hervé Delingette and Grégoire Malandain for helpful discussions and remarks. Thanks also to Mike Brady for his review of the paper. This work was partially supported by Digital Equipment Corporation.

---

[2] Courtesy of Docteur Cutting and David Dean from New-York University Hospital

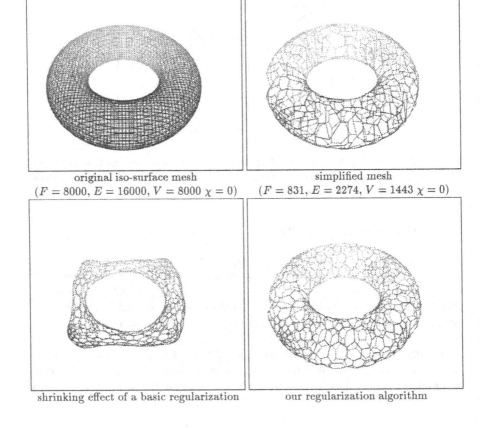

original iso-surface mesh
$(F = 8000, E = 16000, V = 8000 \; \chi = 0)$

simplified mesh
$(F = 831, E = 2274, V = 1443 \; \chi = 0)$

shrinking effect of a basic regularization

our regularization algorithm

Fig. 2. iso-surface of a torus (vertices were removed at random)

References

1. Akio Doi and Akio Koide. An efficient method of triangulating equi-valued surfaces by using tetrahedral cells. In *IEICE Transactions*, January 1991.
2. A. Guéziec and R. Hummel. The wrapper algorithm : Surface extraction and simplification. In *Proceedings of the IEEE Workshop on Biomedical Image Analysis*, June 1994.
3. H. Hoppe, T. De Rose, T. Duchamp, J. Mc Donald, and W. Stuetzle. Mesh optimization. In *Computer Graphics Proceedings, Annual Conference Series*, pages 19–25, August 1993.
4. D. Lehmann and C. Sacré. *Géométrie et topologie des surfaces*. Presses universitaires de France, 1982.
5. W. E. Lorensen and H. E. Cline. Marching cubes: A high resolution 3d surface reconstruction algorithm. *Computer Graphics*, 21(4), July 1987.

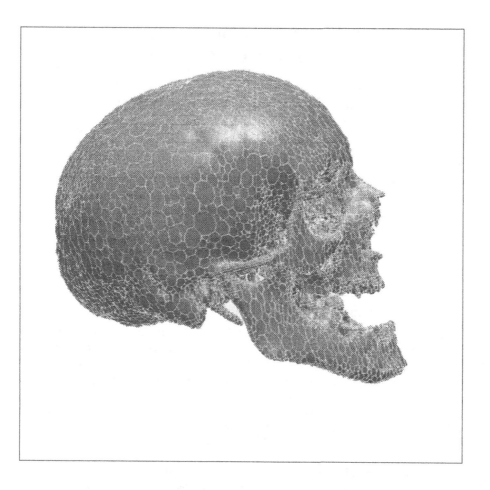

Fig. 3. Simplified and regularized mesh of a skull (vertices were removed in flat areas)

6. O. Monga and S. Benayoun. Using partial derivatives of 3d images to extract typical surface features. *rapport de recherche INRIA*, March 1992.
7. F. P. Preparata and M. I Shamos. *Computational Geometry : an Introduction.* Springer-Verlag, 1985.
8. W. J. Schroeder, J. A. Zarge, and Lorensen W. E. Decimation of triangles meshes. *Computer Graphics*, 26(2), July 1992.
9. J.-P. Thirion and A. Gourdon. The marching lines algorithm : new results and proofs. Technical Report 1881, INRIA, April 1993.
10. G. Turk. Re-tiling polygonal surfaces. *Computer Graphics*, 26(2), July 1992.
11. J. Wilhelms and A. Van Gelder. Topological ambiguities in isosurface generation. Technical Report UCSC-CRL-90-14, CIS Board, University of California, Santa Cruz, 1990.

Deformable Models for Reconstructing Unstructured 3D Data

María-Elena ALGORRI and Francis SCHMITT

Images Department, Télécom-Paris, 46 rue Barrault, 75634 Paris France

Abstract. We propose an algorithmic methodology that automatically produces a simplicial surface from a set of points in $\Re^3$ about which we have no topological knowledge. Our method uses a spatial decomposition and a surface tracking algorithm to produce a rough approximation **S'** of the unknown manifold **S**. The produced surface **S'** serves as a robust initialisation for a physically based modeling technique that will incorporate the fine details of **S** and improve the quality of the reconstruction.

1 Introduction

When choosing an algorithmic approach to reconstruct an unknown surface **S** from a set **P** of unstructured $3D$ points that samples the surface we must consider: 1) what information other than position is available on **P** (curvatures, normals, discontinuities, boundaries), 2) which class of surface is represented by **P** (closed or open, genus number), and 3) how **P** was originated (segmentation of parallel or non-parallel images, $3D$ scanning of an object,...). The constraints that an algorithmic approach imposes on **P** with respect to these three aspects determine the degree of generality of the algorithm.

As medical imaging technology provides larger and more complex databases, two approaches have proven general enough to deal efficiently with the problem of $3D$ reconstruction: 1) local techniques (i.e. marching cubes [1], particle systems [2]), and 2) deformable or physically based models (i.e. geometrically deformable models [3], adaptive meshes [4]).

Local techniques are able to reconstruct arbitrarily complex shapes to a good degree of accuracy. A drawback of these techniques is that they require additional information on the set of $3D$ points other than the position (normals, neighborhood information etc...)., for which some sort of pre-processing might be required. In [5] Hoppe et al. present a marching cubes algorithm modified for reconstructing unstructured $3D$ points rather than sets of $2D$ images which requires a pre-processing stage to estimate the oriented normals of the set of points.

Deformable models such as the $3D$ adaptive meshes in [4] and [6] require no additional information on **P** to reconstruct the underlying surface, but the type of surfaces they can reconstruct is usually limited to being homomorphic to the initial mesh: they start with a generic mesh (usually a sphere or cylinder) which is then deformed to recuperate the shape of **S**. In a post-processing stage some models incorporate holes and borders, or change the topology of the initial mesh [7]. In addition, global models might develop auto-intersections when reconstructing surfaces that fold over themselves or have complex topology. In [2] Szeliski et al. implement a physically based approach in the form of a system of interacting particles to reconstruct arbitrary shapes, but the inital orientations of the particles are crucial for the reconstruction and must be given as input.

Our motivation comes from the possibility of combining local techniques and deformable models to produce a robust reconstruction method that eliminates the hypotheses of additional information on **P** (in local techniques) and of homomorphism to the initial global mesh (in deformable models). We use a local technique to recuperate the initial topology of **P** and build a good initial model for a deformable adaptive mesh.

Problem Definition We address the problem of reconstructing a surface **S'** that approximates an unknown surface **S** using a set **P** of sample points in $\Re^3$ that provides partial information about **S**. We place ourselves in the situation where the set **P** satisfies the following density constraint: for any point s of **S**, its nearest point x∈**P** according to the point to point Euclidean distance in $\Re^3$, is also its nearest point x∈**P** according to the geodesic distance on the surface **S**. This implies that the maximal distance ρ between any two nearest points of **P** must be smaller than any hole, discontinuity or bending of **S**.

2 Model Initialization

The first step of the surface reconstruction algorithm consists of passing from the set **P** to a rough model **S'** containing the main topological characteristics of **S**. The initial model **S'** will then be used to initialize an adaptive mesh that will improve the quality of the reconstruction.

The initialization process takes as input the set **P** of points $x_1, x_2, \ldots, x_n \in \Re^3$, and the sampling step ρ. It performs a partitioning of the space into cubes with edges equal to ρ. In cases where a uniform sampling density can be guaranteed and where the size of discontinuities or holes of **S** is known to be more important than ρ, or when a model of lower accuracy is required, a compression factor can also be specified to increase the size of the spatial cubes. The algorithm then flags the cubes that are occupied by one or more points of **P**.

From the set of flaged cubes we build a cuberille, that is, a surface composed of all the exterior faces that are not shared by any two cubes. The cuberille defines a rough surface **S'** approximating **S**. To build the cuberille we use the surface extraction algorithm proposed by Gordon and Udupa [8] which tracks a closed surface from a set of connected cubes. This eliminates the cubes created by noisy points in the dataset (if they are at a distance $\delta > \rho$ from the data points in **P**). Figure 1a and 1c show two sets **P** of unstructured $3D$ points from the surface of a heart [1] and from a blood vessel [2] taken from two sets of $2D$ segmented images. Figures 1b and 1d show the cuberilles that were extracted from the spatial partitioning and that define the rough surfaces S'.

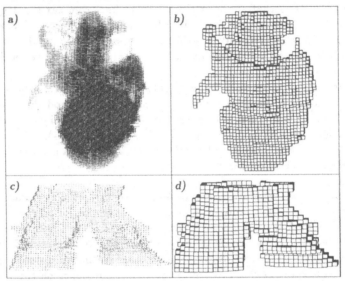

Fig. 1. a) A set **P** of unstructured $3D$ points from the surface of a heart (116,385 points). b) The approximated rough surface **S'** defined by the cuberille (8,202 squares). c) A set **P** of $3D$ points from a blood vessel (8,031 points). d) The extracted rough surface **S'** (6,330 squares).

We systematically triangulate the set of squares by splitting each square by one of its diagonals. We also integrate the information about the created triangles and their adjacencies into a triangulated mesh structure. The stepped surface **S'** of the triangulated cuberille incorporates the topological characteristics of **S** (including holes and discontinuities). It can be directly used as an initialization model for the adaptive mesh algorithm. However, to speed up the convergence of the adaptive mesh, we smooth the surface **S'** using a simple low pass filter. The low pass filter assigns to each triangle vertex a new position that is a weighted average of its old position and the position of its neighbors. Figures 2a and 2c show the systematic triangulations constructed on the rough surfaces **S'** of Figures 1b and 1d. Figures 2b and 2d show the smoothed surfaces **S'** obtained after applying the low pass filter to the initial triangulations.

3 Adaptive Mesh

The second stage of the reconstruction algorithm deforms the initial model **S'** to better conform to **S** and to recover the fine details not incorporated in the

---

[1] Made available by Eric Hoffman at University of Pennsylvania Medical School, and redistributed to us courtesy of Dimitry Goldgof at University of South Florida.

[2] Courtesy of C. Pellot and A. Hermet at INSERM U256, Hôpital Broussais, Paris.

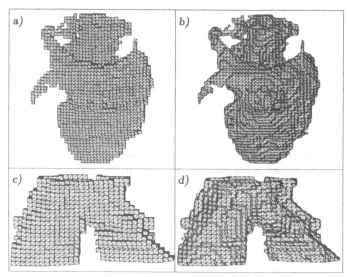

Fig. 2. a),c) The triangulations constructed on the cuberilles of Figures 2b and 2d. b),d) The smoothed surfaces **S'** after applying the low pass filter to the triangulations.

initialization procedure. In order to deform **S'** we will consider it as an adaptive mesh. We retake the mass-spring adaptive mesh model described in [4], [6].

In an adaptive mesh the 3D points are a set of forces that attracts and deforms the surrounding mesh. The mesh is a polyhedral structure and in our case a triangulated mesh. Each triangle vertex in **S'** is a nodal mass, and each triangle side an adjustable spring. Each nodal mass is attached to the data points by an imaginary spring. From the space partitioning scheme we know which data points are inside every cube and the triangles that were originated from it, thus we can establish a fast, local correspondance between **S'** and **P** as follows: for every vertex on **S'**, we search inside the cube from which it originated, and inside its 26-neighboring cubes, the point in **P** that is closest to the considered vertex. This correspondance is re-calculated at every iteration by searching inside the cube containing the point of **P** that was last assigned to a given vertex and inside its 26-neighboring cubes. By controlling the iteration time step δt so that the motion of a vertex remains smaller that ρ, we keep a correct correspondance as the vertices of **S'** move in time through the spatial cubes to adapt to **S**.

3.1 Overview of Dynamic Equations
In the adaptive mesh, the nodal masses react to forces coming from the data-points, and from the springs that interconnect them to ensure a coherent structural movement. Each nodal mass has a dynamic equation of the form:

$$\mu_i \frac{d^2 \mathbf{x}_i}{dt^2} + \gamma_i \frac{d\mathbf{x}_i}{dt} + \sum_{j=1}^{n} \kappa_j (\mathbf{x}_i - \mathbf{x}_j) + \kappa_d (\mathbf{x}_i - \mathbf{x}_d) = 0, \qquad (1)$$

where $\mathbf{x}_i$ is the 3D position $[x_i, y_i, z_i]^t$ of node i at time t, and μ_i and γ_i are the mass and damping values associated to node i. κ_j is the stiffness coefficient of the spring connecting node i to neighboring node j, and κ_d is the stiffness coefficient of the spring connecting node i to the database. We use springs of natural length equal to zero. The set of coupled equations is solved iteratively in time using the explicit Euler integration method until all masses reach an equilibrium position.

Adaptive meshes exhibit different types of behaviour (oscillatory, exponential) depending on the values of their dynamic parameters. By analyzing the stability of the coupled equations we can calculate the optimal values of the global parameters (κ, γ, μ) that ensure a stable, non-oscillatory behaviour of the nodes and optimize the convergence time. This analysis is computationally expensive, therefore, we solve the coupled system of equations using for every equation the values of the parameters that guarantee the stability of that equation when solved independently. That is, we obtain *approximated* parameter values by analyzing the stability of each nodal mass considering its neighboring masses fixed. We have verified experimentally that, in our reconstruction setting, such parameter values approximate well the optimal parameters.

We justify this approximation because: 1) we make the coupling forces on the nodes coming from the interconnecting springs weaker than the forces coming from **P**, and 2) our initial mesh is dense and already close to the data. Therefore, the movement of each node in relation to its neighboring nodes remains small.

Choice of the Parameter Values - The general solution of equation (1) is the sum of two components, a steady-state and a transient component [9].

The steady-state solution represents the final position of the nodal masses. The form of this solution is found by putting $\frac{d^2 \mathbf{x}_i}{dt^2} = \frac{d\mathbf{x}_i}{dt} = 0$ in equation (1)

$$\mathbf{x}_i \big(\kappa_d + \sum_{j=1}^{n} \kappa_j \big) = \mathbf{x}_d \kappa_d + \mathbf{x}_1 \kappa_1 + \mathbf{x}_2 \kappa_2 + \ldots + \mathbf{x}_n \kappa_n, \tag{2}$$

where we want to impose the condition that the final position of $\mathbf{x}_i$ be as close as possible to the database points: $\mathbf{x}_i \approx \mathbf{x}_d$.

We obtain the desired steady-state solution by manipulating the stiffness coefficients $\kappa_j, j = 1, \ldots, n$ of the n springs connected to node i to make their sum smaller than κ_d. This makes the influence of the coupling forces in the system weak relative to the external forces coming from **P**. In our approach we have obtained successful reconstructions by setting the values of κ_j to be between 1 and 2 orders of magnitude smaller than κ_d.

The transient component of the general solution determines the type of dynamics that nodal masses will exhibit. To determine the transient solution we rewrite equation (1) as:

$$\mu_i \frac{d^2 \mathbf{x}_i}{dt^2} + \gamma_i \frac{d\mathbf{x}_i}{dt} + \big(\kappa_d + \sum_{j=1}^{n} \kappa_j \big) \mathbf{x}_i = \mathbf{x}_d \kappa_d + \sum_{j=1}^{n} \mathbf{x}_j \kappa_j. \tag{3}$$

The terms on the right side are the forces acting on node i that depend on the position of the neighboring masses and of the points in $\mathbf{P}$ and are called the driving function. The terms on the left side involve x_i, and its derivatives, and are called the response function. The transient response is determined by solving the characteristic equation of the response function:

$$\mu_i \lambda^2 + \gamma_i \lambda + \left(\kappa_d + \sum_{j=1}^{n} \kappa_j\right) = 0, \tag{4}$$

$$\lambda_{1,2} = -\frac{\gamma_i}{2\mu_i} \pm \sqrt{\left(\frac{\gamma_i}{2\mu_i}\right)^2 - \frac{\left(\kappa_d + \sum_{j=1}^{n} \kappa_j\right)}{\mu_i}}. \tag{5}$$

If the value of the radical term in equation (5) is cancelled, the nodes will move as quickly as possible towards the equilibrium position. The corresponding value of γ_i is called critical damping value or γ_c and its value is equal to

$$\gamma_c = 2\sqrt{\left(\kappa_d + \sum_{j=1}^{n} \kappa_j\right)\mu_i}. \tag{6}$$

Figure 3 shows three results of reconstructing the same surface using varying damping values. The initial adaptive mesh is the filtered surface $\mathbf{S'}$ of Figure 2d (12,660 triangles). In Figure 3a we show the underdamped case, in 3b the critically damped case, and in 3d the overdamped case. In all three cases we let the adaptive mesh evolve for 15 iterations (number of iterations needed for the critically damped case to converge). Both the underdamped and the overdamped cases are still far from convergence after 15 iterations. Figure 4 shows the two final reconstructions obtained for our examples.

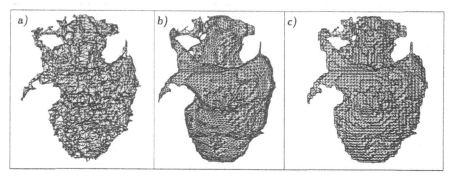

Fig. 3. Reconstruction example using different damping coefficients. a) Reconstruction with $\gamma = \frac{\gamma_c}{10}$. b) Reconstruction using $\gamma = \gamma_c$ where convergence is reached. c) Reconstruction using $\gamma = 5\gamma_c$ the mesh remains close to the initial position.

4 Conclusion

We have presented an algorithm that can automatically reconstruct arbitrary surfaces by using a technique of spatial decomposition and surface tracking as a robust initialization for an adapative mesh model. By combining two popular reconstruction methods we reduce the constraints on $\mathbf{P}$ and obtain a good

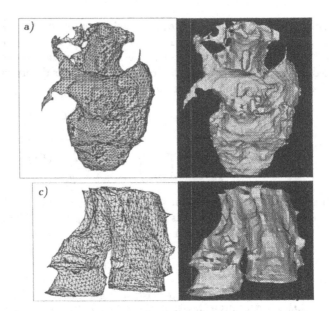

Fig. 4. The results of the reconstruction algorithm. a) The final triangulation of the dog's heart consisting of 16,404 triangles. b) The triangulation of the dog's heart as a shaded image. c) The final triangulation of the blood vessel consisting of 12,660 triangles. d)The triangulation of the blood vessel as a shaded image.

approximation of the surface **S** sampled by a set of dense but unstructured $3D$ points. Because of its flexibility in reconstructing different topologies, our method is a good tool for unsupervised reconstruction after segmentation of a set of images or for visualising the surface of acquired $3D$ points.

References

[1] W. E. Lorensen, H. E. Cline, "Marching Cubes: A High Resolution 3D Surface Construction Algorithm", *SIGGRAPH '87*, Vol. 21, $N°4$, pp. 163–169, 1987

[2] R. Szeliski, D. Tonnesen, D. Terzopoulos, "Modeling Surfaces of Arbitrary Topology with dynamic particles", *Proc. CVPR '93*, pp. 82–87, New York, June 1993

[3] J. V. Miller, D. E. Breen, W. E. Lorensen, R. M. O'Bara, M. J. Wozny, "Geometrically Deformed Models: A Method for Extracting Closed Geometric Models from Volume Data", *SIGGRAPH '91*, Vol. 25, $N°4$, pp. 217–225, 1991

[4] M. Vasilescu, D. Terzopoulos, "Adaptive Meshes and Shells: Irregular Triangulation, Discontinuities, and Hierarchical Subdiv.", *Proc. CVPR'92*, pp. 829–832, 1992

[5] H. Hoppe, T. de Rose, T. Duchamp, J. McDonald, W. Stuetzle, "Surface Reconstruction from Unorganized Points", *SIGGRAPH '92*, Vol. 26, $N°2$, pp. 71–78, 1992

[6] W-C.Huang, D. B. Goldgof, "Sampling and Surface Reconstruction with Adaptive-Size Meshes", *Proc. SPIE Appl. of Art. Intell. X*, Vol. 1708, pp. 760–770, 1992

[7] H. Delinguette, "Modelisation, Déformation et Reconnaissance d'Objets Tridimensionnels à l'aide de Maillages Simplexes", Ph.D. thesis, Ecole Centrale Paris, 1994

[8] D. Gordon, J. Udupa, "Fast Surface Tracking in Three-Dimensional Binary Images", *Computer Vision, Graphics, and Image Processing*, Vol. 45, pp. 196–214, 1989

[9] J. D'azzo, C. Houpis, "Linear Control System Analysis", McGraw-Hill, 1981

Posters II

Segmentation of Brain Tissue from MR Images

T. Kapur – tkapur@ai.mit.edu[1]
W. E. L. Grimson – welg@ai.mit.edu[1]
R. Kikinis – kikinis@bwh.harvard.edu[2]

[1] Massachusetts Institute of Technology, Cambridge, MA 02139, USA
[2] Harvard Medical School, Boston MA 02115, USA

Abstract. Segmentation of medical imagery is a challenging problem due to the complexity of the images, as well as to the absence of models of the anatomy that fully capture the possible deformations in each structure. In this paper, we present a method for segmentation of a particularly complex structure, the brain tissue, from MRI. Our method is a combination of three existing techniques from the Computer Vision literature: adaptive segmentation, binary morphology, and active contour models. Each of these techniques has been customized for the problem of brain tissue segmentation from gradient echo images, and the resultant method is more robust than its components. We present the results of a parallel implementation of this method on IBM's supercomputer Power Visualization System for a database of 10 brains each with 256x256x124 voxels.

1 Introduction

We are interested in the problem of segmentation of brain tissue from magnetic resonance images, which is an interesting and important step for many medical imaging applications (see [1] for examples). In this paper, we present a method that is a combination of existing techniques from Computer Vision that have been customized for the task at hand, including a combination of intensity based classifiers, morphological operators and explicit shape constraints.

2 Background

This section presents background on two of the techniques we cascade in our method: *adaptive segmentation* and *deformable contours*. The third technique, *binary morphology* is a standard image processing operation that is discussed in detail in [2].

2.1 Adaptive Segmentation

Adaptive Segmentation is a recently developed, powerful technique for simultaneous tissue classification and gain field estimation in magnetic resonance images [3]. Traditional intensity based segmentation relies on elements of the same tissue type having MR intensities that are clustered around a mean characteristic value, and relies on each cluster being well separated from other tissue clusters. Most MR scanners, however, have inhomogeneities in the imaging equipment, which give rise to a smoothly varying, non-linear gain field. While the human visual system easily compensates for this field, the gain can perturb the intensity distributions, causing them to overlap significantly and thus lead to substantial misclassification in traditional intensity based classification methods.

In Adaptive Segmentation, a Parzen density function is constructed using training points for each of the tissue classes to be identified, and then an algorithm similar to the Estimation-Maximization algorithm is used to iteratively obtain tissue classification and a gain field estimate. A smoothness constraint on the gain field is imposed in the process. By obtaining an estimate of the gain field, the classifier can normalize the intensities to make classification more robust.

2.2 Deformable Contour Models

A deformable contour is a planar curve which has an initial position and an objective function associated with it. A special class of deformable contours called *snakes* was introduced by Witkin, Kass and Terzopoulos [4] in which the initial position is specified interactively by the user and the objective function is referred to as the *energy* of the snake. This energy of the snake (E_{snake}) is expressed as:

$$E_{\text{snake}} = E_{\text{internal}} + E_{\text{external}} \ . \tag{1}$$

The internal energy term imposes a regularization constraint on the contour as follows:

$$E_{\text{internal}} = \int_s \left(w_1(s)||v'(s)||^2 + w_2(s)||v''(s)||^2 \right) ds \ , \tag{2}$$

where s is arclength, derivatives are with respect to s, and $v(s)$ stands for the ordered pair $(x(s), y(s))$, which denotes a point along the contour. The choice of w_1 and w_2 reflects the penalty associated with first and second derivatives along the contour respectively.

The external energy term in Equation 1 is responsible for attracting the snake to interesting features in the image. The exact expression for E_{external} depends on the characteristics of the features of interest.

Finding a local minima for E_{snake} from equation 1 corresponds to solving the following Euler-Lagrange equation for v:

$$- (w_1 v')' + (w_2 v'')'' + \nabla E_{\text{external}}(v) = 0 \ . \tag{3}$$

with boundary conditions specifying if the snake is a closed contour, or the derivatives are discontinuous at the end points. This equation is then written in matrix form as $Av = F$, where $F(v) = - \nabla E_{\text{external}}$. Here A is a pentadiagonal banded matrix, v is the position vector of the snake, and F is gradient of the external energy of the snake, or the external force acting on it. The evolution equation $\frac{dv}{dt} - Av = F$ is solved to obtain the v that is closest to the initial position. As $\frac{dv}{dt}$ tends to zero, we get a solution to the system $Av = F$.

Formulating this evolution problem using finite differences with time step τ, we obtain a system of the form [5]:

$$(I + \tau A)v^t = v^{t-1} + \tau F(v^{t-1}) \; , \tag{4}$$

where v^t denotes the position vector of the snake at time t, and I is the identity matrix. The system is considered to have reached equilibrium when the difference between v^t and v^{t-1} is below some threshold.

The balloon model for deformable contours is introduces improvements on the snake model [5]. It modifies the the snake energy to include a "balloon" force, which can either be an inflation force, or a deflation force. The external force F is changed to

$$F = k_1 \mathbf{n}(s) + k \frac{\nabla E_{\text{external}}}{\|\nabla E_{\text{external}}\|} \; , \tag{5}$$

where $\mathbf{n}(s)$ is a unit vector normal to the contour at point $v(s)$, and $|k_1|$ is the amplitude of this normal force.

3 Our Method

We constructed a model for the brain based on expert opinion from Harvard Medical School, and this model is implicit in the segmentation method described below. See [1] for details of the model.

Gain Correction: Initially, we use Adaptive Segmentation to correct for the gain introduced in the data by the imaging equipment. We use a single channel, non-parametric, multi-class implementation of the segmenter that is described in [3]. Training points are used for white matter, grey matter, csf and skin, and therefore the resultant tissue classifications correspond to these four classes. The output of this stage is a set of classified voxels.

Removal of Thin Connectors Using Morphological Operations: We use the following sequence of morphological and connectivity operations to incorporate topological information into the tissue-labeled image obtained from Adaptive Segmentation. First we perform an erosion operation on the input with a spherical structuring element with radius corresponding to the thickness of the connectors between brain and the cranium, so that it eliminates connections from the brain to any misclassified non-brain structure. Then we find the largest connected component with tissue labels corresponding to the brain. And as a third step we dilate the brain component obtained in the previous step by a structuring element comparable in size to the one used in the erosion, conditioned on the brain labels in the input image. This corresponds approximately to restoring the boundary of the brain component that were distorted in the erosion step.

The results of this stage is an improved segmentation of the tissue types, which incorporates topological information, and which has removed some of the artifacts due to pure intensity classification.

Extraction of Brain Surface using Balloon Model: The third step in our segmentation algorithm is the use of a modified balloon model to refine the result of the brain tissue estimate obtained using morphological operations since morphology is often unable to remove all connectors from the brain to the cranium. The intuition behind this step is to incorporate substantial spatial information into the segmentation process via the manual initialization of the brain boundary in a few slices and use that to refine the results obtained thus far. We model the brain surface as a set of adjacent boundary contours for each slice of the scanned volume and use deformable contours to find each of these contours.

We customized the balloon model to exploit the estimate of the brain volume created using the first two steps of our segmentation process. Instead of using a fixed predetermined direction for the balloon force by selecting a sign for the factor k_1 in Equation 5 which is independent of the image characteristics, we define a signed balloon force direction vector, B, with one entry per voxel of the input data. The sign at the ith position of vector B indicates whether the voxel i exerts a force along the inward or outward normal to the evolving contour. This vector B is determined using the brain estimate obtained in the previous morphology step. If voxel i is classified as brain tissue at the end of the morphological routines, then B[i] gets a positive sign, so that the voxel pushes the contour in the direction of the normal towards the boundary of the brain estimate, otherwise B[i] gets a negative sign. The image force is:

$$F = k_1 B(s)\mathbf{n}(s) + k\frac{\nabla E_{\text{external}}}{||\nabla E_{\text{external}}||} , \tag{6}$$

where $B(s)$ is the direction of the balloon force exerted by the image at the point $v(s)$ of the contour, and $\mathbf{n}(s)$ is the normal to the local tangent vector to the contour at s. The unsigned constant k_1 is used to determine the magnitude of the balloon force. This force is used with the same evolution equation as before.

4   Results

We have used our segmentation method to successfully segment several gradient echo data sets. Table 1 quantifies our results for 10 data sets, each of 256x256x124 voxels, by presenting a percentage difference in classification of brain tissue generated by our method when compared with the brain tissue volume generated by an expert on the same data. The validation problem is explored in more detail in [1], [3].

Two views from a 3D reconstruction of the results of our segmenter on a representative data set are shown in the top row of Figure 1, and the same views reconstructed from a manual segmentations for the same data set are shown in the bottom row of the figure.

Case #	1	2	3	4	5	6	7	8	9	10
% Difference	4.6	13.6	10.5	12.3	12.0	0.2	0.5	1.5	2.2	9.6

Table 1. Comparison of Brain Volume with Manual Segmentations

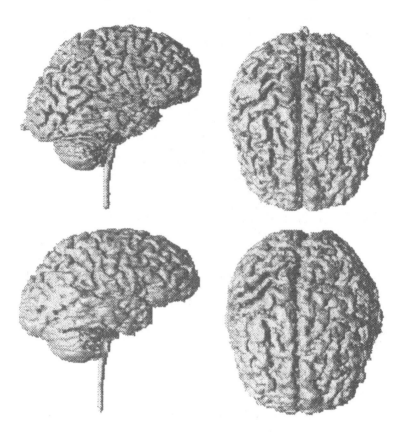

Fig. 1. Results of Our Method (Top Row) vs. Manual Segmentation (Bottom Row)

References

1. T. Kapur. *Segmentation of Brain Tissue from Magnetic Resonance Images.* Master's Thesis, Massachusetts Institute of Technology, Cambridge, MA, 1995.
2. J. Serra. *Image Analysis and Mathematical Morphology.* London:Academic, 1982.
3. W. Wells, R. Kikinis, W. Grimson, and F. Jolesz. Statistical Intensity Correction and Segmentation of Magnetic Resonance Image Data. In *Proceedings of the Third Conference on Visualization in Biomedical Computing.* SPIE, 1994. to appear.
4. A. Witkin, M. Kass, and D. Terzopoulos. Snakes: Active contour models. *International Journal of Computer Vision,* 1(4):321–331, june 1988.
5. L. Cohen. On active contour models and balloons. *Computer Vision, Graphics and Image Processing: Image Understanding,* 53(2):211–218, march 1991.

Shock-Based Reaction-Diffusion Bubbles for Image Segmentation

Hüseyin Tek[1] and Benjamin B. Kimia[1]

Brown University, Division of Engineering, Providence, RI 02912 USA

Abstract. Figure-Ground segmentation is a fundamental problem in computer vision. Active contours in the form of snakes, balloons, and level-set modeling techniques have been proposed that satisfactorily address this question for certain applications, but require manual initialization, do not always perform well near sharp protrusions or indentations, or often cross gaps. We propose an approach inspired by these methods and a shock-based representation of shape. Since initially it is not clear where the objects or their parts are, they are *hypothesized* in the form of fourth order shocks randomly initialized in homogeneous areas of images which then form evolving contours, or *bubbles*, which grow, shrink, merge, split and disappear to capture the objects in the image. In the homogeneous areas of the image bubbles deform by a reaction-diffusion process. In the inhomogeneous areas, indicated by differential properties computed from low-level processes such as edge-detection, texture, optical-flow and stereo, *etc.*, bubbles do not deform. As such, the randomly initialized bubbles *integrate* low-level information, and in the process segment figures from ground. The bubble technique does not require manual initialization, integrates a variety of visual information, and deals with gaps of information to capture objects in an image, as illustrated on several MRI and ultrasound images in 2D and 3D. [1].

1 Introduction

Figure-Ground segmentation is a fundamental problem in computer vision and presents a bottleneck to the recovery of objects from images. Active contours [3], or snakes, are energy minimizing controlled continuity splines which deform under the influence of internal forces, external image forces, and user provided constraints. This technique has proven useful for tracking objects once an active contour, or "snake", has been initialized by the user near the object. There are several problems associated with this approach and some of its problems has been addressed extensively; see [8] for a brief review.

Two excellent approaches have been proposed that address fundamental difficulties with snakes, and inspire our research as presented in this paper. First, Cohen and Cohen [2] introduced the idea of "balloons" as a way of resolving the *initialization* and *stability* problems associated with snakes. They added an "inflation force" to push the snake along the normal to object boundaries, and normalized the image forces to prevent instabilities, which greatly improved the performance of active contours. Despite these improvements, however, certain issues remain unresolved: 1) balloons (as well as snakes) cannot easily handle *topological*

---

[1] The authors gratefully acknowledge the support of NSF under grant IRI-9305630.

changes such as merging or splitting; 2) balloons do not capture sharp *protrusions or indentations* because of arc-length and curvature minimization properties; 3) it is not clear how to choose the *inflation force*: on the one hand, a high value pushes the balloon over the boundary or gaps; on the other hand, a low value will not be sufficient to push the balloon over weak edges; and 4) the balloon method can require extensive user interaction since the user is required to initialize a balloon for each object in the image, see Figure 4.

The second approach was proposed independently by Caselles *et al.* [1] and Malladi *et al.* [6] and views a snake as an evolving contour which is the level set of some surface. The level set approach was proposed by Osher and Sethian for flame propagation [7], introduced to computer vision in [4, 5] for shape representation, and first applied to active contours in [1, 6]. The latter approach considers a curve $\mathcal{C}$ as the zero level set of a surface, $\phi(x, y) = 0$, evolving under constant and curvature deformation modulated by an image based speed term, $S(x, y)$ which is inversely proportional to intensity gradient, $\phi_t + S(x, y)(\beta_0 - \beta_1 \kappa(x, y))|\nabla \phi| = 0$ where β_0 and β_1 are constants and κ curvature of the level set. Unlike snakes, this active contour model is intrinsic, stable, *i.e.*, the PDE satisfies the maximum principle, and can handle topological changes such as merging and splitting without any computational difficulty [1, 6]. Several difficulties remain, however: *1. Symmetric initialization:* This approach works well if the initial contour is placed nearly symmetrically with respect to the boundaries of interest, so that level set reaches object boundaries almost at the same time, otherwise it will cross over due to small but nonzero speed term, Figure 3b. *2. Multiple initialization:* A single level set may not capture the object of interests if the initial contour is embedded in an intermediate object, Figure 3c. *3. Narrow Regions:* The level sets sometimes fail to penetrate into narrow regions. *4. Direction of flow of the level set:* The user has to initially choose a direction of flow for the level set, either outwards or inwards. *5. Gaps on the boundaries:* If there are gaps on the object boundaries, the evolving contour will simply pass over them so that objects represented by incomplete contours are not captured. This is a serious problem in that in realistic medical images there are often gaps of information, *e.g.*, in edges of the ultrasound image of Figure 3e. In this approach, a user is required to place initial level sets in the image. Thus, like snakes and balloons, this approach is also semi-automatic in that extensive interaction is required by a knowledgable user if multiple objects are present in the image. It is highly desirable to remove such interaction and dependencies as much as possible. We now present an approach that addresses some of these difficulties.

2 Reaction-Diffusion Bubbles

In this section, we present an approach for capturing objects in an image which resolves some of the these difficulties. It derives from a shock-based morphogenetic dynamic representation of shape, formed from a reaction-diffusion process for deforming shape equation, $\frac{\partial \mathcal{C}}{\partial t} = (\beta_0 - \beta_1 \kappa)\mathbf{N}$, in the course of which four types of shocks form. A **first-order** shock forms when curvature flows into a curvature extremum and eventually leads to an orientation discontinuity; a **second-order** shock forms when two distinct non-boundary points join, leading to topological changes; a **third-order** shock forms when two separate pieces of the boundary meet along a contour; a **fourth-order** shock forms when an entire closed boundary collapses into a single point. The key idea is to view shape as a morphogenetic sequence [2] in reverse time, Figure 1.

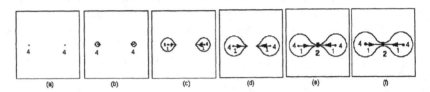

Fig. 1. This figure illustrates a morphogenetic view of shape as being reconstructed from its shock-based representation. First two first-order shocks are born, (a), then these shocks grow and are modified by first-order shocks, (b), (c), and (d). These two parts join at the second order shocks, (e) and the shape finally reconstructed, (f).

Typically, however, the segmentation of shapes in an image is a fundamentally difficult problem, so that complete information about figures as distinct from their background is often not available. Observe that fourth-order shocks represent components of an object, in that their birth initializes evolving contours, which will be modified by other types of shocks. As such, placing a fourth-order shock in an image is tantamount to *hypothesizing* an object component: Image-based information from low-level visual processes is then used to validate, annihilate, or modify these initial hypotheses. The fourth-order shocks in their initial stage of growth resemble "bubbles" which grow, shrink, merge, split, and disappear. When a portion of the boundary of a bubble approaches differential structures, as indicated by measures such as high gradients of intensity (edges), texture, stereo disparity, optical flow, *etc.* , it slows down, while other portions of its boundary deform without inhibition, see [8] for details.

The deformation of bubbles in the reaction-diffusion space involves two extremes: on the one hand, in the reaction process, the bubbles are breakable structures that can easily form singularities, grow into narrow straits, and shrinks onto sharp pointed structures. On the other hand, in the diffusion process, bubbles are cohesive structures that do not easily form singularities, and as such do not easily go through gaps, nor respond to small ripples or noise on the object boundaries. The full space, therefore, represents a spectrum of structures that is captured from the image: the reaction process captures *detailed* structure from *complete* information provided by low-level processes, while the diffusion process captures *coarse* boundary structure from *incomplete* information, *e.g.*, boundaries with small gaps, Figure 2. In addition reaction diffusion interaction also places the captured boundaries in a *hierarchy of significance*.

Experimental results illustrate how the bubble technique deals with problems mentioned earlier, Figures 2, and yields an automatic segmentation of medical images. Contours resulting from the reaction-diffusion process can be traced, grouped, and used to segment the image into meaningful regions, as colored image 4. This framework is extended to 3D in [9], see Figure 2. See [8] for implementation details.

---

[2] Much of the inspiration for this view can be found in Koenderink, Dynamic Shape, 1986

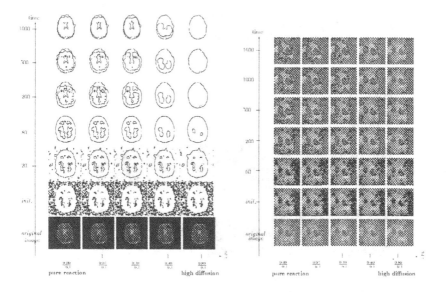

Fig. 2. This figure shows the reaction-diffusion process for MRI and unltrasound images. Each column depicts an evolution from the original image on the bottom row, using a random initialization, converging to the image, on the top row. The left column is evolution by reaction, the right by high diffusion, and the intermediate columns, by combinations. Note the effect of diffusion on gaps and coarse-to-fine structure.

References

1. V. Caselles, F. Catte, T. Coll, and F. Dibos. A geometric model for active contours in image processing. Technical Report No 9210, CEREMADE, 1992.
2. L. D. Cohen. On active contour models. *CVGIP*, 53:211–218, 1991.
3. M. Kass, A. Witkin, and D. Terzopoulos. Snakes: Active contour models. *IJCV*, 1:321–331, 1987.
4. B. B. Kimia, A. R. Tannenbaum, and S. W. Zucker. Toward a computational theory of shape: An overview. In *ECCV*, Antibes, France, 1990.
5. - Shapes, shocks, and deformations, I. *IJCV*, To Appear.
6. R. Malladi, J. A. Sethian, and B. C. Vemuri. Evolutionary fronts for topology-independent shape modelling and recovery. In *ECCV*, pages 3–13, 1994.
7. S. Osher and J. Sethian. Fronts propagating with curvature dependent speed. *Journal of Computational Physics*, 79:12–49, 1988.
8. H. Tek and B. B. Kimia. Shock-based reaction-diffusion bubbles for image segmentation. Technical Report LEMS-138, Brown Unversity, August, 1994.
9. H. Tek and B. B. Kimia. 3D medical image segmentation. Brown U. TR, Jan 95.

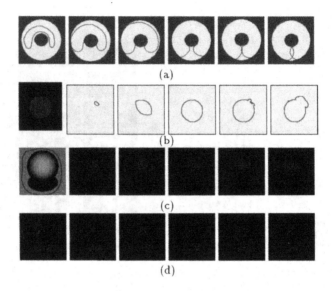

Fig. 3. This figure shows some of the problems associated with active contours: (a) Shows that balloons or snakes cannot handle topological changes. (b) Shows the *nearly symmetric initialization constraint* for level set evolution. (c) Illustrates problems associated with a single level set initialization. (d) The level set will cross over the gaps or low intensity gradient regions.

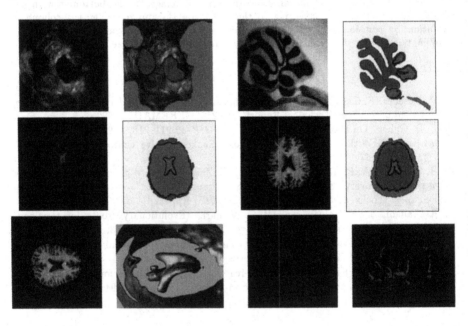

Fig. 4. This figure illustrates the application of bubbles on various images, with the original image on the left, and the segmented image on the right. The last row depicts segmentations of 3D data, with a single slice shown on the left.

MRI Texture Analysis Applied to Trabecular Bone An Experimental Study

Johanne Bezy-Wendling, Alain Bruno, Patrick Reuze

Laboratoire Traitement du Signal et de l'Image, INSERM, Université de Rennes 1, Bat.22
35042 Rennes Cedex, France

Abstract. This paper is aimed at showing the potential interest of texture analysis in Magnetic Resonance images of tissues. In the first section, the texture analysis methods are briefly described : morphological granulometry and the Run Length method. The first one is applied to in vivo images of the wrist and the second one to ex vivo images of vertebrae, in order to characterize the trabecular bone structure. Texture analysis allows to assess information on the trabeculae thicknesses and the sizes of the inter-trabeculae spaces.

1. Introduction

Bone density measurements are usually used to study bone strength which significantly decreases in bone diseases like osteoporosis. However bone mechanical properties are not only depending on bone mass but also related to the structure of trabecular bone, i.e. the architecture of trabeculae. This architecture is of major importance in the evaluation of bone diseases and can be assessed by Magnetic Resonance Imaging (MRI). Quantitative information on trabeculae and inter-trabecular spaces can be obtained by analyzing MR images.

The study of trabecular bone presented in this paper is performed by means of texture analysis methods. Textural components play an important role in medical imaging and texture analysis applied to MR images has a high medical added value : it allows the detection, the quantification and the follow-up of a disease.

In this paper, texture analysis is applied to trabecular bone from two body sites : wrist and vertebrae.

The first section presents the trabecular bone evolution with disease development, the two applications of texture analysis we carried out and, in a second step, the two texture analysis methods we chose to applied (Morphological Granulometry and the Run Length Method). In the second section, the results are discussed and the perspectives are presented.

2. Materials and methods

2.1. Materials

The present study reports two applications. The first one deals with bones located in the wrist (Fig.2) and the second one is on vertebrae (Fig.3). Both applications have in common the image type (MR) and the tissue type (trabecular bone). But they are also quite different : the first application presents the advantage of being an "in vivo" problem, while the second one is still, for now, an "ex vivo" study. Trabecular bone is a site of great interest for the assessment of bone metabolic diseases (like osteoporosis) evolution : it is formed by a three dimensional network of small bone plates, called trabeculae, which are separated by spaces containing red marrow. When the disease develops, trabeculae become thinner, can be perfored and disappear, so that the distance between them - the size of marrow spaces - increase. In the table n°1, the images used in the two applications are described.

First application :	Second application :
Wrist in the coronal plane (Fig.2)	8 Vertebrae in the transversal plane
Bruker MR system 2,4 T	(Fig.3) - MR system 4,7 T - spin echo
gradient sequence - Slice thickness	sequence - Slice thickness 0,5mm -
1,5mm - FOV: 8x8 cm^2 - 256^2 matrix	FOV: 8x8 cm^2 - 512^2 matrix
Resol : 0,3 mm.	Resol : 0,15 mm.
	Vertebrae removed, cleaned, embedded in
	a physiological solution (0,9% NaCl)

Table n°1 : Images used in the two applications of the study.

2.2. Methods

The gray level run length method

This is a well known texture analysis method described in (Galloway,1975) and (Dasarathy,1991). We decided to applied it because of the bone characteristics we wanted to assess : the trabeculae thickness and the inter-trabeculae spaces. These two parameters are both lengths and the Run Length Method is certainly well adapted to compute them.

Mathematical Morphology

Mathematical morphology (Serra,1982) is an important branch of image analysis. In the morphological granulometry method (Chen,1993), the image is considered as a collection of grains with different sizes, and the application of successive openings, with structuring elements becoming larger and larger tends to suppress the image objects (the grains) smaller than the structuring element. Two functions are used to characterize the size distribution : the distribution function and the density function, whose first and second moments are the features generally used in the texture characterization. It is the grainy texture of our particular images that lead us to applied this method.

3. Results

3.1. First application

In the first application we attempted to make the difference between a normal trabecular bone and an osteoporotic trabecular bone, using morphological granulometry. We applied this particular texture analysis method to NMR images of the wrist. Normal trabecular bone contains a great number of trabeculae, giving to the image a grainy and coarse texture. The ROI n°1 (Fig.2) situated in the distal radius, was chosen to represent this kind of bone structure. In the case of bone touched by osteoporosis, trabeculae disappear and marrow spaces extend. A ROI defined in a carpal bone was chosen to represent the osteoporotic process, because it contains a kind of cystic lesion, in which there are no more trabeculae (ROI n°2).

A morphological granulometry was applied to both ROI, with the same sequence of ten flat structuring elements. The distribution function and the density function were locally estimated. Two moments of the density function can be assigned to each pixel: the histogram mean value m and its standard deviation σ. Figure 2 presents the two sets of points obtained when the pixels are represented by their (m_x, σ_x) vector. The classes are kept apart.

Then we classified pixels of both ROIs using the k-nearest neighbors method. We obtained a good classification rate of 94,4% for the radius and 82,2% for the carpal bone when the classified ROIs are the same than those used for the learning and 90,86% for the radius and 61,8% for the carpal bone when the classified ROIs are different.

The co-occurrence matrices method (Conners,1980) was also applied to the ROIs defined on the image. The standard co-occurrence features were computed (standard deviation, homogeneity, contrast, entropy, energy...) and a classification based on the Mahalanobis distance has been applied. The results of this classification were in all the cases lower than the previous ones.

Making the difference between normal trabecular bone and extremely osteoporotic trabecular bone by applying texture analysis methods is obviously an important step in the in vivo study of osteoporosis. However, what we would like to do finally is to assess the development degree of the disease and so to have an accurate quantitative information on the trabecular bone. For this reason, the NMR images of vertebrae used in the second application are very relevant.

3.2. Second application

In this application we worked on eight MR images of vertebrae whose samples are presented on figure 4. Two texture analysis methods were applied to these images : a Markov Random Field model and the Run Length method but the MRF model does not provide interesting results and they are not presented here (Bezy-Wendling,1994). First, the images were binarized. Indeed, it makes the analysis easier without loosing any important information because of the bimodal form of their gray level histogram.

Size of the marrow spaces

We first calculate the Run Length in the four standard directions : 0°, 45°, 90°, 135°. Then, in a second step two important parameters are associated to each pixel:
- the minimum run length over the four directions, lmin,
- the maximum run length over the four directions, lmax.

The first parameter is obviously related to the size of the marrow spaces, given that if the minimum run length has a high value so all the run lengths (of the four directions) are long and thus the pixel belongs to a large cavity. The second parameter is used to underscore the long spaces, what is not so easy with the minimum run length. Indeed, the minimum run length associated to a pixel situated in a long cavity can have a small value and it is not always sufficient to detect long cavities.

It is now possible to assign a gray level to each value of lmin and lmax to get a visual representation of these parameters. Figure 3 shows a lmin map obtained for the vertebra n°2. On this map, the highest gray levels correspond to the largest marrow spaces.

Then, histograms of run lengths have also been calculated to complete the previous representation. Two of these histograms are shown on figure 6. Such histograms represent the number of runs of a certain length.

The mean and the standard deviation of these histograms relate to the size of the marrow spaces and the homogeneity of the image texture and consequently to the bone structure.

Trabeculae thickness

Finally, the run length method is also used to assess trabeculae thicknesses. For a pixel belonging to a trabecula, the minimum length over the four directions is equal to the trabecula thickness. An histogram of the trabeculae thickness can be computed (Fig.5). It clearly shows the vertebrae with the thickest trabeculae and those with the finest ones. This is a very important information for the physicians because it reflects the bone quality.

The run length method gives interesting results for the assessment of two very important characteristics of trabecular bone, which are the trabeculae thickness and the size of the inter-trabeculae spaces. The knowledge of these parameters is of major importance in the trabecular bone structure analysis and also in the evaluation of bone health.

4. Conclusion

An analysis of trabecular bone was performed on MR images, using different texture analysis methods with the aim of characterizing bone structure. Morphological granulometry applied to images of the wrist provided information on the size of bone elements. The Run Length Method provided accurate information on two important characteristics of trabecular bone : trabeculae thickness and marrow spaces size.

The medical interest of the present study consists in the characterization of vertebrae structure which allows the detection of bone diseases (like osteoporosis).

Future works will be based on in vivo images of vertebrae and aimed at analysing not only trabeculae but also marrow in the inter-trabeculae spaces and at linking parameters obtained from the two image types (wrist and vertebrae), all together.

Acknowlegments

The authors thank Dr de Certaines (MR Laboratory of Rennes, France) for his continuous support and Dr Luypert and Dr Allein (Biomedical MR Unit, Brussels, Belgium) for the vertebrae images.

References

(**Bezy-Wendling,1994**) Analyse de Texture, Application de la Modélisation par Champ Aléatoire de Markov et de la Méthode des Longueurs de Plages à des Images R.M.N. de Vertèbres, Rapport de DEA, juillet 1994.

(**Chen,1993**) Classification of Trabecular Structures in Magnetic Resonance Images Based on Morphological Granulometries, Magn. Reson. Med., 1993, 29 : 358-70.

(**Conners,1980**) A theorical Comparison of Texture Algorithms, IEEE Trans. Pat. Anal. Mach. Int., May, 1980, 3 : 204-222.

(**Dasarathy,1991**) Image Characterizations Based on Joint Gray Level-Run Length Distributions, Pattern Recognition Letters, 1991, 12 : 497-502.

(**Galloway,1975**) Texture Analysis Using Gray Level Run Lengths, Computer Graphics Image Processing, June 1975, 4 : 172-179.

(**Serra,1982**) Image Analysis and Mathematical Morphology, Serra J., Academic Press, 1982.

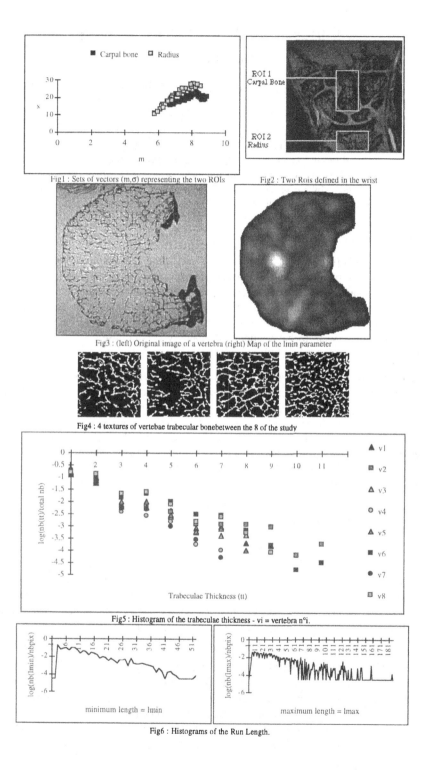

Fig1 : Sets of vectors (m,σ) representing the two ROIs

Fig2 : Two Rois defined in the wrist

Fig3 : (left) Original image of a vertebra (right) Map of the lmin parameter

Fig4 : 4 textures of vertebae trabecular bonebetween the 8 of the study

Fig5 : Histogram of the trabeculae thickness - vi = vertebra n°i.

Fig6 : Histograms of the Run Length.

Object-Based 3D X-Ray Imaging

Ralph. Benjamin

Centre for Biological and Medical Systems, Imperial College, London SW7 2BX, England

Abstract. A form of 3D X-ray imaging is introduced, in which the subject material is represented as discrete "objects". The surfaces of these objects are derived, accurately and in a novel way, from their outlines in about 10 views, distributed in solid angle, and are represented as arrays of miniature triangular facets. The technique is suitable for a number of important applications, and permits dramatic savings in radiation exposure and in data acquisition and manipulation. It is well matched to user-friendly interactive display.

1. Introduction

Prosthetics and other surgical applications - and some physiological ones - need accurate 3D information. The best current technique for this, Computed Tomography (CT) [1], entails very high X-ray exposures and a heavy computational load. CT produces excellent 2D images, but the third dimension depends on interpolation between some tens of slices. Several authors, e.g. [2] have proposed 3D equivalents of CT, but none seem to have found a satisfactory compromise between resolution, signal/noise ratio, and computational load.

In practice, we are not concerned with, say, 10^9 independent voxels, but with a few discrete objects, each comprising a substantial number of voxels. Hence several authors, e.g. [3, 4], have used parallel projection of object outlines, from say 10 distributed views, to define an outer bound to the surfaces of these objects. The resulting representation is inaccurate, and topologically limited, but this scheme restricts the radiation to the volume of interest, and even there reduces it about 1000-fold. Our method, nicknamed "object-3D" [5], retains these benefits, but it uses the information in a novel way, for the precise 3D reconstruction of objects

2. Defining Surface Points

We can use any X-ray system in which the viewing axis can be turned about 2 axes, and the picture is available electrically. (Alternatively we might use 10 fixed sensor arrays and 10 fixed X-ray sources.) Fig. 1 shows three irradiating beams for two sizes of the volume to be examined, defined as a sphere, common to equal conical beams from all the sources. For smaller volumes, the source angles are trimmed down. (Our scheme, unlike conventional systems, yields true 3D positions even with wide X-ray beams; hence we can convert much more of electron-beam energy into *useful* X-rays.)

We treat any volume bounded by a discontinuity in density as an "object". On each projected view, the objects are represented by their edge-extracted outlines - plus any intermediate loci of maximum density gradient - converted into concatenated polynomial splines. Identifying any point on the object's surface on two such outline views defines the 3D location of that point. See Fig. 2. The irradiation of object O by source S_1 generates outline O_1 in image plane I_1, where each picture point defines a ray from S_1. A second source, S_2, generates outline O_2 in image plane I_2. Plane S_1S_2BA, rotated about S_1S_2 to touch O at the extremity E_1, then contains:-

- Rays $S_1 E_1 E_{11}$ and $S_2 E_1 E_{12}$, intersecting at E_1;
- Tangent $A_1 E_{11} B_1$ to O_1, in I_1;
- tangent $A_2 E_{12} B_2$ to O_2, in I_2.

Thus the 3D location of E_1 is defined by its projections in the two image planes. The other extremity, E_2, is similarly defined [6].

Re-entrant features in the objects normally generate two additional local extremities, one concave and one convex, in both views, thus providing the 3D location of two further points. Sharp corners or other singularities can also be identified (See Fig.3.) The more complex the shape, the greater is the number of points required, but the greater is also the number of points generated. At the lower limit, for a very simple object, each pairing of two views defines just two common 3D points, so that n views define $n \cdot (n-1)$ 3D points. 10 views are generally sufficient. Objects changing their tangent angle monotonically through $360°$ intersect the other 9 outlines at 18 common points, spaced at approximately $20°$ of tangent angle. Any inflexions increase the total number of identified points. Considering each segment of an inflexion *as if* it were part of a monotonically curved contour shows that we still create one point per $\pm10°$ of (concave or convex) angular change. However, a sharp corner generates just one additional singular point. Since the points defined on the objects are evenly spread, *in tangent angle*, see Fig. 4, *the point distribution adapts optimally to the size, shape, and complexity of each object.*

3. Establishing a Surface-Mesh Network

The surface points are interconnected by a network of line segments, whose 3D track we can infer from their known end-points and their known projected contours. This network defines the surface as a set of predominantly quadrilateral mesh cells, see Fig.5. Generally the sides of these cells are curved, and their corners are *not* coplanar. Image manipulation is substantially simplified by using "wire-frames", [7] representing curved inter-nodal links by straight lines, and curved surfaces as assemblages of triangular facets. However, to maintain our accuracy, we represent the curved contour segment between two identified surface points, A and B, by a 3-line approximation. This reduces the peak errors to $\pm0.003AB$ in displacement and $\pm 4.25°$ in angle. The 3D positions of A' and B' in Fig. 6, corresponding to the image points A and B, are known, since they are common to two distinct views. The 3D position of the two interpolated points, P" and Q", is then defined by projection onto the plane, through A' B', normal to the plane A' B' B A. The originally 4-sided mesh, between the thick points of Fig.7, is thus represented by 10 triangular facets, and a simple rounded object, with no bumps or dents, by 900 such facets. This yields dramatic savings in computation for image manipulations.

Where an excrescence (or hole) joins an object, the 45 rotating planes, formed by pairings of our 10 views, define the 3D position of 45 points in the transition region. See Fig. 8. The surface of the remainder of the excrescence is formed in the normal way. A point singularity generates 45 coincident point locations, one for each rotating plane. Similarly, singular ridge generates 45 *non-coincident* locations (more if the ridge changes direction by more than 180°). A closed sharp-edged curve generates at least two tangent points on each of the 45 rotating planes.

4.   Multiple Objects.

Overlapping objects are normally resolved in each view, by edge extraction [8]. The identity of a given object, in two distinct views, is confirmed when the rotating plane touches extremities and other key features in both projections at the same time. If $O(p, 1)$, i.e. object p in view 1, cannot be directly identified with $O(p, 2)$, it is identified via intermediate views: $O(p, 1) \rightarrow O(p, x) \rightarrow O(p, y) \rightarrow O(p, 2)$. Provided an object can be resolved in any one view, it can be recognised in all views.

When the source angles just encompass the objects of interest, other objects may be partially included in the spherical volume, irradiated by all 10 sources. On any such "intruding" object, the 3D positions of "common points", derived from pairs of views, are then checked, and the object is notionally terminated, just inside the selected sphere. (However, unlike [3, 4], our method could not reconstruct a smooth cylinder or cone whose extremities lie outside the selected volume.)

Fig.9 is an example of edge extraction by our technique, superimposed on the source X-ray. After proving our concept on computer-generated objects [6], we embedded objects in a foam-plastic sphere, so that they could be rotated to the 10 desired viewing angles. This produced the 3D reconstruction of a bone, shown in Fig. 10.

5. Overview and Conclusions.

1) Object-3D, using standard, 2-axis, digital read-out, X-ray apparatus, can reconstruct objects accurately in 3D
2) It yields dramatic savings in radiation:- The exposure is only that of 10 conventional X-rays of the objects of interest
3) It is efficient in data-acquisition, storage, and processing:-
- It only notes and records *changes* in density or surface slope.
- The format and accuracy of the data is symmetric in 3 dimensions.
4) It is well matched to user-friendly inter-active display:-
- Rotation only entails coordinate conversion for a set of straight-line links.
- Slicing merely involves finding the set of straight lines cut by the slicing plane.
- An object's outline, in any direction of view, merely consists of the relevant edges.(An outline can never lie within a triangular facet.)

Acknowledgements.
        The author owes sincere thanks to Prof. R.I.Kitney for his full support throughout this project, and to a number of past and present research students for the implementation of the scheme: above all to Mr. Simant Prakoonwit for object reconstruction and system integration, and Mr. Ioannis Matalas for edge extraction and representation.

References
1.   Hounsfield, G. N., 1979, Philosl Transacs Royal Soc, A 292, 223 - 232, .

2.   Peyrin, 1985, IEEE Trans. Nucl. Sc. NS-32, 1512 - 1519.

3. Stenstrom, J.R., and Conolly, C.I., 1992 Intnl. Jnl. of Computer Vision, 19, 185-212.

4. Vaullant, R., Faugeras, O., 1989, Internatl. Advanced Robotics Program.

5. Internat. Patent Appl. No. PCT/GB 92/01969, based on U.K. Patent Appl. No. 9122843.

6. Prakoonwit, S., Benjamin, R., Kitney, R.D., 1994, Proc. World Congr. on Medl Phy. and Eng., *Rio*.

8. Woodwark, J., 1986, *Computing Shape*. London: Butterworths, .32-37.

9. Matalas, R. Benjamin, R.D. Kitney, 1994, Proc. 12th Internat. Conf. on Pattern Recogn., Jerusalem

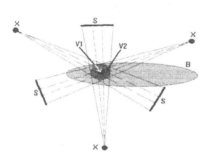

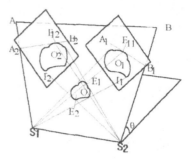

Fig. 1: Sources and sensors, viewing min. and max. target volumes, V_1 and V_2

Fig.2: Locating points common to two views

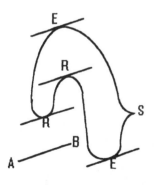

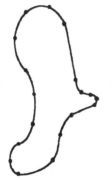

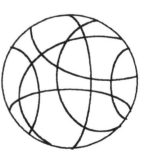

Fig. 3: Types of common pts:
E = end point
R = re-entrant pt.
S = singular pt.
AB = dir^n. of plane

Fig. 4: Self-optimised spacing of points on outline

Fig. 5: Surface mesh

448

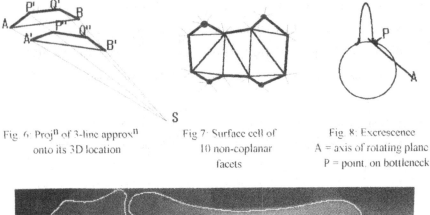

Fig. 6. Proj^n of 3-line approx^n onto its 3D location

Fig. 7. Surface cell of 10 non-coplanar facets

Fig. 8. Excrescence
A = axis of rotating plane
P = point on bottleneck

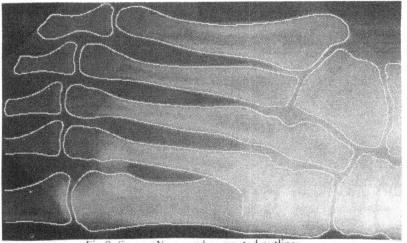

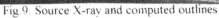

Fig. 9. Source X-ray and computed outlines

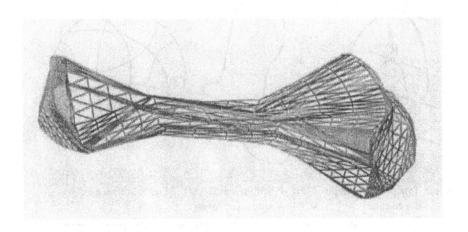

Fig. 10. Reconstruction of phantom bone.

Quantitative Vascular Shape Analysis for 3D MR-Angiography Using Mathematical Morphology

Yoshitaka Masutani, Tsuyoshi Kurihara, Makoto Suzuki and Takeyoshi Dohi

Dept. of Precision Machinery Eng., Faculty of Eng. The University of Tokyo
7-3-1 Hongo, Bunkyo-ku, Tokyo 113 Japan
yos@rieko.pe.u-tokyo.ac.jp

Abstract. Beyond visualization of 3D MR-Angiography, further analysis has been carried out to obtain vascular shape in an anatomically-relevant generalized cone expression, which is suitable for the purpose of surgical simulation. Methods of mathematical morphology were employed for quantitative vascular shape analysis and processing in 3D binary and grayscale data. As a quantitative descriptor of global and local vascular shape, pattern spectrum was applied to detect abnormal vascular shapes like aneurysm and stricture. And 3D methods of radii estimation and thinning were carried out to reconstruct the vasculature. These analysis and processing procedures were examined using phantoms and clinical MRA data.

1 Introduction

Blood vessel was one of the organs hardest to visualize and perceive its shape and structure for its imaging difficulty and shape complexity, although it is one of the most important organs for diagnosis, surgical planning and surgery itself. However in these days, due to progress of medical imaging technology, there already exist several modalities to visualize the blood vessels. Among them, MR(Magnetic Resonance)-Angiography is the best way for its non-invasiveness and ability to obtain functional and phenomenal information. Vasculature in MRA data can be directly visualized using projective methods such as maximum intensity projection method or volume rendering [1]. However, the formed image does never include information of vascular shape explicitly. Even after segmentation, we still have only the shape of vasculature expressed as just an accumulated set of voxels, which is insufficient in further applications like surgical simulation of vessel anastomosis/resection. Alternatively, vascular shape in an explicit geometrical expression is required. As such an anatomically-relevant expression for vascular shape, binary tree expression with vessel radius information(called as generalized cone) is quite popular and certainly standard. Excepting methods using limited projections like biplane angiography, there exist some ways to reconstruct a vascular shape in such expression from 3D medical images like MRA. According to a rough classification, we can consider three ways; (1) 2D sectional image based approach [2] [3] [4], (2) 3D voxel based approach [5] and

(3) deformable model based approach. At this point of time, it seems the most reasonable to apply approach (2) for two major reasons. One is that recently, we can acquire 3D images of thin slice and with no gap easily, at least via an interpolation procedure with already reported algorithms [6]. The other is, no effective method, which is based on deformable models, has not been presented to cope with the vasculature with complex structure or abnormal shapes. In the approach (2) we selected, the vasculature expressed by generalized cone can be reconstructed via 3D thinning, binary tree acquisition and radii estimation in 3D space. The main problems in this approach are: (a) loss of local contrast in original MRA data, (b) noisy shape cleaning while keeping necessary shape, and (c) how to detect and separate abnormal vascular shape like aneurysm. We coped with these problems using quantitative methods of mathematical morphology [7]. Mathematical morphology is one of the most suitable theory which provides quantitative ways to analyze the shape of an object in voxel expression. Morphological method is getting to be recognized also in medical image processing [8]. In this paper, we intend to describe our techniques to obtain vascular shapes both in an anatomically-relevant expression and in a quantitative way from MRA data.

2 Materials and methods

We considered that two procedures are required for our purpose. They are 1) signal level processing, 2) shape level analysis and processing. The former is an application of 3D image processing for the purpose of restoration of the quality of MRA data, for instance, noise reduction, enhancement. Some excellent methods were already reported [9] [10] which act as shape-concious signal processing filter. We employed 3D grayscale opening and closing [11], and 3D median filter for noise reduction. In the latter, we apply methods of 3D binary shape analysis and processing of mathematical morphology. The main roles of this procedure are to extract binary tree structure as the medial axis of vasculature from the voxel-represented shape, and to estimate radii on the medial axis for generalized cone reconstruction. However, abnormality in vascular shape like aneurysm and stricture should be detected before this procedure. Because there exist many cases in which it is difficult to express such shapes in generalized cone expression. Besides, they are absolutely important in diagnosis and surgery. We utilized the pattern spectrum [12] which is the pattern-size descriptor based on mathematical morphology. According to the original definition for pattern spectrum by Maragos, we considered that pattern spectrum can be inspected both globally and locally. The local pattern spectrum is expected to indicate certain abnormality when the vascular shape has local abnormality. The n th component of global pattern spectrum for voxel-represented object X with structuring element B is identical with the original definition, excepting applying in 3D space, and is expressed as

$$GPS(X, B, n) = V[X_{nB} - X_{(n+1)B}] \quad (n \geq 0) \tag{1}$$

where V represents volume of object, X_{nB} represents n times opened shape of X with structuring element B. The local pattern spectrum is

$$LPS(X, B, p, n) = V[W(p) \cap (X_{nB} - X_{(n+1)B})] \quad (n \geq 0) \qquad (2)$$

where p represents local position and $W(p)$ represents a windowing shape for location at p. Between the two procedures signal level processing and shape level processing, a segmentation procedure is required. However, because other organs can not be imaged so clearly in MRA data, it is easier to extract vessel region than in other modalities. We used thresholding with a threshold adjusted interactively. Beside pattern spectrum inspection, we employed binary 3D opening and closing for shape smoothing, our serial processing version of the 3D thinning algorithm by Tsao [13] for binary tree acquisition, 3D radii estimation. The author examined several methods to estimate 3D radius including the conventional estimation which is the radius of the maximum sphere insertable in the position [14]. And we concluded that a method based on average size [12] of local pattern spectrum is better than the conventional way. The one more thing left to be considered here is the shape of structuring element. Though there exist some exceptions, the most vessel sections are real circle. Therefore, it can be reasonable to use the spherical shape of structuring element.

To examine the feasibility of our methods of vascular shape analysis and processing, we prepared two types of data, simulated vascular shape phantoms in binary voxel expression and ,clinical MRA data. The former consists of basic shapes #S1, #S2, noise-appended shapes #S3(#S1+noise), #S4(#S2+noise), abnormal vascular shapes #S5(with aneurysm) and #S6(with stricture). The latter is of cranial MRA data of volunteers by 0.5T MRI, #C1($256\times256\times64$, time of flight, TR=60, TE=11, FA=11) and #C2($256\times256\times128$ phase subtraction, TR=40, TE=15, FA=90). The results of these experiments and discussions for them will be appeared in the next section.

3 Results and discussion

Experiment(1): Global and local pattern spectrum inspection. Figure 1 and 2 show global pattern spectra of basic vascular shapes A(#S1) and B(#S2). Each pattern spectrum is normalized by whole volume of the shape. Globally, each represents the characteristic of each shape. For vascular shape #S1 which is a simple vessel with uniform radii, its pattern spectrum indicated a strong peak. On the contrary, for shape #S2 which consists of truely round cones, nearly equally-distributed components were observed. In local pattern spectrum inspection, no abnormal distribution was observed, as we expected. However, in some cases, the local pattern spectrum indicates some abnormality caused by adjacent thick branch. This can be considered as one of the so-called windowing problem like of other image processing algorithms. To avoid this, the size and shape of window shape W must have been well considered. We utilized a spherical shape of window, of which radius is slightly larger than the maximum size of structuring element of which component is not zero in the global pattern spectrum. For instance, if the maximum size in global pattern spectrum is 10, the radius of window shape proposed is 12. With this window shape, described problems in the local pattern inspection was reduced.

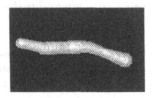 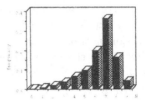

Fig. 1. vascular shape #S1(left), global pattern spectrum of #S1(right)

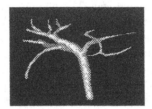 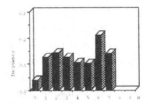

Fig. 2. vascular shape #S2(left), global pattern spectrum of #S2(right)

Experiment(2): Shape smoothing. Shape level smoothing, closing and opening were carried out in this experiment. Voxels were scattered on the surface of basic vascular shapes #S1 and #S2 with a ratio 2.0 shape #S3 and #S4, the smoothing effect was recognized by applying 3D thinning. Figure 3 shows the result of #S3 using closing and opening. For the purpose of noise removal, opening was superior. In the same way, thin branches of #S4 were removed by opening with certain size of structuring element. Thus, the size of structuring regulates the minimum thickness of the smoothed vascular shape like the cut-off frequency of LPF in wave form analysis.

Experiment(3): Shape abnormality detection. The local pattern spectrum indicated a pair of strong peaks, while the window shape covered the volume of aneurysm shape #S5(Figure 4). And the aneurysm shape could be separated by an opening operation with the structuring element of which size is middle of them, which is 12 in Figure 4b). After the separation, the volume of aneurysm shape can be measured easily, it is important in the case of occlusion surgery to estimate the proper volume of occulusion medium. Though any obvious abnormality could not be seen in its local pattern spectrum, stricture could be detected by a discontinuity in the binary tree structure of #S6 obtained after an opening operation with certain size of structuring element. However, it

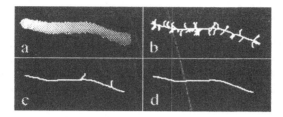

Fig. 3. a) noisy shape #S3, b) skeleton of #S3, c) skeleton of #S3 after closing and d) skeleton of #S3 after opening

is clear that the stricture could have not been detected with smaller structuring element. The problem is that a stricture shape is not defined quantitatively as it is well-defined and easier to judge by inspecting the inner wall of the vessel from the pathological views. Conversely speaking, we can give some quantitative answers using these morphological methods of shape analysis.

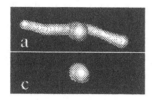
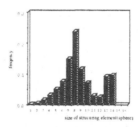

Fig. 4. a) simulated aneurysm #S5, b) pattern spectrum of #S5(right) and c) separated aneurysm from #S5

Experiment(4): Whole vasculature reconstruction. Figure 5 shows the vascular shape of the arteria cerebri includes the willis from the clinical data of MRA (#C1), which was reconstructed in generalized cone expression through descibed methods, and visualized by surface shading method.

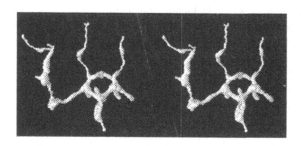

Fig. 5. the reconstructed arteria cerebri from #C1 includeing the willis(a stereo pair)

4 Conclusion

We presented methods based upon mathematical morphology which are effective for the quantitative shape analysis to obtain an anatomically-relevant generalized cone expression of vasculature. Especially, we have shown that local pattern spectrum is a powerful tool to inspect the local characteristics of a vascular shape.

References

1. A. Pommert, et al. Volume Visualization in Magnetic Resonance Angiography. IEEE Computer Graphics and Applications Sep. (1992) 12–13
2. M. Block et al. Quantitative Analysis of a Vascular Tree Model with the Dynamic Spatial Reconstructor. Journal of Computer Assited Tomography 8 (1984) 390–400
3. J. A. Fessler, et al. Object-Based 3D Reconstruction of Arterial Trees from Magnetic Resonance Angiograms. IEEE trans. on Medical Imaging 10 (1991) 25–39
4. Y. Masutani, et al. Development of an Interactive Vessel Modelling System for Hepatic Vasculature from MR-Images. Medical & Biological Engineering & Computing (to appear)
5. G. Székely, et al. Structural description and combined 3-D display for superior analysis of cerebral vascularity from MRA. Proc. of Visualization in Biomedical Computing (1994) 272–281
6. W. E. Higgins, et al. Shape-Based Interpolation of Tree-Like Structures in Three-Dimensional Images. IEEE Trans. on Medical Imaging 12 (1993) 439–450
7. J. Serra Introduction to Mathematical Morphology. Computer Vision, Graphics and Image Processing 35 (1986) 283–305
8. T. Schiemann, et al. Interactive 3D-Segmentation. Proc. of Visualization in Biomedical Computing (1992) 376–383
9. G. Gerig, et al. Line-finding in 2-D and 3-D by multi-valued non-linear diffusion of feature maps. Proc. of DAGM Symposium (1993) 289-296
10. D. Vandermeulen, et al. Local filtering and Global optimisation Methods for 3D Magnetic Resonance Angiography (MRA) Image enhancement. Proc. of Visualization in Biomedical Computing (1992) 274–288
11. S. R. Sternberg Grayscale Morphology. Computer Vision, Graphics and Image Processing 35 (1986) 333–355
12. P. Maragos Pattern Spectrum and Multiscale Shape Representation. IEEE Pattern Analysis and Machine Intelligence 11 (1989) 701–716
13. Y. F. Tsao, et al. A Parallel Thinning Algorithm for 3-D Pictures. Computer Graphics and Image Processing 17 (1981) 315–331
14. Y. Masutani Studies on processing and analysis of vascular shapes in 3D medical images. Master thesis of the university of Tokyo (in Japanese, 1993)

B-Deformable Superquadrics
for 3D Reconstruction

Neveu M., Faudot D., Derdouri B.
LIESIB. Université de Bourgogne
BP 138- 21000 Dijon Cedex- France
email : faudot@satie.u-bourgogne.fr

Abstract

We propose a new model for 3D representation and reconstruction. It is based on deformable superquadrics and parametric B-Splines. The 3D object deformation method uses B-Splines, instead of a Finite Element Method (FEM). This new model exhibits advantages of B-Splines It is significantly faster than deformable superquadrics without loss of generality (no assumption is made on object shapes,).

1. Introduction

Specification of appropriate models for 3D objects reconstruction **and** recognition remains difficult, because of conflicting requirements. Shape reconstruction involves general geometric models without assumptions on objects shapes. Free-form models [1] and generalized splines [2] are well suited to this purpose. Recognition involves data reduction and abstract shape description. Primitives seem better suited, as parts of composite objects that may be expressed with a small set of parameters [3].

Superquadrics [4][5][6] have been recently used to describe smooth objects with a wide range of shapes. A new hybrid model named "deformable superquadrics" was introduced in [3]. It combines global and local parameters into a model that can be modified to allow shape reconstruction and recognition of objects of irregular shapes.

In this paper, we present a new tool for a faster deformation of deformable superquadrics. The superquadric model surface is approximated by a B-spline surface. Modifications of B-spline control points deform the model named "B-deformable superquadrics". We begin with a description of deformable superquadrics. Then, details on B-deformable superquadrics are given, together with comparative performances.

2. Deformable Superquadrics

Let $U = (u,v)$ be a parametric surface, $x(U,t)$ the deformable model in an inertial frame of reference Φ at time t, and ϕ a model-centered reference frame. Positions of a point on the model are given by $X(U,t) = C(t)+R(t)*p(U,t)$. $C(t) = (px\ py\ pz) = q_c$ is the origin of ϕ relative to Φ, $R(t)$ is the rotation matrix, depending on Euler angles $(\varphi, \theta, \psi) = q_\theta$ and $p(U,t)$ denotes the canonical positions of points on the model relative to ϕ. $p(U,t)=s(U,t)+d(U,t)$. $s(U,t)$ is the original superquadric determined its parameters (scale, aspect ratio and squareness) gathered in a parameter vector q_s. $d(U,t)$ stands for deformation, describing shape differences between the original superquadric and the actual one.

Generally, this displacement is expressed by a linear combination of form functions

$$d = Sq_d \tag{1}$$

where S is the form functions matrix and q_d is the vector of degrees of freedom.

The aim is to update the vector of degrees of freedom $q = (q_c, q_\theta, q_s, q_d)$ when matching the model with data. Notice that q_c and q_θ are motion global coordinates, q_s denotes global deformation coordinates and q_d denotes local deformation coordinates. Motion equations are of Lagrangian form

$$M\ddot{q} + C\dot{q} + Kq = g_q + f_q \qquad (2)$$

with M, C, K mass, damping and stiffness matrices, g_q inertial forces and f_q generalized external forces. Under the hypothesis of a null mass matrix, that leads to a model without inertia, at equilibrium as soon as external forces vanish, (2) becomes

$$C\dot{q} + Kq = f_q \qquad (3)$$

Space discretization of the former differential equation is based on Finite Element Method. Time discretization by Euler method computes the vector of freedom degrees q at time $t+\Delta t$ according to the following formula (where Δt is Euler spatial increment):

$$q^{t+\Delta t} = q^t + \Delta t (C^t)^{-1} (f_q^t - Kq^t) \qquad (4)$$

3. B-Deformable Superquadrics

Let us consider the vector q^t in equation (4). Its size is :

$$[\text{gdm}] + [\text{spsize} * (\text{nodes} * \text{dfree})] = \left[\#(q_c) + \#(q_q) + \#(q_s) \right] + \left[\#(q_d) \right] \qquad (5)$$

where gdm denotes the size of coordinates for global motion and deformation, spsize denotes the space size (n for $\Re^n$), nodes is the number of nodes of the model and dfree is the degrees of freedom for each node.

Unfortunatly, deformable superquadrics (DS) converge rather slowly because they use all the nodes of the model together with their degrees of freedom. This yields to solve a large system. A way to solve this problem is to compute a parametric B-Spline approximation of this model [7] as shown hereafter. We name this model **B-Deformable Superquadrics** (BDS).

3.1 Definition

In this model, the initial surface is approximated by a B-Spline surface and motion equation is approximated by another motion equation, at equilibrium as soon as external forces vanish. In this new model local deformation concerns the B-Spline control vertices instead of the DS nodes.

The approximate surface is given by a tensor product of B-spline basis functions and of vertices of a control mesh [8][9] that is computed by least-squares approximation. This approximation of the initial surface leads to a similar system in the motion equations, but with lower size : gdm+spsize*(M+1)*(N+1) instead of gdm+spsize*nodes*dfree where (M+1)*(N+1) denotes the number of control mesh vertices.

Let us point out that motion equation for B-deformable superquadrics takes into account the whole set of surface points, although its minimization leads to solve a smaller system built from control vertices. Indeed, the computation of external forces takes into account the whole surface.

3.2 Control mesh

Given $(P+1)*(Q+1)$ points D_{ij} in 3D space with associated parametric values (ζ_i, η_j), the goal is to compute a mesh of control points V which minimizes distance between B-spline surface and data points [10][11][12]. We look for $(M+1)*(N+1)$ control points V_{mn} of surface S such that S fits points D_{ij} (using least-squares approximation). This problem yields to solve two linear symetric definite positive systems of size $(N+1)$ (resp. $M+1$).

$$\begin{cases} B_\eta B_\eta^T V_\eta = B_\eta D B_\zeta^T \\ \text{et} \\ B_\zeta B_\zeta^T V = V_\eta^T \end{cases} \qquad (6)$$

with D the data matrix, V the unknown matrix, B_ζ is the $(M+1)(P+1)$ matrix of bases $B_m^K(\zeta_i)$ and B_η is the $(N+1)(Q+1)$ matrix of bases $B_n^L(\eta_j)$

3.3 Motion equation with B-Deformable superquadrics

Finite Element Method (FEM) [13], divides continuous space into elements linked together by a finite number of nodes located on their boundary. Nodes displacements are the problem's unknowns. *In our problem, unknowns are control points.*

In the geometric formulation of DS [3], we replace form functions based on FEM by B-Spline functions in formula (1). In our model, we express displacement d as:

$$d = \sum_i \text{diag}(\bar{S}_i) q_i \qquad (7)$$

where $\text{diag}(\bar{S}_i)$ is a diagonal matrix formed from B-spline basis functions and where q_i depend only on time and are known as degrees of freedom or generalized coordinates.

We can write the displacement field as : $d = \bar{S} q_d$ where $\bar{S}$ is the shape matrix, consisting only of B-spline basis functions and where $q_d = (...,q_i,...)^T$ is the vector of degrees of freedom for the BDS built with control points.

Therefore, every formula using the S matrix in the DS model is modified. We replace S by $\bar{S}$ in the M and C matrices, and in the external forces vector F. In the same way, in the elasticity K_{dd} matrix, N_i^j nodal form functions of an element E^j are replaced by B_k^l B-spline functions of a surface patch E^l where i varies from 1 to n, number of nodes associated with E^j, j varies from 1 to nelt, number of finite elements, k varies from 1 to K (B-Spline order) and l varies from 1 to npatch, number of patches.

4. Results

The main advantages of our method concern time computation and memory requirements. The size of the system to solve in the case of DS model is (gdm + spsize * nodes * dfree) whereas it is (gdm + spsize * (M+1) * (N+1)) for the BDS model. We tried two main families of examples.

One when "nodes" (number of nodes) equals to $(M+1) * (N+1)$ (number of vertices). This rarely occurs and is the worst case for our improvement. Both systems have identical sizes and time consumption is approximately the same *only when linear shape* *functions are used* (involving C^0 continuity between elements boundaries). As soon as higher continuity is desired the size of the BDS system is smaller than the DS one.

The general case with "nodes" greater than $(M+1) * (N+1)$. In this case, the BDS system is smaller and the BDS model is faster than the DS model whatever the nodal functions (even linear).

Figure 1 illustrates size of BDS versus size of DS for various continuities and numbers of data points. Figure 2 shows reconstruction times for the same trials. For all these trials, model deformation follows an iterative process that comes to rest as soon as external forces vanish. This criterion ensures a **same degree of accuracy for both BDS and DS reconstruction**.

5. Conclusion

A new model for object representation and reconstruction has been presented. In order to deform the model, it uses B-Spline shape functions that only modify control vertices· Reconstruction appears to have the same accuracy with both models. Ours converges faster. It seems to be more general, because interpolating shape functions used in DS model involve the inclusion of all the nodes of the model. This constraint seems too strong, as nodes are not imposed by the reconstruction process. A least-squares fit seems sufficient. Continuity properties included in DS model are preserved but with faster computation.

References

[1] T.W. Sederberg, S.R Parry, *"Free Form Deformation of Solid Geometric Models"*, SIGGRAPH 1986, vol. 20, n°4, 1986.

[2] G.Farin, *"Curves and surfaces for computer aided geometric Design"*, Academic Press, N.Y., 1988.

[3] D.Terzopoulos and D.Metaxas, *"Dynamic 3D models with local and global deformations: Deformable superquadrics"*, IEEE PAMI, Vol. 13, pp. 703-714, 1991.

[4] A.Barr, *"Superquadric and angle-preserving transformations"*, IEEE Computer Graphics ans Applications, pp. 11-23, Jan. 1981.

[5] A.Pentland, *"Perceptual organization and the representation of naturel form"*, Artificial Intelligence, Vol. 28, pp. 293-331, 1986.

[6] R.Bajscy and R.Solina, *"Three-dimensional objet representation revisited"*, in IEEE First Conference on Computer Vision, London, England, pp. 231-240.

[7] R.Bartels, J.Beatty, and B.Barsky, *"An introduction to splines for use in computer graphics and geometric modeling"*, MorganKaufmann, Los Altos, CA 94022, 1987.

[8] Riesenfeld R.F. *"Applications of B-Spline Approximation to Geometric Problems of Computer Aided Design"*. Syracuse University, PHD 1973.

[9] deBoor C. *"A Pratical Guide to Splines"*. Springer Verlag. New York 1978.

[10] P.Saint-Marc and G.Medioni, *"B-spline contour representation and symmetry detection"*, In 1st ECCV, pp. 604-606, Antibes, France, April 1990.

[11] A. Gueziec *"Reconnaissance Automatique de surfaces et courbes gauches. Application à l'analyse d'images volumiques"*, PhD Thesis . Orsay University, 26 fev 93.

[12] M. Daniel *"Modélisation de courbes et surfaces par des B-splines. Application à la conception et à la visualisation de formes"*, PhD Thesis Nantes University, 12 mai 89

[13] O.C. Zienkiewicz,*"The finite element method in engineering science"*, Third edition. Mc Graw-Hill, London, 1977.

459

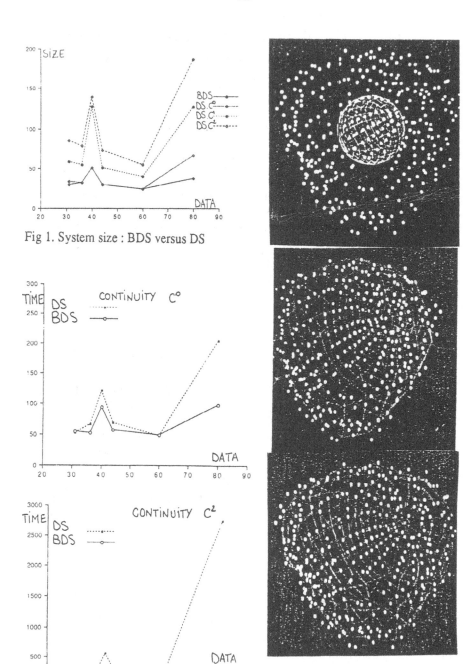

Fig 1. System size : BDS versus DS

Fig 2 Time reconstruction : BDS versus DS

Fig 3. Data points sampled on a tapered-bended superquadric with local random perturbations. From top to bottom : initial model. Reconstruction with DS and BDS models with C^2 continuity.

Modeling 3D Objects with Quadratic Surface Patches: Application to the Recognition and Locating of Anatomic Structures

Ivan Bricault and Olivier Monga

INRIA-Rocquencourt, BP 105, 78153 Le Chesnay Cedex, FRANCE

Abstract. In this paper, we show how to extract reliable informations about the shape of 3D objects, obtained from volume medical images. We present an optimal region-growing strategy, that makes use of the differential characteristics of the object surface, and achieves a stable segmentation into a set of patches of quadratic surfaces. We show how this segmentation can be used to recognize and locate a target sub-structure on a global anatomic structure.

1 Introduction

For a computer vision system, performing tasks of recognition and locating is a major challenge. Achieving these tasks automatically may help in a great number of applications, such as computer-assisted surgery. In the work presented here, we focused on the processing of 3D anatomic structures : we show how to extract reliable informations about their shape, and how these informations can be used to recognize and locate a particular anatomic piece on a bigger structure. These informations consist of a set of patches of quadratic surfaces, that locally approximate relevant parts of the object studied. The main problem is to ensure the stability of the segmentation in quadratic patches. For this purpose, we present a region-growing algorithm that uses the differential characteristics of the object surface. This work is more precisely described in the reference [7].

2 Method

The data involved in this work are volumic images obtained from scanner medical systems. According to the methodology we have developped, the extraction of relevant quadratic patches requires the steps described in the following paragraphs.

2.1 Edge detection and differential computations

We used algorithms described in [3] and [4] to perform the edge detection, and the computation of 2 differential features on the object surface : the *gaussian curvature* and the *gaussian extremality*. The last one has been introduced in [6]; gaussian extremality contains information about extrema of the curvature, for instance about crest lines. These differential features have a major interesting property : they are characteristic of the object shape, and invariant through any rigid displacement.

2.2 Initial segmentation

The initial segmentation of the object surface consists in finding homogeneous patches in term of differential features. Thus, the object is first divided into maximal connected patches such that signs of gaussian curvature and extremality are constant. As a consequence, boundaries between patches correspond to parabolic lines and lines of extremal curvature. Besides, it is necessary to improve this initial segmentation thanks to a few mathematical morphology operators : in particular, an *opening* disconnects parts where the diameter is below the one of the structuring element used.

2.3 Region growing

The segmentation then go on through a region-growing process. The algorithm used is described in [2]; the principle is to merge patches according to quality criteria. This particular algorithm is optimal, in the fact that each step chooses the best possible pair of patches to merge. This is done quickly, thanks to the use of adapted data structures : a dynamic graph of neighbourhood and a priority heap. The quality criteria is obtained from an error computation, during the approximation of the patch by a quadratic surface. The approximation method used is presented in [1]; given the points of a particular patch, we use a least mean square estimation of the best quadratic fitting surface. The search for stability of the region-growing process led us to implement a specific strategy, involving the following features :

- We introduced 2 quality criteria, associated to 2 thresholds allowing a merging :
  1. The *continuity criterion,* for a pair of patches, estimates how well one patch extends the other. To do so, we have chosen to compute the error when approximating one patch by the quadratic surface associated to the other, and vice versa.
  2. The *boundary criterion* estimates the error of approximation by the quadratic surface, for the points located at the boundary of a pair of patches. Thus we can control the quality of the approximation along characteristic parts of the object, such as crest and parabolic lines.
- Thanks to the computation of reference errors, we can specify relative thresholds (that is to say, percentage of tolerance) : we authorize the merging only if the increase of the error after merging is less than a given ratio of a local reference error. Thus we avoid the need for absolute threshold values, that would be dependant of each particular application, in particular when the noise on the data is not homogeneous.

- We divided the region-growing process into various steps, beginning with restrictive thresholds, then allowing more mergings.
- When merging 2 patches of different gaussian nature (an elliptic and a hyperbolic patch), we introduced more restrictive criteria.

2.4 Registration

We now consider 2 images where we can find the same structure, although not in the same position. The segmentation into quadratic surfaces, presented above, helps us to achieve the matching process. We developped a registration algorithm according to the prediction-verification paradigm, with the following main features :

- From a set of matched patches, the displacement (represented by a quaternion) is estimated by superimposing the centroid of a patch and the centroid of the matched patch. This estimation uses a least mean square estimation of the best fitting quaternion (see [1]).
- Once a displacement has been estimated, we try to match a new pair of patches. We search for the pair of patches that are the nearest, according the following vicinity criterion : we compute the error when approximating the first patch by the quadratic surface of the second patch, after displacement; and we compare this error with the error when approximating the first patch by its own quadratic surface. Thus, this criterion is much alike the continuity criterion introduced above. This criterion makes use of the quadratic segmentation information, and is able to discriminate with a great accuracy among the possible matches, according to the position and shape of the different patches.
- For the initial estimation of a displacement, 3 matches are needed. They are guided by the similarity of parameters (eigenvalues and eigenvectors of the quadratic surfaces) for the possible patches.

Here we do *not* tackle the problem of a precise registration. Our aim is to rapidly recognize and locate (approximatively) a particular structure, despite of the following difficulties :

- we want to recognize and locate a particular substructure on a bigger structure; both can have thousands of edge points.
- we have no a-priori information about where the structure should be found.

A more precise registration can follow the one we present; for example thanks to an iterative method using splines (see [5]). This type of methods requires a good enough initial estimate, in order to avoid local minima; thus registration from quadratic segmentation can complete and extend application field for iterative methods.

3 Experimental results : Recognition and locating

We focus on the problem of recognizing and locating a target substructure on a global anatomic structure. The practical application field could be the computer-assisted guidance of a surgical act. Here, a volumic scanner image including 28

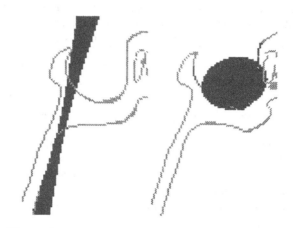

Fig. 1. Eye – 2 sections from the target substructure.

successive sections defines the target substructure (the left eye). Two sections are reproduced figure 1. Using our quadratic patches extraction algorithm, we obtained 5 patches of important size. Our algorithm is then able to match each

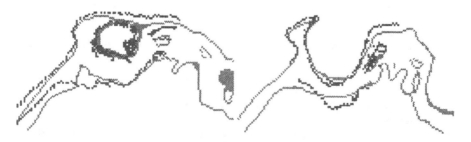

Fig. 2. Grey points : sections from global structure — Black points : sections from target substructure (**eye**) after recognition and locating.

of the 5 patches in the substructure with the corresponding patch in the global structure. The locating result is shown in figure 2. More experimental results can be found in [7].

4 Conclusion

This work is the natural continuation of the ones described in the references [3],[4]. The goal of these works is to define from original data (volume images) a hierarchical sequence of shape representations that may be used at each level to solve a given task such as registration, localization, recognition... In this paper we have adressed the problem set by the determination of intrinsic parametric surface models using the differential characteristics. We used the key idea of reference [1], that is to approximate a surface using quadratic patches thanks to a graph based region growing strategy. Our contributions with respect to [1] are :

- We take into account the differential characteristics of the studied object (gaussian curvature and extremality), for the initial segmentation and during the mergings.
- We implement, thanks to the use of an adapted data structure, a fast optimal region-growing algorithm.
- We introduce merging criteria that are specific (continuity, boundary) and flexible (relative thresholds).
- The relevance and stability of the quadratic segmentation obtained is, as far as we know, without equivalent in previous works. The use of this quadratic information has allowed us to achieve efficient recognition and locating of real anatomic structures.

References

[1] O.D. Faugeras, M. Hebert.: The representation, recognition and locating of 3-D objects. The International Journal of Robotics Research, vol 5 no 3, 1986.
[2] O. Monga.: An optimal region growing algorithm for image segmentation. International Journal of Pattern Recognition and Artificial Intelligence, vol 1, 1987.
[3] O. Monga, R. Deriche, G. Malandain et J.P. Cocquerez.: Recursive filtering and edge tracking : two primary tools for 3D edge detection. Image and vision computing, vol 9 no 4 août 91.
[4] O. Monga, R. Lengagne, R. Deriche.: Extraction of the zero-crossing of the curvature derivative in volumic 3D medical images : a multi-scale approach. IEEE conference in Computer Vision and Pattern Recognition, Seattle (USA), June 1994.
[5] R. Szeliski, S. Lavallée.: Matching 3D anatomical surfaces with non-rigid deformations using octree-splines. IEEE workshop on Biomedical image analysis, Seattle (USA), June 1994.
[6] J.P. Thirion.: The extremal mesh and the understanding of 3D surfaces. IEEE workshop on Biomedical image analysis, Seattle(USA), June 1994.
[7] I. Bricault, O. Monga.: From volume medical images to quadratic surface patches. INRIA Research Report number 2380, September 1994.

A Method of Analyzing a Shape with Potential Symmetry and Its Application to Detecting Spinal Deformity

Seiji Ishikawa†, Hiroyuki Kosaka†, Kiyoshi Kato†, Yoshinori Otsuka‡

†Department of Civil, Mechanical and Control Engineering
Kyushu Institute of Technology
Tobata, Kitakyushu 804, Japan

‡Department of Orthopedic Surgery
National Sanatorium Chiba Higashi Hospital
Nitonacho, Chiba 280, Japan

Abstract   This paper describes a technique for analyzing a shape with potential symmetry which includes approximate symmetry and original symmetry. A technique is proposed for identifying a symmetry axis of a shape with potential axial symmetry by searching for the largest symmetric subset of the shape. It is applied to the axial detection and asymmetry evaluation of Moire topographic images of human backs to automate spinal deformity inspection. Some experimental results are shown and discussion is given.

1 Introduction

Computer vision includes shape analysis of 2D and 3D objects as one of its most important fields of study. Symmetry is a useful index for describing a shape, since it can be employed for object recognition as a global feature and also leads to data compression. A number of automatic symmetry detection algorithms have already been proposed[1,2] which discuss exact symmetry. When practical objects are taken into account, however, one can easily find around himself various asymmetric objects which seem symmetric or suggest original symmetry. A human face is often referred to as a shape with typical mirror symmetry, but asymmetry is found by its careful observation: Many man-made objects have symmetric structure and an accidentally cracked vase, for example, suggests us some kind of original symmetry such as bilateral symmetry. Although symmetric structure had better be identified for their meaningful shape analysis, all the present techniques based on exact symmetry cannot be employed for the purpose. There are very few reports which have ever discussed symmetry identification of such shapes as those having approximate or original symmetry. Marola[3] proposes a technique for defining symmetry axes on 'almost symmetric' shapes. It is only applicable to those 2D shapes that are very close to exact symmetry, however, because of its mathematical nature. Zabrodsky *et al.*[4] decrease resolution of an acquired approximately symmetric image to recover its symmetry, which has effects on a limited range of shapes.

A shape having potential symmetry is defined as a shape which is slightly deformed from exact symmetry or a shape which makes us associate with original symmetry, even if it has not 'approximate' symmetry. This particular paper focuses its attention on potential axial symmetry and a technique is proposed for detecting the axis of potential axial symmetry. This axis is called the potential symmetry axis. It is then applied to automatic human spinal deformity inspection employing Moire topographic images. Experiments are performed on Moire images of children's backs. The axis of potential axial symmetry is detected on each image and asymmetric portions are extracted about it. A numerical index is defined representing the degree of symmetry of a shape and is calculated on the image. Finally, discussion is given based on experimental results.

2 Identifying the axis of potential axial symmetry

In the technique proposed, the original gray image containing an object interested is superposed onto its mirror symmetric gray image and, under rotation and parallel translation, the best match position is searched for in the sense of the minimum difference of gray values between the two images. The difference image at the matched position provides a potential symmetry axis of the object.

A shape on the xy orthogonal coordinate system is denoted by $f(x,y)$, $(x,y) \in R$, where f takes gray values and R is a region on the xy plane. Let the origin O of the xy coordinate system be coincident with the centroid of the region R. With respect to a line $y = x\tan\theta$, shape f receives reflection and the reflected shape is denoted by $f^r(X,Y)$, $(X,Y) \in R^r$. Here R^r is a region on the xy plane and

$$\begin{pmatrix} X \\ Y \end{pmatrix} = \begin{pmatrix} \cos 2\theta & \sin 2\theta \\ \sin 2\theta & -\cos 2\theta \end{pmatrix} \begin{pmatrix} x \\ y \end{pmatrix}.$$

The line $y = x\tan\theta$ is called the reflection axis and, for each $\theta(0 \le \theta \le \pi)$, shape f is reflected around the axis to give f^r. Shape f^r is then superposed onto f by parallel translation so that the difference of the gray values between f and f^r decreases. If the translation vector is denoted by (u,v), the procedure is written as

$$E = \sum_{(x,y) \in R \cup R^r} (f(x,y) - f^r(x+u, y+v))^2 \to \min$$

or

$$E = \sum_{(x,y) \in R} (f(x,y) - f(X,Y))^2 \to \min \tag{1}$$

under $0 \le \theta \le \pi$ and

$$u + v\tan\theta = 0, \tag{2}$$

where

$$\begin{pmatrix} X \\ Y \\ 1 \end{pmatrix} = T \begin{pmatrix} x \\ y \\ 1 \end{pmatrix}, \qquad T = \begin{pmatrix} \cos 2\theta & \sin 2\theta & u \\ \sin 2\theta & -\cos 2\theta & v \\ 0 & 0 & 1 \end{pmatrix}.$$

Equation (2) comes from the fact that, detection of a preferable potential symmetry axis is equivalently achieved through iterating following steps: (i) defining an axis on a given shape, (ii) folding the shape along the axis and calculating the gray value difference between one side of the shape and the other side. Obviously, this excludes parallel translation of shape f^r in the direction of the reflection axis.

Let us define a difference shape $\Delta(x,y)$ by

$$\Delta(x,y) = |f(x,y) - f^r(x+u, y+v)|.$$

In case that $\Delta(x,y) \ne 0$, $\Delta(x,y)$ is always symmetric according to Eq.(2) with respect to the normal bisecting the line segment connecting the centroids of shape f and f^r. When Eq.(1) is realized through the optimal transformation $T^* = T(\theta^*, u^*, v^*)$, the symmetry axis of $\Delta(x,y)$ is defined as the potential symmetry axis of shape f. In case $\Delta(x,y) = 0$, it represents symmetry of shape f, and its axis of symmetry is employed for further analysis. Obviously, $u^* = v^* = 0$ in this situation.

3 Experiment

3.1 Background

Spinal deformity is a serious problem especially for teenagers and doctors employ Moire topographic images of their backs to inspect it. If a subject's spine is normal, the Moire image is symmetric with respect to the middle line of his/her back: If it has some deformity, the Moire image shows asymmetry and the degree of asymmetry is evaluated visually by a doctor. Therefore, for automating this inspection routine, a potential symmetry axis needs be defined on the Moire image of each subject's back. Batouche[5] recovers 3D shape of backs from their Moire topographic images for possible numerical diagnosis of scoliosis and gibbosity, but it is at least time consuming for handling a large number of Moire image data. For primary screening, evaluation based on 2D images is likely to be promising in a practical sense.

3.2 Acquisition of Moire images

The Moire topographic image concerned is taken by a Moire camera, whose lattice plane is adjusted in parallel with the flat plane of a positioner on which a subject rests himself. This adjustment is realized by tilting and panning the Moire camera so that the Moire stripes on a view from the camera finder disappears on the positioner's flat plane. In this situation, a subject stands on the positioner and is asked to stick both of his respective shoulders and pelvis uniformly on it. If the subject is normal, a symmetric Moire image of his back emerges by some trials of positioning: If he has deformity, no positioning efforts succeed in eliminating asymmetry of the image. Then the image is photographed.

3.3 A symmetry index

When the stripes pattern of a Moire image of a subject's back is evaluated its symmetry, a rectangle window is specified on the back with respect to the detected axis and the stripes inside of the window receives the evaluation. The region in the window is denoted by R_w.

An index describing the degree of symmetry is called the symmetry degree and denoted by sd. Index sd is defined by

$$sd = m_{sym} / m,$$

where

$$m_{sym} = \sum_{(x,y) \in R_w} m_{sym}(x,y),$$

$$m_{sym}(x,y) = \begin{cases} 1 ..... |f(x,y) - f(x',y')| \le th \\ 0 ..... |f(x,y) - f(x',y')| > th \end{cases},$$

$$m = \sum_{(x,y) \in R_w} 1 .$$

Here a pixel (x,y) corresponds symmetrically to a pixel (x',y') with respect to a given axis and th is a threshold. Obviously, $0 \le sd \le 1$.

3.4 Experimental results

The Moire topographic image of a subject's back is provided by a photographic film. It is fed into a workstation through an image scanner and transformed into a 256 by 256 digital image with 256 gray levels. The proposed technique is then applied to this image to detect a potential symmetry axis. Here all this image is specified as region R in Eq.(1), though both arms are excepted manually at the moment. The symmetry degree sd is also calculated. Some experimental results are shown in Fig.1. In Fig.1, the left-hand side images show the detected axes of potential symmetry and the specified windows superposed on the original images, whereas the right-hand side images represent asymmetric portions of the Moire stripes. The symmetry degrees are $sd=0.90$ for the case of (a) and $sd=0.88$ for (b), provided that $th=15$. The average elapsed time is about two minutes by Sparc Station 10.

4 Discussion

Eight cases are experimented including the above two and all of them support availability of the proposed technique. The extracted axis of potential symmetry almost agrees with the middle line of the back in every case and asymmetric portions can clearly be observed.

In the two cases of Fig.1, Moire image of case (a) is apparently better than that of (b) in the sense of symmetry. The symmetry degree is, however, not very different between them. This can be understood by comparing those figures of asymmetric portions in Fig.1, which have similarity in the number of asymmetric pixels.

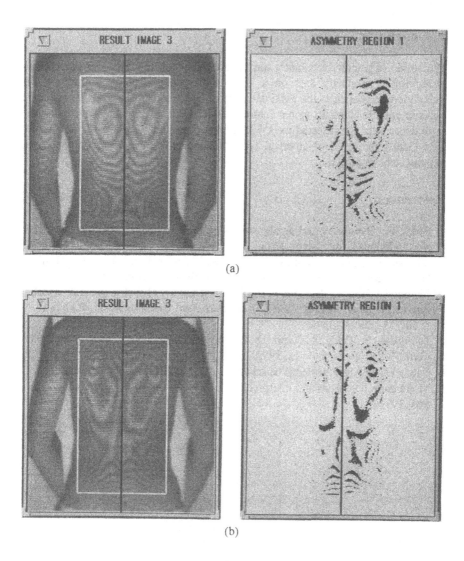

(a)

(b)

Fig. 1 Experimental results.

There are still issues to be solved before putting the symmetry degree into practical use. The value of the symmetry degree depends on the threshold *th* and the specified window size. They relate themselves to some medical knowledge on this spinal deformity inspection and more undeformed/deformed specimens need be employed for specifying those parameters. On the other hand, contrast of a given Moire image also gives influence to the symmetry degree. It needs normalization before proceeding to *sd* calculation, though it is not done in this particular experiment, since gray level histograms show similar distribution among the employed images.

5 Conclusion

The notion of potential symmetry was introduced and a technique was proposed for identifying a symmetry axis on a shape with potential axial symmetry. The technique was applied to the axial detection of Moire topographic images of human backs in order to automate spinal deformation inspection. Experimental results were satisfactory with the detected axes. Asymmetric portions on the back of a subject were clearly indicated. Numerical representation of the degree of symmetry still remains to be improved.

References

1. Eades, P.: "Symmetry finding algorithms", *Computational Morphology*, 41-51, North-Holland, Amsterdam, 1988.
2. Minovic, P., Ishikawa, S., Kato, K.: "Three-dimensional symmetry identification, Part I: Theory", *Memoirs of The Kyushu Inst. Tech.*, **21**, 1-16, 1992.
3. Marola, G.: "On the detection of the axis of symmetry of symmetric and almost symmetric planar images", *IEEE Trans. Patt. Anal. Machine Intell.*, **PAMI-15**, 5, 507-514, 1993.
4. Zabrodsky, H., Peleg, S., Avnir, D.: "Hierarchical symmetry", *Proc. 11 Int. Conf. Pattern Recogn.*, 9-12, 1992.
5. Batouche, M.: "A knowledge based system for diagnosing spinal deformations: Moire pattern analysis and interpretation", *Proc. 11 Int. Conf. Patt. Recogn.*, 591-594, 1992.

Realtime Camera Calibration for Enhanced Reality Visualization *

J.P. Mellor

Massachusetts Institute of Technology, Cambridge, MA 02139 USA
email: jpmellor@ai.mit.edu

Abstract. The problem which must be solved to make realtime enhanced reality visualization possible is basically the camera calibration problem. The relationship between the coordinate frames of the patient, the patient's internal anatomy scans and the image plane of the camera observing the patient must be established. This paper presents a new approach to finding this relationship and develops a system for performing enhanced reality visualization. Given the locations of a few fiducials our method is fully automatic, runs in nearly real-time, is accurate to a fraction of a pixel, allows both patient and camera motion, automatically corrects for changes to the internal camera parameters (focal length, focus, aperture, etc.) and requires only a single video image.

1 Introduction

Enhanced reality visualization is the process process of adding information to a real image. We take a model of the patient obtained from MR or CT data and overlay it on a video image of the patient. The enhanced image effectively provides X-ray vision by displaying those portions of the model which are not visible in the video image in the correct location.

We have developed a novel method for determining the relationship between model and image coordinates using two key insights which simplify the problem.

1. It is not necessary to separate the intrinsic and extrinsic camera parameters for enhanced reality visualization.
2. It is possible to recover depth information from a singe 2D image.

Many of the current enhanced reality visualization systems rely on active sensors such as magnetic trackers and require calibrated cameras. In contrast, our approach uses video information exclusively and does not require a calibrated camera making it particularly well suited for enhanced reality visualization. For a summary of current enhanced reality visualization techniques see [3].

---

* This work was supported in part by ARPA under Rome Laboratory contract F3060-94-C-0204 and ONR contract N00014-91-J-4038.

2 Our Method

2.1 A Perspective Transformation is Enough

The camera calibration problem is typically posed as follows:

$$I = M \begin{bmatrix} \mathcal{R} \\ \mathcal{T} \end{bmatrix} \mathcal{C} \tag{1}$$

Where I is a matrix of image points, M is a matrix of model points, $\mathcal{R}$ is an orthonormal rotation matrix, $\mathcal{T}$ is a translation vector and $\mathcal{C}$ is an internal camera calibration matrix. In general separating the parameters of $\mathcal{R}$, $\mathcal{T}$ and $\mathcal{C}$ is difficult. Unless the individual parameters are needed, there is no reason to separate them.

Camera calibration is often performed as a preliminary step in many applications. A set of camera calibration parameters is recovered and the intrinsic parameters are used for future images. This assumes that the intrinsic parameters are fixed. In general, they are not. They change with the focus and aperture settings. For example, the principle point can shift by 8 pixels or more with adjustments to focus [4]. The effective focal length f also varies with focus and aperture settings. Zoom lenses take this variability to an extreme enabling large changes to f. Lens distortion also varies with changes to focus and aperture [1].

In enhanced reality visualization, we are interested in the total transformation from model to image coordinates. We do not need to separate intrinsic and extrinsic parameters to generate an enhanced reality image. All of the parameters comprising both the intrinsic and extrinsic calibration parameters can be composed into a single 3×4 matrix. Equation (1) can be rewritten as:

$$I = M\mathcal{P} \tag{2}$$

Where M is a matrix of model points in the form $[X\ Y\ Z\ 1]$, I is a matrix of image points in the form $[x\ y\ z]$, x' and y' are the image coordinates of the projection of M onto the image plane and $x' = x/z$, $y' = y/z$. For our purposes finding values for the elements of $\mathcal{P}$ is sufficient. By formulating the problem in this manner we avoid the difficulties associated with decomposing the intrinsic and extrinsic camera parameters. We solve (2) for each image we obtain. Changes in the intrinsic parameters of the camera are inherently captured.[2]

2.2 Depth Information From a Single 2D Image

Even with the simplifications made so far, the problem is still nonlinear. Using spatial features rather than point features enables us to measure a local scale factor at each feature. We use circular fiducials as our spatial features. In essence, we are able to recover $2\frac{1}{2}$D information. The local scale factor s_i is equal to

---

[2] A linear approximation to radial distortion is implicitly modeled. Using 16mm and 25mm lenses of average quality we have found this approximation quite satisfactory. If lens distortion is more severe, a separate correction could be added

the focal length divided by the depth of the feature (f/z_i). The idea of using spatial features to recover a measure of depth is not new, however our use of this information is. Given the local scale factors, solving for $\mathcal{P}$ reduces to a set of three linear equations.

$$x_i' = s_i\,(p_{11}X_i + p_{21}Y_i + p_{31}Z_i + p_{41}) \tag{3}$$

$$y_i' = s_i\,(p_{12}X_i + p_{22}Y_i + p_{32}Z_i + p_{42}) \tag{4}$$

$$1 = s_i\,(p_{13}X_i + p_{23}Y_i + p_{33}Z_i + p_{43}) \tag{5}$$

Where x_i', y_i' and $1/s_i$ are the location and local scale factor of the ith image point and X_i, Y_i and Z_i are the components of the ith model point. Given correspondences between four model and image points (3), (4) and (5) are exactly determined. If more than four correspondences exist the problem is solved in a least-squares fashion by minimizing the following error terms. Where $j = 1 - 3$ and I_{ij} is the jth component of the ith image point $[x_i'\;y_i'\;1]$

$$\|r_j\|_2 = \sum_{i=1}^{n} \left| \frac{I_{ij}}{s_i} - (p_{1j}X_i + p_{2j}Y_i + p_{3j}Z_i + p_{4j}) \right|^2 \tag{6}$$

2.3 Feature Detection

The location and local scale factor of our circular fiducials are recovered using moment calculations.[3] The projection of a circle is an ellipse. Under orthographic projection the centroid of the ellipse corresponds to the projection of the centroid of the circle and the major axis of the ellipse is related to the diameter of the circle by f/z. Under perspective projection these relationships are no longer exact. However for our configuration, a 1cm fiducial viewed from 1m using a 16mm or 25mm lens, the effects of perspective distortion are negligible compared to noise. A more detailed discussion can be found in [3].

2.4 Implementation

The current system is implemented in Lucid Common Lisp and runs on a Sun SparcStation 2 using a VideoPix frame grabber. The two most limiting components are the frame grabber (≤ 4 frames/sec) and the rendering/display system. Depending on the complexity of the model, the renderer may require a minute or more to perform the rendering. Using a simple model, frame rates of $\sim$2hz can be achieved. If the image acquisition and rendering overheads were removed and the rest of the system was optimized, frames rates of $\sim$10-20hz should be achievable without upgraded hardware. Using a C-30 digit signal processing board frame rates of $>$30hz should be achievable.

---

[3] The current implementation utilizes the aspect ratio of the image plane. Of all the camera parameters, the aspect ratio is truly fixed for a given camera/frame grabber combination. In theory, it is possible to perform a self-calibration to recover the aspect ratio when needed. We have not yet implemented this capability.

3 Results

Figure 1 shows some results typical of our method for a geometric object. The locations of the fiducials are accurately known. There are a total of seven fiducials. Three of the images have five in one plane and two in a plane displaced by 1cm. The fourth image has a single fiducial 4cm out of the plane. The image is obtained using a 16mm lens from ~1m. The pillar near the center of the object is 8cm high and is used exclusively for validation purposes. A wire frame corresponding to the edges of the pillar is overlayed on an image. The degree to which the wire frame matches the edges in the image is a measure of the accuracy of our method. The enhancement is accurate well outside the volume enclosed by the fiducials.

Figure 2 shows some results typical of our method for a plastic skull. The locations of the fiducials are determined using a laser scanner [2]. A discussion of this initial calibration can be found in [3]. Given the locations of the fiducials, a model of the skull obtained from CT imaging (shown as black dots) and a video image taken from ~ 1m away with a 25mm lens, the enhanced reality visualizations are generated. There are some slight inaccuracies near the edges of some of the images. The source of this error is currently under investigation. At least some of the error is introduced during the initial calibration.

4 Conclusion

A novel method for enhanced reality visualization has been presented. The method implicitly models the transformation from model to image coordinates and takes advantage of spatial features to obtain a linear system of equations. The method requires only a few fiducials and a single video image. The results are quick and accurate allowing camera parameters such as focus, aperture and zoom to vary dynamically without knowledge of the changes.

References

1. Duane C. Brown. Decentering distortion of lenses. *Photogrammetric Engineering*, 32(3):444–462, 1965.
2. W.E.L. Grimson, T. Lozano-Pérez, G.J. Ettinger W.M. Wells III, S.J. White, and R. Kikinis. An automatic registration method for frameless stereotaxy, image guided surgery, and enhanced reality visualization. In *Computer Vision and Pattern Recognition*, pages 430–436. IEEE, June 1994. Seattle, WA.
3. J.P. Mellor. Enhanced reality visualization in a surgical environment. Master's thesis, Massachusetts Institute of Technology, 1994.
4. Reg G. Willson and Steven A. Shafer. What is the center of the image? Technical Report CMU-CS-93-122, Carnegie-Mellon University, Computer Science Department, April 1993.

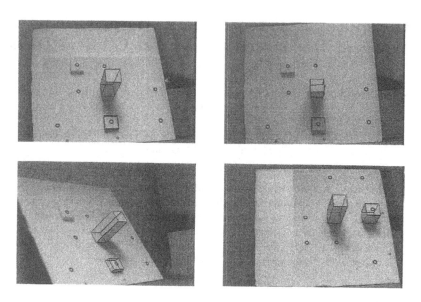

Fig. 1. Some Enhanced Reality Visualizations Using a Geometric Object.

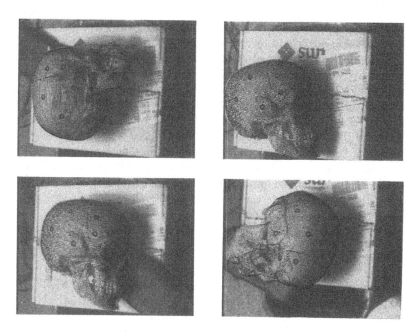

Fig. 2. Some Enhanced Reality Visualizations Using a Plastic Skull.

Computer Assisted Knee Anterior Cruciate Ligament Reconstruction: First Clinical Tests

Vincent Dessenne[1], Stéphane Lavallée[1], Rémi Julliard[2], Philippe Cinquin[1],
Rachel Orti

[1] TIMC-IMAG, Institut Albert Bonniot, 38706 La Tronche Cedex, France
[2] Clinique Mutualiste, 38028 Grenoble, France

Abstract. Anterior Cruciate Ligament reconstruction is a delicate task. An anisometric position of the graft often leads to failure. We propose an original method that allows to position the central part of the ligament graft at the least anisometric sites avoiding an impingement with the femoral notch's roof. The system uses a workstation and a 3D optical localizer. This technique has been validated on 12 patients.

1 Introduction

When the broken ACL has to be replaced, the surgery consists (for most of the surgeons) of making two tunnels, one in the femur notch and one in the tibia, and then to insert and fix a graft (here, the patellar tendon) inside these tunnels. To determine the optimal placement of an ACL graft, the concept of *isometry* has been advocated by many authors to be the main criterion [1]. The graft is assumed to be attached at two points F and T on the femur and the tibia respectively. The anisometry is the residual length variation of the distance between F and T during a flexion-extension (Fig.1). For weak anisometry, the risk of a rupture will be reduced and the knee stability will be improved [2]. In our model, the optimal criterion corresponds to the minimal anisometry between the centers of the tunnels' extremities drilled by the surgeon on the femur notch and the tibia (the graft is roughly a cylinder) [3]. There are many different surgical techniques arguing to obtain near-isometric graft placements, but they all remain controversial. We propose a system which interactively predicts, in real time, the anisometry and the profile of the length variation of the graft, in function of flexion angles, for any point of the femoral notch surface.

2 System

The system we propose uses only per-operative components. The whole system is installed on a cart: a workstation (DEC 5000, Unix) and a 3D optical localizer (Optotrak^{TM}, Northern Digital). The optical localizer is made of 3 linear CCD cameras that detect the position of infra-red emitting diodes with an accuracy of +/- 0.3 mm. The localizer can compute in real time the position and orientation of rigid-bodies made of 6 diodes. The rigid-bodies are water-proof and they can be sterilized with plasma, ethylene oxide or with liquid sterilization chemicals.

3   Method

Many authors have estimated that for all the tibial insertion sites of a reasonable area, the anisometry maps on the femur have similar shapes and values, they are just translated [2][4][5]. In the current version of the system, the surgeon drills the tibial tunnel using the computer system which computes the tibial insertion site according to the *non-impingement* criterion (see step 3). The system is then used to optimize the placement of the femoral tunnel.

First Step: Passive Flexion-Extension. At the beginning of the surgical procedure, the surgeon firmly fixes 2 optical rigid-bodies to the femur and the tibia respectively. These rigid-bodies are used as reference coordinates systems, namely RF and RT. A passive flexion-extension is then applied to the knee by the surgeon (Fig.2). For about 20 to 50 knee positions ranging from maximal extension to maximal flexion, the system stores the location of the coordinate system RT with respect to RF. This gives a set of matrices RTj, $(j = 1 \ldots M)$ (Fig.1).

Second Step: 3D Points Acquisition. The surgeon uses the third rigid-body (RP) to collect some surface points interactively (Fig.3). But before that, the 3D pointer is calibrated easily, using a "pivot technique" that takes about 15 seconds. The surgeon acquires 3 surfaces (each one consists of 20 to 100 points, sizes about 3 cm^2 and is acquired in less than 2 minutes):

- Tibial and femoral surfaces: areas that correspond with all the possible candidates points respectively for the tibial and the femoral attachment sites.
- Femur notch's roof surface: area that could induce collisions with the ligament graft at maximal extension.

Third Step: Tibial Insertion Site Computation. One data modeling step is required before the system can compute the tibial insertion site:

1. Spline interpolations of the tibial and femoral surfaces: for both set (femoral notch surface points and tibial surface points), we initially compute the least-squares planes fitting their points to define two new "intrinsic surface coordinate systems". Their points are interpolated by bicubic spline surfaces and transformed (by mean of transformation matrices) in their intrinstric coordinates systems. Each of the digitized surfaces is small enough to be represented by only one surface patch.
2. Tibial insertion site computation: one of the main problem of ACL reconstruction is the impingement with the femur notch's roof (Fig.1). The main result from experimentations reported in the litterature is that the ACL's lifetime is directly dependant on whether it collides with the roof or not: it is extremely important to avoid any collision. In our system, the graft is considered as a cylinder 10 mm wide: as we have seen before, we modelize it by its central fiber. So, the condition for a non-impingement is that this central fiber is 6 mm away from each point that has been digitized on the roof at step 2. Therefore, the system computes a line having the direction of

the roof length (using an inertia tensor) and so that none of the roof's points is closer than 6 mm to it. The tibial attachment site is the intersection of the tibial surface and this line is worked out.

Fourth Step: Anisometry Map Computation. All the data necessary to optimize our criterion have been acquired or computed.

1. Reconstruction of the 3-D trajectory of T: step 3 gives the coordinates of the tibial attachment point $T_{drilled}$ in RT. Step 1 gives a set of positions RT_j of RT in RF. Simple matrix products give a set of point positions T_j, $j = 1 \ldots M$, in RF. The trajectory of the tibial point $T_{drilled}$ is roughly a portion of a circle.

2. Computation of the femur anisometry map: for each point F of the inter- polated femur spline surface, the system can now compute the predicted ligament length variation curve (in function of flexion angles) and the ani- sometry criterion ANI(F) which is the maximal length variation:

$$ANI(F) = MAX_j \; distance(F, T_j) - MIN_j \; distance(F, T_j) \qquad (1)$$

The *anisometry map* is the projection of ANI(F) on the femur spline's least- square plane. The map is represented as a pseudo-color image (Fig.4).

Fifth Step: Interactive Placement of the Femoral Tunnel. The surgeon can now locate the most isometric point on the femoral surface using any standard sur- gical tool equipped with a fourth rigid-body. For instance, we can equip and calibrate a drill: the surgeon moves the drill and the system computes in real time the intersection point I between the spline femur surface and the drill axis. The point I is displayed on the anisometry map, and the anisometry value ANI(I) and the curve of length variation are displayed. The surgeon can thus easily adjust the position of his tool until it is into a satisfactory region of the anisometry map, and then he can drill the 2 mm femoral tunnel at that point.

4 Clinical Validation

The system has been tested on eight cadaveric specimens: anisometry better than 2 mm could always been obtained. Anatomical results are detailed in [5]. The system has been successfully tested on 12 patients, in open surgery for 3 cases, and under arthroscopy for 9 cases. For the first experiments, we used a conservative approach in which the surgeon used his standard technique, namely the method of Morgan [6], while the system was simply used to measure and study the residual anisometry obtained: it ranged from 1.5 mm to 6.8 mm, with a mean value of 3.0 mm. From these first results, we conclude that the standard technique we used, which is one of the most performant technique at that time, provides a good anisometry in mean, but placements with large anisometry can still occur in some cases. Considering standard devices are not adapted to each individual case, we could expect this result.

5 Discussion

Cost Versus Benefit. Since the purpose is to improve a standard technique, only a long-term study can definitly prove that this improved technique is better than previous ones. However, cost and expected benefit can be analyzed.

1. General cost
   - The system requires less than 10 minutes only during surgery, and about 15 minutes for preparation.
   - The system adds a cumbersome new material in the operating room, but it is easy to move. It is strongly interactive and easy to understand.
   - Adding any system in the orthopaedics surgical room increases the risks of infection. Special care about sterilization techniques must be respected.
   - Such a system only needs a standard computer and a 3D optical localizer: the hardware components of these systems are now cheap.
2. Expected Benefit
   - The system helps to obtain an optimal placement of the graft, that is to increase its lifetime. Contrary to many currently used techniques, the system is not operator-dependant: it is only knee-dependant.
   - The system can help experienced surgeons and may help young surgeons or surgeons who do not perform several ACL reconstructions per week. Our system should anyway help surgeons to acquire experience and knowledge rapidly and in a rational way.

Towards an Easy Single-Tunnel Technique. Some authors do advocate the single-tunnel technique but its realisation is actually not an easy task. The technique we propose is likely to turn this realisation as an easy, fast and accurate one, but we still need to imagine some new material.

6 Conclusion

Anterior Cruciate Ligament reconstruction is a delicate task for which many techniques have been marketed. The system we propose is accurate, non-operator dependant, and it really enables to optimize a defined criterion. It is based on affordable technology, it does not require X-rays or pre-operative imaging. It is very interactive, simple to use. To go any further, a realistic model of the anterior cruciate ligament is necessary. Therefore, we are working on building such a model using elastic models. Although this is already a challenging research, this model will be only a part of a more complex model of the whole knee, that we hope to contribute to build.

References

1. Odensten, M., Guillquist, J.: Functionnal anatomy of the anterior curciate ligament and a rationale for reconstruction. J. Bone and Joint Surg. **67** (1985) 257–261

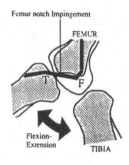

Femur notch Impingement

FEMUR

T F

Flexion-
Extension TIBIA

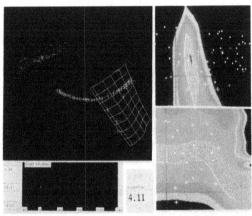

4.11

Fig. 1. the ACL in the knee

Fig.4. the anisometry map and curve

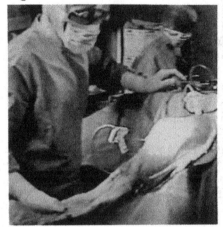

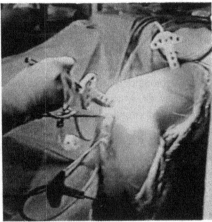

Fig. 2. rigid-bodies, flexion-extension

Fig.3. surfaces and points digitization

2. Fleming, B., Beynnon, B.D. and al.: Isometric versus tension measurements: a comparison for the reconstruction of the anterior cruciate ligament. The American Journal of Sports Medicine **21** (1993) 82–88

3. Orti, R., Lavallée, S. and al.: Computer assisted knee ligament reconstruction. IEEE EMBS Conf. (1993) 936–937

4. Muneta, T., Yamamoto, H. and al.: Relationship between changes in length and force in in vitro reconstructed anterior cruciate ligament. The American Journal of Sports Medicine **21** (1993) 299–304

5. Lavallée, S., Julliard, R. and al.: Reconstruction du ligament croisé antérieur : détermination du meilleur point isométrique fémoral assistée par ordinateur. Orthopédie Traumatologie **4** (1994) 87–92

6. Morgan, C.D., Garrett, J.C. and al.: Transtibial single incision anterior cruciate ligament reconstruction: Arthrex. (1993)·

Extracting 3D Objects from Volume Data Using Digital Morse Theory

Daniel B. Karron * and James Cox [†]

*New York University Medical Center, Department of Surgery
560 First Avenue, New York, New York, 10016
e-mail: karron@nyu.edu, **voice:** 212 263 5210 and
[†]Brooklyn College of the City University Of New York, Department of Computer Science

Abstract. Algorithms that tile isovalued surfaces should produce "correctly" tiled orientable manifold surfaces. Rigorous evaluation of different algorithms or case tables has been impossible up to now because of the lack of a clear and comprehensive theoretical framework. We propose and develop an extension of continuous Morse theory, called Digital Morse Theory. In contrast to applications of Morse theory for a single isovalued surface, we seek to apprehend the data as a whole, independent of isovalue. DMT provides a heuristic to correctly disambiguate tiling decisions. DMT gives insight into topologically correct simplification of a volume data set independent of isovalue. We discuss our preliminary implementation of these ideas, with applications to imaging, segmentation, and navigation of a volume while dynamically changing resolution scale and/or isovalue.

1 Introduction and Motivation

This ongoing work is motivated by the desire to establish a theoretical and practical basis for building "correctly" tiled isovalued surfaces (isosurfaces) in a volume data set. The investigation has led to the development of Digital Morse Theory (DMT), which will allow us to efficiently characterize all possible isosurfaces (up to topological equivalence) over all isovalues, that is, to completely apprehend the volume data, and provide a starting point for physical and model-based reasoning.

Volume data consists of real numbers (from a sampled function) at lattice points in space. The problem is to interpolate the level set (isosurface) corresponding to a specific function value τ (isovalue). We refer to the cubic volume of the lattice in 3 dimensions as a cubel (resp. boxel in 2 dimensions). The lattice vertices are thus connected by cubel edges, with each cubel having eight vertices and sharing each face with an adjacent cubel. Members of the level set lie on the edges that straddle τ at the vertices (one vertex **In**, the other **Out**), and we interpolate a single isovalue "hit" thereon.

In general, the isosurfaces should be oriented manifolds that contain maximal connected sets of data readings that are uniformly either greater than or equal to the isovalue (**In**) or less than the isovalue (**Out**). To define data lattice connectivity, one generally uses the usual 6-adjacency. However, there is a fundamental asymmetry that forces one to extend the notion to 18-adjacency in some cases.

Consider the situation where there are 4 threshold crossings in a cubel face, a cubel face, as in figure 1, 5-8. In this case we have to decide whether to associate the diagonally opposing high (**In**) readings or the diagonally opposing low (**Out**) readings with the same (relative) isosurface interior. We call these choices "knitting rules", see for example [1]. To answer critical questions in object definition, segmentation, and topological connectivity, we need more fundamental insight as to the meaning of tiled isosurfaces [2] [3] [4] [5].

A Morse function is a function that has a finite set of critical points and has a non-singular Hessian at each critical point. The fundamental result of Morse theory says that the topology of the levels sets is invariant between critical values, and that topological changes at the critical values are completely characterized by the Morse data (number of negative eigenvalues of the Hessian) of the corresponding critical points. Similarly, DMT investigates the topological changes in the isosurfaces as the isovalue is varied continuously. This work uses Morse theory in a different setting than Shinawaga *et al* [6] [7], in the sense that our analysis of the density function is independent of the choice of isovalue.

2 Isosurface Algorithms and Axioms.

Many algorithms work by means of a rules encoded into a look-up table [8] [9] [10] [11] [12] [13] [14] [15]. There has yet to emerge a consensus as to how to define topological correctness [16] [3] [4], and various schemes to disambiguate [1] [17] or re-tile [18] the apparently "rare" ambiguous (4-hit face) circumstances have been implemented.

We have formulated a consistent system of 4 axioms to describe a correct set of isosurfaces [19]. Our axioms define the set of isosurfaces up to homeomorphism. Our first three axioms conform to the usual goals of the aforementioned surface construction algorithms. Our fourth axiom specifies the disambiguating knitting rule for the 4 hit faces (described below). The essential point is that any disambiguation rule for 4 hit faces implies a critical point in the density function in this face. The current practice [20] of drawing contour maps omits this critical point information.

3 The SpiderWeb algorithm.

The SpiderWeb algorithm [21] [22] [23] produces a collection of surfaces, each consisting of a triangle tiling (simplicial complex), as does the well-known Marching Cubes algorithm [8] [10]. The SpiderWeb algorithm builds the triangulation for each cubel independently (and thus is highly parallelizable). It creates an "articulating point", which is the spatial mean of a "connected" system of hits within a cubel. Each triangle consists of the articulating point and an adjacent pair of hits from the connected system.

Hit connectivity is defined in a manner similar to digital topology [24]: Two hits are adjacent if they share a common 2 hit cubel face, or are adjacent on a 4 hit face. Path connectivity is the transitive closure of the adjacency relation. The hits on a 4 hit face are separated into two adjacent pairs as follows (see figure 1):

The critical value is the isovalue below which the two line segments defined by the pairs of hits straddling the **Out** vertices have shorter total length than the segments obtained by the pairs straddling the **In** vertices. Above the critical value the diagonally opposed **In** vertices are part of locally (relative to the cubel) separate objects, and thus the pair of hits on the edges incident to each **In** are considered adjacent. At the critical value the two local objects merge. Below the critical value the **In** vertices are part of the same local object interior, and thus the two hits on the edges incident to each **Out** vertex are adjacent.

4 Applying Digital Morse Theory

4.1 Comparing the Knitting Rules.

The first, shown in figure 1, is "Knit High Above τ_{crit}, Knit Low Below", and the second, shown in figure 1, is "Knit Low Above τ_{crit}, Knit High Below". We can see that the first rule is appropriate, since it corresponds to the local topological changes that one would expect when there is only one saddle critical point. By contrast, in figure 1, we get extra local transitions. There are similar problems with other knitting rules. In our subsequent work we justify our choice, in a manner similar to [25].

We collect (in breadth-first fashion) all connected collections of identically valued vertices. For each vertex (or collection) we can recognize an extremum or saddle by examining the edge adjacent vertices. Additionally, a pattern of reversing gradients around the perimeter of a cubel face indicates a saddle (appropriate τ causes 4 hits). Each critical point owns its "basin of attraction". We can now use the natural global relationship between criticalities to build an object spectra, such as indicated in figure 2, and we can include the associated Morse data. In addition, one can now divide the entire range into critical value free intervals and build the isosurfaces for a single (sample) value from each interval, thus representing all possible topologies.

From rectilinear monotonic regions, *i.e.*, where the data lattice values are monotonically increasing or decreasing, we can form "Super" cubels, independently of isovalue (figure 3). Note that Schroeder [26] and Kalvin [27], simplify a tiled surface for a single isovalue. Significant data simplification can now be applied directly to the volume data, independently of the isovalue choice. Further, one can approximately render the volume using super cubels, and then give a more refined rendering of the super cubel volume, as more finely detailed geometric information is needed, independently of the surrounding regions. Using this

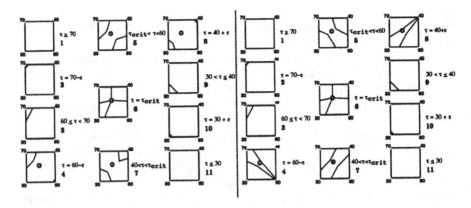

Fig. 1. LEFT:"Knit Kigh Above Knit Low Below" rule. Note that there is only **one** transition discontinuity, at the critical point, at 6, which is as expected by Digital Morse Theory. RIGHT: "Knit Low Above Knit High Below" rule. Note that there are **three** discontinuous transitions, from 3 to 4, at 6, and from 8 to 9.

idea, as well as the aforementioned techniques, we anticipate the development of powerful software tools to visually navigate the data space, at dynamically changing resolution and isovalue. In addition, we can rank criticalities by the size of their associated regions, and eliminate smaller, innessential criticalities relative to a particular resolution scale.

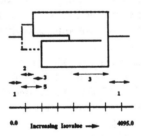

Fig. 2. For every valid isovalue, τ, we can look up what objects exist there, and how many distinct objects are present. This can be an important guide to apprehending a volume. This is a kind of **Reeb Graph**.

5 Summary and conclusions.

Digital Morse Theory (DMT) will provide the ability to completely apprehend volume data lattices independent of any particular isovalue.

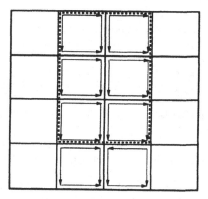

Fig. 3. Monotonic "Super Boxel" hits behave the same way as regular, simple boxels, with only 2 hits possible along entire perimeter, the dashed line.

References

1. G. M. Nielson and B. Hamann, "The Asymptotic Decider: Resolving the Ambiguity in Marching Cubes," in *Proceedings of Visualization 91* (G. M. Nielson and L. Rosenblum, eds.), vol. 2, pp. 83–91, 1991.

2. J. K. Udupa, "Surface Connectedness in Digital Spaces: Theory and Algorithms," Technical Report MIPG188, Medical Image Processing Group, University Of Pennsylvania, Medical Image Processing Group, Department of Radiology, University Of Pennsylvania, Brockley Hall, Fourth Floor, 418 Service Drive, Philadelphia,Pennsylvania, 19104–6021, Oct. 1992.

3. A. V. Gelder and J. Wilhelms, "Topological Ambiguities in Isosurface Generation," tech. rep., University of California at Santa Cruz, 1990.

4. J. Wilhelms and A. V. Gelder, "Topological considerations in isosurface generation: Extended abstract," *ACM Computer Graphics*, vol. 24, pp. 79–86, Nov. 1990.

5. J. Wilhelms and A. V. Gelder, "Octrees for faster isosurface generation," *ACM Transactions on Graphics*, vol. 11, pp. 201–227, July 1992.

6. Y. Shinagawa, T. L. Kunii, and Y. L. Kergosien, "Surface Coding Based on Morse Theory," *IEEE Computer Graphics and Applications*, vol. 11, pp. 66–78, Sept. 1991.

7. Y. Shinagawa and T. L. Kunii, "Constructing a Reeb Graph Automatically from Cross Sections," *IEEE Computer Graphics and Applications*, vol. 11, pp. 44–51, Nov. 1991.

8. W. E. Lorensen and H. E. Cline, "Marching Cubes: A High Resolution 3D Surface Construction Algorithm," *ACM Computer Graphics*, vol. 21, pp. 163–169, July 1987.

9. H. E. Cline, C. L. Dumoulin, H. R. H. Jr., and W. E. Lorensen, "3D Reconstruction of the Brain from Magnetic Resonance Images Using a Connectivity Algorithm," *Magnetic Resonance Imaging*, vol. 5, pp. 345–352, July 1987.

10. H. E. Cline, W. E. Lorensen, S. Ludke, and B. C. T. C. R. Crawford, "Two Algorithms for the Reconstruction of Surfaces from Tomograms," *Medical Physics*, vol. 15, pp. 320–327, May 1988.

11. H. H. Baker, "Building, Visualizing, and Computing on Surfaces of Evolution," *IEEE Computer Graphics and Applications*, vol. 8, pp. 31–41, July 1988.

12. E. Artzy, G. Frieder, and G. T. Herman, "The theory, design, implementation and evaluation of a three–dimensional surface detection algorithm," *Computer graphics and Image Processing*, vol. 15, pp. 1–24, Jan. 1981.

13. J. Bloomenthal, "Polygonization of Implicit Surfaces," *Computer Aided Geometric Design*, vol. 5, pp. 341–355, 1988.

14. A. Wallin, "Constructing Isosurfaces from CT Data," *IEEE Computer Graphics and Applications*, vol. 11, pp. 28–33, Nov. 1991.

15. T. Nagae, T. Agui, and H. Nagahashi, "Orientable Closed Surface Construction from Volume Data.," *IEICE Transaction Inf. and Systems*, vol. E76D, pp. 269–273, Feb. 1993.

16. P. Ning and J. Bloomenthal, "An Evaluation of Implicit Surface Tilers," *IEEE Computer Graphics and Applications*, vol. 13, pp. 33–41, Nov. 1993.

17. A. D. Kalvin, *Segmentation and Surface-Based Modeling of Objects in Three-Dimensional Biomedical Images*. Ph.D. dissertation, New York University, Computer Science Department, 1991.

18. P. Frey and M. Gautherie, "Generation Automatique D'un Maillage 3D Dans Un Ensemble De Voxels: Application à la modèlisation thermique numèrique 3D en thermothèrapie ultrasonore," *Innovation Et Technologie En Biologie Et Medecine*, vol. 12, pp. 428–442, Apr. 1991.

19. D. B. Karron, J. Cox, and B. Mishra, "New findings from the spiderweb algorithm : Toward a digital morse theory," in *Visualization in Biomedical Computing - '94* (R. A. Robb, ed.), no. 2359 in SPIE Proceedings, pp. 643–657, SPIE, SPIE, Oct. 1994.

20. W. M. Snyder, "Contour Plotting," *ACM Transactions on Mathematical Software*, vol. 4, no. 3, pp. 290–294, 1978.

21. D. B. Karron, "The "SpiderWeb" algorithm for surface construction in noisy volume data," in *Visualization in Biomedical Computing '92* (R. A. Robb, ed.), vol. 1808, pp. 462–576, Society of Photo–Optical Instrumentation Engineers, 1992.

22. D. Karron, J. Cox, and B. Mishra, "The SpiderWeb Surface Construction Algorithm for Medical Imaging: Properties of Its Surface," Robotics Laboratory Technical Report, New York University, Computer Science Department, 1992.

23. J. L. Cox, D. B. Karron, and B. Mishra, "The SpiderWeb Algorithm for Surface Construction from Medical Volume Data: Geometric Properties of its Surface," *Innovations Et Technologie en Biologie et Medecine*, vol. 14, pp. 634–656, Nov. 1993.

24. G. T. Herman, "Oriented Surfaces in Digital Spaces," *CVGIP: Graphical Models and Image Processing*, vol. 55, pp. 381–396, Sept. 1993.

25. D. Mumford and J. Shah, "Optimal Approximations of Piecewise Smooth Functions and Associated Variational Problems," *Communications in Pure and Applied Mathematics*, vol. 42, pp. 577 – 685, 1989.

26. W. J. Schroeder, J. A. Zarge, and W. E. Lorensen, "Decimation of triangle meshes," *ACM Computer Graphics*, vol. 26, pp. 65–70, July 1992.

27. A. D. Kalvin and R. H. Taylor, "SuperFaces: Polyhedral Approximation with Bounded Error," Research Report RC19135 (82286), IBM Research Division, IBM Research Division, T. J. Watson Research Center, Yorktown Heights, New York 10598, Apr. 1993.

Towards Realistic Visualization for Surgery Rehearsal

B. Pflesser and U. Tiede and K.H. Höhne

Institute of Mathematics and Computer Science in Medicine (IMDM)
University-Hospital Eppendorf
Martinistraße 52, 20246 Hamburg, Germany
e-mail: pflesser@uke.uni-hamburg.de

Abstract. A method for free-form cutting in tomographic volume data is presented. As a basic data structure, the generalized voxel model is chosen. Removed regions are indicated using attributes. Tools like a "rasp" or a "knife" are presented. Methods for detection and visualization of cut surfaces, both for mapping of original gray values and of color labels for the segmented objects, are discussed. It is claimed that the possibilities of the described method are exceeding those of any surface-based approach.

1   Introduction

So far, systems for rehearsal of surgical interventions are based on traditional computer graphics methods, where an object is represented by its surface only. However, in order to provide a 'look and feel' close to a real dissection, both

- information about the interior of an object, and
- free form cutting

are required. Furthermore, surgical rehearsal requires that any operation may be undone. The first point clearly implies that we need a volume-based approach. For an implementation of free form operations, the following problems have to be solved:

- how can we specify an arbitrarily shaped region in 3D space?
- how do we represent the (partial) objects generated by cutting?
- how do we visualize free form cuts and partial objects?

Several applications for object manipulation have been suggested that are based on the binary-voxel-model [3, 11, 12]. These applications emphasize the definition of objects by performing boolean operations with a user-defined mask. The specification of arbitrarily shaped objects is a less developed subject. Some approaches have been developed by [1, 12, 13]. However, all these applications do not provide the possibility of visualizing information about the interior structure of an object. Therefore, we wanted to establish free form operations in our VOXEL-MAN volume visualization system [5, 6, 8, 9].

VOXEL-MAN already provides a set of tools for object manipulation in a volume representation. For example, objects defined in a previous segmentation step may be removed or added like in an assembly kit, or arbitrary cut planes may be specified. Clearly, these functions are not yet sufficient for our above described goals.

2 Method

2.1 Basic Data Structure

Within the VOXEL-MAN system, anatomical objects are described using a two level data structure [5]. The lower level is a discrete data volume, as obtained from a medical imaging system. In addition, a set of attributes is assigned to every voxel, indicating its membership to anatomical regions under various aspects (e.g. morphology, functional anatomy). This level is equivalent to the previously described *generalized voxel model* [4]. On the upper level, objects and their relations are symbolically described [7].

For achieving the new functionality of representing arbitrarily formed areas within the generalized voxel model we are using an additional voxel attribute, indicating its membership in a cut-out region. In contrast to other attributes this kind of information is not static and object relations have to be updated whenever new areas are specified. This way, the original object information is available at any point of a cut-out region, and all operations can easily be reversed.

2.2 Specification

As an extension of our VOXEL-MAN volume visualization system, we developed different tools for specifying arbitrary regions which are presented in the following. As a first step, geometrical shapes like boxes, spheres or shapes given by a set of polygons can be defined. Of course, this method does not yet allow realistic simulations. Therefore, we developed interactive specification tools which are based on ray traversal procedures. This way, one can define arbitrarily shaped regions within the context of 3D-images.

One of these tools works like a rasp, which is used to peel off voxels at an object surface layer by layer. Its size and shape may be chosen. Fig.1 shows the simulation of a craniotomy where a tumor has been removed using this tool. Another tool works like a scalpel or a saw. It is used to cut away whole regions by specifying a contour, a cutting depth and a cutting direction. The latter may be specified in three different ways:

- viewing direction: the cut follows the direction of the viewing ray and is thus perpendicular to the screen
- surface normal direction: the cut is specified by the surface normal at the position of the cutting tool and is thus perpendicular to the local object surface
- free direction: the direction of the cut is interactively specified by the user.

These tools provide free-form cuts within the volume model. By changing their "sharpness", they can be limited to work for certain objects only.

2.3 Visualization

For the visualization of free-form cuts two problems must be solved: the detection of the surface formed by a cut-away region and a surface normal estimation at these positions. Once the free-form surface is detected and a surface normal has been calculated, either original gray-level data or object colors can be mapped to the shaded-surface display (fig. 2).

Detection of Free-Form-Cut Surfaces A major problem is to decide whether the visible parts of an object are representing a "normal" object surface or a free-form cut. Since the removed region is represented as an individual object in the generalized voxel model, the cut surface is not explicitly represented. Thus, the decision has to be made during ray traversal, depending on whether the voxel preceding the voxel in question belongs to a cut-away region or not. Moreover, it has to be decided whether a laid off surface is a surface of an anatomical object or not. For the latter, the problem of surface normal estimation has to be solved.

Z-Buffer-Gradient Shading For rendering surfaces in tomographic volume data, the grey-level gradient method has proven to be accurate. However, if a cut is to be shaded, this method can not be used because gray-level differences inside an homogeneous object are not related to a surface and more or less randomly distributed. In our first attempt we therefore have implemented a solution that is based on Z-buffer gradient shading.

This method, first proposed by [2], was originally designed for the visualization of binary volumes and calculates the surface normal vectors from the depth image of an object, stored in the Z-buffer. While the basic principle follows that in [10], it is important for our application that the calculation of backward and forward differences of the neighboring pixels is done locally at the free-form cuts. This is restricted to an individual object and is done during projection. This way the algorithm delivers fairly realistic images and the impression of free form cuts can be improved.

3 Conclusion

The novel approach presented in this paper provides the basis for a realistic rehearsal of surgical interventions, which could not be achieved with any surface-based method. We presented a suitable data structure, tools for free-form cutting, and adapted visualization methods.

While the feasibility of this approach could be shown, we consider improvement of the visualization, especially for surface normal estimation, an important next step. A major task for the future is of course also the design of a suitable user interface, which will allow to handle the presented methods in a rather "natural" way.

4 Acknowledgement

We are grateful to all members of our department for valuable discussions. We thank A. Pommert for practical assistance. The original MRI image sequence of the head has been kindly provided by Siemens Medical Systems (Erlangen).

References

1. Arridge, S. R.: Manipulation of volume data for surgical simulation. In Höhne, K. H. et al. (Eds.): *3D-Imaging in Medicine: Algorithms, Systems, Applications*, NATO ASI Series F 60, Springer-Verlag, Berlin, 1990, 289–300.
2. Chen, L. S., Herman, G. T., Reynolds, R. A., Udupa, J. K.: Surface shading in the cuberille environment. *IEEE Comput. Graphics Appl. 5*, 12 (1985), 33–43.
3. Chen, L.-S., Sontag, M. R.: Representation, Display and Manipulation of 3D Digital Scenes and their Medical Applications. *Comput. Vision Graphics Image Process. 48* (1989), 190–216.
4. Höhne, K. H., Bomans, M., Pommert, A., Riemer, M., Schiers, C., Tiede, U., Wiebecke, G.: 3D-visualization of tomographic volume data using the generalized voxel-model. *Visual Comput. 6*, 1 (1990), 28–36.
5. Höhne, K. H., Bomans, M., Riemer, M., Schubert, R., Tiede, U., Lierse, W.: A 3D anatomical atlas based on a volume model. *IEEE Comput. Graphics Appl. 12*, 4 (1992), 72–78.
6. Höhne, K. H., Pommert, A., Riemer, M., Schiemann, T., Schubert, R., Tiede, U., Lierse, W.: Framework for the generation of 3D anatomical atlasses. In Robb, R. A. (Ed.): *Visualization in Biomedical Computing II, Proc. SPIE 1808*. Chapel Hill, NC, 1992, 510–520.
7. Pommert, A., Schubert, R., Riemer, M., Schiemann, T., Tiede, U., Höhne, K. H.: Symbolic modeling of human anatomy for visualization and simulation. In Robb, R. A. (Ed.): *Visualization in Biomedical Computing 1994, Proc. SPIE 2359*. Rochester, MN, 1994, 412–423.
8. Schubert, R., Höhne, K. H., Pommert, A., Riemer, M., Schiemann, T., Tiede, U., Lierse, W.: A new method for practicing exploration, dissection, and simulation with a complete computerized three-dimensional model of the brain and skull. *Acta Anat. 150*, 1 (1994), 69–74.
9. Tiede, U., Bomans, M., Höhne, K. H., Pommert, A., Riemer, M., Schiemann, T., Schubert, R., Lierse, W.: A computerized three-dimensional atlas of the human skull and brain. *Am. J. Neuroradiology 14*, 3 (1993), 551–559.
10. Tiede, U., Höhne, K. H., Bomans, M., Pommert, A., Riemer, M., Wiebecke, G.: Investigation of medical 3D-rendering algorithms. *IEEE Comput. Graphics Appl. 10*, 2 (1990), 41–53.
11. Trivedi, S. S.: Interactive Manipulation of Three Dimensional Binary Scenes. *Visual Comput. 2* (1986), 209–218.
12. Udupa, J. K., Odhner, D.: Fast visualization, manipulation and analysis of binary volumetric objects. *IEEE Comput. Graphics Appl. 11*, 6 (1991), 53–62.
13. Yasuda, T., Hashimoto, Y., Yokoi, S., Toriwaki, J.-I.: Computer system for craniofacial surgical planning based on CT images. *IEEE Trans. Med. Imaging MI-9*, 3 (1990), 270–280.

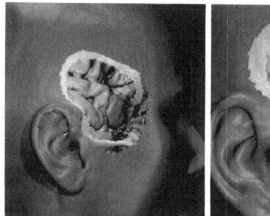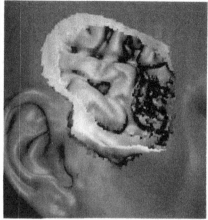

Fig. 1. Simulation of craniotomy. Parts of the skull and soft tissue have been removed laying off a tumor (left). The tumor itself has been peeled off using a "rasp". The cut surface has been shaded using the grey-level gradient method and thus some artefacts occur (right).

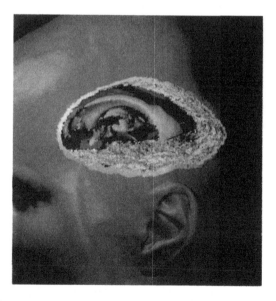

Fig. 2. Free-form cutting. A cut-away region has been defined by specifying a contour and a cutting depth. The cut has been specified to be perpendicular to the local object surface excluding the ventricular system. The cut surface has been shaded using the Z-buffer gradient method.

Segmentation III

Segmentation of 3D Objects from MRI Volume Data Using Constrained Elastic Deformations of Flexible Fourier Surface Models

G. Székely, A. Kelemen, Ch. Brechbühler and G. Gerig

Communication Technology Laboratory
ETH-Zentrum, CH-8092 Zurich, Switzerland
email: szekely@vision.ee.ethz.ch

Abstract. This paper describes a new model-based segmentation technique combining desirable properties of physical models (snakes, [2]), shape representation by Fourier parametrization (Fourier snakes, [12]), and modelling of natural shape variability (eigenmodes, [7, 10]). *Flexible shape models* are represented by a parameter vector describing the mean contour and by a set of *eigenmodes of the parameters* characterizing the shape variation with respect to a small set of stable landmarks (AC-PC in our application) and explaining the remaining variability among a series of images with the model flexibility. Although straightforward, the extension to 3-D is severely impeded by finding a proper surface parametrization for arbitrary objects with spherical topology. We apply a newly developed surface parametrization [16, 17] which achieves a uniform mapping between object surface and parameter space. The 3D model building and Fourier-snake procedure are demonstrated by segmenting deep structures of the human brain from MR volume data.

1 Introduction

Segmentation of anatomical objects from large 3D medical data sets, which result from routine Magnetic Resonance Imaging (MRI) examinations, e.g., represents one of the basic problems of medical image analysis. In some limited applications, segmentation could be achieved with appropriate tools by minimal user interaction [1]. For general applications, however, adequate segmentation cannot be obtained without expert knowledge, requiring tedious manual interaction by a human specialist.

Elastically deformable contour models (snakes) [2] have been proposed as tools for supporting manual object delineation. While such procedures can be extended to 3D [3, 4], their initialization becomes difficult. Most often, the initial guess must be very close to the sought contour to guarantee a successful result [5]. While a careful and time-consuming analysis is acceptable for outlining complex pathological objects, no real justification for such a procedure can be found for the delineation of normal, healthy organs, as needed in radiation treatment planning, for example.

The primary reason for the need of a precise snake initialization is the presence of disturbing attractors in the image, which do not belong to the actual object contour but force the snake into local energy minima. If the deformation of a snake could be limited to shapes within the normal anatomic variation of organs, such local minima could be eventually avoided.

Inclusion of prior knowledge in the image interpretation process can be achieved e.g. by incorporation prior distributions on the variables to be estimated, as proposed by Vemuri and Radisavljevic [6]. Cootes et.al. [7] use an alternative way which parallelly reduces the dimensionality of the object descriptor space. They use active shape models, which strictly restrict their possible deformations according to the statistics of training samples. Object shapes are described by the point distribution model (PDM) [8], which represents the object outline by a subset of boundary points. There must be a one-to-one correspondence between these points in the different outlines of the training set. After normalization, they provide the basis for the statistical analysis of the object shape deformations. The mean point positions and their modes of variation (i.e. the largest eigenvectors of their covariance matrix) are used for delimiting the object deformations to a reasonable linear subspace of the complete parameter space. They propose a slice-by-slice approach for solving 3D shape analysis problems [9]. Similar parametrization based on point-by-point correspondence, but on real 3D models, were proposed for the 3D shape analysis of brain structures by Martin et al. [10].

While the idea of restricted elastic deformation of an average surface model is very promising, the parametrization of shapes by displacement of corresponding points on their surfaces is not a convenient technique. For a large training set containing many different anatomic structures, the generation of this parametrization seems to be very tedious and, because of the lack of a reasonable automatization, can be a source of errors. A similar modal analysis, however, can be performed for other contour parametrization techniques, as for example for the Fourier-parametrization which was originally proposed by Persoon & Fu and Kuhl & Giardina [18, 11]. Staib and Duncan have demonstrated segmentation by parametrically deformable elastic models for 2D outlines [12] and 3D object surfaces [13]. Herein, we propose a novel technique based on modal analysis of the parameter vector of object contours, providing the desirable restriction of elastic deformations. The method uses automatic shape parametrization, thus avoiding the problem of finding corresponding points among different boundaries.

2 Modal analysis of 2D Fourier models

2.1 Parametrization of 2D contours with Fourier descriptors

The contour of a simply connected object (without holes) is represented by a closed curve with coordinates $(x(t), y(t))$, with variable t ranging from 0 to 2π. The coordinate functions can be developed in a Fourier-series. Restricting the series to its first K degrees results in the parametric description

$$\mathbf{r}(t, \mathbf{p}) = \begin{pmatrix} x(t, \mathbf{p}) \\ y(t, \mathbf{p}) \end{pmatrix} = \begin{pmatrix} a_0 \\ c_0 \end{pmatrix} + \sum_{k=1}^{K} \begin{pmatrix} a_k & b_k \\ c_k & d_k \end{pmatrix} \cdot \begin{pmatrix} cos(kt) \\ sin(kt) \end{pmatrix} \quad . \tag{1}$$

The outline is now parametrized by the parameter-vector

$$\mathbf{p} = (a_0 \ldots a_K, b_1 \ldots b_K, c_0 \ldots c_K, d_1 \ldots d_K)^\mathsf{T} .$$

The parameters can be easily calculated from the sampling points of the outline $q_0, q_1, \ldots, q_P$ with $q_0 = q_P$ (we use maximally dense sampling of the boundary, as provided by the image raster). The resulting parametric shape description can be made invariant under similarity transformations by shifting, rotating and scaling according to the actual displacement, orientation and size of the ellipse determined by the first degree terms of the Fourier series. Similarly, the starting point is moved to a canonical position.

2.2 Fourier Snakes

The snake technique as proposed by Witkin et.al. [2] tries to find the position of a curve $r(t, p)$, which minimizes the energy

$$E(p) = E(r(t, p)) = E_I(r(t, p)) + E_D(r(t, p)) .$$

By varying p, the curve deforms itself to minimize the image energy

$$E_I(r) = - \int_0^1 P(r(t, p)) \, dt ,$$

searching for an optimal position in the image, described by the potential P. A typical choice takes P equal to the negative magnitude of the image gradient.

The deformation term $E_D(r)$ is called the internal energy of the snake and serves as a regularization force. It restricts the elongation and bending of the snakes, and normally depends on the first and second derivatives of the curve $r(t, p)$.

Staib and Duncan [12] propose a different energy model, which makes use of the normal direction of the parametrized curve and of the image gradient to achieve a higher selectivity. Normalizing the image potential by the contour length allows contraction and dilation of curves without affecting the energy function.

$$E_I(r(t, p)) = \pm \left(\int_0^{2\pi} \nabla I(r(t, p)) \cdot \dot{r}_\perp(t, p) \, dt \right) \cdot \left(\int_0^{2\pi} \|\dot{r}(t, p)\| \, dt \right)^{-1}$$

The sign of the energy $E_I(r)$ will decide about the polarity of the object.

One has to realize that cutting the Fourier expansion at a finite degree serves already as a regularization, leaving out high frequency variations of the coordinate functions. However, the internal energy still cannot be neglected, basically because of sharp cusps, shown even by low degree Fourier models, and self-crossing problems. Whereas self-crossings of the outline are very hard to detect, discontinuities of the tangent can be evaluated from the curve parametrization. At such location the curvature $\kappa(t_0, p)$ and its derivative $\dot{\kappa}(t_0, p)$ become both infinite. While high curvature of the boundary should not be excluded a priori, the curvature derivative is chosen to indicate discontinuities (see also [12]), providing the following expression for the internal energy of the Fourier-snake

$$E_D(r(t, p)) = \int_0^{2\pi} \dot{\kappa}^2(t, p) \cdot \|\dot{r}(t, p)\|^2 \, dt \tag{2}$$

For the minimization of the total energy function we used the E04JBF routine of the NAG^{TM} library [14], using a quasi-Newton algorithm for finding an unconstrained minimum of a function of several variables.

Initial placement of model contour by Hough transform: A segmentation of
the corpus callosum from grey-valued images based on the deformation of the
average model requires a suitable initialization. Due to the normalization of the
Fourier coefficients, the average model only expresses shape deformations up to
a similarity transformation (translation, rotation and scaling). Therefore, the
initial placement has to provide an optimal match between the model and the
edges in the grey-valued image. The Hough-transform with the rigid template
was chosen to solve this first optimization problem. The goodness of fit was
calculated for a Canny edge map on a relatively large scale, since the rigid
transformation does not allow for elastic shape deformations. Figure 3 illustrates
the result of the Hough-initialization.

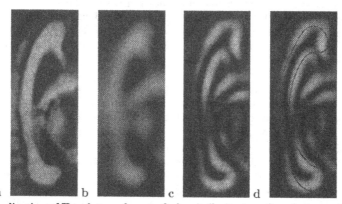

a   b   c   d

Fig. 3. Application of Hough transform to find a similarity transform between the mean
model curve and the gradient magnitude image. Figure **a** shows the original image, **b**
its Gaussian smoothed version ($\sigma = 5$ *pixel*), and **c** the corresponding Canny edge
magnitude image, respectively. In **d**, the optimal fit found by the Hough transform is
overlayed with the edge image.

Segmentation by restricted elastic deformation: After initialization, we apply
a modified version of the Fourier snakes program, which allows only deformations according to the selected eigenmodes. This is nothing else than selecting a
different set of basis functions in place of the harmonics. The restricted variation
is achieved by choosing a subset of eigenmodes, usually the n largest ones, and
calculating the optimization in this linear subspace. Figure 4 illustrates iteration
steps of the optimization procedure on an image not included in the training set.

Sometimes, however, we met difficulties to find the correct contour(see Fig. 5,
e.g.). We found, that the separation of the parameters for the similarity transform and the Fourier coefficients in the model is mainly responsible for this
failure. This separation of rigid and elastic deformation is somewhat artificial,
as they together express fully the biological variations. The quasi-Newton algorithm used by the NAG library routine determines the local optimum nearest
to the initialization, making it extremely sensitive to the initialization, which is
unsatisfactory, since the Hough transform results in only a rough rigid match.

3   Improving Fourier-snake segmentation

Model incorporating full biological variability: We expect for images represent-

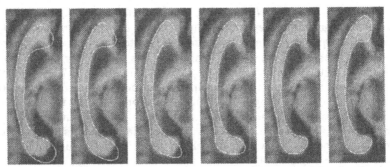

Fig. 4. Iteration steps of the fitting of a Fourier snake restricted by the eigenmodes. The initial placement (left) is calculated by means of a Hough transform. The elastic deformation of the model curve ("Fourier" descriptors up to degree 12) is constrained by the prior information about the normal variability of the corpus callosum, determined from training data.

ing anatomy that the *relative position, rotation, and size* of healthy organs is restricted in a similar way *as their elastic deformation.* If we could define a coordinate system fixed to the anatomy, there would be no reason for a unrestricted similarity transform which precedes the elastic matching. The Fourier descriptors of the organ outlines *originally contain this information,* but we suppress it by normalizing the coefficients. In the case of the corpus callosum, the AC/PC line is a generally accepted, well detectable geometric feature of the mid-sagittal images, which represents such a standard coordinate system. The line from the anterior to the posterior commissure (AC/PC line) has been manually extracted for each image of the training set. After determination of the Fourier coefficients, we apply normalization only for fixing the starting point of the curve parametrization. The standardization of the images, necessary for the determination of the deformation modes, is based on a normalization of the AC/PC line to a e_x unit vector. After that, the same statistical analysis of the test set can be performed as previously explained, providing a mean model (now including its relative position and size to the AC/PC line), and the deformation modes which incorporate the parameters of the similarity transform too.

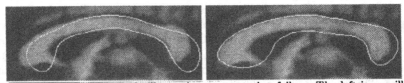

Fig. 5. Segmentation example illustrating segmentation failure. The left image illustrates the initial placement of the model curve (using the Hough transform), theright one shows the segmentation result. The linear subspace was restricted to the largest 12 eigenmodes.

Segmentation: The determination of the AC/PC line now becomes part of the segmentation, since the model is built based on a normalization to these landmarks. Proceeding the segmentation, we first determine the AC/PC line manually. The segmentation is performed by a *coarse to fine* strategy. The flexible model, characterized by the mean contour and the eigenmodes, now incorporates *changes of the position and local deformations* of the generic model, which will be used to achieve a more robust initialization. An initial placement of the curve is performed with a procedure similar to the Hough transform, as described previously. However, we now use a small set of a few dominant modes and calculate the best match in this linear subspace of major deformations. Also the actual segmentation is performed in the homogeneous parameter space of the largest eigenvectors, now choosing a larger number of eigenvectors than in the initialization. Using this seqmentation procedure we achieved perfect results in almost all cases.

4 3D Fourier models of human brain structures

Our general goal is the generalization of the improved 2D procedure to 3D. Unlike the technique proposed by Cootes et al. [7] it will be a true 3-D technique and not based on a combination of 2-D segmentations. The new tool should allow a segmentation of objects in volume data with *minimal, well reproducible human interaction*. This section describes the first steps in this direction, the generation of 3D Fourier models from manually segmented training data, and the use of unrestricted 3D Fourier snakes for elastic matching in grey-valued volume images. As in the previous section, we first summarize the basic mathematics of the 3D Fourier snakes, and then show first results on some MRI brain data. The major problem, finding a *homogeneous parametrization* of surfaces of *arbitrarily shaped objects*, is solved by applying a most recently developed new parametrization technique. It overcomes limitations given by other surface parametrization schemes, e.g. the torus topology presented in [12]. The following description is guided by the example of segmenting deep grey matter structures of the human brain from MR volume data.

4.1 Description of surfaces by spherical harmonic functions

The description of the surfaces of simply connected 3D objects in an orthonormal basis can be performed similarly to the 2D case. The surface will be parametrized by two variables, the θ and ϕ polar parameters, and will be defined by three explicit functions

$$\mathbf{r}(\theta, \phi) = \begin{pmatrix} x(\theta, \phi) \\ y(\theta, \phi) \\ z(\theta, \phi) \end{pmatrix} \quad .$$

We emphasize that this is not a radial function. If we select the spherical harmonic functions (Y_l^m denotes the functon of degree l and order m, see [15]) as a basis, the coordinate functions can be written as

$$\mathbf{r}(\theta, \phi, \mathbf{p}) = \sum_{k=0}^{K} \sum_{m=-k}^{k} \mathbf{c}_k^m \, Y_k^m(\theta, \phi) \quad .$$

The surface is described by the $\{\mathbf{c}_k^m\}$ coefficients, similarly to the 2D case.

In contrast to the 2D case, the *parametrization of a given surface* by the variables θ and ϕ *is far from trivial*. The problem is especially hard for closed surfaces, the case of our primary interest. Brechbühler [16, 17] developed a new method for generating such a parametrization for segmented binary voxel objects by using a first approximation derived from the neighbourhood relationships of the surface nodes. After arbitrary selection of the poles, physical analogy based on the Laplacian equation with Dirichlet border conditions is used to calculate latitude. The longitude is determined similarly, but under cyclic boundary conditions with a 2π discontinuity on the 'date line'. The resulting initial mapping is far from uniform over the sphere, but is a reasonable starting point for a refinement procedure based on non-linear relaxation of the nodes preventing large deformations of the original surface elements, under constraints enforcing exact preservation of the area ratios. This surface parametrization technique is applied for the 3D Fourier-snake segmentation procedure.

One has to realize, that the Fourier-parametrization is just one possibility for the parametric description of contours. Alternative methods, as e.g. deformable superquadrics constructed in ortonormal wavelet bases has also proposed in the literature [6], and can be used for the implementation of elastically deformable parametric models.

4.2 Elastically deformable Fourier surface models

Using the parametric surface description presented previously, the parametrized Fourier-snake concept can be generalized from 2D to 3D. The concept is is similar to the technique proposed by Staib and Duncan [13]. A surface can be arbitrarily sampled based on the variables θ and ϕ (there is no distinguished orientation or position of poles), and the surface energy function can be similarly defined and evaluated as in the 2D case. The image potential can still use the complete (vector-valued) gradient information

$$E_I(\mathbf{r}(\theta, \phi, \mathbf{p})) = \pm \int\int_A \nabla I(\mathbf{r}(\theta, \phi, \mathbf{p})) \cdot \mathbf{n}(\mathbf{r}(\theta, \phi, \mathbf{p})) \, dA$$

where dA is the surface element and $\mathbf{n}$ is the surface normal vector.

We use the internal energy term $E_D(\mathbf{r}(\theta, \phi, \mathbf{p}))$ to avoid sharp discontinuities in the surface normals. The curvature of the surface can be described by the principal curvatures κ_1 and κ_2, which are combined to $\kappa = \sqrt{\kappa_1^2 + \kappa_2^2}$, creating a measure for the curvature of every point on the surface. As in the 2D case, the regularization term will limit its derivative.

After the definition of the total energy, the problem is completely analogous to the 2D case, we have to determine the parameters that generate a surface which minimizes this energy. We used exactly the same minimization procedures as in the 2D case.

4.3 3D segmentation of deep grey matter structures

The training set consists of a collection of 30 3D MRI data volumes of the human brain, were deep grey matter structures (putamen, caudate nucleus and globus pallidus) have been manually segmented. Figure 6 shows a coronal slice through one of the volumes and the outlines of the manually segmented objects. In the case of the putamen and globus pallidus one can see that there is practically

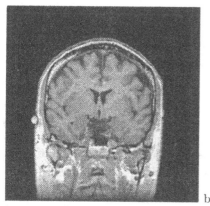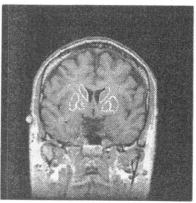

a   b

Fig. 6. Manual segmentation of the putamen, the caudate nucleus and the globus pallidus. The images show a coronal slice from a 3D data set (a) with overlay of the contours of segmented objects (b).

no grey-level evidence to separate the two objects. Only a priori anatomical knowledge will allow their segmentation, which clearly demonstrates the need for model-based 3D segmentation procedures.

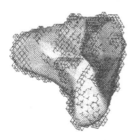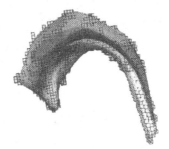

Fig. 7. Parametrized description by spherical harmonics up to degree 8 of the surface of deep grey-matter organs. The putamen is shown on the left, the caudate nucleus on the right. The original voxel object is overlayed as a wireframe structure of the voxel edges.

The modules for 3-D surface parametrization and Fourier description, for the calculation of eigenmodes and for 3D segmentation by restricted elastic deformations are implemented and ready for tests and validation. Preliminary results demonstrate two different procedures of the complete segmentation system:

- Figure 7 illustrates the generation of parametric surface descriptions from binary segmentations. The surfaces of the putamen (left) and of the caudate nucleus (right) use a spherical harmonic approximation up to degree 6 and 8, respectively.
- Figure 8 demonstrates the segmentation of the caudate nucleus from original grey-valued volume data by the 3D Fourier-snake procedure. The initial placement of the model surface was performed using spherical harmonic surface of low degree (degrees 0 . . . 3). For the elastic fit we used spherical

harmonics up to degree 5. 15-20 minutes were needed for the elastic fit of the models on a Sparc10/41 processor.

We are currently calculating the surface parametrization and the description by spherical harmonics of all the 30 segmentations. Based on these results, the deformation eigenmodes for these objects can be determined.

5 Conclusions

Automated, robust segmentation of medical images most often needs a priori anatomical knowledge. Typical cases are the segmentation of healthy organs, which present restricted anatomical variability, or the segmentation of organs if only incomplete evidence for boundaries is given by the grey-valued images, requiring an 'intelligent guess' about the position of the object boundary.

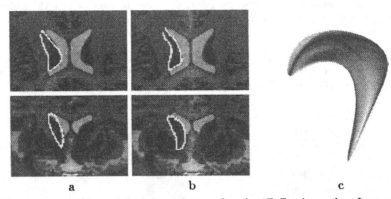

a   b   c

Fig. 8. Segmentation of the left caudate nucleus by 3D Fourier-snakes. Images in column a represent the initial placement of the 3-D model as axial (top) and coronal (bottom) cuts (with spherical harmonics up to degree 3 with 48 parameters). Column b shows the final segmentation result. A graphical display of the elastically deformed model representing the result of the 3-D segmentation is shown to the right (c). The final optimization was based on spherical harmonics up to degree 5 (108 parameters).

Geometric organ models and the statistics of their *normal (expected) variation* seems to offer a promising solution to this problem. We proposed the use of the Fourier parametrization of our models, followed by a statistical analysis of a training set, providing mean organ models and their eigen-deformations. Elastic fit of the mean model in the subspace of eigenmodes restricts possible deformations and finds an optimal match between the model surface and boundary candidates.

We demonstrated the complete procedure with the determination of the outline of the corpus callosum on a 2D MRI slice of the human brain, and presented preliminary results of a full 3D generalization of the Fourier-snake procedure. While the modules are implemented and ready for analysis, we still need to spend effort into the 3D model building.

Our ultimate goal is to provide an automated 3D segmentation procedure that needs only minimal user interaction. This manual interaction would consist of the selection of a few clearly defined landmarks and could therefore be carried out also by non-experts. The segmentation itself would then run fully automatically. Such an elastic deformation procedure restricted by prior knowledge about the deformation range would also find applications in *tracking* problems, where objects once defined with a relatively high expense could be automatically tracked in dynamic images sequences.

Acknowledgement The authors thank Ron Kikinis, Brigham and Women's Hospital, Harvard Medical School, Boston for organizing the MR acquisitions and for discussions in regard to the clinical needs for robust 3D image segmentation. Martha Shenton, Brain Imaging Laboratory, Dept. of Psychiatry, Harvard Medical School, Boston is kindly acknowledged for providing the MR and the manually segmented 3D data.

References

1. G. Gerig, J. Martin, R. Kikinis, O. Kübler, M. Shenton and F. Jolesz, *Automatic Segmentation of Dual-Echo MR Head Data*, Proc. IPMI'91, pp. 175-187, 1991
2. M. Kass, A. Witkin and D. Terzopoulos, *SNAKES: Active contour models* Int. J. Comp. Vision 1(4) pp. 321-331, 1987
3. D. Terzopoulos, A. Witkin and M. Kass, *Symmetry-Seeking Models and 3D Object Reconstruction*, Int. J. Comp. Vision 1(3) pp. 211-221, 1987
4. I. Cohen, L. D. Cohen and N. Ayache, *Using Deformable Surfaces to Segment 3D Images and Infer Differential Structures*, CVGIP: Image Understanding, 56(2), pp. 242-263, 1992
5. W. Neuenschwander, P. Fua, G. Székely and O. Kübler, *Initializing Snakes*, Proc. CVPR'94, pp. 658-663, 1994
6. B.C. Vemuri and A. Radisavljevic, *Multiresolution Stochastic Hybrid Shape Models with Fractal Priors*, ACM Trans. Graphics, 13(2) pp. 177-207, 1994
7. T.F. Cootes, A. Hill, C.J. Taylor and J. Haslam, *The Use of Active Shape Models For Locating Structures in Medical Imaging*, Proc. IPMI'93, pp. 33-47, Flagstaff USA, 1993
8. T.F. Cootes and C.J. Taylor, *Active Shape Models - 'Smart Snakes'*, Proc. British Mach. Vision Conf., Springer-Verlag 1992, pp. 266-275
9. A. Hill, T.F. Cootes and C.J. Taylor, *A Generic System for Image Interpretation Using Flexible Templates*, Proc. British Mach. Vision Conf., 1992, pp.276-285
10. J. Martin, A. Pentland and R. Kikinis, *Shape Analysis of Brain Structures Using Physical and Experimental Modes*, Proc. CVPR'94, pp. 752-755, 1994
11. F.P. Kuhl and Ch.R, Giardina, *Elliptic Fourier features of a closed contour*, CVGIP 18, pp.236-258, 1982
12. L.H. Staib and J. S. Duncan, *Boundary Finding with Parametrically Deformable Models*, IEEE PAMI 14(11) pp.1061-1075, 1992
13. L.H. Staib and J.S. Duncan, *Deformable Fourier models for surface finding in 3D images*, Proc. VBC'92 Conf., pp.90-194, 1992
14. The NAG Fortran Library Manual - Mark 13, 1st Edition, July 1988
15. W. Greiner and H. Diehl, *Theoretische Physik - Ein Lehr- und Übungsbuch für Anfangssemester*, Band 3, Verlag Harri Deutsch, Zürich , pp.61-65
16. Ch. Brechbühler, G. Gerig and O. Kübler, *Surface parametrization and shape description*, Proc. VBC'92 Conf., pp.80-89, 1992
17. Ch. Brechbühler, G. Gerig and O. Kübler, *Parametrization of closed surfaces for 3-D shape description*, to be published by CVGIP:Image Understanding
18. E. Persoon and K.S. Fu. Shape discrimination using fourier descriptors. *IEEE Trans. Systems, Man and Cybernetics SMC*, 7(3):170-179, March 1977.

Liver Definition in CT Using a Population-Based Shape Model

Jennifer L. Boes[1], Charles R. Meyer[1], Terry E. Weymouth[2]

[1] The University of Michigan Medical Center, Department of Radiology,
Kresge III Research Bldg. Box 0553, Ann Arbor, MI 48109
[2] Department of Electrical Engineering and Computer Science,
The University of Michigan, Ann Arbor, MI 48104

Abstract. Organ definition in computed tomography (CT) is of interest for treatment planning and response monitoring. We present a method for organ definition using *a priori* information about shape encoded in a biometric organ model--specifically a liver model--that accurately represents patient population shape information. This model is generated by averaging surfaces from a learning set of liver shapes previously registered into a standard space defined by a small set of landmarks. The model is placed in a specific patient's data set by identifying these landmarks and using them as the basis for model deformation; this preliminary representation is then iteratively fit to the patient's data based on a Bayesian combination of the model's priors and CT edge information, yielding a complete organ surface. We demonstrate this technique on a set of ten abdominal CT data sets and show its effectiveness as a tool for organ surface definition in this low-contrast domain.

1 Introduction

Definition of organ boundaries is necessary to provide volumes and locations for radiation therapy treatment planning, surgical planning, and oncologic monitoring. Unfortunately, manual definition of organ edges is tedious and time consuming, while automatic definition is impeded by low contrast differences between soft tissues in the body. Low-level processes have proved unsatisfactory for organ definition in this domain. Investigators are exploring ways of bringing higher-level information to bear on this task. Blackboard techniques combine information at different levels of abstraction, encoding the statistical properties of the problem only as discrete bits of "expert knowledge" [1]. Deformable template techniques [2,3] construct an "expected" scene and its pixels or edgels are adapted to those of the specific image. Other approaches build "prototypes," such as quadric surfaces, and instantiate them by globally fitting the underlying algebraic parameters in accordance with image properties [4,5]. This paper introduces a method sharing aspects of these approaches. We generate a normalized three-dimensional (3D) geometric model or "template" by averaging surfaces of learning set objects registered using thin-plate splines into a standard space defined by a small set of landmarks. We instantiate the model in a particular data set using these landmark points as the basis of a deformation of the model template. This model is a true representation of the central tendency of the scene analysis sought. Furthermore, the Bayesian "uncertainty" of the fit is encoded in correct biometric fashion, as a true variability of the observed scene analysis over a population learning sample, rather than as a vaguely assumed prior distribution of noise. Fitting the model template to the data set proceeds using a unique combination of local and global computations. We demonstrate this for liver definition in CT data.

2 Population-Based Shape Model Formulation

The modeling method summarized here [6] models a population of shapes in a standard space defined by a set of landmark points. The model incorporates both the 3D mean population shape and statistics representing the variation of the population from the mean. Other work in this area has modeled curves rather than surfaces [7]. To generate the prior statistics for a learning set of objects, we first select a set of identifying landmarks for the object. At least four non-coplanar landmarks provide an affine solution with additional landmarks providing for local shape deformations. After normalization, an averaging of the landmarks from the learning set defines the "standard" space [8] where collection of object statistics occurs. The object surface is identified by manual tracing in the 2D high resolution images of each learning data set; generation of a three-dimensional mesh representing the surface uses these tracings. The user also manually identifies the selected landmarks in the learning data set. The learning set object is transformed into the standard space using thin-plate spline warping [9] based on the landmark sets. A mean surface is generated from the registered object and model using a shape-based interpolation technique. This technique uses a method similar to field strength equipotential surface computation to generate an average surface. Learning set objects are added one at a time to the average model using a weighted interpolation between the two surfaces with weighting based on the number of objects currently in the model. The result is a consistent connected 3D volume average. A measure of the variance of learning set object surfaces from the mean surface is maintained at regularly spaced sample points on the surface. The final model represents the object shape class of the learning set.

3 Model Placement and Fitting in Data Set

The object shape model previously generated is now used for semi-automated object surface definition. First, we place a template model by manually identify the set of organ model landmarks in a patient data set. Thin-plate spline warping deforms the model to this new patient-specific landmark configuration, forming a preliminary model instantiation. Fitting is accomplished by identifying additional highly likely object surface points with which to revise the model fit. These points are identified by using a metric representing object surface probability given a detected edge; this metric, derived in the following section, is a Bayesian formulation combining both priors from the model and evidence from edge detection in a patient data set.

3.1 Derivation of Surface Probability Using Bayesian Formulation of Model Priors and Edge Detector Performance

The derivation in this section uses classical probability theory to combine both model and data set evidence into a metric for model fitting. Assume that we have a volumetric data set containing a single object with surface s. Define e as a detection event of a surface ("edge") detector. We can estimate the *a priori* probability, $P(s)$, that a voxel is on or off the surface using our model. Using Bayes' Theorem we can write the probability that the edge detection event was caused by the existence of the surface as

$$P(s|e) = \frac{P(e|s)P(s)}{P(e)} = \frac{P(e|s)P(s)}{P(e|s)P(s) + P(e|\overline{s})\,P(\overline{s})} \tag{1}$$

where $P(e) = P(s)P(e|s) + P(\overline{s})P(e|\overline{s})$ by the rule of elimination when $P(s) + P(\overline{s}) = 1$. $P(e|s)$ is the probability of e given the existence of a surface and $P(e|\overline{s})$ is the probability of e given no surface present. Given a sample space of decision points consisting of defined object and non-object points, we can compute $P(e|s)$ as the fraction of object points and $P(e|\overline{s})$ as the fraction of non-object points at which the edge detector goes off. In receiver operating characteristic (ROC) analysis $P(e|s)$ is the true-positive fraction (TPF) and $P(e|\overline{s})$ the false-positive fraction (FPF) of the edge detector. Then we write

$$P(s|e) = \frac{TPF\,P(s)}{TPF\,P(s) + FPF\,P(\overline{s})} = \frac{\frac{TPF}{FPF}}{\frac{TPF}{FPF} - 1 + P(s)^{-1}} \tag{2}$$

The true positive fraction to false positive fraction ratio, TPF/FPF, is a performance metric of the surface detector. A ratio of one indicates an edge detector that has no real information to contribute to the problem, a condition equivalent to random guessing. Larger ratios indicate higher edge detector confidence.

Points with high values for $P(s|e)$ are most likely to be part of the object boundary and will be used as additional landmarks for fitting the model surface to the object. Computation of this function requires that we first instantiate the model in a patient data set; computation of three-dimensional maps of the "priors", P(s), uses the instantiated model and computation of the edge detector performance characteristic, TPF/FPF, uses edge detection results.

3.2   Model Priors

It is straightforward to calculate the three-dimensional probability distribution predicted by a model instantiation, $P(s)$. We assume a model generated from a learning set that is large enough to permit the assumption of a normal distribution of component surfaces from the model mean. The *a priori* surface probability, *P(s)*, is then defined for a range of normal distances from the surface mean given the standard deviation at that particular location on the model surface. A probability map is computed for each voxel in the volumetric data set; this 3D map is the prior probability of the location of the object boundary in a particular data set given a particular learning set from which the model was computed.

3.3   Edge Detector Performance Characteristic

We have developed a method for approximating a likelihood function L(*edge detector side measures*) that estimates *TPF/FPF*, the edge detector performance characteristic, for use in the combined probability equation. The parameters of this function are measures that can be easily computed from the volumetric data set. These measures-- for example gradient magnitude, edge length, or intensity--are potentially correlated to detector performance. For tractability the function is restricted to a maximum variate order of five and is specific to the object, edge detector, and image source. We have chosen to use a robust edge detector due to its ability to function well in low-contrast images. We compute the performance of the edge detector, not as a single general measure, but as an object-specific measure. Both likelihood ratio and side measures are computed for local regions in a data set with known object edge locations. A polynomial L fitting this data is then estimated using the least-mean-square error method. The resulting polynomial and error can then be analyzed to determine the relative strength and importance of the side measures in the likelihood function. A reduced rank function is selected that uses a minimum number of well-correlated parameters to model the ratio *TPF/FPF* for the particular object.

3.4 Implementation of Model Fitting

The technique described here generates an object surface definition using the previously derived probability measures as a basis for a series of incremental updates on the 3D model placed in a data set. This is in contrast to other techniques that attempt to link edge fragments or surface patches into a complete 3D object definition. Using the model provides for the definition of a complete object boundary, even in low-contrast regions providing little or no additional evidence.

The basic strategy for model fitting is the identification of additional "good" points with which to update the fit. First, a user manually identifies the set of landmarks in the data set and an initial placement of the model is done. Next, we identify additional points with which to augment the initial set. The measure which we compute for point selection is the previously derived $P(s|e)$. An initial threshold is selected for $P(s|e)$; points above this value are selected to use in revising the model fit. These points are matched to points on the surface of the currently instantiated model. Matching is done to vertices of the model mesh using a shortest distance criteria. This subset of homologous point pairs is then used in model fitting. The fitting method uses a point-to-point thin-plate spline warping on the identified set of homologous point pairs to improve the local aspects of the liver representation. After an iteration has been completed, the $P(s|e)$ threshold is revised and additional points are considered for fitting parameters. This continues until the threshold reaches an absolute threshold on acceptable evidence which has been identified by experimentation to yield a minimal number of errors in point selection.

4 Experimental Results

Our tests use CT data both for model definition and for liver fitting. Software for model visualization, placement and fitting was implemented using the Application Visualization System (AVS) software package (AVS, Inc. Waltham, Mass.)

The liver model was generated from a learning set consisting of fifteen abdominal contrast enhanced CT studies (GE 9800; GE Medical Systems, Milwaukee). Each randomly selected CT study consists of a complete volumetric set of liver images showing no significant abnormality, as determined by a radiologist. We manually identified the liver surface. We also selected six non-coplanar landmarks that could be easily identified manually in most liver studies: (a) dome center, (b) inferior tip, (c) most lateral extent of left lobe, (d) & (e) points on right side and posterior of right lobe, and (f) gall bladder neck. The liver shapes were transformed into the standard space and averaged to generate a normal liver population shape model (Fig. 1). To visualize the potential descriptiveness of this model we have color coded the model mean surface to represent the standard deviation in millimeters with a maximum average deviation of 13.3 mm, approximately 10% of the maximum liver dimension.

We computed the object specific measures *TPF* and *FPF* for the liver in five studies consisting of 128x128 CT contrast enhanced contiguous images spaced on 1 cm centers reduced to byte data using a consistent window and level value of 256 and 127 Hounsfield units. Gradient and edge calculations are done in the highest resolution image dimension. Size 16x16 pixel regions provide sufficient statistics for *TPF/FPF* functional approximation; error analysis shows a strong correlation with the gradient. This function, specific to the liver, CT, and robust edge detector is shown in Fig. 2. Very low and very high contrast edges within the liver region are downplayed by this function while medium contrast edges are highlighted (Fig. 4a).

The fitting technique has been applied to a set of ten data sets (same resolution as above). The model is placed into a patient-specific data set using manual identification of the landmark set (Fig. 3) and then probability map computations are completed; two-dimensional cross-sections of 3D maps for $L(g)$, $P(s)$, and $P(s|e)$ are illustrated (Fig. 4). A progression from preliminary instantiation to final result is also shown (Fig. 5). The 2D intersection of the model surface with a single image illustrates the action as additional parameters are added to the model instantiation. One measure of the fit between the current instantiation and the desired surface definition is the ratio of non-overlapping volumes between the two objects to the total desired volume. Fig. 6 illustrates how this value changes over the update iterations. The dotted line is the case in Figs. 3-5. A linear error measure, average standard deviation between model and surface, has final values of 4-13 mm with an average reduction of 6 mm. As demonstrated, the update technique improves the initial fit.

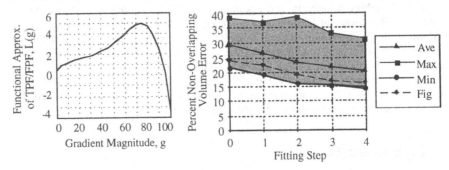

Fig. 2. Edge likelihood functional approximation for liver-CT-robust edge detection over 5 CT cases.

Fig. 6. Volumetric error percent as a function of iteration showing maximum, minimum, and average plots for 10 test cases. Dotted line is for Figs. 3-5.

5 Discussion and Conclusions

The population-based shape model and Bayesian approach to fitting detailed here offer a promising method for complete object surface definition in low-contrast data sets. Several areas of work are suggested by the results shown here. Landmark selection is a significant factor in the ability of the model to accurately represent a general class of surfaces and could be improved. Further analysis of statistics of an overselection of landmark locations would help determine the statistically important landmarks for accurate liver modeling [8]. Object classification is also an issue in accurate modeling. The liver model here models normal anatomy. When diseased livers are added to this set, the question of whether one or multiple models will be required must be explored. Finally, model fitting metric, point selection and update method are also issues. The likelihood ratio we estimate contributes evidence to the fitting metric, but a more sensitive metric would be helpful. In particular, a 3D spatially varying metric in the standard space would be more sensitive and accurate. Point selection strategy currently uses a threshold; possible alternatives would include adding points to the model one at a time. Finally, model deformation is presently defined using a point-to-point mapping between homologous points pairs; work currently being done to allow surface points additional degrees of freedom to roam over a region of the model surface would provide for a smooth deformation function with no artificially high bending energy regions. In conclusion, this modeling method is capable of representing the true variation of a population of non-rigid shapes and this fitting method solves the problems of missing boundary segments in low contrast data sets by using the model information more heavily in areas in which data sets provide only minimal information and using underlying data information more heavily in areas in which this information is known to be valid.

Acknowledgments

Thanks to F. Bookstein for motivating this use of thin-plate splines. Thanks to DEC for providing access to a 3000/500x Alpha for swift program development and execution. Work supported in part by NIH Grant No. 1R01CA52709-01A1.

References

1. S. Tehrani, T.E. Weymouth: "Knowledge-Guided Left Ventricular Boundary Detection," Proceedings of Computer Vision and Pattern Recognition, 342-347 (1989)
2. R. Bajcsy, R. Lieberson, M. Reivich: "A Computerized System for the Elastic Matching of Deformed Radiographic Images to Idealized Atlas Images," Journal of Computer Assisted Tomography 7, 618-625 (1983)
3. M.I. Miller, G.E. Christensen, Y. Amit, U. Grenander: "Mathematical textbook of deformable neuroanatomies," Proc. Natl. Acad. Sci. U.S.A. 90, 11944-11948 (1993)
4. D. Terzopoulos, D. Mataxas: "Dynamic 3D models with local and global deformations: deformable superquadrics," IEEE Trans. on Pat Anal and Mach Intel 13, 703-714 (1991).
5. L.H. Staib, J.S. Duncan: "Boundary finding with parametrically deformable models," IEEE Trans. on Pattern Analysis and Machine Intelligence 14, 1061-75 (1992)
6. J.L. Boes, P.H. Bland, T.E. Weymouth, L.E. Quint, F.L. Bookstein, C.R. Meyer: "Generating a Normalized Geometric Liver Model Using Warping," Investigative Radiology 29, 281-286 (1994)
7. C.B. Cutting, F.L. Bookstein, B. Haddad, D. Dean, D. Kim: "A spline-based approach for averaging three-dimensional curves and surfaces," Proceedings of the International Society for Optical Engineering 2035, 29-41 (1993)
8. F.L. Bookstein, *Morphometric tools for landmark data: geometry and biology* (Cambridge University Press, Cambridge, 1991)
9. F.L. Bookstein, "Principal Warps: Thin-plate splines and the decomposition of deformations," IEEE Trans. Pattern Analysis and Machine Intelligence 11, 567-585 (1989)

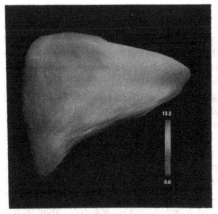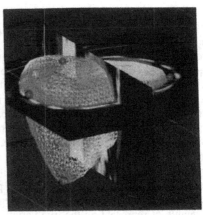

Fig. 1. Liver model (6 landmarks, 15 livers) with standard deviation in mm from mean surface encoded in surface color from blue at zero deviation to red at 3.3 mm.

Fig. 3. Three-dimensional view of liver model placed into patient data set after user identification of six landmarks which are shown as red spheres.

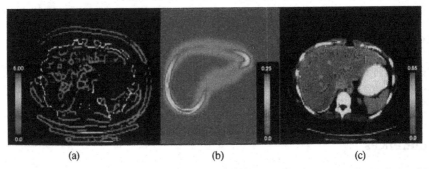

(a)   (b)   (c)

Fig. 4. Evidence applied to the liver boundary definition problem (cross-sectional views of 3D maps): (a) likelihood ratio, TPF/FPF, (b) model surface location probability, P(s), (c) liver surface probability given a detection event, P(sle).

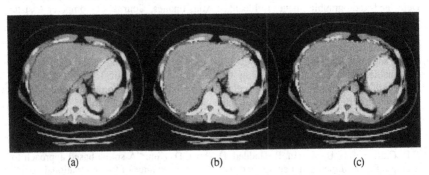

(a)   (b)   (c)

Fig. 5. Visualization of liver model (cross-sectional views of 3D surface) in several stages in the organ definition process: (a) initial placement, (b) after two iterations, (c) after final fitting step. Yellow points are used to update model fit.

Retrospective Correction
of MRI Amplitude Inhomogeneities

Charles R. Meyer [1]

Peyton H. Bland[1]

James Pipe [1,2]

[1]Department of Radiology, University of Michigan, Ann Arbor, MI 48109-0553

and

[2]Currently: Harper Hospital, Wayne State University, Detroit, MI

This work supported in part by
NIH 1R01 CA52709-03 and 1F32 CA09309-01A1

Please address all correspondence to C. R. Meyer, Department of Radiology,
Box 0553, University of Michigan Hospitals, Ann Arbor, MI 48109-0553,
email: chuck.meyer@med.umich.edu.

Abstract

MRI data sets are corrupted by multiplicative inhomogeneities, often referred to as
nonuniformities or intensity variations, that hamper the use of quantitative analyses.
The use of adiabatic pulses can remove the inhomogeneity effects on transmit, but
coil and patient parameters still affect reception. We describe an automatic technique
that not only improves the worst corruptions such as those introduced by surface
coils, but also corrects typical inhomogeneities encountered in routine volume data
sets such as head scans without generating additional artifact. Because the technique
uses only the patient data set, the technique can be applied retrospectively to all data
sets, and corrects both patient independent effects such as rf coil design, and patient
dependent effects such as tissue attenuation and dielectric-induced resonances experienced in high field MRI. Patient dependent attenuation effects are also encountered in
x-ray computed tomography. All of the above are examples of multiplicative
inhomogeneities which result in low spatial frequency corruption of acquired volume
data sets. While we concentrate on MR in the remainder of the paper, the algorithms
and techniques described are directly applicable to CT as well. Following such
corrections, region of interest analyses, volume histograms, and thresholding
techniques are more meaningful. The value of such correction algorithms may
increase dramatically with increased use of high field strength magnets and associated
patient-dependent rf attenuation and resonance effects.

Key Words: Inhomogeneity correction, intensity correction, background correction,
uniformity correction, retrospective, image processing.

Introduction

MRI rf-coil field strength inhomogeneities yield variations on the order of 30% in image amplitude variations in newer head coil designs on 1.5 T magnets. While variations of this magnitude usually have no effect on diagnostic accuracies, they do cause significant problems for volume thresholding, segmentation, and statistical clustering tasks, particularly where it is desirable to differentiate gray from white matter [1]. Moreover the possible migration of clinical MRI to higher field strengths with associated rf penetration and resonance problems remain significantly problematic [2,3]. There are many published techniques to ameliorate the effects of inhomogeneities, especially for applications involving MRI surface coils. Most of the published retrospective techniques have the property of assisting only the worst cases [4,5,6]. Because of inappropriate spatial frequency separation assumptions, their application in less dramatic cases often induces more inhomogeneity than originally present. Techniques utilizing separate phantom acquisitions [7,8,9,10] require that the corrupting effects are patient independent, and the phantom scan is obtained with the same scanner acquisition parameters as the patient's. Another technique uses a body coil acquisition to correct limited field-of-view surface coil acquisition [11]. More recently Moyher modeled the field strength variations associated with known coil geometries and used the results for intensity corrections [12]. Ideally only the patient's volume data set from a single acquisition should be used to correct for both patient-independent effects such as rf field strength based on coil geometry, and patient-dependent effects such as attenuation and dielectric resonance. With these goals in mind we introduce significant extensions beyond those recently published [13] which reduce both user interaction and hypersensitivity. The extensions include the use of an inhomogeneity-tolerant, preliminary segmentation technique, and increased region of support for calculation of the inhomogeneity function through the simultaneous use of many different tissue segments and three dimensional (3D) modeling functions.

The use of a relatively new segmentation algorithm, referred to in the remainder of this paper as LCJ-segmentation [14], and a novel method of modeling the segmented data set, allows computation of stable estimates of the corrupting process using only the patient's data set. The estimate is then used to correct the global effect. Since the published LCJ-segmentation algorithm description is widely available, only a brief review follows.

LCJ-segmentation is an iterative process consisting of thresholding the 3D gradient magnitude of the volume data set to form hypotheses of homogeneous volumes, and then checking the validity of each hypothesis by fitting the volume's amplitudes with a polynomial function of 3D coordinates, $f(x,y,z)$. For each hypothesized volume if the resulting model residual compares favorably with noise, the volume is considered to be homogeneous, i.e. truly a single volume, is labeled as such, and no further processing of that specific volume ensues. However if the residual is too large, the homogeneous hypothesis for the defined volume is rejected, and the algorithm iterates by lowering the threshold on the gradient magnitude further, thus eventually selecting smaller, and thereby potentially more homogeneous volumes for further checking. In the hypothesis checking process the intensities of voxels within each volume are fit with a polynomial consisting of terms up to some predetermined maximum variation order (mvo), typically 4 or less. The segmentation process ceases when the remaining unfit volume hypotheses are too small to yield an overdetermined solution to the fitting polynomial. The small volumes remaining unfit, as well as those regions not examined because their gradient magnitudes were above the selected thresholds, result in uncommitted voxels in the segmentation when the process finishes. In summary the LCJ-segmentation yields conservative estimates of homogeneous volumes within 3D data sets whose intensities are well fit by local, low-order polynomial functions of position. The process is capable of segmenting data sets affected by low-spatial frequency corrupting processes such as rf field inhomogeneities in MRI and beam-hardening in CT, precisely because the fitting polynomial includes terms beyond the usual constant term.

It is reasonable in the general sense, and certainly in the computer vision context that led to the original development of the LCJ algorithm, to treat every volume as an independent entity with its own local polynomial. But for data sets from medical acquisition systems we expect image intensities of a particular tissue histology to have the same intensity independent of spatial location. Since inhomogeneities in the acquisition system typically corrupt intensities in a slowly varying fashion over the whole data set, a more reasonable phenomenological modeling approach to use within the LCJ algorithm when operating on the log of CT or MRI modulus data sets would be to use the same function to globally fit all volumes with one polynomial except for a unique constant offset term for each different volume hypothesis. Because the described corrupting processes are multiplicative, the logarithm of the intensity data is modeled by a constant term for each unique volume, and a global, additive inhomogeneity function. It is this notion and associated implementation that is the major innovation we demonstrate. The problem here is cast in a least mean square error (lmse) formulation with a single solution that can be computed without iteration after the initial LCJ-segmentation of the data set has been completed.

Methods

All data sets were submitted to the LCJ-segmentation algorithm using a polynomial fit of mvo = 4. Before forming the 3D gradient magnitude of the intensity data, the intensity data was smoothed in the high resolution plane of the scanner via convolution with a box-car window whose size was chosen to mimic the out-of-plane acquisition window width. Thus the 3D gradient magnitude operation was performed on data sets with nearly isotropic partial volume effects to remove directional gradient bias. Following LCJ-segmentation, the log intensities of the successful volume hypotheses, hereafter referred to as volume segments, were collectively modeled by a global corrupting polynomial including unique constants, one for each volume segment, i.e.

$$\bar{o} = A\,\bar{m} + \bar{e}.$$

Here $\bar{o}$ is the N-by-1 observation vector of N log intensities, A is the N-by-p matrix of input Cartesian coordinates, their powers, and their associated cross-terms according to the mvo selected, $\bar{m}$ is the corrupting model's p-by-1 vector consisting of model coefficients to be determined, and $\bar{e}$ is the N-by-1 error vector. More specifically

$$\bar{o} = [\, i_{11}\, i_{12}\, \cdots\, i_{1k_1}\, |\, i_{21}\, i_{22}\, \cdots\, i_{2k_2}\, |\, \cdots\,]'$$

where i_{jk} is the k th of k_j log intensities (or amplitudes, depending on what is observed) in volume j out of a total of M volumes, $'$ is the transpose operator, and

$$A = \begin{bmatrix}
x_{11}^n & y_{11}^n & z_{11}^n & x_{11}^{n-1}y_{11} & \cdots & 1 & 0 & \cdots & 0 \\
x_{12}^n & y_{12}^n & z_{12}^n & x_{12}^{n-1}y_{12} & \cdots & 1 & 0 & \cdots & 0 \\
\vdots & \vdots & \vdots & \vdots & \ddots & \vdots & \vdots & \cdots & \vdots \\
x_{21}^n & y_{21}^n & z_{21}^n & x_{21}^{n-1}y_{21} & \cdots & 0 & 1 & \cdots & 0 \\
x_{22}^n & y_{22}^n & z_{22}^n & x_{22}^{n-1}y_{22} & \cdots & 0 & 1 & \cdots & 0 \\
\vdots & \vdots & \vdots & \vdots & \ddots & \vdots & \vdots & \cdots & \vdots \\
x_{Mk_M}^n & y_{Mk_M}^n & z_{Mk_M}^n & x_{Mk_M}^{n-1}y_{Mk_M} & \cdots & 0 & 0 & \cdots & 1
\end{bmatrix}$$

where x_{jk} is the x-axis Cartesian coordinate of the k th point in the j th volume corresponding to the locus of the observation i_{jk}. Moving from left to right each row contains all of the powers of x_{jk}, y_{jk}, and z_{jk}, and the appropriate cross terms associated with the chosen mvo up to and including the ellipsis. Columns to the right of the ellipsis are associated with a particular volume. Thus there are M columns corresponding to M volume segments from the initial LCJ segmentation. Counting from the ellipsis to the right, column j, corresponding to volume j, is set to 1.0 while the remaining columns are set to 0. This formulation of the matrix A affects only one constant term corresponding to the appropriate volume in the model vector v, where

$$\bar{m} = [\, a_1\, a_2\, \cdots\, a_{p-1}\, |\, c_1\, c_2\, \cdots\, c_M\,]'$$

where a_n is the n th coefficient of the mvo model consisting of p terms, and c_j is the constant term associated with volume j. For example if there were 3 separate volumes, and we choose the fitting polynomial to be mvo=2 (and thus p=10), the row in A for the fourth voxel coordinate in the third volume would look like

$$[\, x_{43}^2\ y_{43}^2\ z_{43}^2\ x_{43}y_{43}\ x_{43}z_{43}\ y_{43}z_{43}\ x_{43}\ y_{43}\ z_{43}\ 0\ 0\ 1\,]$$

while the model vector would look like

$$\bar{m} = [\, a_1\, a_2\, a_3\, a_4\, a_5\, a_6\, a_7\, a_8\, a_9\, c_1\, c_2\, c_3\,]' .$$

The solution for $\bar{m}$ is obtained from the standard singular value decomposition of the matrix A which results in $A = u\, s\, v'$ where u and v are orthonormal matrices of left and right handed eigenvectors corresponding to the associated eigenvalues in the diagonal matrix s [15]. The model is computed as

$$\overline{m} = v\,s^+\,u'\,\overline{o}.$$

where s^+ is the generalized, or pseudoinverse of s. Additional details regarding the formation of the inverse and the behavior of the residuals as a function of rank for differing mvo models can be obtained from Meyer, *et al.* [16].

The preliminary LCJ-segmentation algorithm was implemented using the Fortran77 programming language in AVS 5.0 modules (Advanced Visual Systems, Inc., Waltham, MA) on a DEC3000/500x OSF1/AXP workstation. The LCJ-segmentation was typically performed on normalized, unsigned byte, linear data sets, e.g. MRI volumetric modulus data, using residual fitting criteria dependent on the modality and noise artifacts present in the data. An initial simple region of interest statistical analysis is sufficient to determine the residual criterion for the LCJ segmentation. By selecting a region containing the desired noise characteristics, the user can control the outcome of the segmentation. For example if the data set contains significant cardiac noise "splattered" in the phase encoding direction, by selecting the residual criterion from a region unaffected by the motion splatter, i.e. low noise, the resulting segmentations will contain only regions of the same, or lesser, noise, thus rejecting regions containing phase noise splatter.

In computing the model of the corrupting polynomial, each voxel's intensity, 3-space coordinates, and segment number for all voxels in all LCJ-segmented regions were written to an ASCII file. Model computations were performed using Matlab 4.0 (Mathworks, Natick, MA) running on a Sun Sparc 2 workstation. Segmented volumes were randomly subsampled in order to keep the total number of observations in the neighborhood of 4000-5000 points. The mvo of the corrupting function was chosen to be either 2 or 4 as determined by expected spatial complexities in the physical imaging configuration. The ability of polynomials of mvo 2 through 4 to remove spatial nonuniformities in MRI has already been demonstrated [10]. In addition the model vector representing the corrupting multiplicative process computed from the log of the observation vector was chosen to have a zero constant coefficient at the spatial centroid of the observations, to yield a corrective gain of unity for the centroid. The correction of the acquired data set was produceded by subtracting the computed corrupting model polynomial from the previously log transformed input data and exponentiating the result.

Results

The following results have been computed retrospectively using only patient data sets according to the methods described above, and are shown in image groupings of the original and corrected data sets where the gray scale images are presented at *exactly* the same window and level contrast settings for both sets.

The first data set shown in Fig. 1 results from the use of GE's general purpose flexible surface coil applied to MRI breast imaging in a 1.5T Signa. The patient was lying prone in the magnet. Both cardiac and respiratory gating were applied to reduce motion artifacts. The phase encoding direction was chosen to be left-right. The surface coil was used for both transmission and reception. Due to the spatial complexity of the rf coil configuration, a corrupting function of mvo=4 was chosen and computed. The left hand column contains the original scan intensity images shown for slice 6 (top row), slice 10 (middle row) and slice 14 (bottom row) from a 19 slice acquisition spaced at 0.9 cm intervals. The middle column contains the homogeneous volumes used for computational support of the corrupting function derived from preliminary LCJ-segmentation shown at the same 3 slice locations. Volume segments are gray scale coded according to individual segment number. Segments shown with the same gray scale are connected in three space. The right hand column contains images taken from the same slice locations in the corrected volume data set

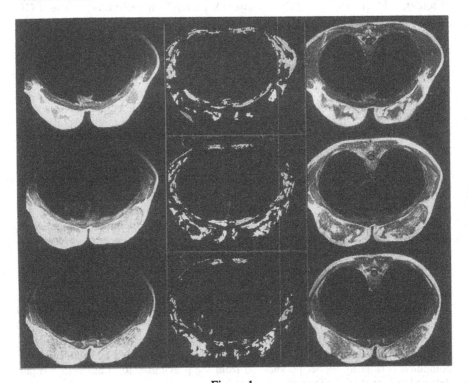

Figure 1.

Note that the corrected images in the right-hand column are significantly superior to the original acquisition shown in the left-hand column. Also note the stability of the correction near the posterior body wall. The average coefficient of variation for 4448 voxels across different segments was reduced from 37% in the original data set to 14% in the corrected volume. By way of comparison, Moyher's corrections were applied to *uniform* head phantoms imaged with phased array surface coils designed for imaging the temporal mandibular joint. For imaging with only one of the two coils she reports reducing the coefficient of variation from 92% to 10%, and from 79% to 12% for the more complex two coil case [12].

The next data set shown in Fig. 2 is an MRI head study of a patient with a large left hemisphere infarct. Again the 3 rows of images represent the superior (top row), midbrain (middle row), and base of cerebellum (lower row). Columns left of center are associated with the original data acquisition, and columns right of center are associated with the corrected data. The central column displays the difference between the two adjacent columns: immediately to the left is the uncorrected, acquired, T1-weighted image set, while immediately to the right of center is the corrected T1-weighted set. As before the window/level settings for the three central gray scale columns are *exactly* the same, with the exception that the level of the difference images has been adjusted such that zero difference yields black (cursor, central image). A narrow window was chosen to emphasize differences. The outermost two columns display cluster labels corresponding to "gray matter" (gray) and CSF (white) obtained from a global trivariate, histogram-based clustering (HICAP) of the uncorrected (left-most column) and corrected (right-most column) data volumes [17]. The trivariate

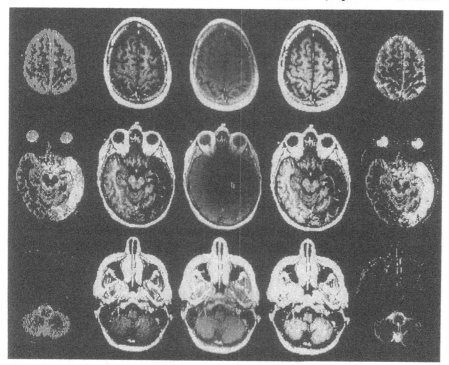

Figure 2.

clustering algorithm used proton density and T2-weighted volume data sets (single spin-echo acquisition, TE=30/90 ms, TR=3000 ms), and a T1-weighted image (separate spin-echo acquisition, TE=20ms, TR=500ms) set. The same correction function, i.e. that computed from the T1-weighted data set's white matter volume segment, was applied to each of the trivariate sets. Observe that the clustering from the uncorrected set significantly overestimates the quantity of gray matter at the periphery at all levels due to the fall-off of signal intensities and resultant incorporation of the CSF peak into the gray matter peak. Note that classification of the eye's vitreous as CSF is obtained only in the corrected data set. Differentiation between CSF and gray matter is obtained only in the corrected set from the regions at the vertex and base. Such corrections of vertex and base can be made only if the data is treated as a continuous, 3D set. The coefficient of variation for 3759 white matter voxels was reduced from 10% in the original data set to 8% in the corrected volume.

The axial data sets were acquired using a 1.5 T GE Signa using a "bird cage" rf head coil for reception and the body coil for transmission. Voxel size was $(0.8 \text{ mm})^2$ x 7 mm. Since the nonuniformity was expected to be moderate due to the use of body coil for transmission and the head coil for reception, polynomial mvo=2 was chosen for the corrupting function. Inspection of the maximum and minimum of the resulting corrupting function indicated a 30% maximum variation over the region of the head extending from the vertex to the base of the cerebellum. While the variation was greatest in the cranial-caudal direction, significant variation was also noted at the midbrain periphery. This data set is especially interesting due to the rapid decrease in signal intensity in the region of the infarct. Other techniques that make inappropriate frequency assumptions, e.g. ref. [6], would cause overshoot in the correction of normal brain near the infarct, and undershoot in the correction of the infarct nearest the boundary with normal brain.

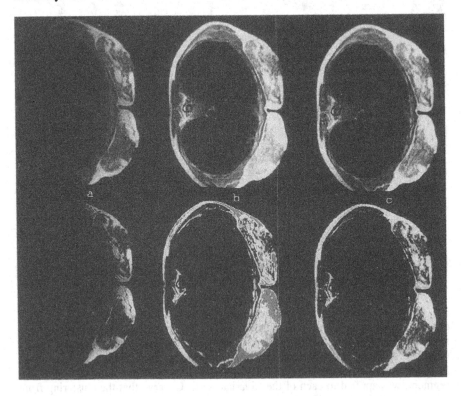

Figure 3.

Figure 3 demonstrates further improvements obtained by cluster/constant merging. The left column (a) is from the original data set, the middle column (b) is the result of the correction presented in Fig. 1, and the right column (c) is the result of merging clusters in the modeling process. Images in the top row are gray scale images of slice 12 presented at higher contrast than Fig. 1, and images in the bottom row are grayscale coded, uniformly thresholded versions of the upper row. In the original LCJ algorithm the number of separate segments was determined by spatial separation, i.e. each volume hypothesis that passed the uniformity check was assigned a separate volume identification number. Thus if N such volumes resulted from the initial LCJ segmentation, then N constant terms were created in the polynomial model used for refitting the dataset amplitudes in the inhomogeneity modeling algorithm. But after realizing that some of the larger volumes are artifically divided into smaller ones by the gradient thresholding process, and that there are relatively few different tissue histologies contributing to an imaged volume, we noted that the stability of the correction algorithm could be improved by merging segments corresponding to the same tissues and thus reducing the degrees of freedom for the same mvo model. The retrospective test for which segments should be merged is the same as that used in standard statistical clustering, i.e. the cluster means, i.e. the resultant constants, are not significantly different. Since the global model residual is also computed the test is trivial to implement. The result of merging segments corresponding to constants less than 2 times the root mean square (rms) model error from each other is shown in Fig 3. The improved uniformity obtained in both breasts is obvious in the right column's images. In this process 19 segments were merged into a total of 10. The average coefficient of variation of the result remained unchanged at 14%, but small average differences taken over the whole volume do not reflect important local changes such as those demonstrated in Fig. 3.

Discussion

Here we show that through the use of LCJ preliminary segmentation, 3D inhomogeneity modeling functions of $2 \leq mvo \leq 4$, and the simultaneous use of multiple 3D volume segments, we can routinely compute accurate, stable estimates of corrupting functions for a wide range of imaging geometries. Required *a priori* user inputs for the entire process are limited to 1) choosing the upper limit on the preliminary polynomial fitting residual to accept a volume segment hypothesis in the LCJ procedure, and 2) choosing the mvo of the global corrupting polynomial estimate. Choice of mvo is primarily driven by anticipated complexity in the spatial distribution of the inhomogeneity. For cases of suspected smooth, symmetric behavior such as those encountered in MR head imaging mvo=2 appears ideal. Increasing mvo to 4 allows for correction of more spatially complex inhomogeneities, but carries the potential penalty of reduced stability in regions not well represented, i.e. undersampled. Random subsampling of intensities in the preliminary volume segments is well tolerated as long as sampling of the corrupting process is approximately uniformly distributed over the region of support. Clamping, or limiting the correcting function to a predetermined maximum was not necessary for the cases presented. However such clamping may be necessary for cases where the preliminary segmentation yields a limited or spatially skewed region of support and the resulting extrapolation of the correcting function is ill behaved.

Acknowledgments

The authors would like to express their gratitude to Shih-Ping Liou and Ramesh Jain for their assistance and discussions in implementing the LCJ-segmentation. In addition we would like to thank Digital Equipment Corporation for access to a DEC3000/500x OSF/1 AXP for program development and execution.

References

1. Kohn MI, Tanna NK, Herman GT, et al: Analysis of brain and cerebrospinal fluid volumes with MR imaging, Part I. Radiology (1991) 178:115-122.
2. Foo TK, Hayes CE, Kang YW: Reduction of RF penetration effects in high field imaging. Mag Reson Med (1992) 23:287-301.
3. Carswell H: Ultrahigh-field MRI shows clinical promise. MR, The Newsmagazine of Magnetic Resonance (1993 July/Aug) 3:7-8
4. Lufkin RB, Sharpless T, Flannigan B, Hanafee W: Dynamic-Range Compression in Surface-Coil MRI. AJR 147:379-382, 1986.
5. Zanella FE, Lanfermann H, Bunke J: Automatic correction of the signal intensity of surface coils: Clinical application and relevan. Radiologe (1990) 30(5):223-7.
6. Haselgrove J, and Prammer M: An algorithm for compensation of surface-coil images for sensitivity of the surface coil. Mag Res Imag (1986) 4:469-472.
7. Wicks DA, Barker GJ, Tofts PS: Correction of intensity nonuniformity in MR images of any orientation. Magn Reson Imaging (1993) 11(2):183-196.
8. Listerud J, Lenkinski RE, Kressel HY, Axel L: The correction of nonuniform signal intensity profiles in magnetic resonance imaging. J Digital Imaging (1989) 2(1):2-8
9. Axel L, Costantini J, Listerud J: Intensity correction in surface-coil MR imaging. Am J Roentgenol (1987) 148(2):418-420.
10. Tincher M, Meyer CR, Gupta R, Williams DM: Polynomial modeling and reduction of RF body coil spatial inhomogeneity in MRI. IEEE Trans Med Imag (1993) 12(2):361-365.
11. Brey WW, and Narayana PA: Correction for intensity falloff in surface coil magnetic resonance. Medical Physics (1988) 15(2):241-245.
12. Moyher SE, Vigneron DB, Dillon W, Wald LL, and Nelson SJ: High resolution imaging of the brain using surface coils and an intensity correction algorithm. Proc. SMR (1994) 1:9.
13. Dawant BM, Zijdenbos AP, and Margolin RA: Correction of intensity variations in MR images for computer-aided tissue classification. IEEE Trans Med Imag (1993) 12(4):770-781.
14. Liou SP, Chiu AH, and Jain RC: A parallel technique for signal-level perceptual organization. IEEE Trans PAMI (1991) 13:317-325.
15. Nobel B, and Daniel JW: Applied Linear Algebra (1988: Prentice Hall, Englewood Cliffs, NJ) p. 348.
16. Meyer CR, Bland PH, Pipe J: Retrospective correction of intensity inhomogeneities in MRI. IEEE Trans Med Imag (1995) 14(1).
17. Wharton SW: A generalized histogram clustering scheme for multidimensional image data. Pattern Recognition (1983) 16(2):193-199.

Design of New Surface Detection Operators in the Case of an Anisotropic Sampling of 3D Volume Data

Chafiaâ Hamitouche[1], Christian Roux[1] and Jean Louis Coatrieux[2]

[1] Département Image et Traitement de l'Information
Télécom Bretagne, BP 832, 29285 Brest Cedex, France
[2] Laboratoire de Traitement du Signal et de l'Image, Université de Rennes I, France

Abstract. Medical imaging systems do not provide direct volume information. These data are generally a result of stacking-up 2D slices, with a resolution in the plane of the slice higher than the one perpendicular to the slice. The volume data is anisotropic. The objective of this paper is to provide an original way to design surface detection operators taking into account the anisotropic aspect. Two approaches are studied and illustrated by examples: signal processing and elaboration of continuous anisotropic model.

1 Introduction

The objective of medical imaging is to provide spatial information as accurate as possible for diagnosis and therapy purpose. Localization of the structures without ambiguity can only be achieved thanks to 3D data volume. The introduction of a third direction helps definitely more for the comprehension and the quantification of the manipulated objects. But, on the other hand, it generates some specific problems. For rapidity reasons, the slices are quite distant from each other. The size of the processed data is important unlike their representation, which can be considered as a less open problem since many efforts have been devoted in elaborating algorithms for 3D visualization [1]. 3D data acquisition is characterized by three parameters (fig.1) the dimension of the pixel d, the thickness of the slice e and the distance between slices i. The volume data is said to be isotropic if the voxel is cubic ($d = e = i$); it is said to be anisotropic when the voxel is parallelepipedic. The anisotropic coefficient ω is defined as the relationship between the resolution in the plane (X, Y) and the resolution in the Z direction.

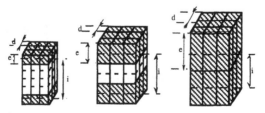

Fig. 1. 3D anisotropic data (4 slices are to be interpolated: $\omega=4$)

A rigourous 3D analysis [2] should take into account the spatial inhomogeneity. Traditionally, the dimensions of the voxel are adjusted by interpolation [3] which brings no new information even though the data volume is significantly increased. In this paper, a more original approach is proposed to handle this problem. It concerns an integration of anisotropic characteristics in the processing operators in order to work only on the original images. We will focus on the segmentation operators using surface detection. An extension to other operators can be done in a similar manner. Two approaches (signal processing, new model) can be followed, each of them will be developped and illustrated by examples.

2 Introduction of anisotropic characteristics in surface detection operators

2.1 The signal processing approach

In the sequel, we assume that the gray-level voxels $f_d(i, j, k)$ are obtained by integration and sampling of the continuous, physical image $f(x, y, z)$ (fig. 2).

- *Integration* :

$$f(x, y, z) \rightarrow f(x, y, z) * f_I(x, y, z) = f_1(x, y, z)$$
$$f_I(x, y, z) = \prod_{[-\frac{1}{2}, +\frac{1}{2}]}(x) \cdot \prod_{[-\frac{1}{2}, +\frac{1}{2}]}(y) \cdot \prod_{[-\frac{e}{2}, +\frac{e}{2}]}(z) \tag{1}$$

where:

* indicates the convolution product, and $\prod_{[-\frac{a}{2}, +\frac{a}{2}]}(x) = \begin{cases} 1 & \text{if } x \in [-\frac{a}{2}, +\frac{a}{2}] \\ 0 & \text{otherwise} \end{cases}$

- *Sampling* : $f_d(i, j, k) = f_1(i, j, \omega k) = \int_{i-\frac{1}{2}}^{i+\frac{1}{2}} \int_{j-\frac{1}{2}}^{j+\frac{1}{2}} \int_{\omega k - \frac{e}{2}}^{\omega k + \frac{e}{2}} f(u, v, w) \, du \, dv \, dw$

where, the sampling rate is normalized to 1 in the X and Y directions, and equal to ω in the Z direction. The f_I operator in (1), imposed by the physical process of acquisition, can be interpreted as an anti-aliasing filter used to limit the frequency spectrum bandwidth before sampling [4] [5]. The anisotropic correction can be delt with in the signal processing framework when considering the 1D case (the 2D and 3D cases follow easily from this). The $1D$ case is illustrated in figure 2, where we notice that the bandwidth of F_I (the frequency response of the integrator $f_I(x)$) is unfortunately too large to avoid completely the aliasing spectrum, when sampling $f(x)$ at the rate ω. A stronger pre-filtering can be obtained using $\omega < e$.

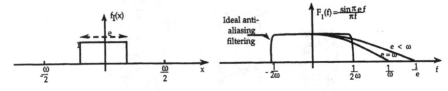

Fig. 2. Effect of integration followed by a sampling of a continuous signal

The linear processing being done is characterized by a 3D impulse response in the continuous domain. One can obtain [6] a discrete linear processing by using a discrete mask, by sampling a mask defined in the continuous domain. Let us consider the Fourier Transform (FT) $H(f)$ of a continuous mask $h(t)$. The filtering equation is: $Y(f) = X(f).H(f)$ where $X(f)$ and $Y(f)$ are the FT of the input and output signals respectively.

Let us consider an ω-step discretization $x_\omega(n) = x(n\omega)$ of the signal $x(t)$ and a discretization of the mask at the same rate, $h_\omega(n) = h(n\omega)$. We have :

$$FT((x_\omega * h_\omega)(n)) = \left[\frac{1}{\omega}\sum_n X\left(f + \frac{n}{\omega}\right)\right] \cdot \left[\frac{1}{\omega}\sum_n H\left(f + \frac{n}{\omega}\right)\right] = S(f) \quad (2)$$

If the supports of $X(f)$ et $H(f)$ are both included in the interval $]-\frac{1}{2\omega}, +\frac{1}{2\omega}[$ then we have : $\forall f \in]-\frac{1}{2\omega}, +\frac{1}{2\omega}[\quad S(f) = \frac{1}{\omega^2}X\left(f + \frac{n}{\omega}\right)H\left(f + \frac{n}{\omega}\right) = \frac{1}{\omega^2}Y(f)$

For the study of this result in the 3D case with a continuous mask $h(x, y, z)$, where, the sampling rate equals 1 along X and Y and ω along Z, we shall use a discrete mask thanks to the separability property of the Fourier transform : $h_{d,\omega}(n, m, l) = \omega h(n, m, \omega l)$. The a priori isotropic feature of the image in the continuous domain leads to consider the same spectral characteristic for the three spatial frequencies f_x, f_y and f_z.

Clearly, two reasons can prevent us from obtaining a discrete linear processing equivalent to the continuous one :

• The sampling rate of the data is too low in the Z direction. Consequently, before any processing, the information is heavily damaged by the aliased spectrum.

• The bandwidth of the designed operator in the continuous domain is too large to let its sampled version be equivalent. In order to cope with these problems, we shall try to limit the action of the operator, in the frequency domain, to the only band which can be used by the signal.

In the following, we present a way to overcome this difficulties using the approximation of the ideal linear derivation operator $H(f) = 2\pi i f$. If we consider the structure of the filter corresponding to a "weakly filtered" gradient using : $H(z) = \frac{(z - z^{-1})}{2\delta}$: δ being the sampling rate. This allows us a good approximation of the derivation operation along f_x and f_y (figure 3.a), but along f_z the result is less satisfying (figure 3.b). In the latter case we could search a polynomial form $H_1(z)$ with a higher order to better approximate the derivation as indicated in figure 3.c.

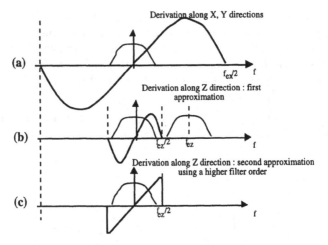

Fig. 3. Two possible approaches for compensation

3 Approach based on the definition of a continuous anisotropic model

This approach is made from a new continuous $3D$ surface model. Two operators will be infered: the moment based operator [7] and the Zucker's operator [8] that can be applied in the anisotropic case.

The idea is to express the problem using an ellipsoidal window instead of a spherical window in order to adapt to information deficiency in the direction corresponding to the weakest sampling. Using a spherical window in this case can result in using too little information in the Z direction. Thus, we propose to state the problem by substituting this window by a "sufficiently extended" ellipsoidal window in the Z direction (Fig. 4).

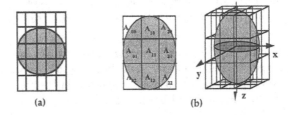

Fig. 4. Using a spherical window (a)
and an ellipsoidal window (b) on anisotropic data

3.1 The moment based operator

3D isotropic moment based operator. The trade-off between edge detection and localization is not always satisfied by the classical detection operators.

The elaboration of a $3D$ surface detection operator based on geometrical moments is motivated mostly by the need for accuracy in locating the surface and for performance. The model of the considered surface in the isotropic case (figure 5) is a plane cutting a sphere in two pieces: the background and the object at level **a** and **a** + **b**. The normal to this plane is defined by the angles α and β. This plane is located at a distance **h** from the origin of the sphere. The objective is to use the geometrical moments up to second order to determine these parameters. The moments of order $p + q + r$ of a continuous function $f(x, y, z)$ are defined by :

$$M_{pqr} = \iiint x^p \, y^q \, z^r \, f(x, y, z) \, dx dy dz$$

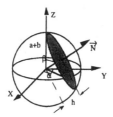

Fig. 5. Ideal surface model

After a mathematical development which consists in calculating moments and resolving a system of equations, the parameters are given by:

- *the orientation :*

$$\tan \alpha = \frac{M_{010}}{M_{100}} \qquad \tan \beta = \frac{\sqrt{M_{100}^2 + M_{010}^2}}{M_{001}} \tag{3}$$

- *the sub-voxel localization (translation) :*

$$h = \frac{1}{4M_b^3} \left[\left(5M_{200} - R^2 M_{000}\right) M_{100}^2 \right.$$
$$+ \left(5M_{020} - R^2 M_{000}\right) M_{010}^2 + \left(5M_{002} - R^2 M_{000}\right) M_{001}^2$$
$$\left. + 10 \left(M_{001} M_{010} M_{011} + M_{001} M_{100} M_{101} + M_{100} M_{010} M_{110}\right) \right]$$

$$M_b = \sqrt{M_{100}^2 + M_{010}^2 + M_{001}^2} \tag{4}$$

- *the contrast :*

$$b = \frac{4}{\pi} \frac{M_b}{\left(R^2 - h^2\right)} \tag{5}$$

3D anisotropic moment based operator. In the anisotropic case with a coefficient $\omega > 1$, an ellipsoid is defined by :

$$x^2 + y^2 + \frac{z^2}{\omega^2} \leq R^2$$

where (x, y, z) are defined in the local coordinate system. Origin is in the center of the window, R is the disk radius of the central plane $(z = 0)$.

The geometrical transformation: $x' = x$, $y' = y$, $z' = z/w$, allows us to keep the same formula for the parameters that characterize the surface. All the calculations done in the isotropic case can be generalized to make a new set of masks for a given window size and an anisotropic coefficient ω. The calculation of the moments is done in an ellipsoidal window, with every elementary parallelepiped having its own contribution. To take this contribution into account, the weighting functions (correlation masks) C_{xyz} have to be calculated.

The mask C_{010} can be obtained from C_{100} by symmetry, C_{011} from C_{101} and C_{020} from C_{200} by using the following rotations:

$$C_{010} = C_{100} \cdot M_{R_z}(90°), \quad C_{101} = C_{110} \cdot M_{R_y}(-90°), \quad C_{020} = C_{200} \cdot M_{R_z}(90°),$$

where :

$$M_{R_z}(\xi) = \begin{pmatrix} \cos \xi & \sin \xi & 0 \\ -\sin \xi & \cos \xi & 0 \\ 0 & 0 & 1 \end{pmatrix} \quad M_{R_y}(\psi) = \begin{pmatrix} \cos \psi & 0 & -\sin \psi \\ 0 & 1 & 0 \\ \sin \psi & 0 & \cos \psi \end{pmatrix}$$

Performance evaluation. Studying the performance of this anisotropic operator consists in studying the discretization and the noise effects. An anisotropic plane, passing through the center $(h = 0)$ of the central elementary parallelepiped is built, which is separating the volume into two parts $a = 50$ and $a+b = 100$. The construction accuracy is $\frac{1}{20}$ with an anisotropic coefficient variable $(\omega = 2, \omega = 3,$ ...). α and β which characterize the orientation of the plane, are variables :α varying from $0°$ to $355°$, β from $5°$ to $175°$ with an incremental step of $5°$. Thus, it is sufficient to estimate these parameters and calculate the resulting errors. The errors representations obtained in the deterministic case with an anisotropic coefficient $\omega = 3$ are shown in figure 6. In presence of additive Gaussian noise, several tests have been performed, demonstrating the robustness of the operator and the efficiency of the mask's approximation. The obtained results are shown in figure 7. This study shows that in terms of RMS (Root Mean Square) error, the translation error h is about $\frac{2}{100}$ of the elementary parallelepiped, the contrast error about 4 % of the contrast b. In estimating the angles α and β, the error is approximately $0.3°$. This remains true in presence of an additive Gaussian noise.

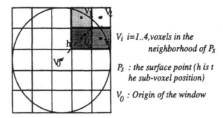

V_i $i=1..4$, voxels in the
neighborhood of P_s

P_s : the surface point (h is t
he sub-voxel position)

V_0 : Origin of the window

Fig. 8. Contrast distribution on P_s neighbors with respect to their position (2D)

Results. Several experiments have been conducted. They include the comparison between the interpolation followed by segmentation with the isotropic operator framework versus the segmentation with the anisotropic operator followed by interpolation. The tests have been performed on an anisotropic $84 \times 84 \times 61$ slice CT scan corresponding to a proximal end of the radius. The pixel dimension within the plane is $d = 0.42$ and the thickness of the slice $e = 1.5$. So, the anisotropic coefficient $\omega = 4$. Figure 9.a-b depicts the resulting 3D segmentation using the two frameworks described above. We display here the 3D rendering of the external surface of the segmented structure by means of direct volume rendering [9]. Figure 10 shows the result within 3 slices of the anisotropic dataset.

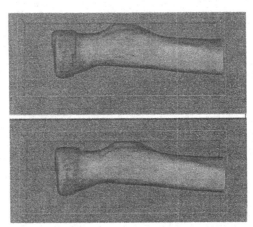

Fig. 9. Interpolation-segmentation with isotropic operator (a)
Segmentation with anisotropic operator-Interpolation (b)

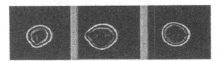

Fig. 10. 3 segmented anisotropic slices (10, 30, 50)

3.2 Zucker and Hummel's anisotropic operator

Similarily to the moments based operator, we propose to take into account the spatial inhomogeneity by reformulating the identification problem using an ellipsoidal window. In this purpose, we search the plane passing through the center of the ellipsoid and which the best approximates the surface.

Determination of continuous masks in the ellipsoidal domain. In order to simplify the notations, the calculations will be made in 2D space. The generalization to the 3D is trivial. Let the 2D ellipse $\mathcal{E} = \left\{ (x,y) \ / \ \left(\frac{x}{R}\right)^2 + \left(\frac{y}{\omega R}\right)^2 \leq 1 \right\}$

Thus, we want to find the orientation θ which minimizes:

$\iint_{\mathcal{E}} | \ I(x,y) - M_\theta(x,y) \ |^2 \ dx dy$, where: $M_\theta(x,y) = \begin{cases} 1 & \text{if } (x,y) \in \mathcal{E}_{+1} \\ -1 & \text{if } (x,y) \in \mathcal{E}_{-1} \end{cases}$

by using, if possible, the proposed solution in the spherical domain $(\mathcal{D})$. $\mathcal{E}_{-1}$ and $\mathcal{E}_{+1}$ correspond to the background and the object respectively. We denote by $\text{Arg min}_\theta \ \mathcal{A}$, the θ value which minimizes $\mathcal{A}$. Let $\dot{\theta}^*$ be the solution in the spherical domain :

$$\dot{\theta}^* = \text{Arg min}_\theta \iint_{\mathcal{D}} | \ \dot{I}(\dot{x},\dot{y}) - \dot{M}_{\dot{\theta}}(\dot{x},\dot{y}) \ |^2 \ d\dot{x} d\dot{y}$$

is approximated by :

$$\dot{\theta}^* = \tan^{-1}\left(\frac{\dot{b}}{\dot{a}}\right) \qquad \dot{a} = \dot{I}(\dot{x},\dot{y}) \cdot \dot{\Phi}_{\dot{x}}(\dot{x},\dot{y}) \qquad \dot{\Phi}_{\dot{x}}(\dot{x},\dot{y}) = \frac{\dot{x}}{\sqrt{\dot{x}^2 + \dot{y}^2}}$$

$$\dot{b} = \dot{I}(\dot{x},\dot{y}) \cdot \dot{\Phi}_{\dot{y}}(\dot{x},\dot{y}) \qquad \dot{\Phi}_{\dot{y}}(\dot{x},\dot{y}) = \frac{\dot{y}}{\sqrt{\dot{x}^2 + \dot{y}^2}}$$

To do this, it's sufficient to consider the geometric transformation $\begin{cases} \dot{x} = x \\ \dot{y} = \frac{y}{\omega} \end{cases}$ from the initial ellipsoidal domain to a spherical domain.

It can be shown that the masks in the ellipsoidal domain are given by :
$\Phi_x(x,y) = \dot{\Phi}_x(x, \frac{y}{\omega}) \qquad \Phi_y(x,y) = \frac{1}{\omega} \cdot \dot{\Phi}_x(x, \frac{y}{\omega})$

In the 3D case, with an ω-anisotropic Z direction, the masks become :

$$\Phi_x(x,y,z) = \frac{x}{\sqrt{x^2+y^2+\left(\frac{z}{\omega}\right)^2}}, \ \Phi_y(x,y,z) = \frac{y}{\sqrt{x^2+y^2+\left(\frac{z}{\omega}\right)^2}}, \ \Phi_z(x,y,z) = \frac{\left(\frac{z}{\omega}\right)}{\sqrt{x^2+y^2+\left(\frac{z}{\omega}\right)^2}}$$

Determination of discrete masks. The corresponding numerical processing is obtained by using the discrete masks obtained by sampling of Φ_x, Φ_y and Φ_z according to an anisotropic grid. Note that Zucker et al [8] have not taken into account the spherical neighborhood in the discrete case. It would have been better to first find a weighting function (correlation masks) representing the volume contribution of every voxel in the sphere before convolving with the basis functions Φ_x, Φ_y and Φ_z approximated by masks in the $n \times n \times n$ discrete neighborhood.

Actually, by using the Zucker operator as it is described in the literature, an error is done in considering a cubic neighborhood instead of a spherical one taken in the continuous case. When using a spherical neighborhood in the discrete case, the obtained results are better than the ones obtained from the commonly used operator. A better segmentation is consequently achieved [2].

3.3 Conclusion

An original way to design some surface detection operators suitable in the case of an anisotropic sampling of 3D volume data set has been proposed following two approaches. A 3D segmentation of anisotropic medical structures using a suitable moment-based 3D edge detection has been achieved. This operator uses a new surface model. It allows efficient and accurate surface estimation directly on anisotropic data without performing any interpolation preprocessing. This paper emphasizes the fact that the design of discrete operators must take into account the same sampling characteristics as the 3D data set that has to be processed. The operators as those based on moments, integrates intrinsically the operation of averaging, contrary to the Deriche's operator [6]. Futur work will adress the design of such operators directly in the discrete domain using Canny like optimality criteria.

References

1. Todd Evins, T. : A survey of algorithms for volume visualization. Comput. Graphics, Vol 26, No 3, pages 194-201, August 1992
2. Hamitouche, C. : Analyse d'images médicales tridimensionnelles : Application à l'extraction de structures anatomiques. Ph.D. Thesis, University of Rennes I, Nov. 1991
3. Kochanek, D.H.U. and Bartels, R.H. : Interpolating Splines with Local Tension, Continuity, and Bias Control. Comput. Graphics, Vol 18, pages 33-41, July 1984
4. Crochiere, R.E. and Rabiner, L.R. : Interpolation and Decimation of digital signals-A tutorial review. Proceedings of the IEEE, Vol. 69, pages 300-331, March 1981
5. Mintzer, F. : On $Half - band$, $Third - band$, and $N^t h - band$ FIR Filters and their design. IEEE Trans. on Acoustics, Speech, and Signal Processing, Vol.ASSP 30, pages 734-738, Oct. 1982
6. Deriche, R. : Using Canny's criteria to derive a recursively implemented optimal edge detector. International journal of computer vision, pages 167-187, 1987
7. Luo, L.M., Hamitouche, C., Dillenseger, J.L., Coatrieux, J.L. : A moment based three-Dimensional surface operator. IEEE Trans. on Biomedical Engineering, Vol. 40, No 7, pages 693-703, July 1993
8. Zucker, S.W., Hummel, R.A. : A three dimensional edge operator. IEEE PAMI Vol 3, No 3, pages 324-331, May 1981
9. Jacq, J.J. : Rendu volumique direct multi-objets. Implémentation et application à l'imagerie médicale. Sept. 1994

Augmented Reality II

Modelling Elasticity in Solids Using Active Cubes – Application to Simulated Operations

Morten Bro-Nielsen[12]

[1] INRIA Epidaure group, 2004, route des Lucioles,
06902 Sophia Antipolis cedex, France
[2] Institute of Mathematical Modelling
Technical University of Denmark, Bldg. 321
DK-2800, Lyngby, Denmark
e-mail: bro@imm.dtu.dk

Abstract. This paper describes an approach to elastic modelling of human tissue based on the use of 3D solid active models - active cubes [2] - and a shape description based on the metric tensor in a solid. Active cubes are used because they provide a natural parameterization of the surface and the *interior* of the given object when deformed to match the object's shape. Using the metric tensor to store the shape of the deformed active cube the elastic behaviour of the object in response to applied forces or subject to constraints is modelled by minimizing an energy based on the metric tensor. The application of this approach to modelling the elastic deformation of human tissue in response to movement of bones is demonstrated.

1 Introduction

The purpose of simulated operations is to enable a surgeon to experiment with different surgical procedures in an artificial environment. Applications include the training of surgeons and for practice before difficult operations.

Generally, simulated operations may be separated into two distinct but overlapping processes: visualization of the actual surgical procedure using artificial scapels etc.; and modelling the results of operations. The latter is used in particular for determining the results of craniofacial surgery to remove craniofacial deformations. The purpose of a simulated operation system in this case is to evaluate and visualize the results of operations on the overall facial shape of the patient. Although relatively few craniofacial operations are performed each year, their impact can be profound; in some cases changing the life of an individual. Simulation of the results is not only important for the surgeon, because such operations are difficult, but also to demonstrate to the patient and relatives the potential results of the often painful surgery and the long, slow recovery

Previously, simulated operations have been performed using surface models. For example, Caponetti et.al. [3] used a surface model reconstructed using the occluding contours in two x-rays to simulate bone surgery. Surgical reconstruction of the skull, where the skull is cut into several pieces and subsequently assembled into a new shape, has been modelled by several teams [5, 8, 9, 12].

They all used surface models, although Delingette et.al. [5] connected the surface of the bones and the surface of the skin with 'muscles' defined as a 3D structure, thereby obtaining a pseudo-3D model. In some cases, the influence of bone movement on facial features has been modelled. Yasuda et.al. [12] used an approximate method to put soft tissue onto the skull after surgery, based on the thickness of the soft tissue before the operation. Delingette et.al. [5] used the 'muscles' referred to above to model the deformation of the face. In both cases, the approach only supported a restricted set of operations, relevant to their application, and in the latter involved operator intervention for application of 'muscles'.

The approach proposed here involves complete 3D modelling of the *solid* - as opposed to *surface* - structure of the object. It is quite general, and is for example able to model elastic deformation of soft tissue in response to applied forces and constraints such as moved bones. An example of a simulated operation involving movement of the jaw is used to illustrate the results.

An extension of the Snake family of active models called active cubes [2] is used to model the shape of the given object. Active cubes parameterize a 3D solid shape and differ from previously proposed active models [7, 4] by having nodes in the interior of the object they model. Performing simulated operations, that include cutting into the model, is straightforward with active cubes because of the interior nodes. Intuitively, a cut corresponds to deleting the connection between two nodes on the surface of the active cube. For a surface model, a cut creates a hole in the model; with an active cube, the revealed interior nodes become new boundary nodes that model the interior bared by the cut.

Interior nodes also make active cubes suitable for modelling the 3D elastic behaviour of solids. Because the parameterization of the active cube is inherent in its structure, deforming an active cube to match a given object, provides a simple discrete parameterization of the object in curvilinear coordinates. After deformation of the active cube to match the 3D object, the equilibrium shape is stored in the active cube using the metric tensor [6, 10]. The metric tensor stores distances and angles and is therefore useful as a measure of shape. It has been used previously for shape description in [1, 10]. Elastic deformation of the head is modelled using an energy measure based on the metric tensor. When constraints or forces are applied to the active cube, energy minimization techniques can be used to determine an equlibrium shape which is a compromise between the original shape of the object and the constraints applied to it. This is used in practice to simulate the elastic deformation of soft tissue due to movement of included bones.

2 Modelling Object Shape with Active Cubes

To model the 3D data set, a 3D active cube [2] is used. An active cube is a parameterization of a subspace of the data space $\mathcal{R}^3$ defined by $v(r,s,t) = (x(r,s,t), y(r,s,t), z(r,s,t))$, where $(r,s,t)\epsilon([0,1]^3)$. By discretizing this subspace, a 3D mesh of nodes is defined in the subspace defined by $node_{ijk} = (il, jm, kn)$ where (l, k, m) are the discretization steps used.

To control the deformation of the active cube an energy function is defined:

$$E(v) = \int_0^1 \int_0^1 \int_0^1 E_{int}(v(r, s, t)) + E_{ext}(v(r, s, t)) dr ds dt \qquad (1)$$

where E_{int} is the internal energy of the net, that controls the shape and structure of the net and E_{ext} is the energy due to external and image forces.

The role of the internal energy term is to preserve the rigid structure of the node mesh, to smooth irregularities on the surface, and to force the active cube to contract. The internal energy can be defined straightforwardly using first and second order derivatives:

$$\begin{aligned} E_{int}(v) = &(\alpha(|v_r|^2 + |v_s|^2) + |v_t|^2)) \\ &+ (\beta(|v_{rr}|^2 + |v_{ss}|^2 + |v_{tt}|^2 + (\gamma(2|v_{rs}|^2 + 2|v_{rt}|^2 + 2|v_{st}|^2))) \end{aligned} \qquad (2)$$

where subscripts signifies partial derivatives and α, β and γ are coefficients controlling the first and second order smoothness of the net. The internal energy has the same form and functionality as that used with other active models of the Snake family [7, 4]: the first derivatives control contraction, and the second derivatives control bending and twisting.

The external energy is designed to attract the active cube to image objects which, in this context, are assumed to have high image intensities. Because of the solid structure of the active cube, the external energy is not defined using edge data which is usually used for surface/contour models. Instead the actual image data is used. The general form is:

$$E_{ext}(v(r, s, t)) = \omega f[I(v(r, s, t))] + \qquad (3)$$
$$\frac{\rho}{|\mathcal{N}(r, s, t)|} \sum_{p \in \mathcal{N}(r,s,t)} \frac{1}{\|v(r, s, t) - v(p)\|} f[I(v(p))]$$

$$f[I(v(r, s, t))] = \begin{cases} h[I_{max} - \overline{I(v(r, s, t))}_n] & for\ internal\ nodes \\ h[I(v(r, s, t))] & for\ boundary\ nodes \end{cases}$$

where ω and ρ are weights, $\mathcal{N}(r, s, t)$ is the neighbourhood of the node (r, s, t) not including the node itself, $\overline{I(v(p))}_n$ is the mean intensity in a $n \times n \times n$ cube, I_{max} is the maximum image intensity and h is an appropriate scaling function.

This energy is basically a sum of two terms: the first is a function of the image intensity at the current node; the other is the weighted contributions from the neighbouring nodes. f is defined differently for internal and boundary nodes because of the different roles assigned to these two groups of nodes. Internal nodes are attracted to volumes with high intensities corresponding to image objects, whereas boundary nodes are repulsed from the same volumes. In practice, the boundary nodes limit the contraction of the active cube which is caused by the internal energy and the internal nodes. Energy minimization is performed locally using an improved version of the finite difference Greedy algorithm [2, 11].

3 Shape Quantification

In order to model the elastic deformation of the active cube with a given shape as a reference, a quantification of the shape must be determined. A practical quantification measure is the metric tensor, or the first fundamental form, of a solid [1, 10], which is a 3 by 3 matrix defined by $G_{ij}(v(p)) = \frac{\partial v}{\partial p_i} \cdot \frac{\partial v}{\partial p_j}$ where p_i is the i'th element of the parameter vector p. The metric tensor stores the shape of a solid defined by distances and angles.

The parameterization of the active cube is a manifold with codimension 0, meaning that the dimension of the parameter and image space is the same. The shape of a manifold with codimension c is described by c curvature tensors and the metric tensor [6, 10]. As the codimension is 0, only the metric tensor is needed. The metric tensor is also known in elasticity theory as the Right Cauchy-Green tensor.

4 Elastic Deformation

In order to handle elastic deformations of the active cube from a reference object shape, the following energy measure is defined to quantify the shape deviation from the reference shape G^o [10]:

$$E_{Shape}(v) = \int_0^1 \int_0^1 \int_0^1 \sum_{i,j=1}^3 w_{ij}(G_{ij} - G_{ij}^o)^2 dr ds dt \qquad (4)$$

where w_{ij} are weights determining the influence of the different tensor components.

When constraints or forces are applied to the active cube, the equilibrium shape of the active cube is determined by minimizing the shape energy E_{Shape} under the given constraints.

5 Simulating Operations

This section applies the framework presented above to model the movement of bone structures in a human body. First, an artificial example is used to illustrate the procedure; then the movement of the jaw in a CT scan is shown.

The active cube model is used to model the shape of the object, and the metric tensor is used to quantify the reference shape and changes to this. The general procedure is the following:

1. Deform an active cube to model the object.
   The active cube is initialized around the object and contracts to model it.
2. Determine the equilibrium shape using the metric tensor.
3. Fix the position of nodes in the active cube which are positioned in image voxel labelled as bone.
   Fixing the position, means that subsequent elastic deformation will not be applied to these nodes. This way, only the soft tissue will move elastically.

4. Determine the bones to be moved. Move the corresponding active cube nodes to the required new position.

5. Using the final position of the bone nodes as constraints, minimize the E_{Shape} energy.

5.1 Experimental Results

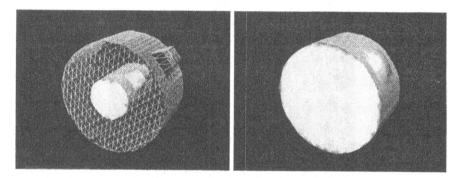

Fig. 1. Left: The active cube after initial movement modelling the test object and movement of hard tissue. Right: The resulting active cube after the elastic behaviour of the soft tissue has been simulated.

First results with an artificial example illustrates the simulated operation algorithm. The example is supposed to illustrate an orthogonal slice of a leg, of which a piece of bone is moved outwards from its reference position.

First, an active cube was allowed to deform to match the reference shape of the test data set. A 3D rendering of the active cube after the first initial movement of the bone is shown in figure 1. Because the elastic energy minimization has not been applied yet the soft tissue is just moved outwards, corresponding exactly to the movement of the bone. Figure 1 shows the result after elastic deformation has been modelled using energy minimization under the constraints posed by the bones. This clearly demonstrates the elastic behaviour of the soft tissue in response to the bone movement.

Figure 2 shows an active cube after having contracted around a CT scan of a head. To simulate an operation, the jaw was moved approximately 1 cm outwards horizontally. Figure 2 shows the active cube after the initial movement corresponding to figure 1. Figure 2 shows the result after energy minimization. In figure 2/bottom it is possible to see how the movement has influenced the soft tissue. Notice the inward contraction of the soft tissue on the cheek because of the elongation of the face.

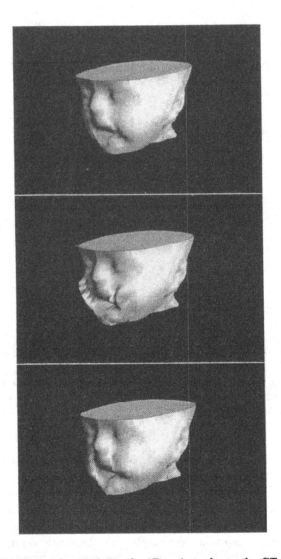

Fig. 2. Top: The result after applying the 3D active cube to the CT scan of a head. Middle: Active cube after the initial movement of the jaw. Bottom: Active cube after elastic deformation under constraints of jaw movements.

6 Conclusion

A approach to modelling elastic deformations in 3D solid objects has been proposed. Using the active cube introduced in [2], the solid 3D structure has been modelled, providing a curvilinear, discrete parameterization of the object.

The active cube subsequently provided the basis for quantizing the shape of the object using the metric tensor. Using an energy measure based on the metric tensor, elastic deformations have been modelled successfully.

Simulation of an operation involving movement of bone in a human head allows the user to perceive the elastic deformation of the patient's soft tissue.

In general we believe that using 3D solid models for operation simulation and 3D solid shape measurement has considerable promise. Simulated operations involving movement of bone have been demonstrated here. However it is obvious that simulated operations that include cutting into the pseudo-patient also require 3D solid models to enable visualization both of the interior of the patient and the actual elastic behaviour of the patient's soft tissue during cutting.

Using 3D solid active cubes increases the computational complexity of the algorithms; but the time required is not prohibitive. In the case of modelling the head, the deformation of the active cube to match the head took 15 minutes on a SGI Indigo II using an inefficient program. Modelling the elastic deformation of the soft tissue after movement of the jaw was performed in less than 1 minute. In practice, extracting the jaw was the most time-comsuming process.

References

1. K.A. Bartels, A.C. Bovik and C.E. Griffin: *Spatio-temporal tracking of material shape change via multi-dimensional splines*, Proc. IEEE Workshop Biomedical Image Analysis, Seattle, USA, pp. 110-116, June 1994
2. M. Bro-Nielsen: *Active nets and cubes*, submitted to CVGIP: Image Understanding, 1994
3. L. Caponetti and A.M. Fanelli: *Computer-aided simulation for bone surgery*, IEEE Computer Graphics & Applications, November, pp. 86-92, 1993
4. L. D. Cohen and I. Cohen: *Finite-element methods for active contour models and balloons for 2-D and 3-D images*, IEEE Trans. Pattern Analysis and Machine Intelligence, vol. 15, no. 11, pp. 1131-1147, 1989
5. H. Delingette, G. Subsol, S. Cotin and J. Pignon: *A craniofacial surgery simulation testbed*, INRIA Tech. Rep. 2199, 1994
6. M.P. Do Carmo: *Differential geometry of curves and surfaces*, USA, Prentice-Hall, 1976
7. M. Kass, A. Witkin and D. Terzopoulos: *Snakes: Active contour models*, Int. J. of Computer Vision, vol. 2, pp. 321-331, 1988
8. J. Satoh, H. Ciyokura, M. Kobayashi and T. Fujino: *Simulation of surgical operations based on solid modelling*, in T. L. Kunii: *Visual computing, Integrating computer graphics with computer vision*, Tokyo, Springer Verlag, pp. 907-916, 1992
9. R.H. Taylor: *An overview of computer assisted surgery research at IBM T.J. Watson research center*, in *Innovation et technologie en biologie et medecine*, 1992
10. D. Terzopoulos: *Deformable models*, The Visual Computer, vol. 4, pp. 306-331, 1988
11. D. J. Williams and M. Shah: *A fast algorithm for active contours and curvature estimation*, CVGIP: Image Understanding, vol. 55, no. 1, pp. 14-26, 1992
12. T. Yasuda, Y. Hashimoto, S. Yokoi and J-I. Toriwaki: *Computer system for craniofacial surgical planning based on CT images*, IEEE Trans. Medical Imaging, vol. 9, no. 3, pp. 270-280, 1990

Automated Extraction and Visualization of Bronchus from 3D CT Images of Lung

Kensaku MORI[1], Jun-ichi HASEGAWA[2], Jun-ichiro TORIWAKI[1],
Hirofumi ANNO[3] and Kazuhiro KATADA[3]

[1] Faculty of Engineering, Nagoya University, Furo-cho, Chikusa-ku,
Naogoya-shi 464-01, Japan
E-mail : mori@toriwaki.nuie.nagoya-u.ac.jp
[2] School of Computer and Cognitive Sciences, Chukyo University, 101 Tokodate, Kaizu-cho,
Toyota-shi,470-03, Japan
[3] School of Health Sciences, Fujita Health University, 1-98 Dengakugakubo, Kutsukake-cho,
Toyoake-shi, Aichi 470-11, Japan

Abstract. In this paper we present a procedure to extract bronchus area from 3D
CT images of lung taken by helical CT scanner and to visualize it as a 3D shaded
image. The extraction procedure consists of 3D region growing with the parameters adjusted automatically and is performed fast by using 3D painting algorithm.
The result is visualized by computer graphics workstation, and the bronchus is
observed from the inside just like a simulated bronchus endoscope freely without
any pain. We call this way of visualization "navigation" .

1 Introduction

Nowadays we can take high quality of X-ray CT (Computed Tomography) images which
cover wide area of human body in short time by using a helical (spiral) scan type CT
scanner or an ultra fast CT scanner. It is particularly important that by those high-speed
CT a kind of three dimensional (3D) image consisting of a large number of 2D cross
sections (slices) will be taken even in screening. This means that more than thirty slices
must be examined for every patient by a doctor working for screening[1]. Computer
aids, in particular a kind of automated diagnosis system is strongly desired to reduce
this load. The authors first developed a 3D image processing procedure to automatically
detect lung cancer lesions, using a thin slice helical scan CT images [2][3][4].

In order to realize automated diagnosis, it is important to recognize each organ in
lung separately, in particular, blood vessels and bronchi recorded in CT images. On a 2D
slice, cross sections of bronchi and blood vessels often appear as circumscribed shadows
which are likely to be confused with small cancer shadows. Therefore, to distinguish
vessels and bronchi from lung cancer lesions with reasonable accuracy is indispensable
to automatically detect lung cancer with the high recognition rate, keeping the false
alarm rate low enough. There is no report about processing of bronchus shadow because
the contrast of bronchus of CT images is very low.

Also important is to visualize both of original 3D X-ray CT images and processed
results. Although there are many reports concerning displaying outside views of 3D
objects extracted by image processing[5], very few about demonstrating inside views
of such objects as if they were observed from the inside. We consider that techniques

for viewing the inside of a 3D object are very useful to examine each component in 3D chest X-ray CT images from the diagnostic viewpoint because it makes possible to do endoscope simulation.

In this paper we present a procedure to extract bronchus area from 3D CT images of lung taken by helical CT scanner and to visualize it as a 3D shading image. The extraction procedure consists of 3D region growing with the parameters adjusted automatically. The result is visualized by employing a shading model of computer graphics. In this procedure we can observe the bronchus from the inside just like a simulated bronchus endoscope. We also travel inside the displayed bronchus freely by manipulating mouse cursor. We call this way of visualization "navigation". This simulation will make it possible to observe very thin bronchi without any pain.

After the features of a bronchus image are described in Section 2, a procedure of automated extraction of a bronchus area from 3D chest X-ray CT images is presented in Section 3. In Section 4, two methods to visualize 3D structure of the bronchus are explained, the outside view and "bronchus endoscope simulation" or "navigation". Finally in Section 5, we show results of applying these methods to real 3D chest CT images.

2 Features of a Bronchus Area in X-ray CT Images

In this section, we briefly summarize features of a bronchus image.

The bronchus has a pipe structure with air inside it. Starting from the end of trachea, it extends in lung with branching repeatedly like a tree. Because its wall is very thin and inner area is filled with air, the contrast of the bronchus image is very low. If the bronchus runs across the slice vertically, its section on a slice is observed as an approximately circular ring, but its border is often very vague. CT values in the inside of bronchus are lower than those of the wall of it. This suggests that the volume inside the bronchus (which we call bronchus area in this paper) can be extracted by following those areas in which the CT value is low and surrounded by walls of relatively higher CT values. An example of the bronchus image seen on a slice is given in Fig. 1.

3 Automated Extraction of Bronchus Area

3.1 Basic Idea

We extract the bronchus area as thin volumetric areas in 3D space instead of extracting the wall of the bronchus as curved surfaces. We perform this by tracing voxels with relatively low CT values corresponding to air. This process is regarded as a kind of region growing procedure. The process is controlled so as not to proceed across voxels with relatively high CT values corresponding to the wall. A starting point of tracing and the criterion to merge a new area to the bronchus should be selected carefully.

3.2 Outline of Procedure

The procedure consists of the starting point selection, repetition of the region growing with the threshold accommodation, and the bronchus area extraction (Fig. 2).

Selection of Start Point The method proposed here is basically a region growing in 3D space. An inside point of trachea is used as the starting point. The trachea area is extracted by thresholding.

Repetitive Region Growing

3-D Painting Algorithm : A kind of 3D region growing method ("painting") was developed to extract the bronchus area. This paint algorithm is performed by the line-by-line mode along three axes in 3D space to reduce the computation time.

Optimization of the Threshold Value : To use the above 3-D painting algorithm, we must determine the threshold value to distinguish the bronchus wall area and the inside of the bronchus area, or to decide whether a current voxel is merged to the colored area or not.

An iterative procedure is employed as follows : The initial painting is performed using a relatively low threshold value, and the number of voxels extracted as the bronchus area is counted. Then the painting and counting are iterated with the threshold value T increased by an appropriate increment ΔT. When the number of extracted voxels increases explosively, the iteration is terminated. We regard the result just before this explosion as the bronchus area we desire.

4 Visualization of the Bronchus area

The outside view is constructed by the voxel data manipulation system presented in [6] using extended VC algorithm, parallel projection and Gouraud shading[7]. We generate an image from the extracted result of the bronchus as if it were observed from the viewpoint inside the bronchus. This is regarded as a simulation of bronchus endoscopic observation.

First, the surface (polygon) data of the bronchus inner wall is constructed from the 3D binary voxel data of the bronchus area. Secondly, the normal vector of each polygon is calculated for shading. Finally, the shaded polygons are displayed at an arbitrary viewing position and direction. The bronchus endoscopic simulation can be done by displaying such shaded images with changing the viewing position and direction continuously as presented. Basically the procedure similar to the one in the outside view is utilized with Marching Cubes Algorithm (MCA)[8], perspective projection and the Gouraud Shading method.

5 Navigation

By changing a viewpoint continuously in the space inside the bronchus area, we have a moving image sequence giving the feeling that we navigate the 3D space freely along the wall of the bronchus. This was realized by using a fast CG workstation. The direction and the speed of navigation is controlled by a mouse cursor. The viewer's position can be selected arbitrarily and can jump to any place. The current location of a viewer is found by another picture shown in the window of the same frame.

6 Experiment

We applied the methods mentioned above to real 3D CT images taken by a helical (spiral) type of CT scanner (Toshiba TCT-900S). Specification of images is shown in Table 1. No specific preprocessing such as smoothing, interpolation or extraction of the lung area was used in this experiment.

Extraction of Bronchus Area Examples of slices and the processed results are shown in Fig. 3, a shaded 3D display of the extracted bronchus area in Fig. 4. Computation time is about 1 minutes for one case including all processing by SUN SPARCstation10/51.

Visualization of the Bronchus Area The outside view and the inside view are shown in Fig. 4 and 5, respectively. Fig. 5 is a scene of navigation. During navigation a user can find his current position in the bronchus by a white point moving in the bronchus shown in the window at the upper right corner of a picture. Rendering speed was about 0.45 sec. for one picture (by Silicon Graphics IRIS Crimson Reality Engine).

7 Discussion

7.1 Medical Use of the Result

The bronchus area extracted here corresponds to the volume of air filling the real bronchus. Still it surely provides morphological information of the bronchus of each patient with reasonable accuracy. The bronchus was extracted satisfactorily until the depth of the fifth or sixth branch. The outside view from an arbitrary direction is extremely useful to understand global and local shape of the bronchus. If some malfunction such as tracheostenosis or bronchiostenosis exists, physician will find how long the bronchiostenosis region is and how severe is the abnormality. Fig. 4(c) and 5(c) show an example of such abnormal case.

The inside view and navigation provide a new tool to visualize 3D images for diagnosis. The navigation is considered as a kind of simulation of the bronchus endoscope. Although pictures generated here keep only morphological information, it has advantages over a real endoscope. First it can proceed to the bronchus further than an endoscope. Second the navigation can start at an arbitrary position and move to any direction. If bronchiostenosis exists, a real endoscope cannot proceed further. Thirdly, the navigation in computer can be tried as many times as needed without giving any pain to a patient. Fourth quantitative features can be extracted by computer such as the length of the bronchiostenosis region.

The bronchus area extracted here is also useful for computer aided diagnosis of lung cancer. For instance, false alarm will be greatly decreased by differentiating each other the bronchus, blood vessels and other massive shadows observed on each slice exactly.

7.2 Visualization

In this experiment we developed two methods to display processed results of 3D images : shaded surfaces of the outside view of objects and the inside view with navigation. The latter is especially useful for organs of pipe-like structure. All of these were implemented with the combinations of existing CG techniques. This technique of navigation shows a new intelligible way to visualize 3D medical images in that free movement of the viewpoint like a bronchus endoscopic simulation becomes available.

As was stated in 7.1, we can observe such a thin bronchi that the real bronchus endoscope can not reach. We can enter into bronchus from any point. These suggest new image interface for medical doctors. Also, it is expected to calculate feature vectors such as the length of a branch, angles between branches, and the radius of bronchus. We are now to developing these measuring functions in the near future. Improvement of spatial resolution is required for further use of quantitative measurement. For example, abnormal protrusion of the surface by 0.5 ~ 1mm height should be detected to find small tumors.

8 Conclusion

In this paper, we presented a method for automated extraction of the bronchus area from 3D chest X-ray CT images and display of 3D forms using the extracted results. We applied the proposed method to real 3D chest CT images and confirmed that it worked satisfactorily. We performed "navigation inside the bronchus" or simulation of a bronchus endoscope basing upon the bronchus area extracted above and techniques for generating the inside scene of a 3D object. It was shown that this visualization could generate the inside view of the bronchus area very well. Extraction of very thin bronchus remains to be studied in the future. Furthermore applications are expected to be extended to larger number of cases.

Acknowledgments : Authors thank to the member of their laboratory in Nagoya University for their collaboration. Parts of this research were supported by the Grant-In-Aid for Scientific Research from the Ministry of Education, the Grant-In-Aid for Cancer Research from the Ministry of Wealth and Welfare, and Special Coordination Funds for Promoting Science and Technology from the Science and Technology Agency, Japanese Government.

References

1. S. Yamamoto, M. Senda, Y. Tateno, T. Iinuma, T. Matsumoto, and M. Matsumoto : "Image Processing for Computer Aided Diagnosis in the Lung Cancer Screening System by CT (LSCT)", Trans. IEICE, **J76-D-II**, 2, pp.250-260 (Feb. 1993) (in Japanese)
2. J. Hasegawa, K. Mori, and J. Toriwaki, H. Anno, K. Katada : "Automated extraction of lung cancer lesions from multi-slice chest CT images by using three- dimensional image processing" Trans. IEICE, **J76-D-II**, 8, pp.1578-1594 (Aug. 1993) (in Japanese).
3. K. Mori, J. Hasegawa, J. Toriwaki, H. Annno, K.Katada : "A Procedure with Position-variant Thresholding and Distance Transformation for Automated Detection of Lung Cancer Lesions from 3-D chest X-rayt CT images", Medical Imaging Technology, **12**, 3, pp.216-223 (May 1994) (in Japanese)
4. J.Toriwaki : "Study of Computer Diagnosis of X-ray and CT Images in Japan - A Brief Survey", Proceedings of the IEEE Workshop on Biomedical Image Analysis, pp.155-164 (June 1994)
5. "Special Issue on Volume Visualization", The Visual Computer, **6**, 1 (Feb. 1994)
6. E. Kitagawa, T. Yasuda, S. Yokoi, and J. Toriwaki : "An Interactive Voxel Data Manipulation System", Proceedings of 3rd IEEE international Workshop on Robot and Human Communication, pp.204-209 (Jul. 1994)
7. Gouraud, H., "Continuous Shading of Curved surfaces", IEEE Trans. on Computer, C-**20**(6), pp. 623-629 (June 1971)
8. Lorensen W.E. and Cline H.E., "Marching Cubes : A high resolution 3D surface construction algorithm", Computer Graphics, **21**, 4, pp.163-169 (Apr. 1986)

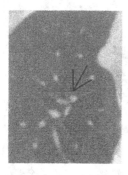

Fig. 1. An example of bronchu area on a X-ray CT image

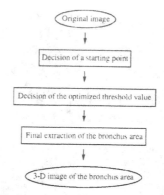

Fig.2. Whole procedure of bronchus area extraction

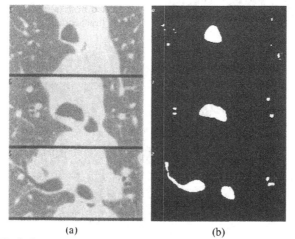

(a) (b)

Fig.3. Processing results (only three slices are displayed) (a) original image (b) results of bronchus area extraction (white areas)

Table 1. Specificatoin of images

	Pixels	Slices	Thickness (mm)	Speed (mm/sec)	Reconstruction Pitch (mm)
Data1	512x512	62	2	2	1
Data2	512x512	62	2	2	1
Data3	512x512	62	2	2	1
Data4	512x512	62	2	2	1
Data5	512x512	79	5	2.5	1

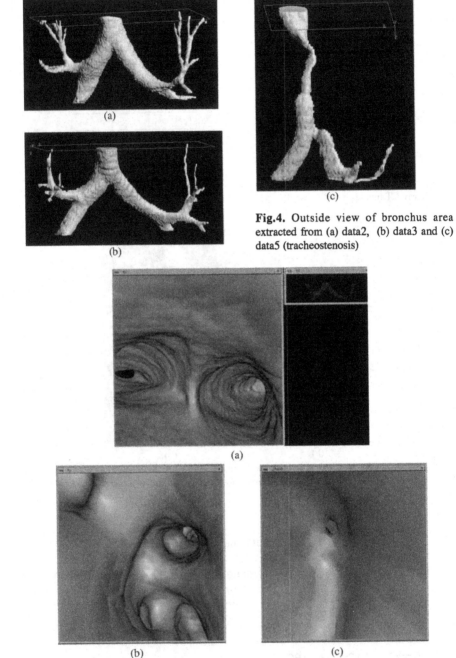

(a)

(b)

(c)

Fig.4. Outside view of bronchus area extracted from (a) data2, (b) data3 and (c) data5 (tracheostenosis)

(a)

(b)

(c)

Fig. 5. Examples of scene in simulation of (a) a view of the first branching point (data2), (b) a view of other branching point of bronchus (data2) and (c) tracheostenosis part (data5).

Virtual Reality as an Operative Tool During Scoliosis Surgery

Bernard Peuchot[1], Alain Tanguy[2] and Michel Eude[3]

[1] LASMEA CNRS URA 1793, Les Cézeaux, 63177 Aubière, France
[2] Centre Hospitalier Universitaire, Hôtel-Dieu, BP 69
63003 Clermont-Ferrand, France
[3] C.U.S.T, Les Cézeaux, BP 206, 63174 Aubière, France

email : peuchot@le-eva.univ-bpclermont.fr

Abstract. As a three-dimensional deformity, scoliosis receive a three-dimensional correction as well. Several limitations with the current techniques do not allow for this goal to be accomplished. Evaluation of vertebral displacements while corrective forces are taking place is the first step to know precisely what the surgery accomplishes. We have already reported on a method based on video tracking of vertebral displacements using high precision algorithm.

Such a method allowed the surgeon to watch vertebral displacements occuring through the 3D positioning of vertebral model on a monitor by the side of the surgeon. The main drawback is the need for the surgeon to distract his attention from the operative field to get a plane view of a screen.

We propose to use a new approach of virtual reality to superpose a 3D "transparent" vision of the vertebra directly on the surgeon operative view. This method uses a dedicated apparatus to produce an augmented reality 3D view projected directly in the operative field improving reality perception of the operative field.

1 Introduction

Scoliosis is a deforming process which disturbs the normal spinal alignment through one or several curves. Being a three-dimensional deformity, it should get a three-dimensional correction as well. Surgical maneuvers are performed to realign the spine as best as possible and certainly correctives forces induce three-dimensional displacements of the vertebrae included in the curve -and even outside the curve-. However, we have no means to assess these displacements so that the correction obtained does not match the specific three-dimensional deformity we have to treat. In fact, posterior spinal standard exposure gives to the surgeon a limited view of vertebral anatomy and this partial visualization does not allow for a precise evaluation of positioning in space. Also such a partial visualization of vertebral anatomy may create difficult or even dangerous situations : pedicular identification with potential injury to the spinal cord or the roots, penetration depth or direction for any implants in the spine which may be dangerous for the vessels. Of course, we could get intra-operative X-rays but this gives only 2D evaluation which is far from the more and more refined pre-operative imaging techniques available to the surgeon to elaborate mentally the surgery to be performed. In the present state of the art, there is a growing discrepancy between precise pre-operative knowledge and surgical "rusticity" where visual feeling for a "good" correction combined with post-operative X-ray documentation is all we get for 3D appreciation of the correction.

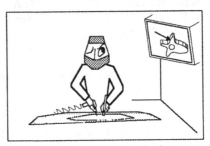

Fig.1. Poor 2D Vision "feeling"

The aim of our study is to give intra-operatively to the surgeon a 3D anatomical view of vertebrae of interest without the constraints of restricted surgical exposure. We use a dedicated apparatus to produce an augmented reality 3D view projected directly in the operative field improving real perception of the operative field.

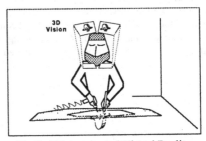

Fig.2. 3D Augmented Virtual Reality

2 Vertebral Displacements Measurement By Video Tracking

As previously reported elsewhere, we use a method based on the principle of three dimensional telemetry from a single perspective view [1] which had to be adapted to various requirements. Without additional surgery, small pellets are strongly fixed to the vertebrae to be tracked which geometry has been determined by pre-op analysis (TDM, MRI or 3D Xrays). This last point must be tacken in account as it is critical for patient X-rays exposure. We are presently looking for as less as possible standard X-ray exposure to onbtain an accurate 3D reconstruction. The use of a C-arm to locate the pellets at the beginning of the procedure from two views is satisfactory.

By the knowledge of the geometry of the pellets it is then possible to locate these vertebrae in space from the modification in their perspective view from a single video camera. We use inverse perspective algorithm which is very standard in imaging field.

We have improved the operability of the system by automatic detection of the pellets and the accuracy of the measurement by precise localisation of these pellets (0.1 pixels) and optimal modelization of the acquisition system. A camera virtual equivalent model where all the characteristics are modelized through a very precise calibration grid provides precise measurements tacking in account all optical distortion and electronical disturbances. Subpixel detectors using grey levels response have been developped. Such methods give excellent results for the detection of every grid intersections or spots[2] (about 0.01 pixels).

This method has been validated on vertebral specimens which can be moved in any direction. Reproducibility and measurement accuracy are quite good for the purpose of the method (less than 1 mm in depth).

3 Standard 2D Display Limitations

Pure displacements measurement values would not be very practical for the surgeon and would not say much to him. We translated the numerical data into the positioning of a vertebral model constructed from pre-operative analysis.

On a monitor placed by the side of the surgeon, a video view of the operative field is displayed and vertebral 3D models are adjusted to the vertebrae in the field. This first design of vertebral positioning display has been used experimentally but we never tried to use it operatively as its limitations had already prompted more fascinating solutions.

Two limitations had to be overcome :
- the need for the surgeon to distract its attention from the operative field to watch the monitor
- the 2D perception on the monitor.

4 Virtual Reality Enhancements

The development of Virtual Reality focused on eliminating the discontinuity in the perception by the surgeon of the operative situation when he wants to get access to 3D modelization. 3D modelization should then placate the operative field and gives a perfect illusion of it. This is very precisely the field of virtual reality and the interaction expected between virtual reality and the perception of the real situation is called augmented reality.

We explored the existing solutions :
- All of them use head mounted displays which are cumbersome and unconfortable for the surgeon,
- They need a precise tracking of the surgeon head and of the objects under observation which is quite expensive and potentially sources of errors,
- None of them are able to produce high luminous virtual images which could be perceived in the high lighted operative field.

We came to the following prerequisites for our own solution :
- no apparatus at all on the surgeon's head,
- same sensory process as the natural perception of the operative field (no geometrical distorsion, good luminosity for the 3D virtual images),
- perfect matching between 3D synthetic images and real view.

The surgeon points out the vertebra of interest which precise 3D position is determined from camera pellets detection. This position by itself gives the area where computer binocular images must be visualized. There is no need the follow the surgeon sight as we know the position of what he is looking at.

The components of our prototype (Fig.3) include:
- a VGA LCD color panel of medium resolution to visualise the left and right model images
- a high intensity lamp to illuminate this panel
- two semi-transparent mirrors to partially reflect the 3D model image with unobstructed view of the operative field
- a single video camera to observe the vertebrae in the field

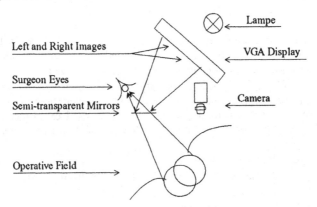

Fig.3. Prototype block-diagram

Specific procedures and reference objects are used to calibrate all these components to get a good matching between the 3D scene and the 3D virtual images.

This first prototype, as shown Fig.4, gives us a full satisfaction :
- the main parameters of human vision have been taken in account to get a good perception of the reality and comfortable observation : 3D eyes location, viewing direction and observation distance. This gives the location of the scene under observation, that is, in the present case, the operative field.
- a binocular image of the model is calculated with the convergence of the right and left views precisely on the operative field. This gives not only a 3D stereoscopic view but also a correspondance between the virtual image and the real image of the operative field.
- the left and right images of such a 3D Vision System have be provided with high luminosity to be visible in the operative field itself. The quality of these images is very satisfactory and provide good informations to the observer.

With our approach, in Real operative situation a 3D "transparent" vision of the vertebra is superimposed on the surgeon operative view. We have developped a prototype using a vertebral model located in space by some spots observation. This application establishes the good superposition between the specimen and its computer virtual model.

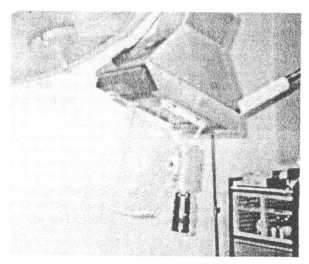

Fig.4. Prototype photgraph in operative situation

Prerequisites for practical intra-operative use have been fulfilled : it is no more invasive for the patient than the surgery itself but for the implantation of small pellets, it can be monitored at some distance from the operative field, minimizing the risk of sepsis and interferences with the surgical procedure. For the surgeon, the use of the system is as simple as looking through a binocular.

In the present state of development, the weakest point is the complete diagnosis assessment of the deformity. In fact, the precision obtained by pre-op analysis is very critical in the knowledge of the geometry of the vertebrae to be tracked. We have to be aware of the necessary reduction of X-rays doses, of the limited access to MRI and certainly, we will have to come with some responses to this.

5 Prospective

Many advantages can be expected from the introduction of such an operative tool especially in the field of surgical scoliosis management :
- knowledge of the correction in progress of a scoliotic curve during surgery allows for the necessary adjustments to obtain an optimal reduction. Thus, the reduction obtained will not be left to the surprise of post-operative roentgenogram. Further analysis will be possible on the effectiveness of surgical instrumentations and on the distribution of intervertebral rigidity inside various types of curves. The use of specific hardware can lessen conciderably the response time.

- safety during the placement of any surgical implants, particularly pedicular fixation. It is of special interest to note that information given by virtual reality reduces the use of intra-operative X-rays which is safe both to the patient and the surgeon.
- restriction in the extent of operative exposure because virtual reality introduce "tranparent" vision of hidden aspects of the spine.

Virtual reality can be introduced in the operating room during spinal surgery. It seems a promizing method to extend the three-dimensional knowledge from pre-operative imaging to intra-operative perception by the surgeon with a possible real time ajustement to vertebral displacements. Of course, the virtual reality is useful to show some hidden aspects of the spine and/or the operating instruments positioning.

References

1. Peuchot B., Tanguy A., Saint-André M.: Video tracking of vertebral displacement for intra-operative evaluation of scoliosis correction. Principles and methods. International Symposium on 3-D Scoliotic Deformities, Edition de l'Ecole Polytechnique de Montréal, (Juin 1992) 38-41

2. Peuchot B. : Camera virtual equivalent model. 0.01 pixel detectors. Special issue "3D Advanced Image Processing in Medicine" in Computerized Medical Imaging and Graphics, Vol.17, Number 4/5, 1993.

We acknowledge the financial support of "LA FONDATION DE L'AVENIR"

Neurosurgical Guidance Using the Stereo Microscope

P.J. Edwards[1], Dr. D.L.G[1]. Hill, Dr. D.J.Hawkes[1],
R. Spink[2], Dr. A.C.F Colchester[3],
Mr A. Strong[4], Mr M. Gleeson[5]
p.edwards@umds.ac.uk

[1] Dept. of Radiological Sciences, UMDS,
Guy's Hospital, London SE1 9RT, U.K.
[2] Leica, Heerbrugg, Switzerland.
[3] Dept. of Neurology, UMDS.
[4] Neurosurgical Unit, Maudsley Hospital, London.
[5] ENT surgery, UMDS.

Abstract. Many neuro- and ENT surgical procedures are performed using the operating microscope. Conventionally, the surgeon cannot accurately relate information from preoperative radiological images to the appearance of the surgical field. We propose that the best way do this is to superimpose image derived data upon the operative scene. We create a model of relevant structures (e.g. tumor volume, blood vessels and nerves) from multimodality preoperative images. By calibrating microscope optics, registering the patient in-theatre to image coordinates, and tracking the microscope intra-operatively, we can generate stereo projections of the 3D model and project them into the microscope eyepieces, allowing critical structures to be overlayed on the operative scene in the correct position. We have completed initial evaluation with a head phantom, and are about to start clinical evaluation on patients. With the head phantom a theoretical accuracy of 4.6mm was calculated and the observed accuracy ranged from 2mm to 5mm.

1 Introduction

The prevalence of MR, CT and MRA imaging has dramatically increased the amount of 3D information about a patient's anatomy and pathology that is available to the surgeon preoperatively. However the display of this information as slices printed onto radiographic film is frequently difficult to relate to the appearance of the surgical field. Consequently, there has been considerable interest in developing surgical guidance systems that register the coordinate system of a 3D surgical localiser to image coordinates. This enables the surgeon to view the position of a pointer or tool that is inserted into the wound overlayed onto reformatted or rendered versions of the radiological images displayed on a computer monitor in the operating room[1, 2, 3].

For this type of image guidance the surgeon must look away from the surgical field to view the images. We believe that, when a microscope is being used, projecting relevant radiological information into the eyepiece of the microscope can provide the surgeon with the information they need more conveniently. The principle of superimposing data on real optical scenes (head-up displays) has been used for many applications[4].

The idea of overlaying image information on the intra-operative scene is not new. As early as the 1930's Steinhaus used X rays of gunshot injuries to locate the embedded bullet. A sheet of glass was placed over the patient and a light source positioned in such a way that its reflection appeared at the site of the bullet[5].

The injection of image data into the operating microscope has also been reported. Simple models, such as tumor outline derived from CT/MR slices, have been overlayed on the microscope view for image guidance, using ultrasound localisation[6, 7] or a fixed geometry with respect to a stereotactic frame[8].

Our objectives were to build a functional model of a microscope that could accurately overlay 3D preoperative information onto the surgical field and to demonstrate that the overlay remains accurate when the microscope is moved.

2 Methods

In order to overlay stereo perspective projections of image data in the microscope field of view in the correct position the following steps are required:

1. Microscope Calibration - Calibration of the microscope optics using a reference object.

2. 3D Model Construction - Identification of relevant features from preoperative scans.

3. Patient Registration - Matching image and patient coordinates using point pairs and/or skin surface matching.

4. Microscope Tracking - Use of a 3D localiser to track the position and pose of the microscope.

5. Stereo Projection - Stereo perspective projection of relevant structures selected by the surgeon onto the current microscope view.

Once these steps have been achieved, the microscope may be moved as desired and the overlayed information will be updated to represent the current view.

2.1 Microscope Calibration

The process of microscope calibration introduces many of the concepts used throughout this paper, and as such deserves some attention. The basic aim of the calibration process is to produce a matrix that will project any 3D point relative to the microscope's frame onto a pixel position in the injected image.

The use of an LED based 3D localiser is central to several components of this project. The coordinates obtained from this system will be referred to as 'room coordinates' in the following discussion.

Firstly, a calibration object consisting of a perspex pyramid with numerous (44) accurate calibration points marked on it is placed within the working field of the localiser. A pointer is used to obtain the room coordinates of all 44 calibration points and a rigid body transformation matrix from calibration to room coordinates is calculated by the method of Arun et al[9] using the SVD algorithm[10]. This matrix we call $R_{r \leftarrow c}$ (calibration to room coordinate transformation). The calibration object must not be moved at this point.

Secondly, the microscope is positioned so that the calibration object can be seen through both eyepieces. Its position and pose are recorded by a frame of LEDs securely mounted to the main body. The relative positions of these LEDs are known and recorded as a series of coordinates which define a system of axes fixed with respect to the microscope's main lens. This coordinate system we call 'microscope coordinates'. The positions of these LEDs in room coordinates gives us the matrix $R_{m \leftarrow r}$ (room to microscope coordinate transformation), also by least squares SVD. Multiplying these matrices together ($R_{m \leftarrow r} R_{r \leftarrow c}$) allows us to calculate the positions of the calibration points in microscope coordinates.

Finally, the locations of these calibration points in the eyepiece view are marked with an overlayed cursor. Using homogeneous coordinates[11] a projection matrix can be calculated which projects any point in microscope coordinates onto the position where it appears in the overlayed display, as we desired.

Separate projection matrices, P_m^L and P_m^R, are obtained for each eyepiece. This process is rather laborious, but thankfully only needs to be done once for a particular microscope arrangement. It would be fairly straightforward to automate the identification of each calibration point, for example by placing LEDs at every point.

2.2 3D Model Construction

In order to obtain information about tumour volume, bone, blood vessels and nerves for a real patient it is necessary to register multiple image modalities, such as MRI, CT and MRA. Much work has been done to establish methods for registering these images, by our group and others, using such techniques as stereotactic frames, fiducials, anatomical landmarks, surface matching and voxel based methods[12, 13].

Once the images are registered, the important features must be delineated and labelled, either by hand with computer assistance or using an automated segmentation tool. A simple 3D model of this information is then constructed from these data. Purposes the description of blood vessels and nerves is given as a series of centre points with associated diameters. Tumour outline and bone are represented as a series of surface points.

The graphical representation of this model for our current system consists of single colour ribbons for the linear structures and contour lines for surfaces. The point descriptions are first sorted for distance from the microscope lens to enable correct hidden line removal. A simple representation was chosen as the surgeon requires a simple, uncluttered display which does not complicate image interpretation or cause confusion between reality and graphical reconstruction. Experimentation with the intra-operative graphics will be a major part of the continuation of this project.

For our initial experiments a phantom consisting of a model skull with artificial internal structures was used and a single modality image (CT) was taken.

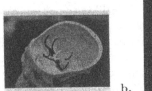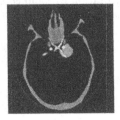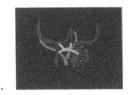

a.   b.   c.

Fig. 1. Example of model construction with skull phantom.
a. Photograph of the skull phantom.
b. Single slice from the CT scan.
c. Example perspective projection of the 3D model.

2.3 Patient Registration

The initial position of the patient relative to the room may be calculated by marking either fiducials, or anatomical landmarks on the skin surface with the 3D pointer. These points, which will previously have been marked in the registered images, give us the transformation from image coordinates to room coordinates. This is the transformation $R_{r \leftarrow i}$ (image to room coordinate transformation). This can be further refined by matching a large number of points on the skin surface to a surface extracted from the images[14].

After draping these points will normally no longer be available, so subsequent movement of the patient will invalidate the registration. With an LED based localisation system it may be possible to attach LEDs firmly to the patient, and for example fixed to a Mayfield clamp, in order to track any movement. Alternatively, after registration, points may be marked on the patient's skin or, after exposure of the skull, on the bone. For our initial system we assumed the head was rigidly clamped and did not move.

2.4 Microscope Tracking

This part of the process is simply performed by recording the room coordinates of the LEDs on the microscope frame as it is moved around. From this we obtain the transformation matrix $R_{m \leftarrow r}$ as described for the calibration process.

2.5 Stereo Projection

Each projection is calculated as follows:

$$P_t^R = P_m^R R_{m \leftarrow r} R_{r \leftarrow i} \tag{1}$$

$$P_t^L = P_m^L R_{m \leftarrow r} R_{r \leftarrow i} \tag{2}$$

where P_t^R and P_t^L are the total projection transformations for the right and left eyepieces and the other terms are as defined in Sections 2.1 and 2.3. If there is little or no patient movement the only matrix that will change is $R_{m \leftarrow r}$ - i.e. the microscope position and pose.

Each of the points in the model is projected by P_t^R and P_t^L onto its position in the eyepiece displays. The different structures are given separate colours for identification. The projection is calculated separately for each eye and the two displays are driven by separate PCs and video converters.

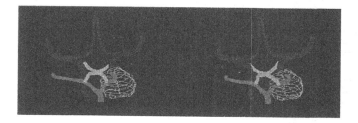

Fig. 2. Example stereo projection of the 3D model.

2.6 The Equipment

The microscope on which the system is mounted is a Leica M690 with an FM2 stand. The localiser is currently a PIXSYS 2000, using a pointer and a frame of LEDs mounted on the microscope body, both of which were custom made. The optical arrangement involves a stereo mounting, again custom made by Leica, which enables two Citizen LCD projectors to inject images into the microscope via a beam splitter. Each projector is driven by a separate PC. This arrangement can be seen in Fig. 3.

3 Error Analysis

There will be sources of error in each stage of this system. The calibration process could in principle be performed many times to reduce any random errors. The sources of error during calibration arise from the accuracy in locating the LEDs and marking the calibration object points, both with the 3D localiser and in the overlayed display. The component due to the last two sources will mean that random calibration errors could be reduced by increasing the number of sample points. The errors in locating LEDs may also have a systematic element. The

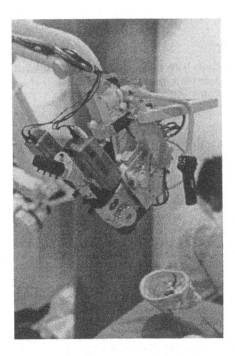

Fig. 3. Arrangement of the equipment showing microscope, projectors and the LED frame.

analysis of random errors due to LED location will be pursued below in the discussion of microscope tracking.

The 3D model construction will have errors associated with the registration of different imaging modalities for a true clinical application. For our single CT example with the head phantom the errors should be of the order of the slice thickness which was 2mm.

Patient registration will depend on the accuracy with which surface points can be located. The errors due to the rotational and translational parts of the rigid body transformation have been derived[15]. As an example the error for 6 points on the surface of a 113mm radius sphere when each of the points has standard deviations of 1mm at the surface in each ordinate (comparable to the localisation system) gives errors of 0.7mm for translation and 0.7mm for rotation about the centroid of the points. This should be a reasonable approximation for our skull phantom. Errors in point location will be greater for a real patient, due to uncertainty in location, skin movement etc. We would estimate the errors in location of each surface point to be about 2-3mm in clinical practice.

The microscope is tracked using 7 LEDs placed at the corners of a 250mm U-shaped frame and the centres of the three sides. Assuming the quoted accuracy of point location (1mm) the errors in translation from this configuration are negligible (0.4mm). For rotation the errors in the Euler angles Θ_x, Θ_y, Θ_z, are given by[15]:

$$\sigma(\Theta_x) = \sigma_k/(\sum_i (y_i^2 + z_i^2))^{1/2}$$

$$\sigma(\Theta_y) = \sigma_k/(\sum_i (z_i^2 + x_i^2))^{1/2}$$

$$\sigma(\Theta_z) = \sigma_k/(\sum_i (x_i^2 + y_i^2))^{1/2}$$

Where x_i, y_i, z_i are the coordinates of the points i relative to the centroid and σ_k is the error in point location in each of the axes (1mm). This gives us the values 0.00363, 0.00327, 0.00243 for the errors in each of these angles. These correspond to errors of 2.7mm, 2.4mm and 1.8mm respectively at the distance of the microscopes focal point of 750mm.

The errors in projection come directly from the calibration process. We are less interested in the level of discrepancy in the actual display than in the meaning of this discrepancy in patient coordinates. Combining the errors we have calculated gives an overall standard deviation of 4.6mm for our head phantom.

Another source of error is non-linearity of the microscope optics. The perspective projection is not entirely accurate as there will be a distortion of 3-5% of the visual field at the periphery. For a 50mm field of view this would correspond to an error of 1.5-2.5mm. It would be straightforward to model and correct for this distortion, though this remains to be done.

The accuracy of this entire system could be improved in a number of ways. The calibration process could be made more accurate by performing a number of calibrations for different microscope positions to reduce random errors arising from microscope tracking. The tracking could be improved by adding more LEDs to the frame or perhaps by averaging a number of readings of LED positions. The localiser technology is also improving, so that accuracies of less than 0.5mm in LED location should be possible. Patient registration could be improved by marking more points or the use of surface matching techniques[14].

The eventual goal of the system is an accuracy of the order of 1mm. Since this is the current limit of CT or MR image slice thickness, we could not expect to do much better than 1mm. For the rest of the system we are close to this goal, and methods for reducing the errors further are outlined above.

4 Results

We performed an initial test of the 3D model derived from the CT scan of the skull phantom. This involved the calculation of the perspective of a photograph of the phantom by marking reference points visible in both the photograph and the CT image. The same projection of the 3D model was then overlayed on the photograph, with the result that can be seen in Fig. 4. The model was seen to be accurate from a number of different perspectives.

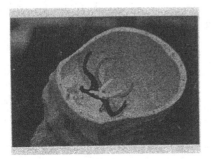

Fig. 4. Superimposition of a projection of the 3D model onto a photograph of the phantom.

Despite the optical arrangement in the microscope being less than optimal (poor contrast and excessive light level in the displays) we have been able to demonstrate that image data can be superimposed accurately for our skull phantom. The optics have now undergone improvements and the stereo effect is markedly better. Figure 5 shows photographs taken through the microscope to demonstrate the accuracy. Full measurements of the accuracy have yet to be performed, but the overlay appeared to be within 5mm in the worst case and 2mm for movements within 30° of the calibration and registration positions. These qualitative estimates of the accuracy are in good agreement with the calculated errors.

a. 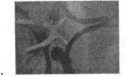   b.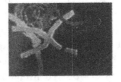

Fig. 5. Views through the microscope showing the accuracy of alignment.
a. View of the skull phantom through the microscope eyepiece.
b. View of projected data through the microscope eyepiece.

The overlays would be updated as the microscope moved in 0.5 to 1 secs, the limiting factor being the rate at which the localisation system could provide coordinates.

5 Discussion

We have developed a system which enables image data about critical structures to be superimposed on the microscope field of view in the correct position. Our advances on previous work [6, 8] include the use of multicolour graphics and accurate stereo projection of a true 3D model. The ability to view different structures, extracted from multiple image modalities, is clearly advantageous. Hidden line removal and stereo projection provide depth perception, showing the 3D relationship between image structures and the patient in-theatre.

We also propose the interactive use of the operative view in order to improve on the image data. Where landmarks are seen to differ from the overlayed view these differences can be marked and the image model updated accordingly. A non-rigid representation will be necessary where tissue has deformed, either naturally or as a result of the surgical procedure. A project has recently begun at U.M.D.S. to examine possible uses of deformation to improve the accuracy of image guidance.

We will be producing an accurately machined geometric phantom that will be scanned using both MRI and CT. Inherent precision measurements will be made on all aspects of the system, including multimodality image registration, MR image distortion, LED location and optical distortion as well as the overall accuracy of the superposition. A clinical evaluation is also about to begin. This will examine the accuracy of the system in theatre, the effectiveness of the stereo overlay on a real operative scene and the clinical value of the complete system.

Further work will include an extensive examination of the visualisation system and the surgeon's interaction with it. Overlays, or head-up displays (HUDs), have been studied in detail for many applications[4]. Our work will look at the specific problems associated with surgical applications as well as the use of stereo projections and HUDs.

We believe that stereo projection into the operating microscope will provide the surgeon with information in the most convenient way and also offers an opportunity to explore the effectiveness of deformable models in image guided surgery.

References

1. Reinhardt, H.F, Horstmann, G.A., Gratz, O.: Sonic Stereometry in Microsurgical Procedures for Deep-Seated Brain Tumours and Vascular Malformations. Neurosurgery **32**(1993) 51-57
2. Adams, L., Gilsbach, Krybus, W., Meyer-Ebrecht, D., Mösges, R.M, Schlöndorff, G.: CAS - A Navigation Aid for Surgery. 3D Imaging in Medicine. NATO ASI series.
3. Colchester, A.C.F., Zhao, J., Henri, C., Evans, R.J., Roberts, P, Maitland, N., Hawkes, D.J., Hill, D.L.G., Strong, A.J., Thomas, D.G.T., Gleeson, M.J., Cox, T.C.S.: Craniotomy Simulation and Guidance Using a Stereo Video Based Tracking System. Vis. Biomed. Comp., Robb, R.A., SPIE **2359** (1994) 541-51

4. Weintraub, D.J., Ensing, M.: Human Factors in Head-Up Display Design: The Book of HUD University of Michigan, May 1992
5. Steinhaus, H.: Sur la Localisation au Moyen des Rayons X. Comptes Rendus de L'Academie des Science **206**(1938) 1473-5
6. Roberts, D.W., Strohbehn, J.W., Hatch, J.F., Murray, W., Kettenberger, H.: A Frameless Stereotaxic Integration of Computerized Tomographic Imaging and the Operating Microscope. J. Neurosurg. **65**(1986) 545-9
7. Friets, E.M., Strohbehn, J.W., Hatch, J.F., Roberts, D.W.: A Frameless Stereotaxic Operating Microscope for Neurosurgery. IEEE Trans. Biomed. Eng. **36** no.6 (1989) 608-617
8. Kelly, P.J., Alker, G.J., Goerss, S.: Computer-Assisted Stereotactic Laser Microsurgery for the Treatment of Intracranial Neoplasms. Neurosurgery **10**(1982) 324-331
9. Arun, K.S., Huang, T.S., Blostein, S.D.: Least-Squares Fitting of Two 3-D Point Sets. IEEE Trans. P.A.M.I. **9** no.5 (1987) 698-703
10. Press, W.H., Teukolsky, S.A., Vetterling, W.T., Flannery, B.P.: Numerical Recipes in C, 2nd Edition, Cambridge University Press 1992
11. Foley, J., van Dam, A., Feiner, S., Hughes, J.: Computer Graphics, 2nd Edition, Addison Wesley 1990
12. Hill, D.L.G., Hawkes, D.J., Crossman, J.E., Gleeson, M.J., Cox, T.C.S, Bracey, E.E.C.M.L., Strong, A.J., Graves, P.: Registration of CT and MR Images for Skull Base Surgery Using Point-Like Anatomical Features. Br. J. Radiology **64**(1991) 1030-35.
13. Hill, D.L.G., Hawkes, D.J., Harrison, N., Ruff, C.F.: A strategy for Automated Multimodality Registration Incorporating Anatomical Knowledge and Imager Characteristics. In: H.H. Barrett, A.F. Gmitro, eds. Information processing an medical imaging. Lecture notes in computer science 687 Springer-Verlag, Berlin (1993) 182-196
14. Henri, C.J., Colchester, A.C.F., Zhao, J., Hawkes, D.J., Hill, D.L.G., Evans, R.L.: Registration of 3D Surface Data for Intra-Operative Guidance and Visualization in Frameless Stereotactic Neurosurgery. Submitted to CVRMed '95
15. D.J.Hawkes, B.P.: The Accuracy of 3D Image Registration Using Point Landmarks. Technical report RS94/1 and submitted for publication.

Author Index

Lecture Notes in Computer Science

For information about Vols. 1–832
please contact your bookseller or Springer-Verlag